Current
Diagnosis & Treatment

A *Quick* Reference for the General Practitioner

THIRD EDITION

Current

Diagnosis & Treatment

A *Quick* Reference for the General Practitioner

THIRD EDITION

Edited by

James O. Woolliscroft, MD

Professor of Internal Medicine
University of Michigan Medical School
Chief of Clinical Affairs
University of Michigan Hospitals
Ann Arbor, Michigan

Springer Science+Business Media, LLC

CM CURRENT MEDICINE

Developmental Editor: Bill Edelman
Editorial Assistant: Nicole Winkler
Layout: Vanessa Ray
Illustrator: Wiesia Langenfeld
Assistant Production Manager: Simon Dickey

Originally published by Current Medicine, Inc., Philadelphia, Pennsylvania in 2001

ISBN 978-1-57340-158-6 ISBN 978-1-4684-0614-6 (eBook)
DOI 10.1007/978-1-4684-0614-6
ISSN 1083-9658

Although every effort has been made to ensure that the drug doses and other information are presented accurately in this publication, the ultimate responsibility rests with the prescribing physician. Neither the publishers nor the authors can be held responsible for errors or for any consequences arising from the use of the information contained herein. Products mentioned in this publication should be used in accordance with the manufacturer's prescribing information. No claims or endorsements are made for any drug or compound at present under clinical investigation.

Manufactured in Canada

5 4 3 2 1

Section Editors

AIDS & Infectious diseases

Powel H. Kazanjian, MD
Associate Professor
Department of Internal Medicine
University of Michigan Medical School
Director, HIV/AIDS Treatment Program
Ann Arbor, Michigan

Alternative medicine

Sara L. Warber, MD
Lecturer
Department of Family Medicine
University of Michigan Medical School
Co-Director, University of Michigan
Complementary and Alternative Medicine
Research Center
Ann Arbor, Michigan

Cardiology

Ragavendra R. Baliga, MD
Assistant Professor
Department of Cardiology
University of Michigan Medical School
Staff Physician, University of Michigan
Ann Arbor, Michigan

Dermatology

Bruce R. Nelson, MD
Director, Cutaneous Surgery and Oncology
Department of Dermatology
University of Texas Health Science Center
Houston, Texas

Contributors

Melissa A. Bogle, MD
Resident
University of Texas Health Science Center
Houston, Texas

Rajani Katta, MD
Assistant Professor
Department of Dermatology
Baylor College of Medicine
Houston, Texas

Jaime A. Tsehen, MD
St. Joseph DermPath
Houston, Texas

Endocrinology & Metabolic disorders

Robert W. Lash, MD
Clinical Assistant Professor
Mediclab
University of Michigan Medical School
Ann Arbor, Michigan

Gastroenterology & Hepatology

Joseph C. Kolars, MD
Associate Professor
Department of Medicine
Mayo Medical School
Consultant, Mayo Clinic
Rochester, Minnesota

General medicine

Brent C. Williams, MD, MPH
Associate Professor
Department of Internal Medicine
University of Michigan Medical School
Ann Arbor, Michigan

Contributors

Kym E. Orsetti, MD
Clinical Assistant Instructor
Department of Internal Medicine
University of Michigan Medical School
Ann Arbor, Michigan

Sean K. Kesterson, MD
Clinical Assistant Instructor
Department of Internal Medicine
University of Michigan Medical School
Ann Arbor, Michigan

Scott L. Furney, MD
Clinical Assistant Instructor
Department of Internal Medicine
University of Michigan Medical School
Ann Arbor, Michigan

Robert D. Ernst, MD
Clinical Assistant Instructor
Department of Internal Medicine
University of Michigan Medical School
Ann Arbor, Michigan

Hematology & Oncology

Scott D. Gitlin, MD
Assistant Professor
Department of Internal Medicine
University of Michigan Medical School
Ann Arbor, Michigan

Nephrology

Frank C. Brosius III, MD
Associate Professor
Department of Internal Medicine, Nephrology
University of Michigan Medical School
Director, Nephrology Training Program at
University of Michigan
Ann Arbor, Michigan

Contributors

Crystal Gardner-Martin, MD
Adjunct Clinical Instructor
Department of Internal Medicine-Division of Nephrology
University of Michigan Medical School
Ann Arbor, Michigan

Rajnish Dhingra, MD
Lecturer
Department of Internal Medicine-Division of Nephrology
University of Michigan Medical School
Ann Arbor, Michigan

Neurology

Linda M. Selwa, MD
Clinical Associate Professor
Department of Neurology
University of Michigan Medical School
Ann Arbor, Michigan

Pulmonary disorders

Cyril M. Grum, MD
Professor
Department of Internal Medicine
University of Michigan Medical School
Associate Chair and Professor, University of Michigan
Ann Arbor, Michigan

Contributor

Jeffrey E. Terrell, MD
Assistant Professor
Department of Otolaryngology-Head and Neck Surgery
University of Michigan Medical School
Ann Arbor, Michigan

Rheumatology & Muscular disorders

Mark A. McQuillan, MD, FACP
Clinical Assistant Professor
Department of Internal Medicine
University of Michigan Medical Center
Ann Arbor, Michigan

Preface

The preface to the first edition of the *Handbook of Current Diagnosis and Treatment* in 1996 set forth the purpose of the book as assisting modern physicians to meet the challenge of information management. "Maintaining knowledge of current diagnostic and therapeutic developments, specifically for clinical problems encountered less frequently, can be a formidable task. *Current Diagnosis and Treatment* is specifically structured to facilitate the busy clinician's access to current information on a wide variety of diseases. It is not designed to provide detailed explanations, but rather to remind the physician who needs to 'brush up' on the diagnosis and management of a clinical entity." This purpose remains as true for the third edition as it was for the first.

Our commitment to a "user friendly," clinically relevant reference for primary care physicians and other members of the health care team is expressed in the consistent layout of each disease chapter. We organized and placed information similarly within each disease spread to enhance ease of use. While antithetical to standard textbooks, the presence of "white space" in many sections reflects this goal of maintaining consistency for ease of use.

Our commitment to providing current information resulted in the addition of a new feature on Alternative Medicine in this edition. Increasingly, patients are using alternative and complementary therapies along with traditional medicine. We have included information on alternative therapies for diseases in which your patients might be availing themselves of these options.

As always, my goal, and that of the section editors is to provide you with concise, relevant, and current information in a readily accessible format. We sincerely hope that this goal is met and that this volume will facilitate your clinical care.

James O. Woolliscroft, MD
Ann Arbor, Michigan

Contents

Contents

P

R

S

T

U

V

W

Appendix

Contents by specialty

AIDS

Cardiology

Dermatology

Endocrinology & Metabolic disorders

Contents by specialty

Gastroenterology

General medicine

Contents by specialty

Contents by specialty

Nephrology

Neurology

Pulmonary disorders

Rheumatology & Muscular disorders

Figure acknowledgments

We gratefully acknowledge the publishers and individuals who allowed us to use the following figures and tables.

Page 4. Figure adapted from Kokko JP: Disorders of fluid, volume, electrolyte, and acid-base balance. In *Cecil Textbook of Medicine*. Edited by Bennet JC, Plum F. Philadelphia: WB Saunders; 1996:543–551.

Page 22. Table adapted from Ewing JA: Detecting alcoholism: the CAGE questionnaire. *JAMA* 1984, 252:1905–1907.

Page 22. Figure adapted from Bradley KA: The primary care practitioner's role in the prevention and management of alcohol problems. *Alcohol Health Res World*, 1994 18:97–104.

Page 28. Figure adapted from Hicks TC, Timmcke AE: Fissure in ano. In *Shackelford's Surgery of the Alimentary Tract*, edn. 3. Philadelphia: WB Saunders; 1991:286–293 and Barnett JL, Raper SE: Anorectal disease. In *Textbook of Gastroenterology*, edn. 2. Edited by Yamada T. Philadelphia: JB Lippincott; 1995:2036–2037.

Page 28. Figure reproduced from Barnett JL: Diseases of the anus. In *Gastroenterology and Hepatology: The Comprehensive Visual Reference: Colon, Rectum, and Anus*, vol. 2. Edited by Feldman M, Boland CR. Philadelphia: Current Medicine; 1996.

Page 58. Figure reproduced from Wong F, Blendis L: Cirrhosis: ascites and spontaneous bacterial peritonitis. In *Gastroenterology and Hepatology: The Comprehensive Visual Reference: The Liver*, vol. 1. Edited by Feldman M, Maddrey WC. Philadelphia: Current Medicine; 1996.

Page 72. Table adapted from Barry WJ, *et al.*: The American Urologic Association Symptom Index for benign prostatic hyperplasia. *J Urol* 1992, 148:1549–1557.

Page 80. Figures adapted from Smith DE, *et al.*: Itraconazole versus ketoconazole in the treatment of oral and oesophageal candidosis in patients infected with HIV. *AIDS* 1991, 5:1367–1371.

Page 94. Figure adapted from Ho-Yen DO: The epidemiology of post viral fatigue syndrome. *Scott Med J* 1988, 33:368–369.

Page 102. Figure adapted from Swash M, Oxberry J (eds.): *Clinical Neurology*. Edinburgh: Churchill Livingstone; 1991:188–204.

Page 120. Figure adapted from Kupfer DJ: Lessons to be learned from long-term treatment of affective disorder. *J Clin Psychiatry* 1991, 52(suppl):12–16.

Page 128. Figure adapted from Besser GM, Bodansky HJ, Cudworth AG: *Clinical Diabetes: An Illustrated Text*. London: Mosby-Wolfe, an imprint of Times Mirror International Publishers; 1995.

Page 134. Figure courtesy of M. Scaglia, MD.

Page 194. Figures courtesy of R. Burney, Ann Arbor, MI.

Page 222. Figure courtesy of Professor A. Grossman, Department of Endocrinology, St. Bartholomew's Hospital, London, UK.

Page 228. Figures adapted from Slade AKB, Saumarel RC, McKenna WJ: The arrhythmogenic substrate—diagnostic and therapeutic implications: hypertrophic cardiomyopathy. *Eur Heart J* 1993, 14:84–90.

Page 232. Figure adapted from Frier BM, Fisher M (eds.): *Hypoglycaemia and Diabetes*. London: Edward Arnold; 1993.

Page 244. Figure adapted from Whitehead WE, Engel BT, Schuster MM: Irritable bowel syndrome: physiological and psychological differences between diarrhea-predominant and constipation-predominant patients. *Dig Dis Sci* 1980, 25:404–413.

Page 260. Figure courtesy of Dr. John Smith, Director, Essex Regional Immunology Service Tenovus Laboratory. Southampton General Hospital.

Page 262. Figure reproduced from Lee WM: Acute liver failure. In *Gastroenterology and Hepatology: The Comprehensive Visual Reference: The Liver*, vol. 1. Edited by Feldman M, Maddrey WC. Philadelphia: Current Medicine; 1996.

Page 272. Figures adapted from Ramsay M, *et al.*: The epidemiology of measles in England and Wales. *Commun Dis Rep* 1994, 4:R141–R145.

Page 296. Figure adapted from Scolar A, French P, Miller R: *Myobacterium avium intracellulare* infection in the acquired immunodeficiency syndrome. *Br J Hosp Med* 1991, 46:295–300.

Page 320. Figure adapted from Wasnich RD: Epidemiology of osteoporosis. In *Primer on the Metabolic Bone Diseases and Disorders of Mineral Metabolism*, edn 3. Edited by Favus MJ. Philadelphia: Lippincott-Raven; 1996:250.

Page 324. Figure adapted from Tsuchiya R: Resection of cancer of the pancreas—the Japanese experience. *Baillières Clin Gastroenterol* 1990, 4:431–434.

Page 340. Figure adapted from Gay NJ, *et al.*: Age specific antibody prevalence to parvovirus B19: how many women are infected in pregnancy? *Commun Dis Rep* 1994, 4:R104–R107.

Page 360. Table adapted from Norton D, McLaren R, Exton-Smith AN: *An Investigation of Geriatric Nursing Problems in the Hospital*. London: National Corporation for the Care of Old People; 1962.

Page 378. Figure adapted from Stansby G, *et al.*: Atherosclerotic renal artery stenosis. *Br J Hosp Med* 1993, 49:388.

Page 404. Figures adapted from Miller E, *et al.*: Rubella surveillance to June 1994. *Commun Dis Rep* 1994, 4:R146–R152.

Page 416. Table adapted from Cooper-Patrick L, Crum RM, Ford DE: Identifying suicidal ideation in general medical patients. *JAMA* 1994, 272:1757–1762.

Page 434. Figure adapted from Franklyn JA, Sheppard MC: Thyroid nodules and thyroid cancer—diagnostic aspects. *Baillières Clin Endocrinol Metab* 1988, 2:767.

Page 436. Table adapted from Heatherton TF, Koziowski LT, Frecker RC, Fagerstrom KO: The Fagerstrom test for nicotine dependence: a revision of the Fagerstrom tolerance questionnaire. *Br J Addict* 1991, 86:1119–1127.

Page 448. Figure reproduced from *MMWR Morb Mortal Wkly Rep* 1992, 41:58.

Page 448. Figure reproduced from *MMWR Morb Mortal Wkly Rep* 1990, 39:421–423.

Page 452. Figure adapted from Kennedy DH: Extrapulmonary tuberculosis. *Update* 1983, 27:671–684.

Page 476. Table adapted from U.S. Preventive Services Task Force: *Guide to Clinical Preventive Services*, edn 2, 1996: 74; and ACOG Committee Opinion Number 152, *Recommendations on Frequency of Pap Test Screening*. March 1995.

How to use this book

This book provides current expert recommendations on the diagnosis and treatment of all major disorders throughout medicine in the form of tabular summaries. Essential guidelines on each of the topics have been condensed into two pages of vital information, summarizing the main procedures in diagnosis and management of each disorder to provide a quick and easy reference.

Each disorder is presented as a "spread" of two facing pages: the main procedures in diagnosis on the left and treatment options on the right.

Listed in the main column of the **Diagnosis** page are the common symptoms, signs, and complications of the disorder, with brief notes explaining their significance and probability of occurrence, together with details of investigations that can be used to aid diagnosis.

The **left shaded side column** contains information to help the reader evaluate the probability that an individual patient has the disorder. It may also include other information that could be useful in making a diagnosis (*e.g.*, classification or grading systems, comparison of different diagnostic methods).

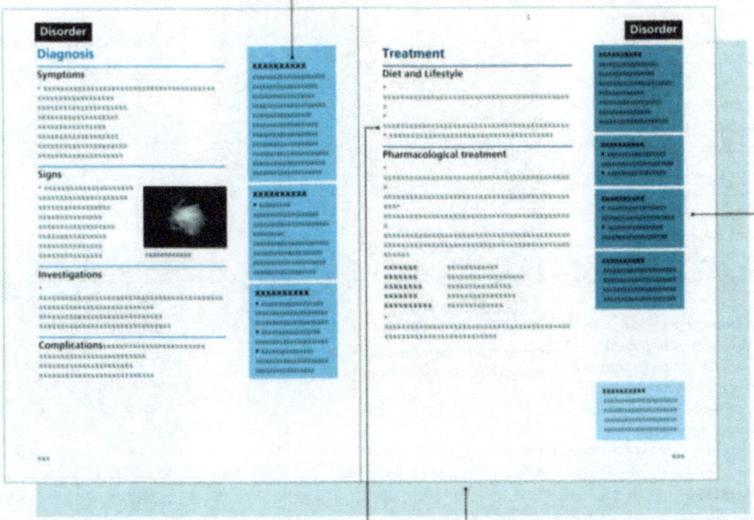

On the **Treatment** page, the main column contains information on lifestyle management and nonspecialist medical therapy of the disorder, with general information on specialist management when this is the main treatment.

Whenever possible under "Pharmacological treatment," guidelines are given on the standard dosage for commonly used drugs, with details of contraindications and precautions, main drug interactions, and main side effects. In each case, however, the manufacturer's drug data sheet should be consulted before any regimen is prescribed.

The main goals of treatment (*e.g.*, to cure, to palliate, to prevent), prognosis after treatment, precautions that the physician should take during and after treatment, and any other information that could help the clinician to make treatment decisions (*e.g.*, other nonpharmacological treatment options, special situations or groups of patients) are given in the **right shaded side column**. The key and general references at the end of this column provide the reader with further practical information.

Achalasia

Diagnosis

Symptoms

• Typically gradual in onset and present for an average of 2 years before diagnosis [1,2].

Dysphagia: usually perceived with both solid food and liquids.

Retrosternal chest pain: intermittent and variable duration, often related to eating.

Weight loss.

Regurgitation.

Nocturnal cough: related to regurgitation and aspiration.

Signs

• Usually no signs are manifest.

Evidence of weight loss: more advanced cases.

Investigations

Radiography (plain film, erect): may show absence of air in gastric fundus or dilated esophagus with air-fluid level.

Radiography (barium swallow): shows delayed passage of contrast through cardia, absence of peristalsis (although "tertiary waves" may be prominent), or esophageal dilatation with "bird-beak" narrowing in the distal esophagus.

Upper gastrointestinal endoscopy: often normal but necessary to exclude competing diagnoses such as malignancy [2]; retained food or fluid may be encountered; increased resistance to passage of endoscope through cardia may be apparent.

Esophageal manometry: required for definitive diagnosis; shows impaired relaxation of lower esophageal sphincter and absent peristalsis; may show prominent nonperistaltic (synchronous) contractions in esophageal body or elevated tonic pressure of lower esophageal sphincter [3].

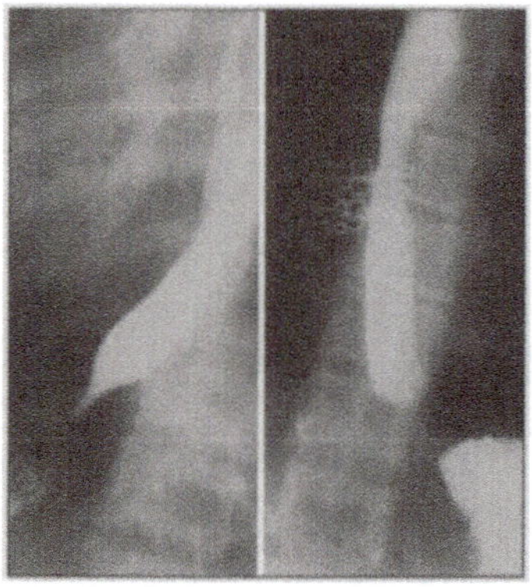

Classic "bird-beak" distal esophagus (*left*) and delay of barium swallow due to spasm (*right*).

Complications

Respiratory complications: *e.g.*, cough, aspiration pneumonitis, in 10% of patients.

Esophageal carcinoma: possibly a late complication; very unusual.

Malnutrition.

Differential diagnosis

Benign or malignant esophageal stricture.

Acid reflux with esophageal spasm.

Gastric or other malignancy at cardia.

Aortic aneurysm compressing cardia.

Chagas' disease.

Hollow visceral neuropathy.

Etiology

• The underlying cause of the defect in the inhibitory innervation of the esophageal body and lower sphincter is unknown.

• Occasionally achalasia will occur as a paraneoplastic process; an occult malignancy should be considered promptly, particularly in older patients.

Epidemiology

• The annual incidence of achalasia is 1 in 100 000 adults.

• The male : female ratio is equal; achalasia may appear at any age in adult life.

• Although achalasia is more common in adults, the occurrence in children is well documented.

Diagnostic pitfalls

• The clinical features and radiography of "classic" achalasia are so characteristic that the existence of less typical presentations is not always appreciated; awareness of the following helps to minimize diagnostic errors:

Early symptoms in some patients resemble those of gastroesophageal reflux.

Abnormalities on barium swallow are sometimes subtle, so the diagnosis of achalasia is easily missed.

Minor inflammation of the mucosa may be diagnosed as esophagitis at endoscopy when food retention in the esophagus is significant.

Prokinetic agents (*e.g.*, metoclopramide, cisapride) may cause achalasia-like symptoms by increasing lower esophageal sphincter tone.

Treatment

Diet and lifestyle

• Until mechanical dilation is achieved, advise a mechanical soft diet with ingestion of meats and other solid food only if it has been ground into fine pieces.

Pharmacological treatment

• Patients obtain some relief from pharmacotherapy when mechanical treatment is not an option. Nifedipine (10–20 mg) or isosorbide dinitrate (5–10 mg), 30 to 45 minutes before meals, provides variable improvement in symptoms.

Nonpharmacological treatment

Endoscopic dilation of the lower esophageal sphincter

• Endoscopic myotomy via balloon dilation (*e.g.*, Rigiflex Balloon; Microvasive, Boston, MA) is the procedure of choice [3,4].

• Local injection therapy with botulinum toxin (80–100 units) is also considered, particularly in high-risk patients , but may require repeat treatments.

• Dysphagia is relieved in about two-thirds of patients after one attempt; a second attempt is usually worthwhile if the first attempt was unsuccessful.

• Complications include esophageal perforation in 5% of patients; surgical repair is not always needed.

Surgery

• Myotomy through the thorax or abdomen or as a "minimal-access" procedure should be pursued if the endoscopic approach is unsuccessful.

Treatment aims

To restore acceptable swallowing.

Prognosis

• Relief of dysphagia and retrosternal pain can be achieved in >80% of patients.

Follow-up and management

• Symptomatic gastroesophageal reflux occurs in 5%–10% of patients after successful dilatation or cardiomyotomy; treatment with an H2 receptor antagonist or proton pump inhibitor is usually successful.

Key references

1. Howard PJ, et al.: Five year prospective study of the incidence, clinical features and diagnosis of achalasia in Edinburgh. *Gut* 1992, **33**:1011-1015.
2. Richter JE: Esophageal motility disorders. *Curr Practice Med* 1998, **1**:741–749.
3. Parkman HP, et al.: Pneumatic dilatation or esophagomyotomy treatment for idiopathic achalasia: clinical outcomes and cost analysis. *Dig Dis Sci* 1993, **38**:75-85.
4. Spechler SJ: American Gastroenterological Association medical position statement on treatment of patients with dysphagia caused by benign disorders of distal esophagus. *Gastroenterology* 1999, **117**:229–233.

Acid-base disorders

Diagnosis

Symptoms
• There are few symptoms associated with acid-base disorders.

Signs
• Signs are generally nonspecific and of limited help diagnostically.

Metabolic acidosis
Hyperventilation (including Kussmaul respiration).
Altered mental status, shock: in severe cases.

Metabolic alkalosis
Hypovolemia: may be associated with metabolic alkalosis.

Respiratory acidosis
Altered mental status (CO_2 narcosis): dilated retinal vessels, papilledema.

Respiratory alkalosis
Tingling of hands, feet, perioral area.
Tetany: in severe cases.

Investigations

All acid-base disorders
Electrolytes, blood urea nitrogen, creatinine, glucose.
Arterial blood gas: if clinically indicated.

Metabolic acidosis
Calculation of serum anion gap [Na - (Cl + HCO_3)].
Calculation of urinary anion gap [(Na + K) - Cl].
Serum ketones, lactate.
Toxicology: salicylates, methanol, ethylene glycol, paraldehyde.

Metabolic alkalosis
Urine chloride.

Respiratory acidosis
• *See* All acid-base disorders *above*.

Respiratory alkalosis
• *See* All acid-base disorders *above*.

Complications
• Most complications are secondary to the underlying disorder (*e.g.*, diabetic ketoacidosis, asthma exacerbation).

Metabolic acidosis
Diminished cardiac output leading to hypotension, decreased tissue perfusion, shock.

Metabolic alkalosis
Volume contraction, hypokalemia.

Respiratory acidosis
Hypoxemia, coma.

Respiratory alkalosis
Tetany, seizures: rare.

Differential diagnosis
Not applicable.

Etiology

Metabolic acidosis

Increased anion gap: diabetic ketoacidosis, alcoholic ketoacidosis, lactic acidosis, renal failure, salicylates, toxins (*see* Investigations).

Normal anion gap: gastrointestinal fluid losses (negative urinary anion gap)—diarrhea, small intestine losses, ureterosigmoidostomy.

Renal tubular acidoses (positive urinary anion gap).

Other causes: parenteral hyperalimentation, potassium sparing diuretics, rapid volume expansion, acetazolamide.

Metabolic alkalosis

U_{Cl} <10 mmol/L: these disorders are associated with hypovolemia and respond to saline infusion; etiologies include, vomiting, nasogastric suction, villous adenoma, diuretics, hypercapnia.

U_{Cl} >20 mmol/L: these disorders are unresponsive to saline infusion; etiologies include mineralocorticoid excess (various causes), severe hypokalemia (not diuretic induced), hypercalcemia, alkali ingestion.

Respiratory acidosis

Ventilatory failure (sedation, cardiac arrest, pulmonary disease, neuromuscular disease, CNS lesions).

Respiratory alkalosis

Hyperventilation (anxiety, CNS lesions, high altitudes, severe liver disease, febrile illnesses, salicylates, pregnancy).

Epidemiology
Not applicable.

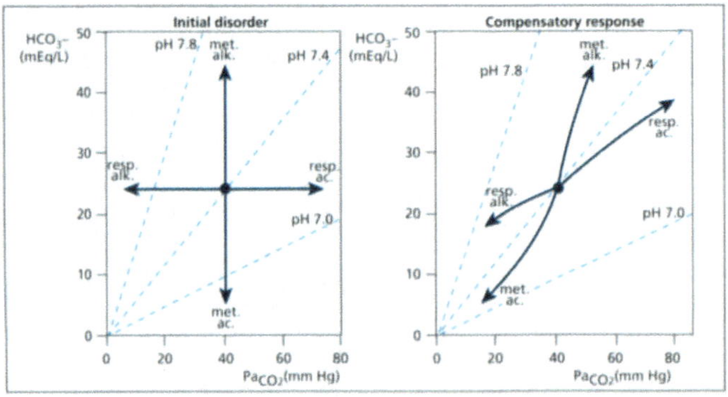

Acid-base disorders initially alter serum concentrations of either HCO_3 (in metabolic disorders) or Pa_{CO_2} (respiratory disorders), leading to changes in arterial pH (*left*). Over time, compensatory mechanisms will shift serum pH back toward a pH of 7.4 (*right*). met. ac.—metabolic acidosis; met. alk.—metabolic alkalosis; resp. ac.—respiratory acidosis; resp. alk.—respiratory alkalosis.

Treatment

Diet and lifestyle

• Patients with chronic diseases such as type I diabetes and asthma should by encouraged to comply with medical regimens.

Pharmacological treatment

Metabolic acidosis

• Treatment of the underlying disorder (*e.g.*, diabetic ketoacidosis or sepsis) includes the following:

Alcoholic ketoacidosis: typically corrects with normal saline and glucose infusion.

Diarrhea/gastrointestinal losses: normal saline and electrolyte replacement (especially potassium).

Renal failure: HCO_3 >15 mEq/dL—no therapy required; HCO_3 <15 mEq/dL (without uremia)—oral alkali; severe acidosis with uremia—hemodialysis.

Toxins: supportive care for all patients; salicylates: hemodialysis for concentrations >100 mg/dL; methanol, ethylene glycol—usually requires hemodialysis.

Alkali therapy: most studies show no significant benefit; may be worthwhile in profound acidosis to keep arterial pH from falling below 7.1; do not use alkali to correct pH to normal.

Metabolic alkalosis

U_{Cl} <10 mmol/L: gastric losses—normal saline infusion; diuretic induced—normal saline infusion, potassium replacement.

U_{Cl} >20 mmol/L: treat underlying disorder (*e.g.*, adrenal disease); potassium replacement.

Respiratory acidosis

Ventilatory support; treat underlying disease; trial of naloxone if narcotic overdose is suspected.

Respiratory alkalosis

Treat underlying disorder; hyperventilation secondary to anxiety may be treated by breathing into a paper bag.

Treatment aims

To restore normal acid-base status.

To replace fluid and electrolytes.

To treat underlying disorder.

Prognosis

Generally good, but depends on underlying disorder.

Follow-up and management

Avoidance of precipitating events.

Ongoing treatment of underlying disorders.

Useful equations for calculating compensatory responses

Metabolic acidosis

For every 1.0 mEq/dL fall in HCO_3, Pa_{CO_2} will decrease 0.8 mm Hg.

Metabolic alkalosis

For every 1.0 mEq/dL rise in HCO_3, Pa_{CO_2} will increase 1.4–1.7 mm Hg.

Respiratory acidosis

Chronic: for every 10 mm Hg rise in Pa_{CO_2}, HCO_3 will increase 3.5–4.0 mEq/dL.

Respiratory alkalosis

Chronic: for every 10 mm Hg fall in Pa_{CO_2}, HCO_3 will decrease 4.0–5.0 mEq/dL.

• Simple compensatory mechanisms move pH back toward (but not all the way to) 7.4 (see figure). If this rule appears to be violated, look for a mixed disorder with two primary abnormalities.

General references

Haber RJ: A practical approach to acid-base disorders. *West J Med* 1991, **155**:146–151.

Kokko JP: Disorders of fluid, volume, electrolyte, and acid-base balance. In *Cecil Textbook of Medicine*. Edited by Bennet JC, Plum F: Philadelphia: WB Saunders; 1996:543–551.

Levinsky NG: Acidosis and alkalosis. In *Harrison's Principles of Internal Medicine*. Edited by Isselbacher KJ, Braunwald E, Wilson JD, *et al*. New York: McGraw-Hill; 1994:253–262.

Preuss JG: Fundamentals of clinical acid-base evaluation. *Clin Lab Med* 1993, **13**:103–116.

Diagnosis

Symptoms

Social embarrassment: concern about appearance, even in cases that may be inconspicuous to the observer.

Pain: from inflammatory papules, pustules, and cysts.

Signs

• Distribution is usually limited to the face, upper back, and chest, but acne can occur over the entire back and extend to the proximal arms in more severe cases.

• **Papules, pustules, nodules, and cysts;** lesions may be excoriated.

• **Oily skin.**

• **Scars.**

• **Comedones: open (blackheads) or closed (whiteheads).**

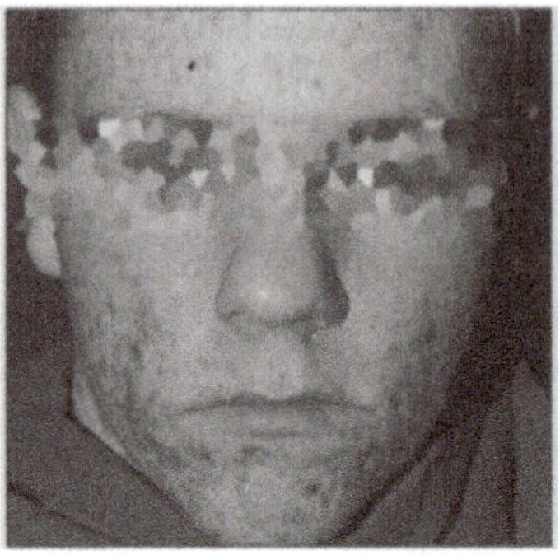

Moderate to severe facial acne. (*See* Color Plate.)

Lesions can be divided into noninflammatory and inflammatory.

Acne category	Comedones	Papules/pustules	Nodules
Noninflammatory:			
Mild	Few	Occasional	None
Inflammatory:			
Mild	Few to many	Few to several	None
Moderate	Few to many	Several to many	Few to several
Severe	Few to many	Extensive	Many

Investigations

• Acne is a clinical diagnosis.

Culture: may be helpful to identify gram-negative folliculitis unresponsive to conventional acne treatment.

Biopsy: may be used to rule out other diseases in cases with an atypical presentation.

• Women with severe acne resistant to standard therapy or associated with hirsutism or menstrual irregularities may have underlying endocrine abnormalities; often the work-up is normal, but polycystic ovaries and ovarian or adrenal tumors may be present and need to be excluded.

Complications

Scarring: from resolving lesions; "ice-pick" scarring or depressed atrophic plaques; occaisionally scars can be hypertonic/keloidal.

Hyperpigmented macules: from resolving lesions, especially in patients with pigmented skin.

Aggressive cutaneous basal cell carcinomas/thyroid carcinomas: prone to develop in patients who have had superficial x-ray irradiation for treatment of acne in the past; such patients should be closely followed and educated.

Differential diagnosis

Rosacea
Episodic facial flushing; lesions can be telangiectatic, granulomatous, papular, or pustular (in any combination).

Perioral dermatitis
Combination of eczematous patches and inflammatory papules around the mouth, most commonly in women.

Steroid acne
Multiple monomorphous inflammatory papules or pustules. Can occur from application of fluorinated topical steroids (especially on face) or in patients on systemic steroids (on chest, back, and shoulders).

Drugs
Can cause acneiform eruption, especially phenytoin and lithium.

Halogenoderma
From iodide, bromide, or chloride.

Gram-negative folliculitis
May occur after long-term use of oral antibiotics; culture useful to differentiate from acne.

Excoriated acne
Can be incorrectly diagnosed as impetigo or factitial dermatitis.

Pyoderma faciale
Rapid development of indurated erythema and fluctuant abscesses on the face of young women.

Tuberous sclerosis
Angiofibromas often misdiagnosed as acne.

Acne fulminans
Severe sudden onset of painful inflammatory nodules mainly on the chest and back of adolescent boys; may be associated with leukocytosis, arthralgias, fever, and ulceration of the nodules.

Etiology

Defective keratinization that obstructs follicular outflow channels.

Increased sebum production (controlled by androgenic hormonal stimulation).

Inflammation: *Propionibacterium acnes* converts sebum into fatty acids that cause an inflammatory response within the follicle, leading to hyperkeratinization and enhanced follicular plugging.

Epidemiology

• Acne is the most common skin disease in the United States.

• 85% of those between the ages of 12 and 25 years are affected.

• Peak incidence is between ages 16 and 18 years.

Treatment

Diet and lifestyle

• Diet appears to have little effect on acne.

• Long-term exposure to chlorinated hydrocarbons, coal tar, machine oils, greases, lubricating oils, and dioxin can cause acneiform lesions.

• Pomade oils and comedogenic cosmetics should be avoided.

Pharmacological treatment

• Most treatments require 4 to 6 weeks before clinical improvement occurs.

Hormonal treatment: triphasic norgestimate, 35 g ethinyl estradiol oral contraceptive pills. For use in females with acne that has a significant hormonal influence.

Spironolactone: 50–100 mg daily; side effects may include teratogenicity, menstrual spotting, electrolyte imbalances (potassium).

For mild acne: topical treatment

Standard dosage	*Benzoyl peroxide,* 2.5%–10%. *Tretinoin,* 0.025%, 0.05%, 0.1% cream; 0.01%, 0.025% gel; 0.05% solution. Apply a thin layer nightly as tolerated. *Tretinoin microsphere* 0.1% gel; use nightly as tolerated. *Adapalene* 0.1% gel; use nightly as tolerated; may be less irritating than tretinoin. *Azelaic acid* 20% cream; apply thin layer up to twice daily.
Contraindications	None.
Special points	*Retinoic acid:* needs to be increased as tolerated; many patients experience an initial flare-up of their acne; may increase photosensitivity; sunscreens should be encouraged. *Azelaic acid:* monitor for hypopigmentation.
Main drug interactions	None.
Main side effects	Drying, irritation, excessive skin peeling.

For mild acne: topical antibiotics

Standard dosage	Clindamycin, 1% solution, gel, or lotion; erythromycin, 2% ointment, gel, or solution; tetracycline; benzamycin; apply thin film to affected areas twice daily.
Contraindications	None.
Main drug interactions	None.
Main side effects	Local irritations; gels tend to be drying, ointments make skin feel "oily."

For moderate acne: oral antibiotics

Standard dosage	Tetracycline, 500 mg once daily to twice daily. Minocycline, 50 mg once daily to 100 mg twice daily. Doxycycline, 100 mg once daily to twice daily. Enteric coated erythromycin, 333 mg three times daily. Erythromycin stearate, 500 mg once daily to twice daily.
Contraindications	*Tetracycline, minocycline, doxycycline:* pregnant women and children <12 years old.
Special points	Tetracycline must be taken on an empty stomach; minocycline and doxycycline must be taken with food.
Main drug interactions	*Erythromycin:* inhibits cytochrome P-450, may interact with any medication metabolized by P-450 (*e.g.*, cisapride).
Main side effects	Oral antibiotics may increase incidence of vaginal yeast infections.

For moderate or severe acne

Standard dosage	Isotretinoin, 0.5 to 1 mg/kg of body weight daily for 20 weeks.
Contraindications	Pregnancy, preexisting hepatic disease, hypertriglyceridemia.
Special points	Female patients in child-bearing years must use two forms of effective contraception 1 month before, during, and 1 month after treatment.
Main drug interactions	Concomitant use with tetracycline, minocycline, or doxycycline may increase risk for pseudotumor cerebri.
Main side effects	Drying of skin and mucosa, elevated liver enzyme and triglyceride levels, myalgias, teratogenicity.

Treatment aims

To reduce inflammatory lesions.
To prevent scarring and embarrassment.

Other treatments

Exfoliants (salicylic acid, alpha-hydroxy acids), triamcinolone injected into inflammatory papules, chemical peels, and cyst incision and drainage.
Treatment of postinflammatory hyperpigmentation and acne scarring: dermabrasion, microdermabrasion, chemical peels, laser resurfacing, and punch grafting of acne scars.

Prognosis

Excellent with spontaneous remission after several years.
Excellent for nodulocystic acne treated with isotretinoin.
• Acne sometimes persists into adulthood.

Follow-up and management

• Follow-up is crucial because rate of response to first-line agents is slow.
• Patient education is key to success.
• Isotretinoin should be considered early in severe cases unresponsive to first-line agents to prevent severe scarring.

General references

Brown SK, Shalita AR: Acne vulgaris. *Lancet* 1998, **351**:1871–1876.

Jansen T, Plewig G: Acne fulminans. *Int J Dermatol* 1998, **37**:254–257.

Leyden JJ: Therapy for acne vulgaris. *N Engl J Med* 1997, **336**:1156–1162.

Lucky AW: Hormonal correlates of acne and hirsutism. *Am J Med* 1995, **98**:S89–S94.

Pochi PE: The pathogenesis and treatment of acne. *Ann Rev Med* 1990, **41**:187–198.

Pochi PE, *et al.*: Report of the consensus on acne classification. *J Am Acad Dermatol* 1991, **24**:495–500.

Acne rosacea

Diagnosis

Symptoms

Episodic facial flushing.

Social embarrassment: concern about appearance.

Signs

Skin findings

• Distribution of skin findings is usually limited to the midface (nose, cheeks, chin, and central forehead); it may occasionally involve the neck and chest.

• The disease occurs in stages:

Episodic facial flushing.

Persistent erythema/edema.

Telangiectasias.

Papules/pustules.

Sebaceous gland hypertrophy.

Rhinophyma.

Ocular findings

• Occur in as many as 50% of patients with rosacea and are the presenting sign in 20%.

Pain/photophobia/foreign body sensation.

Blepharitis.

Recurrent chalazia.

Conjunctivitis.

Contact lens intolerance.

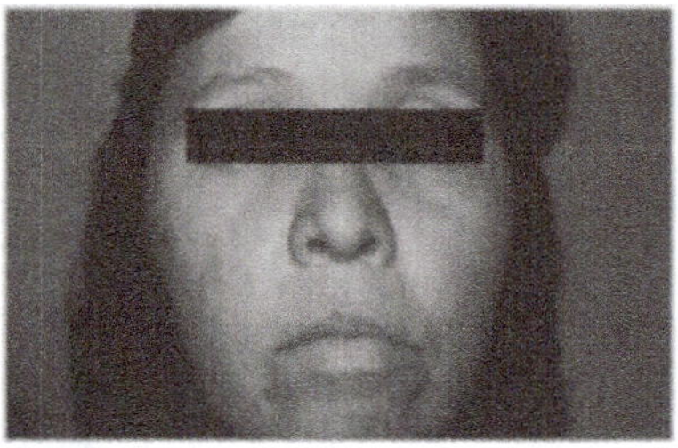

Classic acne rosacea. (*See* Color Plate.)

Investigations

Careful history: needed to identify possible precipitating factors (*e.g.*, drug use, sun exposure, stress, diet, alcohol ingestion).

Culture: may be helpful to identify gram-negative or staphylococcus folliculitis, tinea facei.

Biopsy: may be used to rule out other diseases (systemic lupus erythematosus, sarcoidosis) in patients with an atypical presentation.

Complications

Skin

Rhinophyma: disfiguring hypertrophy of the nose.

Peau d'orange skin: inflamed and thickened edematous skin with large pores, resembling the surface of an orange.

Ocular

Corneal scarring (rare).

Differential diagnosis

Rebound rosacea

Seen in patients applying topical steroids. Involves much wider area of the face and sometimes the neck, ears.

Can see atrophy from steroid applications.

Systemic lupus erythematosus (SLE): butterfly rash can mimic rosacea; other evidence of SLE includes oral mucosal involvement, hair loss, photosensitive dermatitis, arthritis, systemic symptoms.

Seborrheic dermatitis: pustules uncommon; scaling with erythema on face and scalp; no flushing.

Acne vulgaris: occurs in younger patients. Comedones are the primary lesion of acne vulgaris but are typically absent in rosacea.

Gram-negative or staphylococcus folliculitis.

Tinea facei: suspect in patients who have unilateral rosacea. KOH preparation of scale useful to make diagnosis.

Etiology

Unknown, possibly multifactorial.

Vascular disorder in which flushing leads to edema that produces papules, pustules, and eventual fibrosis.

• The following may also play a role:

Demodex infestation: produces folliculitis similar to rosacea; mites often found at the surface of the hair follicle.

Sun exposure: may act as a trigger factor via infrared heat.

Helicobacter pylori: prevalence is higher among rosacea patients.

Epidemiology

• It affects 10%–20% of the adult population; 30%–50% of people >40 years of age.

• Rarely seen in children and blacks persons.

• Women are more likely to be affected than men, but disease often more severe in men.

Treatment

Diet and lifestyle

• Patients should eliminate factors known to trigger flushing: heat, alcohol, hot liquids, spicy foods, certain cosmetics.

Pharmacological treatment

For mild rosacea: topical treatment

Standard dosage	Metronidazole, 0.75% gel, cream, lotion; 1% cream. Topical erythromycin or clindamycin, in concentrations from 0.5% to 2.0%; apply to affected areas twice daily. Sunscreens, preferably broad-spectrum UVA plus UVB with SPF of 15 or higher.
Contraindications	None.
Main side effects	Mild irritation, gels tend to be drying, creams may feel "greasy."
Special points	Metronidazole has its greatest effect on papules and pustules. It does not appear to alter telangiectasias or flushing. Topical steroids are contraindicated in the treatment of rosacea.

For moderate rosacea: oral antibiotics

Standard dosage	Tetracycline, 500 mg once daily to twice daily. Doxycycline, 100 mg once daily to twice daily. Enteric-coated erythromycin, 333 mg three times daily. Erythromycin stearate, 500 mg once daily to twice daily.
Contraindications	*Tetracycline, doxycycline:* pregnancy and children <12 years old.
Main drug interactions	*Erythromycin:* inhibits cytochrome P-450, may interact with any medication metabolized by P-450 (*e.g.*, cisapride).
Main side effects	Any oral antibiotic may increase the incidence of vaginal yeast infections. *Tetracycline, doxycycline:* gastrointestinal effects, photosensitivity, risk for pseudotumor cerebri (rare). *Erythromycin:* gastrointestinal effects.
Special points	Tetracycline must be taken on an empty stomach; doxycycline must be taken with food.

For severe rosacea

Standard dosage	Isotretinoin, 0.5 to 1 mg/kg of body weight daily.
Contraindications	Pregnancy, preexisting hepatic disease, hypertriglyceridemia.
Main drug interactions	Concomitant use with tetracycline, minocycline, or doxycycline may increase risk for pseudotumor cerebri.
Main side effects	Drying of skin and mucosa, elevated liver enzyme and triglyceride levels, myalgias, teratogenicity.
Special points	Female patients in childbearing years must use two forms of effective contraception 1 month before, during, and 1 month after treatment. Serum pregnancy, lipoprotein levels, and liver function tests must be monitored monthly.

Alternative medicine

Recommended use: none.

Common use: B vitamins, especially riboflavin; b complex, 100 mg/day.

Caution: vitamin B_2, B_6, and B_{12} may worsen some rosacea; avoid niacin.

Treatment aims

To reduce the number and severity of lesions.

To induce and/or maintain a remission.

Other treatments

For women flushing through menopause: estrogen replacement therapy, clonidine.

For *H. pylori* in the stomach: oral amoxicillin, metronidazole, and bismuth subsalicylate in combination.

Vascular laser of telangiectatic vessels.

Carbon dioxide laser, dermabrasion, or surgical excision for rhinophyma.

Prognosis

Rosacea is a condition that usually responds to therapy even though it cannot be cured.

Follow-up and management

• Patient education is key to success.

• All patients with progressive rosacea should be evaluated by an ophthalmologist.

General references

Browning J, Proia A: Ocular rosacea. *Surv Ophthalmol* 1986, **31**:145–158.

Dahl MV (ed.): Perspectives. In *Current Concepts in Acne and Rosacea: A Symposium at the American Academy of Dermatology*. Orlando: Mark Dahl and Associates; 1996:8–14.

Wilkin JK: Rosacea: pathophysiology and treatment. *Arch Dermatol* 1994, **130**:1448.

Fitzpatrick TS, *et al.*: *Dermatology in General Medicine*, edn 4. New York: McGraw-Hill; 1993:727–735.

Tackett-Fletcher W, Roberts K: Rosacea. *J Geriatr Nurs* 1999, **20**:44–47.

Thiboutot DM: Acne rosacea. *Am Fam Physician* 1994, **50**:1691–1697.

Actinic keratoses

Diagnosis

Symptoms

• Usually asymptomatic.

Mild local tenderness or pruritus: occasionally.

Signs

Papules: 1–2-mm hyperkeratotic erythematous rough papules on the sun-exposed surfaces of the skin; can be >1 cm in diameter and pigmented as well; occasionally can present as a "cutaneous horn" (*i.e.*, hypertrophic actinic keratoses); often more difficult to see clinically but are easily identified by touch.

Actinic keratoses of the lower lip (actinic cheilitis): presents as a diffuse, ill-defined rough scaling of the vermilion border of the lip.

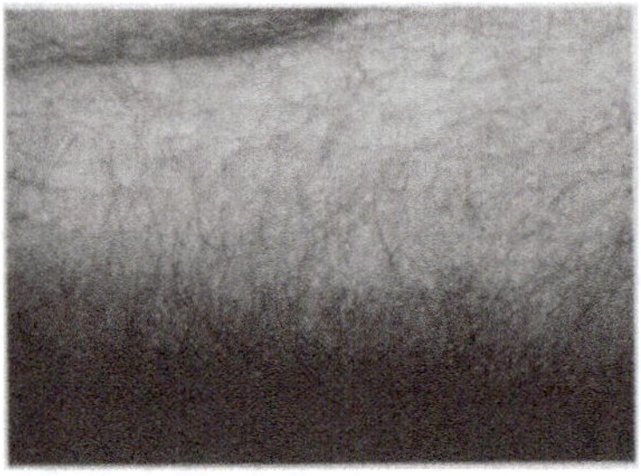

Actinic keratoses. (*See* Color Plate.)

Investigations

Asymptomatic actinic keratoses

• Clinical diagnosis: treated without biopsy confirmation; biopsy is indicated if condition does not respond to treatment.

Symptomatic or hypertrophic actinic keratoses

Skin biopsy: performed at the initial visit or empirical treatment with close follow-up. Biopsy is done if there is no response to treatment to rule out the possibility of an invasive squamous cell carcinoma. If ulceration or induration is present, then a biopsy is mandatory.

• Actinic keratoses are, in fact, squamous cell carcinomas in situ, and it follows that they evolve into squamous cell carcinomas, which in turn may become quite invasive and even metastasize; a high index of suspicion with sound clinical judgment is warranted when evaluating and treating these precancerous lesions.

• It is equally important that a well-experienced dermatopathologist interpret the biopsy specimens It is often necessary to perform deeper sectioning of the specimen to rule out invasive squamous cell carcinoma.

Complications

Squamous cell carcinoma: evolution of an actinic keratosis into an invasive squamous cell carcinoma is of special significance with regard to actinic cheilitis because squamous cell carcinomas of the lower lip have a high metastatic potential.

Differential diagnosis

Seborrheic keratosis.

Verruca vulgaris.

Benign lichenoid keratosis.

Squamous cell carcinoma.

Inverted follicular keratosis: irritated seborrheic keratosis that may look very similar to squamous cell carcinoma histologically.

Etiology

• Causes include long-term UV light exposure, radiograph irradiation, artificial UV light from tanning booths, and polycyclic aromatic hydrocarbon exposure.

• Injury from UV light exposure can select for the clonal expansion of mutated chromosomal *P53* tumor suppressor oncogenes, which can give rise to both actinic keratoses and squamous cell carcinomas.

• Sunlight acts as both an initiator and promoter of nonmelanoma skin cancers.

Epidemiology

• Individuals with blonde hair and blue eyes and persons with a history of childhood freckling are at an increased risk to develop actinic keratoses.

• More than 50% of elderly fair-skinned individuals in hot and sunny climates are affected.

• There is an increased propensity to develop actinic keratoses as well as squamous cell carcinomas in renal transplant recipients and other immuno-suppressed patients.

Treatment

Diet and lifestyle

• Actinic keratoses develop on the exposed surfaces of the skin as a result of long-term sun exposure.

•Increased incidence is associated with occupations such as farming or ranching, outdoor sports and hobbies, and tanning.

•A low-fat diet may decrease the incidence of actinic keratoses in patients with a history of nonmelanoma skin cancer.

Pharmacological treatment

•Prevention of further lesions is key: use daily sunscreen with an SPF of 15 or higher, wear protective clothing, avoid sun exposure.

Topical

Standard dosage — Topical 5-fluouracil, 1% or 5% cream applied twice daily for 3–4 weeks as tolerated.
Tretinoin may enhance the efficacy of 5-fluorouracil when used in combination.

Contraindications — Previous sensitivity.

Main drug interactions — None.

Main side effects — Painful erosions and erythema can be expected; contact dermatitis may occur.
Photosensitivity.

Oral

Standard dosage — Acitretin, 30 mg daily.

Contraindications — Childbearing potential, preexisting hepatic disease, hypertriglyceridemia.

Special points — Decreases occurrence of actinic keratoses and squamous cell carcinomas in high-risk patients (*e.g.*, renal transplant recipients); effectiveness ceases when medication is stopped. Teratogenic potential is present for up to 3 years after drug cessation (and possibly longer).

Main side effects — Drying of skin and mucosa, elevated liver enzyme and triglyceride levels, myalgias, teratogenicity.

Cryotherapy

Open spray technique with a freeze time of 5–10 seconds or, alternatively, the dipstick method.

Surgical treatment

• Superficial dermabrasion, curettage, laser abrasion, and chemical peeling have been effective forms of treatment, especially when there is extensive involvement of the skin with actinic keratoses.

Treatment aims

To prevent the evolution of actinic keratoses into invasive squamous cell carcinomas by early recognition and treatment and judicial biopsies when indicated.

Prognosis

• In a healthy immunocompetent person, actinic keratoses may spontaneously regress, remain unchanged, or may progress into an invasive squamous cell carcinoma.

• It is difficult to ascertain the exact percentages of malignant transformation; two studies with a 1-year time course reported malignant conversion rates between 0.25% and 20%.

• It is nearly impossible to predict the lifetime risk in patients with literally hundreds of actinic keratoses (*i.e.*, risk per lesion).

Follow-up and management

• Clinically suspected actinic keratoses that are unresponsive to treatment must undergo biopsy to rule out the possibility of invasive squamous cell carcinoma.

• Patients with multiple actinic keratoses are at an increased risk to develop melanoma and nonmelanoma skin cancers and should be monitored at 3–6-month intervals.

General references

Callen JP, *et al.*: Actinic keratoses. *J Am Acad Dermatol* 1997, **36**:650–653.

Drake LA, *et al.*: Guidelines of care for actinic keratoses. *J Am Acad Dermatol* 1995, **32**:95–98.

Marks R: Solar keratoses. *Br J Dermatol* 1990, **122 (suppl 35)**:49.

McKenna DB, Murphy GM: Skin cancer chemoprophylaxis in renal transplant recipients: 5 years of experience using low-dose acitretin. *Br J Dermatol* 1999, **140**:656–660.

Odom R: Managing actinic keratosis with retinoids. *J Am Acad Dermatol* 1998, **39**:574–578.

Vitasa BC, *et al.*: Association of non-melanoma skin cancer and actinic keratosis with cumulative solar ultraviolet exposure in Maryland water-men. *Cancer* 1990, **65**:2811–2817.

Ziegler A, *et al.*: Sunburn and *p53* in the onset of skin cancer. *Nature* 1994, **372**:773–776.

Acute crystal synovitis

Diagnosis

Symptoms

• Symptoms develop rapidly, often becoming maximal within 4–12 hours of onset.

• Usual sites are knee or wrist for pseudogout and first metatarsophalangeal joint, mid- or hindfoot, knee, or wrist for gout [1].

• Usually, only one or a few joints are involved; polyarticular attacks occur in < 10%.

Severe pain: "worst ever."

Stiffness, tenderness, swelling.

Fever and systemic upset: particularly with large- or multiple-joint involvement.

Signs

Overlying erythema: later desquamation.

Red hot joint: *i.e.*, periarticular and articular inflammation; always suggests crystals or sepsis.

Tense effusion, increased warmth, marked joint-line and periarticular tenderness, restricted movement with stress pain: *i.e.*, florid synovitis.

Pyrexia: possible confusion, especially in elderly patients.

Turbid or blood-stained aspirated fluid: high cell count, >95% polymorphs.

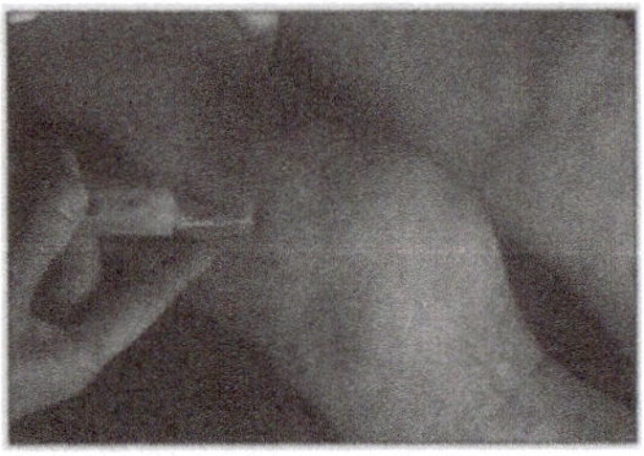

Turbid synovial fluid aspirated from acute knee synovitis due to gout. (*See* Color Plate.)

Investigations

Diagnostic: synovial fluid analysis

Compensated polarized light microscopy: usual method of crystal identification: monosodium urate crystals: strong (negative) birefringence, needle-shaped, 2–25 µm long, easily identified; calcium pyrophosphate dihydrate crystals: weak (positive) birefringence, rhomboid, 2–10 µm long, more difficult to identify; other crystals (cholesterol, oxalate, injected steroid) rare.

Gram stain and culture: essential to exclude sepsis.

Supportive but nondiagnostic

Radiography: to detect chondrocalcinosis (pseudogout); osteophyte, sclerosis, cysts, joint-space narrowing (pseudogout, gout); para-articular erosion (gout); although characteristic, such changes are not always present.

ESR, CRP measurement: usually raised.

Serum uric acid measurement: often but not always raised in gout.

Disease associations

• These should be considered after diagnosis and acute management.

Metabolic screening: calcium, alkaline phosphatase, ferritin, magnesium; if patient is aged <55 years or has polyarticular chondrocalcinosis (pseudogout).

Urea (blood urea nitrogen), creatinine measurement: for renal impairment in primary or secondary gout.

Lipoprotein measurement, liver function tests: in primary and alcohol-associated gout.

Complications

Cluster attacks: one attack triggers attacks at other sites.

Joint rupture: with associated soft-tissue inflammation.

Nerve entrapment: due to acute soft-tissue swelling (most often median nerve).

Differential diagnosis

Septic arthritis: sepsis usually superimposes on abnormal, previously symptomatic joint.

Other crystal synovitis.

• Acute crystal synovitis and septic arthritis may coexist [2].

• More than one crystal type may be present ("mixed crystal deposition").

Etiology

Causes of primary gout

Inherited renal undersecretion of uric acid (in most patients).

Inherited overproduction of uric acid (rare).

Obesity, excess alcohol intake (mainly beer).

Inherited crystal nucleation or growth-promoting tissue factors.

Causes of secondary gout

Chronic diuretic treatment.

Chronic renal impairment.

Lead poisoning (in "moonshine" drinkers).

Causes of pseudogout

Sporadic isolated chondrocalcinosis, pyrophosphate arthropathy (osteoarthritis subset).

Familial predisposition (unusual).

Metabolic predisposition (rare): hemochromatosis, hypomagnesemia, hyperparathyroidism, hypophosphatasemia.

Triggering factors

Local trauma, intercurrent acute illness, surgery, initiation of drug treatment, *e.g.*, allopurinol (gout), thyroxine (pseudogout), parenteral fluids, joint lavage.

• "Shedding" of preformed (previously asymptomatic) crystals initiates acute attack (controversial).

Epidemiology

• Crystal synovitis is the most common cause of acute monoarthritis in middle-aged and elderly patients.

• Before the age of 65 years, more men than women present with gout (mainly primary).

• After the age of 65 years, as many men as women present with gout (mainly secondary).

• Patients with pseudogout are predominantly elderly, with as many men as women.

• Pseudogout is rare in patients aged <55 years (suggests familial or metabolic predisposition).

Treatment

Diet and lifestyle

- No special precautions are necessary in pseudogout.
- Avoidance of high-purine foods may be helpful in gout.

Pharmacological treatment

Oral NSAIDs

- Simple analgesics may be effective with other treatments, but quick-acting NSAIDs are generally preferred (*see* Gout *for further details*) [1,3].

Colchicine

- Colchicine is effective in any crystal synovitis, but it should be used only for very resistant attacks because of toxicity [1].

Standard dosage	Colchicine, 1 mg, then 0.5 mg orally every hour until pain controlled or side effects develop (maximum, 6 mg) in first 24 hours; then maximum dose of 0.6 mg 3 times daily.
Contraindications	Renal or hepatic impairment, dehydration.
Special points	Never given parenterally; not to be given again within 7 days. (Note: i.v. colchicine is hazardous.)
Main drug interactions	None.
Main side effects	Severe nausea, vomiting, watery diarrhea.

Intra-articular steroids

- Steroids are indicated for problematic attacks (large joints, polyarticular involvement, elderly ill patient) or if oral agents are contraindicated.
- They usually reduce synovitis within 24–48 hours.
- The dose should be varied according to joint size; doses listed here are for the knee [3].

Standard dosage	Methylprednisolone, 60 mg. Triamcinolone hexacetonide, 60 mg. Triamcinolone acetonide, 60 mg.
Contraindications	Coexistent sepsis.
Special points	Aseptic technique and single-dose vial should be used.
Main drug interactions	None.
Main side effects	Facial flushing, local skin or fat atrophy (mainly fluoridated steroids), exacerbation of pain (temporary), sepsis (rare).

Nonpharmacological treatment

Local physical measures

- The following are the first line of treatment and must be done early:

Aspiration: to reduce intracapsular hypertension (often temporary).

Local heat or cold: may ameliorate pain and swelling.

Resting support (possibly with splinting): to ease symptoms.

Elevation: to reduce edema.

Early rehabilitation (active movement, mobilization, graded exercise): to maintain muscle and range of movement.

- Prolonged immobilization should be avoided: regular passive movement should punctuate assisted rest.

Lavage

- Lavage is indicated for the following:

Coexistent sepsis.

Florid, large joint synovitis unresponsive after 48 hours to aspiration, steroid injection, and oral medications.

Large loculated effusion (inhibiting effective aspiration).

Treatment aims

To relieve pain.

To reduce intra-articular hypertension.

To avoid muscle wasting or capsular restriction.

Prognosis

- Acute attacks resolve spontaneously, even without treatment, within 1–3 weeks.
- Although prolonged florid synovitis is potentially detrimental, most episodes improve with no apparent lasting damage.
- Incomplete recovery of muscle strength or bulk is the most common problem.

Follow-up and management

- Long-term interventions should be instituted only after an acute attack of gout has settled.
- Metabolic screening for pseudogout should be undertaken if appropriate.
- Patients with associated chronic pyrophosphate arthropathy should be advised about alteration of adverse mechanical factors, reduction in obesity, appropriate exercise, and use of symptomatic agents.

Key references

1. Star VL, Hockberg MC: Prevention and management of gout. *Drugs* 1993, **45**:212–222.
2. Baer PA, Tenenbaum J, Fam AG, Little H: Coexistent septic and crystal arthritis: report of four cases and literature review. *J Rheumatol* 1986,**13(3)**:604–607.
3. Tan N, Lertratanakul W, Barr WG: Acute gouty arthritis: modern approaches to an ancient disease. *Postgrad Med* 1993, **94**:73–75;78;83–84.
4. Fam AG: Calcium pyrophosphate crystal deposition disease and other crystal deposition diseases. Curr Opin Rheumatol 1992, 4(4):574–582.
5. Jensen PS: Chondrocalcinosis and other calcifications. *Radiol Clin North Am* 1988, **26(6)**:1315–1325.

Acute respiratory distress syndrome

Diagnosis [1] (*formerly called* Adult respiratory distress syndrome)

Symptoms

Dyspnea: variable severity, developing abruptly or gradual onset some days after initial insult.

Signs

Respiratory distress: labored breathing, intercostal retractions.

Tachypnea: rapid and shallow.

Warmth and peripheral vasodilatation.

Signs of pulmonary edema: on auscultation.

Other signs of underlying disease.

• Cyanosis may be apparent.

Investigations

Chest radiography: for bilateral pulmonary infiltrates; to confirm pulmonary edema in presence of predisposing condition.

Pulmonary artery catheterization: to measure pulmonary capillary wedge pressure (normally <18 mm Hg) to exclude cardiogenic edema.

Arterial blood gas analysis: refractory hypoxemia unresponsive to increased inspired oxygen concentration (partial arterial oxygen pressure <70 mm Hg breathing 40% oxygen, arterial-alveolar oxygen tension ratio <0.25); low total respiratory compliance (<30 mL/cm H_2O).

Fiberoptic bronchoscopy and lavage or biopsy, upper respiratory tract cultures, CT and nuclear imaging, specialized blood tests (*e.g.*, plasma amylase): to establish underlying condition and assess presence of multisystem organ failure.

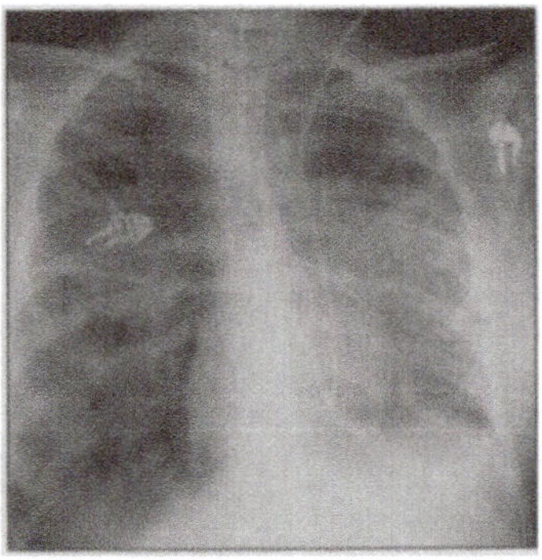

Typical chest radiograph appearance of established acute respiratory distress syndrome, showing pneumothoraces, position of endotracheal tube, intercostal chest drains, and pulmonary artery flotation catheter.

Complications [2]

Death.

Multisystem organ failure: especially renal failure.

Sepsis.

Shock.

Barotrauma: from mechanical ventilation (*e.g.*, pneumothorax).

Debilitation after intensive care: survivors usually recover fully within 12 months [3].

Differential diagnosis

• The diagnostic criteria exclude other diagnoses.

• Hemodynamic pulmunary edema must be excluded.

Etiology [4]

• The etiology follows severe systemic and pulmonary insults including:

Shock.

Sepsis.

Bacterial, viral, or drug-induced pneumonia.

Burns.

Aspiration of gastric contents.

Inhalation of toxic fumes.

Trauma.

Oxygen toxicity.

Disseminated intravascular coagulation.

Massive hemorrhage or multiple transfusion.

Pre-eclampsia.

Embolism: thrombotic, fat, or amniotic fluid.

Acute pancreatitis.

Head injury.

Various drugs and i.v. drug abuse.

Transplantation (lung or bone marrow).

Epidemiology

• Acute respiratory distress syndrome has an incidence of ~1.5 cases per 100 000 persons in the United States, although cases of acute lung injury not meeting the diagnostic criteria occur much more often.

• The prevalence varies according to the predisposing illness (2%–25%).

Pathophysiology

• Acute respiratory distress syndrome causes damage to capillary endothelial cells and alveolar epithelial cells resulting from the activation of many humoral and cellular events.

• It is uniformly characterized by increased permeability of the alveolar-capillary membrane, leading to pulmonary edema.

• Deranged cellular use of oxygen occurs as part of the syndrome and may result in widespread multiorgan failure of variable severity.

Treatment

Diet and lifestyle

• Patients need nutritional support by parenteral or enteral route while on the ventilator.

Pharmacological treatment [5–7]

• Underlying conditions should be fully investigated and steps taken to correct any reversible disorders.

• Nosocomial infection and sepsis should be managed aggressively.

• Vasopressor, inotropic, and chronotropic agents should be used to support circulation and urine output.

• Enteral nutrition should be given when possible.

Nonpharmacological treatment [5–7]

• The involvement of multiple organ systems in the disease process means that supportive measures are not confined to the respiratory system.

• All patients with severe lung injury and established acute respiratory distress syndrome should be managed in the intensive care unit.

• Full respiratory and invasive hemodynamic monitoring and urinary catheterization are often needed.

Respiratory support

• Endotracheal intubation and mechanical ventilation is almost always necessary; it should be instituted early in the course.

• The aim is to maintain oxygen saturation at ~90% using continuous positive airways pressure applied via a face mask or mechanical ventilation.

• New techniques (*e.g.*, pressure-controlled or inverse-ratio ventilation) are aimed at recruiting collapsed alveoli while reducing peak airway pressures (and therefore the risk of barotrauma) and raising mean airway pressures (thereby improving oxygenation).

• Oxygenation may be be improved by turning patients (supine/prone).

Cardiac and circulatory support

• The aim is to maximize oxygen delivery to tissues.

• Hemoglobin should be maintained at or above 10–12 g/dL, with a hematocrit >30%.

• Cardiac output and oxygen delivery may need to be optimized by the judicious manipulation of filling pressures and the use of inotropic drugs. The routine use of a pulmonary artery catheter however is discouraged.

Fluid balance

• The aim of manipulating fluid balance is to reduce circulating volume as much as possible in an effort to reduce further extravasation of edema into the alveoli.

• Pulmonary capillary wedge pressure should be maintained at 8–12 mm Hg.

• Diuretics may be needed to maintain urine output >0.5 mL/kg/h and to reduce intravascular volume.

Prevention

• No measures have been documented to prevent acute respiratory distress syndrome.

Treatment aims

To provide definitive treatment (if available) for the underlying condition.

To support affected systems, *e.g.*, respiratory and cardiovascular, until spontaneous resolution occurs, by optimizing oxygen delivery.

Prognosis

• Mortality depends on the underlying condition and is reported to be 40%–70%.

• 90% of survivors recover 90% of their premorbid lung function after 12 months and suffer little or no respiratory impairment.

• Supportive treatments carry appreciable morbidity (*e.g.*, pneumothorax, renal failure).

• Survivors are invariably debilitated after the prolonged stay in intensive care.

Follow-up and management

• The aim of follow-up is to maximize recovery from the effects of both the initial illness and the adult respiratory distress syndrome.

• Attention to physical rehabilitation, with nutritional advice, physical therapy, and controlled exercise when appropriate, is needed for patients.

Key references

1. Bernard GR, *et al.*: The American-European Consensus Conference on ARDS: definitions, mechanisms, relevant outcomes, and clinical trial coordination. *Am J Respir Crit Care Med* 1994, **149**:818–824.
2. Wyncoll DA, Evans TW: Acute respiratory distress syndrome. *Lancet* 1999, **354**:497–501.
3. McHugh LG, *et al.*: Recovery of function in survivors of the acute respiratory distress syndrome. *Am J Respir Crit Care Med* 1994, **150**:90–94.
4. Hudson LD, *et al.*: Clinical risks for development of the acute respiratory distress syndrome. *Am J Respir Crit Care Med* 1995, **151**:293–301.
5. Kollef MH, Schuster DP: The acute respiratory distress syndrome. *N Engl J Med* 1995, **332**:27–37.
6. Artigas A, Bernard GR, Carlet J, *et. al.*: The American-European Consensus Conference on ARDS, part 2: ventilatory, pharmacologic, supportive therapy, study design strategies, and issues related to recovery and remodeling. Acute respiratory distress syndrome. *Am J Resp Crit Care Med* 1998, **157(4 pt 1)**:1332–1347.
7. Luce JM: Acute lung injury and the acute respiratory distress syndrome. *Crit Care Med* 1998, **26(2)**:369–376.

Addison's disease (primary adrenal insufficiency)

Diagnosis

Symptoms

• Onset is usually insidious.

Dizziness and syncope.

Weakness, fatigue, weight loss: common.

Nausea, diarrhea: in ~50% of patients.

Increase in normal skin pigmentation: may appear well tanned (without tan lines).

Mental changes (especially depression).

Acute back pain: rare finding; limited to some patients with bilateral adrenal hemorrhage.

Signs

Postural hypotension: typically unresponsive to i.v. fluids.

Hypotension: usually systolic blood pressure <110 mm Hg.

Generalized pigmentation: common; extensor and exposed skin should be checked.

Buccal pigmentation: usually manifest with generalized pigmentation.

Scar pigmentation: only scars occurring after onset of Addison's disease.

Signs of organ-specific autoimmune disease: *e.g.*, vitiligo, thyroid disease.

Hyponatremia: inability to excrete water due to mineralacorticoid (aldesterone) deficiency raised antidiuretic hormone concentration, and glucocorticoid effect on renal tubule (common).

Hyperkalemia: usually mild (normal in 40% of patients).

Family history of autoimmune endocrine diseases.

Hypercalcemia: in 10% of patients.

Hypoglycemia: sometimes seen in children or undernourished patients.

Investigations

Serum cortisol measurement: ideally should be done at 8 a.m. but valid results can also be obtained under stressful conditions. Values <7 μg/dL are most often associated with adrenal insufficiency. 7–18 μg/dL is indeterminate, and values >18 μg/dL are unlikely to represent Addison's disease. (Note: cortisol levels in the afternoon and evening are normally <7 in healthy individuals.)

Plasma corticotropic hormone (ACTH) measurement: concentration usually >80 ng/L in primary adrenal failure; low values for both cortisol and ACTH suggest pituitary disease (sample must be collected in the appropriate tube, put on ice, centrifuged, and frozen immediately).

Electrolytes.

Cosyntropin stimulation test: cosyntropin, 250 μg i.v.; cortisol measured at 0, 30, and 60 minutes (normal result: any value >20 μg/dL); the same test using 1 μg of cosyntropin may be more sensitive [1].

Blood count and film: eosinophilia, macrocytosis with coexistent vitamin B_{12} deficiency, normocytic anemia after volume replacement.

Chest radiography: to check for tuberculosis. (*See* etiology.)

Insulin hypoglycemia test: can be used to differentiate primary from secondary adrenal failure. Potentially dangerous, and usually unnecessary. Under control conditions, 0.1 U/kg insulin is injected and serum glucose is monitored until <40 mg/dL. Samples for cortisol and ACTH measurement are drawn at baseline, during, and 30 and 60 minutes after hypoglycemia.

Complications

Death: if diagnosis missed, if patient not given extra steroids in stress situations, or if replacement steroids not taken; hydrocortisone *must* be given before thyroxine when hypothyroidism and Addison's disease coexist (Schmidt's syndrome) to prevent exacerbation of adrenal insufficiency by thyroid hormone.

Associated autoimmune endocrine failure: vitamin B_{12} deficiency, hypothyroidism, type 1 diabetes mellitus, hypoparathyroidism.

Differential diagnosis

Secondary (pituitary) adrenal insufficiency: low ACTH and cortisol response to insulin-induced hypoglycemia.

Other causes of pigmentation: *e.g.*, hemochromotosis, ectopic ACTH.

Etiology

Autoimmune adrenalitis.

Tuberculosis (infrequently seen): whole-gland involvement, calcification on radiography or CT.

• Rare causes include the following, with 80%–90% of both adrenals affected:

Adrenal hemorrhage: usually in anticoagulated or septicemic patients.

Drugs: *e.g.*, ketoconazole, suramin.

HIV-related adrenalitis.

Metastases.

Sarcoidosis.

Hemochromatosis.

Adrenoleukodystrophy.

Amyloidosis.

Congenital adrenal hyperplasia.

Epidemiology

• The incidence of Addison's disease is estimated to be 40–60 in one million.

• The female:male ratio is 2:1.

Treatment

Diet and lifestyle

• Patients should always carry appropriate identification (*e.g.*, wallet card, bracelet, or necklace) and have access to an "emergency pack" (hydrocortisone, 100-mg ampule, with saline solution, needle, and 2-mL syringe).

• Patients and partners should be taught how to give an i.m. injection in case the patient is unable to take oral steroids.

• Patients should be educated about the need for extra hydrocortisone in case of illness or physical stress.

Pharmacological treatment

For acutely ill or hypotensive patients

• If the diagnosis is suspected, prompt diagnostic and therapeutic steps should be taken.

• In previously undiagnosed disease, blood should be drawn for cortisol, ACTH, and thyroid function tests.

Hydrocortisone, 100 mg i.v. bolus.

0.9% saline 1-L bolus initially in 1 hour followed by 0.9% saline infusion.

Glucose i.v. bolus to correct hypoglycemia.

• Inotropic agents are usually unnecessary and are rarely effective [2].

Continued treatment

Acute treatment	Hydrocortisone, 100 mg i.m. every 8 hours until clinical improvement; patients in intensive care units or on anti-coagulants can be treated by 100 mg in 50 mL saline solution at 2 mg/h i.v. infusion.
Contraindications	None.
Special points	When conscious and taking fluids orally, most patients can be converted to oral hydrocortisone; typical replacement dose is 20 mg every morning and 5 mg at bedtime. Prednisolone and dexamethasone sometimes used instead. Patients receiving large doses of hydrocortisone do not usually require mineralocorticoid replacement. Patients on standard oral replacements with hydrocortisone may need fludrocortisone for mineralocorticoid replacement (50–100 mg every day).
Main drug interactions	None.
Main side effects	Short-term treatment at these doses rarely has side effects, but glucose intolerance may occur.

Treatment aims

To alleviate symptoms and restore circulating mineralocorticoid and corticosteroids to physiological levels.

Prognosis

• Patients have a normal life expectancy if adequately treated.

• Adrenal function is rarely recovered.

Follow-up and management

• Electrolytes should be monitored periodically and with illness.

• Plasma renin activity may be monitored 2 hours after fludrocortisone dose.

Key references

1. Oelkers W, Diederich S, Bahr V: Diagnosis and therapy surveillance in Addison's disease: rapid adrenocorticotrophin (ACTH) test and measurement of plasma ACTH, renin activity, and aldosterone. *J Clin Endocrinol Metab* 1992, **75**:259–264.
2. Werbel SS, Ober, KP: Acute adrenal insufficiency. *Endocrinol Metab Clin North Am* 1993, **22**:303–328.

Diagnosis

Definition

• AIDS is defined by progressive immunodeficiency without another cause, manifest by various conditions, including the following:

Opportunistic infections

Viral: cytomegalovirus.

Bacterial: *Mycobacterium avium-intracellulare,* disseminated *M. tuberculosis,* recurrent *Salmonella* spp., pneumococcus.

Fungal: *Candida albicans, Cryptococcus neoformans, Histoplasma capsulatum, Aspergillus* spp.

Protozoan: *Pneumocystis carinii,* cryptosporidia, microsporidia, isospora, *Toxoplasma gondii, Leishmania* sp.

Unusual tumors

Kaposi's sarcoma.

Non–T-cell lymphoma.

Invasive cervical carcinoma.

Neurological manifestations

AIDS dementia complex.

Vacuolar myelopathy.

Progressive multifocal leukoencephalopathy.

Symptoms

• Skin rashes (persistent and severe herpes simplex or zoster infection) occur during the midstage of infection.

Skin rash, temperature, pharyngitis, lymphadenopathy (seroconversion illness): in 50% of patients.

Unexplained diarrhea, fever, dyspnea, focal neurological signs, minor opportunistic infections: particularly oral candidiasis and oral hairy leukoplakia.

Signs

Skin rash.

Lymphadenopathy.

Oral candidiasis, oral hairy leukoplakia: in pre-AIDS.

Opportunistic infection: in AIDS.

Investigations

• In the asymptomatic phase, the diagnosis can be made only by HIV testing.

HIV test: antibodies to HIV (usually occurring within 3 months of exposure) measured by enzyme-linked immunosorbent assay, confirmed by Western blot analysis.

CD4 lymphocyte count: used to assess immune function; normal value ~800×10^6/L; patients with <500×10^6/L have recurrent bacterial infections; patients with <200×10^6/L are at risk for developing opportunistic infections. Useful for determining prophylaxis against *P. carinii* and *M. avium.*

Direct measurement of viral load using polymerase chain reaction: useful for predicting disease progression and monitoring antiviral therapy.

Complications

Not applicable.

Differential diagnosis

Congenital immunodeficiency.

Iatrogenic immunodeficiency: *e.g.*, after bone-marrow transplantation.

HIV-antibody–negative CD4 lymphopenia: rare; different epidemiology from HIV infection.

Etiology

• AIDS is caused by infection by HIV.

• HIV leads to a progressive fall in T-helper (CD4) cells and a failure of T-cell proliferation after antigenic stimulation, even by T cells uninfected by HIV.

Epidemiology

• Geographically, three patterns of disease are seen:

North America and Western Europe

• Transmission in men having sex with men, intravenous drug users, heterosexual transmission, and transmission vertically or among recipients of blood products (patients with hemophilia who received blood products between 1975 and 1984).

• In the United States and United Kingdom, transmission among men having sex with men is declining and the number of heterosexual people and intravenous drug users is increasing.

Sub-Saharan Africa

• The disease is predominantly a heterosexual epidemic, with major transmission vertically and through blood products.

Asia

• An explosive increase in numbers is occurring, mainly by heterosexual transmission.

Treatment

Diet and lifestyle

• No special precautions are necessary.

Pharmacological treatment

• Combination antiviral therapy, highly active antiretroviral therapy (HAART) with a triple-drug regimen, is indicated for patients with a significant HIV viral load or decreased CD_4 cell count. A triple drug regimen using two nucleoside agents with a third agent, either a protease inhibitor or non-nucleoside agent, is indicated.

Nucleoside agents

Standard dosage	Zidovudine, 200 mg 3 times daily.
Contraindications	Bone-marrow suppression.
Special points	Use as part of multidrug regimen.
Main drug interactions	Drugs with similar toxic profile.
Main side effects	Bone-marrow suppression, headache, occasionally myopathy.

Didanosine (ddI)

Standard dosage	Didanosine, 200 mg twice daily.
Contraindications	Previous pancreatitis, peripheral neuropathy.
Special points	Part of multidrug regimen.
Main drug interactions	Given in alkaline buffer, which may reduce absorption of compounds needing acidification in the stomach.
Main side effects	Pancreatitis, peripheral neuropathy.

Stavudine

Standard dosage	Stavudine, 40 mg twice daily.
Contraindications	Pre-existing peripheral neuropathy.
Special points	Part of multidrug regimen.
Main drug interactions	None known.
Main side effects	Peripheral neuropathy, lactic acidosis.

Lamivudine (3TC)

Standard dosage	150 mg twice daily.
Contraindications	None.
Special points	Use with zidovudine or D4T.
Main side effects	Gastrointestinal upset.
Side-effect	Hypersensitivity reaction.

Protease inhibitors

Standard dosage	Inbinavir, 800 mg 3 times daily. Ritonavir, 600 mg twice daily. Fortovase 1200 mg twice daily. Nelfinavir, 750 mg 3 times daily. Amprenavir, 1200 mg twice daily.
Contraindications	Terfenedine, multiple drug interactions.
Special points	Use with nucleoside agents.
Main side effects	Nephrolithiasis, gastrointestinal toxicity.
Short-term side effects	Nephrolithiasis, gastrointestinal toxicity.
Long-term side effects	Lipodystrophy, dysglycemias, central adiposity, cervicofacial fat pad.

Alternative medicine

Recommended use: none.

Common use: astragulus (*Astragulus membranaceus*); echinacea (*Echinacea pupura*); St. John's wort (*Hypericum perforatum*); bitter melon (*Momordica charantia*); Cats claw (*Uncaria tomentosa*); SPV-30 (extracted from an evergreen tree).

Caution: St. John's wort reduces blood levels of antiviral drugs; echinacea is contraindicated.

Treatment aims

To suppress viral replication.

To prevent immunological decline and increases CD4 cell count.

To prolong life.

Prognosis

• 60% of patients progress to AIDS within 10 years of seroconversion in the absence of antiviral therapy.

• 5% remain well, with no evidence of immunological deterioration at this time.

• HAART prolongs life and reduces opportunistic infections.

Follow-up and management

• Patients should have CD4 counts and viral load measured 4 times a year to determine antiviral efficacy.

• Patients with CD4 counts <200 × 10⁶/L should receive *P. carinii* pneumonia prophylaxis; those with CD4 counts <75 × 10⁶/L should receive *M. avium* complex prophylaxis.

General references

Deeks SG, Smith M, Holodney M, Kahn JO: HIV-1 protease inhibitors: a review for clinicians. *JAMA* 1997, **277**:145–153.

Doran CM: New approaches to using antiretroviral therapy for the management of HIV infection. *Ann Pharmacother* 1997, **31**:228–236.

Emmons W: Accuracy of oral specimen testing for human immunodeficiency virus. *Am J Med* 1997, **102**:15–20.

Lewis JS II, Terieff CM, Coulston DR, Garrison MW: Protease inhibitors: a therapeutic breakthrough for the treatment of patients with human immunodeficiency virus. *Clin Ther* 1997, **19**:187–214.

Sheppard HW, Ascher MS: The natural history and pathogenesis of HIV infection. *Annu Rev Microbiol* 1992, **460**:533–564.

Weissman IL: AIDS: the whole body view. *Curr Biol* 1993, **30**:766–769.

AIDS-related lymphoma

Diagnosis

Symptoms

• Lymphoma B symptoms may be difficult to differentiate from other symptoms of HIV infection and AIDS.

Persistent, unilateral, and enlarging nodes: <50% of patients.

Cough, shortness of breath.

Abdominal pain.

Headaches, focal neurological deficits.

Painful and ulcerated mucosal lesions.

Localized indurated skin nodule.

Weakness, weight loss, night sweats, fever.

Signs

Enlarged discrete rubbery nodes in neck, axillae, or groin.

Hepatosplenomegaly.

Enlarged retroperitoneal adenopathy.

Increased intracranial pressure, papilledema, focal neurological signs.

Mass involving unusual site: *e.g.*, pericardium, testicle, oral mucosa.

Anemia, pyrexia, petechiae.

Investigations

Biopsy: to type lymphoma.

Complete blood count: baseline for treatment.

CT of chest, abdomen, and pelvis.

Lumbar puncture: high incidence of CSF involvement.

MRI, CT, CT-guided biopsy: of solitary brain lesion to detect cerebral lymphoma.

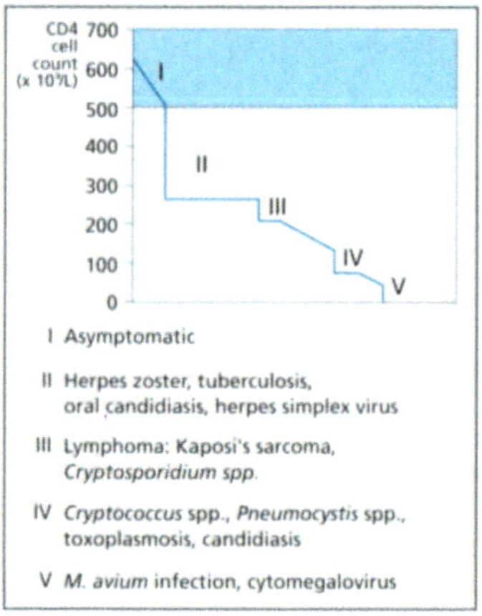

Relationship of CD4 cell count to clinical condition.

Complications

Poor bone-marrow reserve: because of infections or drugs.

Many opportunistic infections.

Differential diagnosis

Nodal

Persistent generalized lymphadenopathy.

Extranodal

Oral aphthous ulcers, Kaposi's sarcoma.

Cerebral toxoplasmosis.

Systemic

Fever of unknown origin, *Mycobacterium avium-intracellulare* or *M. tuberculosis* infection, HIV infection, drug reactions.

Etiology

Non-Hodgkin's lymphoma

• HIV-related immunosuppression may occur secondary to Epstein–Barr virus or other cytokines.

• Non-Hodgkin's lymphoma is seen in other immunosuppressed states: Wiskott–Aldrich syndrome (congenital), organ-transplant recipients.

Epidemiology

• Non-Hodgkin's lymphoma accounts for 3% of AIDS-defining diagnoses in HIV-positive patients; it is the AIDS-defining diagnosis in 60% of those in whom it occurs.

• It usually occurs with a low CD4 count ($<200 \times 10^6$/L).

• It is seen equally in all risk groups.

• It is the most common AIDS-related malignancy in heterosexuals.

Pathology

B-cell non-Hodgkin's lymphoma

High grade: 90% small, noncleaved cells (65% immunoblastic, 25% Burkitt).

Low grade: occasionally, not related to AIDS.

Treatment

Diet and lifestyle

• No special precautions are necessary.

Pharmacological treatment

• Specialist supervision is needed.

• Discussion of treatment options with the patient is vital.

• Patients with good performance status and high CD4 counts are treated by conventional CHOP chemotherapy (cyclophosphamide, vincristine, adriamycin, prednisolone) or short-course high-dose multiple-agent regimens; traditional non-AIDS regimens may cause worsening of prognosis in poor-risk AIDS patients.

• Patients with poor performance status, low CD4 counts ($<100 \times 10^6$/L), and previous AIDS-defining diagnoses can receive low-dose CHOP or vincristine and bleomycin with steroids.

• CNS prophylaxis with intrathecal methotrexate is important because CNS involvement is frequent.

• All chemotherapy is immunosuppressive, depresses bone-marrow function, and may precipitate infection.

Treatment aims

To avoid overwhelming infection in good-risk patients receiving high-dose chemotherapy.

To maintain quality of life.

Other treatments

Radiotherapy

• This is useful in palliative treatment of nodal masses unresponsive to chemotherapy or when chemotherapy is not possible.

External-beam radiotherapy for localized extranodal sites: *e.g.*, lymphoma of tonsil.

Whole-brain radiation therapy for cerebral lymphoma.

Bone-marrow support

With colony-stimulating factors.

Prognosis

• The median survival is <6 months (worse than for non–HIV-related non-Hodgkin's lymphoma, stage for stage).

• Factors associated with poor prognosis include having AIDS before diagnosis of lymphoma, poor performance status (<70% Karnofsky), having a CD4 count $<100 \times 10^6$/L.

• 50% of patients die of non-Hodgkin's lymphoma, 50% of AIDS-related problems.

• Burkitt's lymphoma responds better to chemotherapy than immunoblastic lymphoma does.

• The median survival for cerebral lymphoma is 4–8 weeks.

Follow-up and management

• Patients should be provided with psychological support and continuing care.

General references

Ioachim HL, *et al.*: Acquired immunodeficiency syndrome associated lymphomas. Clinical, pathologic, immunologic, and viral characteristics of 111 cases. *Hum Pathol* 1991, **22**:659–673.

Sandler AS, Kaplan L: AIDS lymphomas. *Curr Opin Oncol* 1996, **8**:377–385.

Straus DJ: Human immunodeficiency virus–associated lymphomas. *Med Clin North Am* 1997, **81**:495–570.

Alcohol problems

Diagnosis

Classification

• Alcohol problems may be classified into several types of decreasing severity: dependence, abuse, and hazardous drinking (*see* Figure) [1].

Alcohol dependence: presence of physical tolerance; history of withdrawal symptoms; persistent desire or lack of success in efforts to cut down; reduction in social, occupational, or recreational activities attributable to alcohol; or continued use despite knowledge or experience of undesirable effects.

Alcohol abuse: recurrent alcohol use resulting in a failure to fulfill major role obligations (work, family, school) in potentially hazardous situations (*e.g.*, driving) or resulting in legal difficulties.

Hazardous drinking: drinking pattern that places patient at increased risk but has not yet resulted in problems. Patients who regularly drink three or more drinks daily (one or more drinks daily if elderly), or who drink five or more drinks per occasion (three or more if elderly) should be considered at risk [1].

Symptoms

A "yes" response to one or more questions from the following alcoholism evaluation (CAGE) identifies patients who are likely to be abusing or dependent on alcohol [2].

CAGE questionnaire

1. Have you ever felt you should Cut down on your drinking?
2. Have people *A*nnoyed you by criticizing your drinking?
3. Have you ever felt bad or Guilty about drinking?
4. Have you ever taken a drink first thing in the morning (*E*ye-opener) to steady your nerves or get rid of a hangover?

• Patients with one or more positive responses should be further evaluated with a detailed alcohol history.

Signs

Unexplained elevation of hepatic transaminase levels or macrocytosis.

• Cardiac, neurological (including cognitive) systems should be evaluated through history and physical examination.

Investigations

• A detailed alcohol history is essential for all new patients and periodically thereafter, and among patients in whom an alcohol problem is suspected; areas to be included are:

Family history of alcohol problems.

Age of onset of drinking.

Amount and frequency of alcohol use.

Changes in role functioning (occupational, social, familial).

Concomitant substance abuse.

Laboratory studies: none are routine. In patients suspected of a chronic moderate or severe alcohol problem, hepatic and renal chemistry tests, complete blood count, and folate and magnesium levels should be obtained.

Complications

Social morbidity: disruption of family relationships and occupational and social functioning.

Trauma, including motor vehicle accidents, physical fights, and drowning.

Physical illness: such as hypertension, acute and chronic liver disease, cardiovascular disease, cancer, and morbidity from withdrawal syndromes.

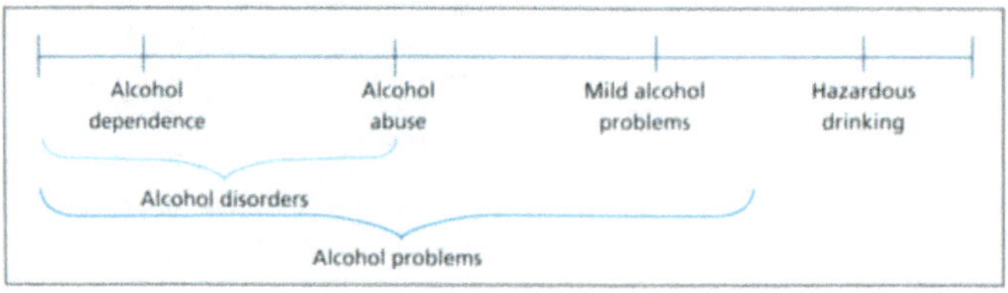

Spectrum of problems related to alcohol use.

Differential diagnosis

• Complications or consequences of alcohol problems are often mistaken for primary rather than secondary problems (*e.g.*, trauma from motor vehicle accidents), or viewed as outside the purview of primary care physicians and therefore not mentioned by the patient, or not investigated by the practitioner (*e.g.*, job loss, marital difficulties).

• Psychiatric symptoms such as depression, insomnia, and anxiety are often clues to underlying alcohol problems.

Etiology

• Risk factors for alcohol problems include:

Male gender.

Heavy drinking in teenage years.

Drinking regularly before age 16 years.

Psychiatric illness.

History of antisocial behavior.

Alcoholic relatives.

Northern European ethnicity.

Some Native American groups.

Epidemiology

Alcohol abuse and dependence

11%–20% of patients in general medicine practice.

20% of emergency department patients.

Hazardous drinking

20% of people who drink.

20% of women in gynecology practices.

Alcohol problems among the elderly [3]

Largely unrecognized problem.

5% of community-dwelling elderly.

20% of medically hospitalized patients.

• Because of polypharmacy, the elderly are at particular risk for adverse drug-alcohol interactions (*e.g.*, benzodiazepines, antidepressants, NSAIDs, oral hypoglycemics).

1989 alcohol-related health care costs among the elderly: $233 million.

Treatment

Diet and lifestyle

Alcohol abuse and dependence

• Referral to alcoholism treatment programs or self-help groups (*e.g.*, Alcoholics Anonymous) is a mainstay of therapy; practitioners should identify a colleague who can recommend the most appropriate programs for individual patients based on availability, patient preferences, insurance coverage, and cost.

• Letters, phone calls, and follow-up appointments from primary care practitioners may help motivate patients to remain in treatment.

Hazardous drinking

• Effective, brief, office-based interventions include the following:

Recommending decreasing drinking to moderate levels, which may improve compliance, for patients who are not abusers or dependent.

Setting specific drinking goals (amount, frequency) mutually with the patient.

Associating physical problems (macrocytosis, transaminase elevation) with alcohol use.

Motivated patients may benefit from programs aimed at developing controlled drinking habits (*e.g.*, DrinkWise, Moderation Management).

Pharmacological treatment [4]

May be useful adjuncts to behavioral therapy in chronic alcohol abuse or dependence, usually after acute withdrawal and detoxification, to maintain sobriety; usually reserved for recurrent, severe problem drinkers or for impulsive drinkers who drink on the spur of the moment, then drink to excess.

Disulfiram

Standard dosage	250–500 mg daily for 1–2 weeks, then 250 mg daily, for several months to years; tablets are crushed in water with a water "chaser," at least 12 hours after the last drink.
Contraindications	Heart disease, psychosis, chronic liver disease, pregnancy, inability to comprehend or comply with therapy; use with caution in diabetes, hypothyroidism, seizure disorders, and nephritis.
Special points	Attendance in treatment program or self-help group (*e.g*, Alcoholics Anonymous) is mandatory; monitor liver transaminases after 1–2 weeks of therapy, then every 2–4 weeks thereafter; monitor complete blood count and "SMA-12" chemistries every 6 months. Treatment of disulfiram-ethanol reaction (flushing, headache, dyspnea, nausea, vomiting; cardiovascular collapse in severe cases) is largely symptomatic and supportive.
Main drug interactions	Phenytoin levels increase in patients on disulfiram. Reduce disulfiram dose to 250 mg three times per week and monitor phenytoin levels. Disulfiram increases levels of coumarin anticoagulants and barbiturates.
Main side effects	Severe side effects (other than the disulfiram-ethanol reaction) are rare; most common side effect is somnolence, usually improved after 10–14 days of therapy; other reported side effects include rash and hepatitis.

Naltrexone [4]

Pure opiate antagonist demonstrated in short-term trials to enhance abstinence from alcohol.

Standard dosage	50 mg daily, usually for 12 weeks. First dose after 7–10 days abstinence from opiates; to assure opiate abstinence, naloxone challenge test should be given prior to first dose.
Contraindications	Demonstrated or suspected opiate use; liver disease (transaminases > 4 times normal or elevated bilirubin, acute hepatitis, liver failure).
Special points	Simultaneous participation in treatment program or self-help group is mandatory; monitor liver function tests monthly; can precipitate severe opiate withdrawal.
Main drug interactions	Opiate agonists (including medications for cough and cold, diarrhea, and pain).
Main side effects	Nausea and/or vomiting, headache; hepatotoxic at high doses.

Treatment aims

To achieve complete abstinence from alcohol abuse and dependence.

• Controlled drinking is not a recommended treatment goal.

To limit drinking or abstinence in hazardous drinking.

Other treatments

• Acute withdrawal syndromes should generally be managed in inpatient settings.

• Benzodiazepines are the mainstay of therapy.

• Mild cases can be managed as outpatients with careful follow-up.

• Future agents, currently in clinical trials, include nalmefene (opioid antagonist) and acamprosate (GABA analogue).

Prognosis

• 60%–80% of patients without severe dependence in treatment programs are drinking without problems 1–2 years later.

• 5%–20% of problem drinkers treated in abstinence-oriented programs are eventually without drinking problems.

Follow-up and management

• Primary goal of follow-up is to prevent or identify relapse.

• Family/peer support is critical for long-term success.

• Periodically review need for maintenance counseling, for successfully abstinent as well as refractory patients.

Information on Alcoholics Anonymous

Check local number in white pages; (212) 870-3400; or at web site: www.alcoholics-anonymous.org.

Key references

1. Bradley KA: The primary care practitioner's role in the prevention and management of alcohol problems. *Alcohol Health Res World* 1994, **18**:97–104.
2. Ewing JA: Detecting alcoholism: the CAGE questionnaire. *JAMA* 1984, **252**:1905–1907.
3. Fink A, Hays RD, Moore AA, Beck J: Alcohol-related problems in older persons. *Arch Intern Med* 1996, **156**:1150–1156.
4. Swift RM. Drug therapy: drug therapy for alcohol dependence. *N Engl J Med* 1999, **340**:1482–1490.

Allergic rhinitis

Diagnosis

Symptoms

History of nasal stuffiness or congestion, rhinorrhea, post nasal drip, itchy nose, sneezing, itchy or watery eyes, decreased or loss of smell and taste, sore throat, headaches or pain over paranasal sinuses. May have history of recurrent sinus infections, asthma, or atopic dermatitis.

Symptoms may be seasonal or chronic. Common seasonal allergens include trees, grasses, and ragweed. Perennial allergens include fungi and molds. Common indoor allergens include fungi, dust mites, cockroaches, and animals such as cats, rats, and guinea pigs. Latex, especially in the health care setting, may be an allergen.

Signs

Swollen, pale nasal mucosa often present but not specific for allergic rhinitis. Nasal mucosa may be erythematous. Clear, watery mucus is typical. "Allergic salute"—upward nasal rubbing. "Allergic shiners"—dark lower eyelid skin.

Investigations

Skin prick testing: determines if patient has IgE antibodies to the antigen but must be correlated with history because positive skin test results with no attendant respiratory complaints are common.

Intradermal dilution testing: routinely used; provides information regarding appropriate starting doses for immunotherapy.

Specific in vitro antigen testing (often referred to as RAST): used for patients who cannot tolerate skin testing or when there is concern about abnormal skin reactivity.

Eosinophilia on nasal smears: may assist in differentiating allergic from infectious rhinitis.

Complications

Sinusitis.

Sleep disturbances due to chronic nasal obstruction.

Asthma: evidence supports treatment of allergic rhinitis to improve asthma control.

Differential diagnosis

Vasomotor rhinitis

Cerebrospinal fluid leak.

Nasopharyngeal structural lesions.

Nasal polyps.

Etiology

IgE mediated release of histamine and proinflammatory mediators resulting in sneezing, itching, rhinorrhea, and nasal congestion.

Epidemiology

Affects about 20% of U.S. population.

Often associated with atopic dermatitis and asthma.

Treatment

Diet and Lifestyle

Allergen avoidance is the starting point for treatment. However, this is frequently difficult because of the ubiquitous presence of the allergen, such as molds, or unwillingness to eliminate carpeting or part with a pet, such as a cat.

Pharmacological treatment

H_1 antihistamines reduce sneezing, itching, and rhinorrhea. Generally they do not eliminate nasal congestion. They are less efficacious in perennial rhinitis in which nasal congestion often predominates.

Decongestants (α-adrenergic agonists). Topical agents provide rapid and more complete relief compared to systemic therapy. Prolonged (>7 days) use of topical agents may result in rhinitis medicamentosa with protracted nasal congestion.

Cromolyn is efficacious and has few adverse effects.

Topical nasal steroids are efficacious for control of nasal symptoms. Ocular symptoms will often persist because the effect is local on the nasal mucosa.

Systemic steroid bursts (7 to 10 days) are occasionally indicated in patients with severe symptoms not responding well to other therapies.

Immunotherapy based on history and skin testing. While a chronic therapy, the value of this approach has been clearly documented for numerous pollen, dust mite, and cat dander allergies.

Nonpharmacological treatment

Saline sprays to sooth nasal irritation.

Treatment aims

Control symptoms.

Prognosis

- Depends on allergen.
- Should be able to achieve symptomatic control with seasonal therapy only or immunotherapy plus medications.

Follow-up and management

Depends on severity and frequency of symptoms.

General references

Barnes PJ: Therapeutic strategies for allergic diseases. *Nature* 1999, 402: B31–B38.

Durham SR, Walker SM, Varga EM, *et. al.*: Long-term clinical efficacy of grass-pollen immunotherapy. *N Engl J Med* 1999, **34441**: 468–475.

Greisner WA III, Settipane RJ, Settipane GA: Natural history of hay fever: a 23-year follow-up of college students. *Allergy Asthma Proc* 1998, **19(5)**:271–275.

Naclerio R, Solomon W: Rhinitis and inhalant allergens. *JAMA* 1997, **278**:1842–1848.

Alopecia

Diagnosis

Symptoms and signs

• Alopecia is a clinical sign and needs to be classified as either scarring or nonscarring before an accurate diagnosis can be made. The distinction is also important because scarring alopecia is generally permanent.

Causes of alopecia

Scarring

Lichen planopilaris; kerio (tinea); folliculitis decalvans; dissecting cellulitis; chronic cutaneous lupus; trauma; scleroderma; congenital causes; alopecia neoplastica (metastatic carcinoma).

Nonscarring (diffuse)

Androgenetic alopecia; telogen effluvium; anagen effluvium; hyperthyroidism/ hypothyroidism; systemic lupus.

Nonscarring (patchy)

Alopecia areata; trichotillomania; tinea capitis; secondary syphilis; traction alopecia.

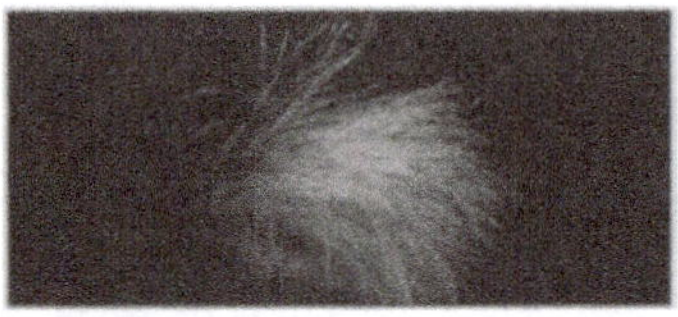

Alopecia areata, with deficient melanin in area of regrowth. (*See* Color Plate.)

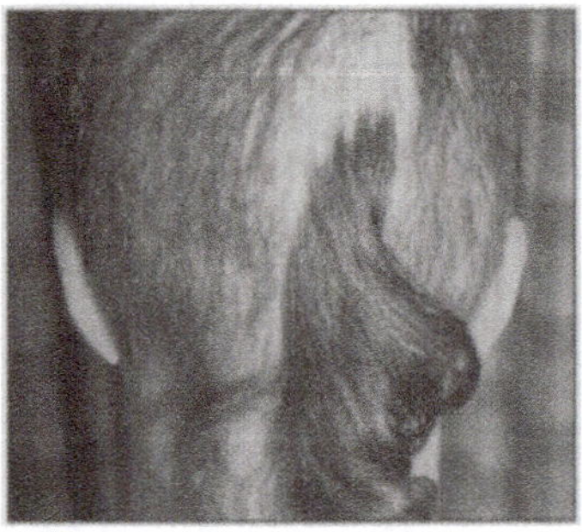

Spared pony tail growth in trichotillomania. (*See* Color Plate.)

Androgenetic alopecia

• Males present with a receding anterior hair line, especially in the parietal regions, which results in an M-shaped recession. Alopecia may involve the posterior crown. In contrast, females usually experience a more diffuse pattern of hair loss, which often begins at the part line. In young women with androgenetic alopecia, signs of virilization such as clitoral hypertrophy, acne, and facial hirsutism should be sought to rule out endocrine dysfunction.

Alopecia areata

Localized "ring shaped" area of nonscarring alopecia: hallmarked by short, tapered "exclamation point" hairs.

Pitted or onychodystrophic nails: may be present.

Alopecia totalis (entire scalp) or alopecia universalis (entire body surface): may occur in rare instances.

Gray or depigmented hair: often appears in regrowth.

Trichotillomania (traumatic alopecia)

Incomplete nonscarring hair loss: hairs of unequal length in alopecic areas; most patients deny (or are unconscious of) pulling out hairs.

Lichen planopilaris

Lichen planus of the scalp: often no lichen planus elsewhere; scarring alopecia with perifollicular erythema and keratotic papules.

Chronic cutaneous lupus erythematosus

Scarring alopecia with follicular prominence and plugging: may or may not be associated with systemic disease.

Investigations

Biopsy of affected area: specimen should be taken from the active edge (biopsy specimens taken from long-standing scarred regions are often nondiagnostic); may be diagnostic in alopecia areata, lichen planopilaris, and chronic cutaneous lupus; reveals follicular hemorrhage and empty follicles in trichotillomania.

Fungal scrapings: often negative in kerion; can be helpful in tinea capitis along with culture; must include hairs in scraping of scalp.

Hormone studies: in women with hair loss and evidence of increased androgens.

Complications

Severe scarring.

Squamous cell carcinomas: in areas of scarring alopecia from lupus (rare).

Differential diagnosis

Not applicable.

Etiology

Alopecia areata

Autoimmune; rarely may be associated with thyroid disease.

Androgenetic alopecia

Increased expression of androgen receptors and/or changes in androgen metabolism of the scalp hair follicles. Heredity is polygenic.

Trichotillomania

Psychological stresses.

Chronic cutaneous lupus

Autoimmune.

Epidemiology

Alopecia areata

• 75% of patients present before age 25 years.

• Patients with Down syndrome, positive family history of alopecia areata, or atopy appear to be more prone; no consistent HLA genotypes have been identified.

Androgenetic alopecia

• May begin any time after puberty in males; often fully expressed by the forties. Females are affected later; approximately 40% present in the sixth decade.

Trichotillomania

• Patients are predominantly female.

Chronic cutaneous lupus

• Appears to be more common in black women.

Fungal infections

• *Microsporum* spp. infection is associated with animal contact and usually affects children.

• *Trichophyton tonsurans* is the most common cause of tinea capitis in the United States and usually occurs in school-age children.

Treatment

Diet and lifestyle

- Iron deficiency may lead to diffuse alopecia.
- Sudden weight loss may precipitate telogen effluvium.
- Lifestyle stressors may exacerbate trichotillomania.

Pharmacological treatment

Alopecia areata

- Alopecia areata usually resolves spontaneously, but some cases may be resistant to treatment.
- Potent topical steroids, intralesional steroids, topical irritants or allergens, and topical minoxidil have all been used successfully.
- Systemic steroids or cyclosporine have been effective but are often not used because of side effects.

Standard dosage	Clobetasol propionate, 0.05% solution applied twice daily. Triamcinolone acetonide, 10 mg/mL intralesionally every 2–4 weeks.
Contraindications	Local infection, atrophy.
Special points	Potent topical steroids: used over a large area can result in systemic absorption.
Main drug interaction	None.
Main side effects	Local steroid atrophy, systemic steroid absorption.

Androgenetic alopecia

- There is no highly effective therapy to prevent the progression of androgenetic alopecia. Finasteride (1 mg daily) is an oral 5-alpha-reductase type II inhibitor, currently approved for use in males only. May cause loss of libido, erectile dysfunction, and a 50% decrease in prostate-specific antigen levels. Hair growth will regress if therapy is stopped. Discontinue use if no results are seen after 6–12 months.

Standard dosage	Topical minoxidil 2% and 5% topical solution; apply twice a day for >32 weeks. The 5% solution shows significantly more hair regrowth than the 2% solution but may cause facial hair growth in females.
Contraindications	None.
Special points	Helpful in reducing rate of hair loss or partially restoring hair in some patients. Frontal-bitemporal recession often fails to respond. Therapy must be continued or hair loss recurs.
Main drug interaction	None.
Main side effects	None.

Trichotillomania

Psychiatric counseling, pimozide, selective serotonin reuptake inhibitors.

Chronic cutaneous lupus

Emphasize sun protection.

Antimalarial therapy is often used by specialists for the treatment of extensive disease.

Standard dosage	Intralesional triamcinolone, 10 mg/mL. Clobetasol propionate, 0.05% solution.
Contraindications	None.
Special points	Topical or intralesional steriods are only local treatments; they do not affect systemic disease.
Main drug interaction	None.
Main side effects	Atrophy, systemic absorption.

Treatment aims

To arrest and reverse pathological hair loss.

To prevent scarring.

Other treatments

- Several antiandrogens (spironolactone, cyproterone acetate, flutamide, and cimetidine) have been reported to be useful in the treatment of androgenetic alopecia.

Prognosis

Alopecia areata

- 50% of patients will have complete regrowth of localized areas in 1 year; one-third of patients never regrow hair.
- Poor prognostic indicators as follows: early onset, severe initial involvement, total alopecia for >1 year, nail dystrophy, ophiasis pattern (alopecia around periphery of scalp).

Androgenetic alopecia

Usually gradual progression of hair loss over years to decades.

Trichotillomania

Good with appropriate psychiatric treatment.

Follow-up and management

Follow-up should be often in all diseases mentioned except androgenetic alopecia patients, who can be followed up every 6–12 months or more frequently depending on the treatment

General references

Cather JC, *et al.*: Finasteride—an update and review. *Cutis* 1999, **64**:167–172.

Price VH: Treatment of hair loss. *N Engl J Med* 1999, **341**:964–973.

Sawaya ME: Clinical updates in hair. *Dermatol Clin* 1997, **15**:37–43.Shapiro J, Shabnam M: Alopecia areata: diagnosis and management. *Int J Dermatol* 1999, **38(1)**:19–24.

Sperling LC, Mezebish DS: Hair diseases. *Med Clin North Am* 1998, **82**:1155–1169.

Tosti A, Piraccini BM: Androgenic alopecia. *Int J Dermatol* 1999, **38(1)**:1–7.

Anal fissure

Diagnosis

Symptoms

Burning or tearing perianal pain: while defecating, often accompanied by small amounts of bright red blood on the tissue paper or surface of the stool.

Signs

Linear ulcer: in the distal portion of the anus; most typically located in the posterior midline. Fissures may also occur in the anterior midline, particularly in women. These are best seen by direct visualization of the distal anus after spreading the buttocks. Linear ulcers in the lateral quadrants are atypical for simple fissures, and other diseases such as Crohn's disease, rectal trauma, or sexually transmitted disease should be considered.

A hood of granulation tissue (*i.e.*, a sentinel tag): often seen at the distal margin of fissures, outside the anus; should prompt closer examination for a linear ulcer.

A hypertrophied anal papilla: often palpable as a large grain of rice on digital examination just proximal to the ulcer.

Investigations

Direct inspection: best method to see anal fissure.

Anoscopy: often painful and may traumatize the area of ulceration.

• Atypical or nonhealing ulcers should be carefully examined for associated disease such as inflammatory bowel disease, malignancy, or infection; sigmoidoscopy with careful visualization of the proximal mucosa and biopsy of the ulcer should be considered in these situations.

Complications

Chronic ulcer.

Constipation.

Persistent bleeding.

Differential diagnosis

Crohn's disease.

Hidradenitis suppurativa.

Carcinoma.

Syphilis.

Tuberculosis.

Hemorrhoid.

Perianal abscess.

Anal trauma.

Etiology

• Higher resting anal sphincter pressure with an abnormally brisk contraction after defecation is found in patients prone to anal fissures; the fissure is often initiated by passage of a large, hard stool and then perpetuated by the increased tone and contraction reflex after defecation.

Epidemiology

Common, particularly in young and middle-aged adults.

• Fissures occur equally in women and men.

Treatment

Diet and lifestyle

• Patients should be placed on a high-fiber diet to achieve soft stools.

• Patients should take sitz baths twice daily to promote healing.

Pharmacological treatment

• Stool softening agents (*e.g.*, synthetic mucilloids or psyllium preparations) should be titrated at a dose that will minimize straining and achieve 1-2 soft bowel movements each day. A typical starting dose consists of one heaping tablespoon (*e.g.*, Metamucil) in 8 oz of water once or twice each day with advancement in the dose frequency every 3-4 days until the desired effect is realized. The patient should be instructed to drink the preparation immediately after mixing and informed that a few days of increased flatus or bloating is commonly experienced at the start of therapy.

• Topical emollients with local anesthetics (*e.g.*, benzocaine, witch hazel) may be used to relieve symptoms; patients should be instructed to apply these preparations locally twice daily as needed for symptom control.

• Topical nitroglycerin 0.2% applied to the anus by finger tip twice daily for 6 weeks; results in healing 60% of patients with chronic posterior anal fissures [2].

• Botulinum toxic injection (20 units) into the internal anal sphincter; results in healing more than 90% of patients with chronic anal fissures [2,3].

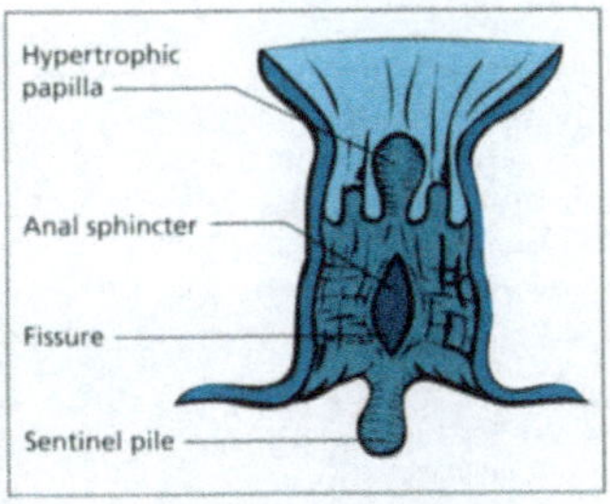

The classic chronic anal fissure triad includes the hypertrophic anal papilla, anal fissure, and sentinel skin tag. The fissure margins may appear fibrotic and slightly undermined, and exposed internal sphincter muscle fibers may be visible.

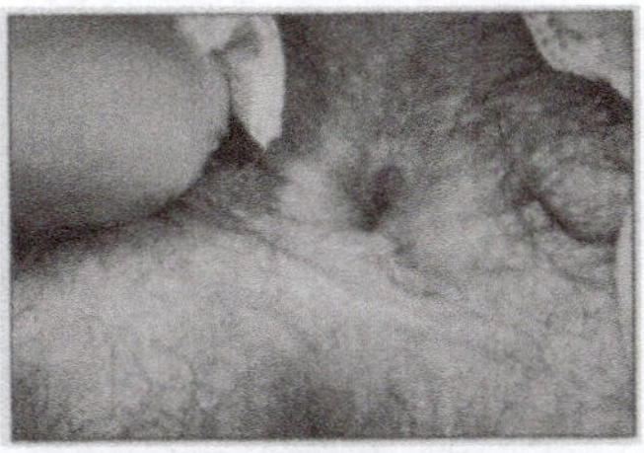

Typical fissure in ano located in the posterior midline. (*See* Color Plate.)

Treatment aims

To reduce pain and bleeding.

Other treatment options

• Chronic fissures that are refractory to the approaches previously mentioned often require a surgical procedure to reduce the internal sphincter tone; this is best achieved by a lateral subcutaneous internal anal sphincterotomy, which is typically performed as an outpatient procedure; manual dilation is an alternative approach.

Prognosis

• Anal fissures often require 4-6 weeks of medical therapy before complete healing is achieved; surgery, when required, has a cure rate in excess of 90%.

Follow-up and management

• The accurate diagnosis of a benign anal fissure is ultimately confirmed by the response to treatment; patients should be seen in clinic until the problem is resolved and to monitor for other possible diagnoses (*see* Differential diagnosis).

Key references

1. Barnett JL, Raper SE: Anorectal disease. In Textbook of Gastroenterology, edn 3. Edited by Yamada T. Philadelphia: JB Lippincott; 1999:217–220.
2. Brisinda G, et al.: a comparison of injections of botulinum toxin and topical nitroglycerin ointment for the treatment of chronic anal fissure. *N Engl J Med* 1999, **341**:65–69.
3. Maria G: A comparison of botilinum toxin and saline for the treatment of chronic anal fissure, *N Engl J Med* 1998, **338**:217-220.

Anemia, aplastic

Diagnosis

Symptoms

• Symptoms and signs are due to and relate to the severity of the peripheral blood pancytopenia.

Fatigue, shortness of breath on exertion, headache, palpitation: symptoms of anemia.

Easy bruising and petechiae, gum bleeding, buccal hemorrhage, visual disturbance due to retinal hemorrhage: symptoms of thrombocytopenia.

Mouth and tongue ulcers, white coating on buccal mucosa, odynophagia, fever: symptoms of infection due to leukopenia.

History of jaundice: may indicate posthepatitic aplasia or associated paroxysmal nocturnal hemoglobulinuria.

Signs

• Bleeding manifestations are usually more common than infection.

Pallor.

Ecchymoses, petechiae of skin and mouth, retinal hemorrhage.

Fever.

Mouth and tongue ulceration, thrush.

Pharyngitis, pneumonia.

Skin and perianal sepsis.

Skeletal, skin, and nail anomalies; short stature: may occur in congenital aplastic anemia.

• Spleen, liver, and lymph nodes are not enlarged.

Investigations

Complete blood count and examination of blood film: show pancytopenia (isolated cytopenias may occur in early stages), macrocytosis, toxic granulation of neutrophils.

Reticulocyte count: shows absolute reticulocytopenia.

Bone-marrow aspiration and biopsy: shows hypocellular bone marrow, no abnormal infiltration, no increase in reticulin, low number of or no colony-forming cells; cytogenetic studies to exclude preleukemia; in Fanconi's anemia, cultured peripheral blood lymphocytes show increased chromosomal breaks with DNA cross-linking agent (*e.g.*, diepoxybutane).

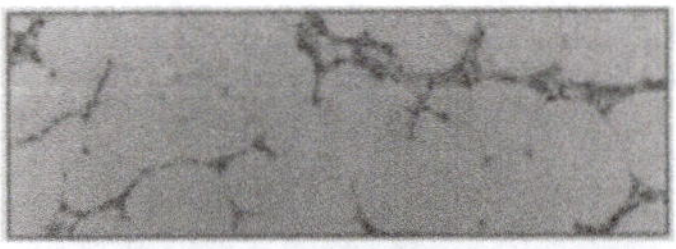

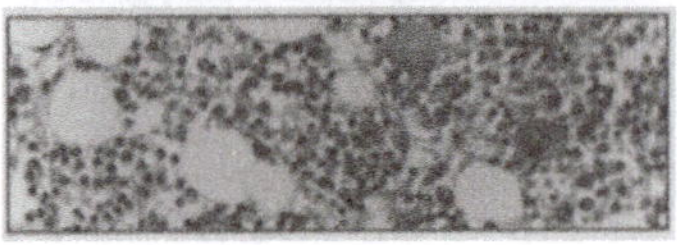

Aplastic anemia bone marrow (*top*), normal bone marrow (*bottom*).

Ham's test and urine hemosiderin analysis: classically negative in aplastic anemia and positive in paroxysmal nocturnal hemoglobulinuria (PNH), but a small proportion of PNH cells can be detected in up to 30% of patients with aplastic anemia.

Liver function tests and viral studies: to detect antecedent hepatitis; test for hepatitis A, B, and non-A, non-B (hepatitis C); Epstein–Barr virus; cytomegalovirus; and parvovirus B19 (parvovirus classically causes pure erythrocyte aplasia and can also cause pancytopenia associated with hemophagocytosis).

Chest and sinus radiography: to evaluate for the presence of infections.

Hand and forearm radiography: may be abnormal in congenital aplastic anemia.

Abdominal ultrasonography: to exclude splenomegaly; anatomically displaced or abnormal kidneys in Fanconi's anemia.

Complications

Failure of random donor platelet transfusions to increase recipient's platelet count, increased bone-marrow graft rejection potential: due to sensitization to non-HLA antigens from multiple blood transfusions.

Late clonal evolution to myelodysplastic syndrome or acute myeloid leukemia in 10% of patients with aplastic anemia or paroxysmal nocturnal hemoglobulinuria in 10% of patients who have not had transplantation.

Differential diagnosis

Hypoplastic myelodysplastic syndrome or hypoplastic acute myeloid leukemia in adults.

Hypoplastic acute lymphoblastic leukemia in children.

Hairy cell leukemia.

Other bone-marrow infiltration: *e.g.*, lymphoma, carcinoma, myelofibrosis.

Anorexia nervosa.

Severe infection: *e.g.*, tuberculosis, overwhelming gram-negative or gram-positive sepsis.

Systemic lupus erythematosus.

Etiology

Congenital causes

Fanconi's anemia, dyskeratosis congenita.

Acquired causes

Idiopathic: in 75% of patients.

Drugs: *e.g.*, NSAIDs, gold, chloramphenicol, sulfonamides.

Chemicals: benzene, organic solvents, aniline dyes.

Viruses: hepatitis A, B, or non-A, non-B (hepatitis C), and other as yet unidentified viruses; Epstein–Barr virus.

Paroxysmal nocturnal hemoglobinuria: 25% of patients later develop aplastic anemia.

Rare causes

SLE, pregnancy.

Epidemiology

• The annual incidence in the United States is 2–8 per million.

• The male:female ratio is equal.

• Two peaks are seen in the age incidence for men: 15–25 years and >60 years; one peak for women: >60 years.

Treatment

Diet and lifestyle

• If neutrophils count is <0.5×10^9/L, food should be well cooked and fresh fruit washed before consumption.

Pharmacological treatment [1,2]

• Drugs are indicated for patients ineligible for bone-marrow transplantation.

• High-dose corticosteroids should be avoided because of toxicity (infection, hypertension, diabetes, avascular necrosis of bone) and lack of convincing benefit in aplastic anemia.

• Drugs that affect platelet function (aspirin, NSAIDs, glycoprotein II/III inhibitors) or that may cause aplastic anemia must be avoided.

Antilymphocyte globulin (ALG) or antithymocyte globulin (ATG)

• Horse ATG should be used initially.

Standard dosage	ATG, 10–20 mg/kg daily for 8–14 consecutive days followed by alternate-day therapy for another 14 days, or 40 mg/kg/day for 4 days equally effective.
Contraindications	Hypersensitivity or severe systemic reaction to test dose, active infection, hemolytic paroxysmal nocturnal hemoglobinuria, SLE.
Special points	Central line infusion to prevent thrombophlebitis; platelet transfusion before each dose; low-dose prednisone to prevent serum sickness.
Main drug interactions	None.
Main side effects	Anaphylaxis or allergic reactions (during infusion); serum sickness (7–14 days after starting treatment).

Cyclosporine

• Cyclosporine can be used after ALG, in combination with ALG, or as a single agent.

Standard dosage	Cyclosporine, 12 mg/kg/day orally for 3–6 months.
Contraindications	Renal or liver impairment, breast-feeding.
Special points	Drug blood concentration, blood pressure, renal and liver function must be monitored regularly.
Main drug interactions	Erythromycin, ketoconazole, aminoglycosides, vancomycin, amphotericin B, rifampin, phenytoin.
Main side effects	Nephrotoxicity, nausea, tremor, hypertension, hypertrichosis, gum hypertrophy, hepatotoxicity.

Oxymetholone

• Oxymetholone is now used after ALG and cyclosporine rather than as a single agent.

Standard dosage	Oxymetholone, 2.5 mg/kg orally daily (0.5–1 mg/kg daily for Fanconi's anemia).
Contraindications	Liver impairment, breast and prostate cancer, pregnancy; caution in children (behavioral problems) and elderly men (prostatic hypertrophy).
Special points	Serum cholesterol concentration must be monitored.
Main drug interactions	Other potentially hepatotoxic drugs, *e.g.*, erythromycin, rifampin, ketoconazole, cyclosporine.
Main side effects	Reversible cholestatic jaundice, liver tumors, and peliosis hepatitis with long-term use, virilization in females, acne.

Alternative medicine

Recommended use: Stinging nettle (*Urtica dioica*); Yellow dock (*Rumex crispus*).

Common use: Dong quai (*Angelica sinesis*); ginseng (*Panax ginseng*); Spirulina.

Caution: none.

Treatment aims

To provide good supportive care (critical for survival of patient).

To treat fever promptly (broad-spectrum i.v. antibiotics), routine oral antifungal prophylaxis.

Other treatments

Allogeneic bone-marrow transplantation: treatment of choice for patients who have severe aplastic anemia, are aged <45 years, and have an HLA-identical sibling donor.

Bone-marrow transplantation from an HLA-matched volunteer donor: if patient has very severe aplastic anemia, is aged <30 years, and has no HLA-identical sibling [3,4].

• Hematopoietic growth factors such as granulocyte colony-stimulating factor (CSF), granulocyte macrophage-CSF, interleukin-3, and interleukin-6 have little effect in aplastic anemia, apart from a transient increase in neutrophil count in some patients. Serious toxicity may occur in aplastic anemia patients [5].

Prognosis

• After bone-marrow transplantation from an HLA-identical identical sibling, at least 70%–80% of patients are long-term survivors and can be considered cured of their disease.

• Response to antilymphocyte globulin or cyclosporine occurs in 50%–70% (rarely before 3–6 months), but relapse and later clonal disorders may occur.

Follow-up and management

• Long-term monitoring is needed for clonal disorders and relapse.

Key references

1. Young NS: Acquired aplastic anemia. *JAMA* 1999, **282**:271–278.1
2. Young NS, Barrett AJ: The treatment of severe acquired aplastic anemia. *Blood* 1995, **85**: 3367–3377.
3. Soutar RL, King DJ: Bone marrow transplantation. *BMJ* 1995, **310**:31–36.
4. Tsai TW, Freytes CO: Allogenic bone marrow transplantation for leukemias and aplastic anemia. *Adv Intern Med* 1997, **42**:423–451.
5. Marsh JCW, *et al.*: Haemopoietic growth factors in aplastic anemia: a cautionary note. *Lancet* 1994, **344**:172–173.

Anemia, megaloblastic

Diagnosis

Symptoms

• Many patients have no symptoms; the disease is suspected on routine blood count.

Dyspnea on exertion, tiredness, headache.

Painful tongue.

Paraesthesias in feet, difficulty walking: vitamin B_{12} deficiency only.

Infertility.

Signs

Pallor of mucous membranes: if hemoglobin concentration <9 g/dL.

Mild jaundice.

"Beefy red" glossitis.

Signs of vitamin B_{12} (B_{12}) neuropathy: if present.

Investigations [1,2]

General

Blood count: raised mean cell volume (>100 fL), reduced erythrocyte count, hemoglobin, and hematocrit; low reticulocyte count; reduced leukocyte and platelet counts (in severely anemic patients).

Blood film: shows oval macrocytes, hypersegmented neutrophils (>5 nuclear lobes).

Bone-marrow analysis: in severely anemic patients, the bone marrow is hypercellular with increased proportion of early cells, many dying cells, megaloblastic erythroblasts, giant and abnormally shaped metamyelocytes, and hypersegmented megakaryocytes.

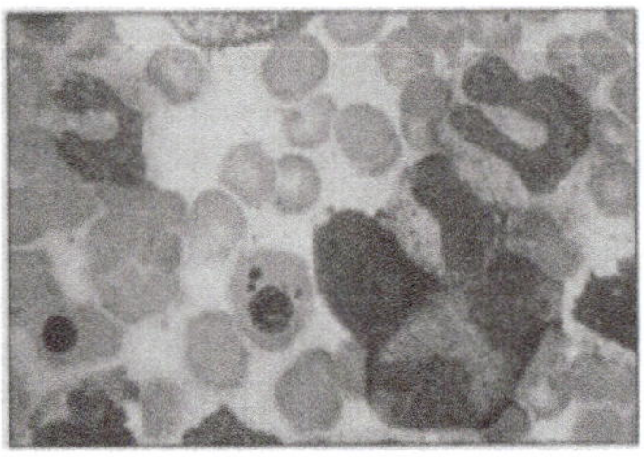

Bone marrow with megaloblastic anemia. (*See Color Plate.*)

Serum indirect bilirubin and lactic dehydrogenase measurement: concentrations raised.

Direct Coombs test: complement only, positive in some patients.

Tests for disseminated intravascular coagulation or intravascular hemolysis: positive in some patients.

Tests for B_{12} or folate deficiency: serum B_{12} low in B_{12} deficiency, normal or slightly low in folate deficiency; serum folate normal or raised in B_{12} deficiency, low in folate deficiency; erythrocyte folate normal or low in B_{12} deficiency, low in folate deficiency.

Deoxyuridine suppression, serum homocysteine and methylmalonic acid measurement: additional tests performed in some laboratories for B_{12} or folate deficiency [3].

Special

Diet history: to exclude veganism, low folate intake.

Schilling test: for B_{12} absorption.

Serum analysis: for intrinsic factor and parietal cell antibodies.

Fiberoptic endoscopy: for gastric biopsy, exclusion of gastric polyps, carcinoma in pernicious anemia.

Contrast radiography: to detect gastric atrophy, neoplasm (pernicious anemia), or small intestinal lesions.

Endoscopy and jejunal biopsy: if gluten-induced enteropathy is suspected in patients with folate deficiency.

Complications

Neuropathy: due to B_{12} deficiency.

Neural tube defects in fetus: risk reduced by folate treatment.

Carcinoma of stomach: in pernicious anemia.

Differential diagnosis

Other causes of macrocytosis [1,2]
Alcoholism, liver disease, hypothyroidism, aplastic anemia, myelodysplasia, acute myeloid leukemia, myeloma, reticulocytosis, drugs.

Other causes of megaloblastic anemia
Nitrous oxide anesthesia.
Transcobalamin II deficiency.
Antifolate drugs: methotrexate, pyrimethamine (reversed by folinic acid), co-trimoxazole.
Drugs inhibiting DNA synthesis: cytosine arabinoside, hydroxyurea, 6-mercaptopurine, azathioprine, 5-fluorouracil.
Congenital abnormalities of B_{12} or folate metabolism.
Congenital abnormalities of DNA synthesis: *e.g.*, orotic aciduria.

Etiology

Causes of B_{12} deficiency [1]
Diet deficiency: *e.g.*, in vegans.
Pernicious anemia.
Congenital intrinsic factor deficiency.
Total or subtotal gastrectomy.
Atrophic gastritis, gastric bypass.
Blind loop syndrome.
Ileal resection or abnormality: *e.g.*, Crohn's disease.
HIV infection.
Drugs: *e.g.*, metformin.
Specific malabsorption with proteinuria.
Fish tapeworm.

Causes of folate deficiency [1,2]
Dietary deficiency: poor-quality diet, goat's milk, specialized diets.
Malabsorption: gluten-induced enteropathy, tropical sprue, congenital.
Increased turnover: pregnancy, prematurity, hemolytic anemias, myelofibrosis, widespread inflammatory or malignant diseases.
Increased losses: congestive heart failure, hemodialysis or peritoneal dialysis.
Uncertain: anticonvulsant treatment.

Epidemiology

• The occurrence of megaloblastic anemia relates to diet (*e.g.*, in Hindu communities, where veganism is common; poor people, in whom dietary folate intake is reduced).
• For pernicious anemia, the peak age of incidence is 60 years.
• The female:male ratio is 1.6:1.

Treatment

Diet and lifestyle

• The quality of the diet must be increased in patients with dietary folate deficiency.

Pharmacological treatment [1,2]

For B_{12} deficiency

Standard dosage	Cyanocobalamin, 1 mg i.m. daily (week 1), 1 mg twice weekly (week 2), 1 mg weekly for 4 weeks, and then 1 mg monthly.
Contraindications	Rare hypersensitivity.
Special points	No evidence suggests that more frequent doses are needed for B_{12} neuropathy.
Main drug interactions	None.
Main side effects	Gout and significant hypokalemia a few days after commencing treatment.

For folate deficiency

Standard dosage	Folic acid, 1–5 mg/d until complete hematologic recovery, then 1–5 mg/d as needed.
Contraindications	B_{12} deficiency, malignancy (unless deficiency is clinically important).
Special points	B_{12} deficiency must be excluded because B_{12} neuropathy could be precipitated or aggravated.
Main drug interactions	None.
Main side effects	None.

• Folic acid should be used as prophylaxis in pregnant women (300–400 µg daily; 5 mg daily if previous neural defect in fetus) and also in renal dialysis recipients.

• In women of childbearing age, folate intake should be increased to at least 400 µg daily by diet or folate supplement.

• For premature babies (birth weight <1500 g), folic acid, 1 mg daily, is indicated.

Alternative medicine

Recommended use: Stinging nettle (*Urtica dioica*); Yellow dock (*Rumex crispus*).

Common use: Dong quai (*Angelica sinesis*); ginseng (*Panax ginseng*); Spirulina.

Caution: none.

Treatment aims

To correct anemia by replenishing body stores of vitamin.

To correct underlying disease.

To restore normal neurological status (B_{12} deficiency).

Other treatments

• Packed red blood cell transfusion should be used only if essential: removal of equivalent volume of plasma in patients with congestive heart failure.

Prognosis

• Prognosis depends mainly on the underlying cause.

• Life expectancy is reduced slightly in patients with pernicious anemia because of the risk of carcinoma of the stomach.

Follow-up and management

• Patients with pernicious anemia should have annual clinical review and blood count.

• Routine endoscopy is not recommended.

• Patients having total gastrectomy or ileal resection need prophylactic cyanocabalamin, 1 mg every 3 months, from the time of surgery for life.

Key references

1. Anthony AC: Megaloblastic anaemias. In *Hematology. Basic Principles and Practice*. Edited by Hoffman R, *et al.* New York: Churchill Livingstone; 2000: 446–485.
2. Zittoun J, Zittoun R: Modern clinical testing strategies in cobalamin and folate deficiency. *Semin Hematol* 1999, **36**:35–46.

Anemia, pernicious

Diagnosis

Definition

Malabsorption of vitamin B_{12} (cobalamin) due to lack of normal intrinsic factor production by the stomach.

Symptoms

• Symptoms often not apparent (vitamin B_{12} deficiency or atrophic gastritis may be an incidental finding).

• When present, symptoms are usually due to anemia or complications of vitamin B_{12} deficiency.

Shortness of breath, lethargy.

Sore tongue: glossitis in 50% of patients.

Parasthesias: due to peripheral neuropathy; classic "stocking-glove" distribution.

Gait disturbance: due to myelopathy (subacute combined degeneration of spinal cord).

Depression, impaired memory.

Loss of taste.

Signs

Mucosal pallor: reflecting anemia.

Glossitis.

Mild splenomegaly.

Signs of other organ-specific autoimmune disease: *e.g.*, hypothyroidism.

Peripheral sensory neuropathy with absent reflexes.

Pyramidal or long-tract neurological signs; loss of joint position sense.

Investigations

Hematology: for macrocytic anemia (mean corpuscular volume >100 fL), leukopenia or thrombocytopenia, hypersegmented neutrophils on blood film.

Bone-marrow analysis: megaloblastic changes with maturation arrest.

Liver function test: increased bilirubin due to ineffective erythropoiesis.

Serum vitamin B_{12} measurement: to detect low concentrations (normal, >160 ng/L).

Schilling test: abnormal part I test using ^{58}Co-labeled vitamin B_{12} (<10% urinary excretion); part II corrects to normal after administration of intrinsic factor.

Serum gastrin measurement: raised concentration in pernicious anemia (normal <100 pmol/L).

Gastric analysis: shows achlorhydria.

Endoscopy and biopsy: for atrophic gastritis on endoscopy and histological assessment of stage of gastritis.

Complications

Gastric carcinoid and enterochromaffin cell hyperplasia: associated with reflex rise in serum gastrin due to reduced gastric acid; 2%–9% prevalence of gastric carcinoid in patients with pernicious anemia [1].

Gastric carcinoma: 1%–7% increased risk in patients with pernicious anemia [2].

Peripheral sensory neuropathy, subacute combined degeneration of spinal cord: affects pyramidal tracts, causing spastic paraparesis and bladder involvement, and dorsal columns, causing sensory ataxia and impaired joint position sense.

High-output cardiac failure, myocardial ischemia: in severe anemia.

Dementia.

Differential diagnosis

Type B chronic gastritis related to *Helicobacter pylori* infection.

Other causes of vitamin B_{12} deficiency: *e.g.*, dietary deficiency in vegans, terminal ileitis (Crohn's disease), terminal ileal resection, blind loop syndromes, small bowel diverticula or bacterial overgrowth, postgastrectomy states, pelvic irradiation.

Etiology

• Pernicious anemia is an organ-specific autoimmune disease, with a strong association with other organ-specific autoimmune diseases, especially thyroid disease.

Epidemiology

• Pernicious anemia occurs more often in female patients than in male.

• Pernicious anemia is common in all races and countries.

Immunology

• Antigastric parietal-cell antibodies (probably involved in pathogenesis) occur in 70%–90% of patients, anti-intrinsic factor antibodies in 50%–70%.

• Antibodies have been shown to be directed against membrane-bound hydrogen/potassium ATPase pump, resulting in blockade of hydrochloric acid secretion and correlating with concentrations of gastric parietal-cell antibodies.

Treatment

Diet and lifestyle

• No special precautions are necessary for uncomplicated disease except for avoidance of extreme isometric exercise.

Pharmacological treatment

Standard dosage	Hydroxocobalamin, 1 mg i.m. 6 times in 2–3 weeks, then 1 mg every 3 months.
Contraindications	None.
Special points	Can cause initial hypokalemia and folate deficiency in patients with marked vitamin B_{12} deficiency; chloride and folic acid supplements are advisable.
Main drug interactions	None.
Main side effects	None.

Alternative medicine

Recommended use: Stinging nettle (*Urtica dioica*); Yellow dock (*Rumex crispus*).

Common use: Dong quai (*Angelica sinesis*); ginseng (*Panax ginseng*); Spirulina.

Caution: none.

Treatment aims

To prevent neurological complications.

To correct anemia.

Prognosis

• Despite the small risk of gastric carcinoid or carcinoma, life expectancy is little altered in patients with uncomplicated disease [1,2].

• Gastric carcinoids have a good prognosis, with no reported cases of carcinoid syndrome in these patients and a low reported incidence of local or regional spread.

Follow-up and management

• The cost of endoscopic surveillance has been shown to outweigh the benefit of screening for the few patients who are found to have unsuspected malignancy; it should probably be reserved for patients who develop symptoms.

• Regular vitamin B_{12} supplementation in outpatients must be ensured.

Key references

1. Born K, *et al.*: Gastric endocrine cell hyperplasia and carcinoid tumors in pernicious anemia. *Gastroenterology* 1985, **88**:638–648.

2. Lechago J, Correa P: Prolonged achlorhydria and gastric neoplasia: is there a causal relationship? *Gastroenterology* 1993, **104**:1554–1557.

Aneurysm & arteriovenous malformation

Diagnosis

Symptoms

Seizures.

Headache: dull frontal or sudden and severe thunderclap headaches.

Visual field deficits.

Diplopia.

Hemiparesis.

Cognitive dysfunction.

Lethargy or coma (*see* Intracerebral hemorrhage).

Signs

Third nerve compression with pupillary dilatation and ptosis (internal carotid artery or posterior communicating artery aneurysm).

Fourth cranial nerve palsy (anterior communicating artery compression).

Cavernous sinus syndrome with ophthalmoparesis and facial numbness.

Reduced visual acuity or visual field deficits.

Hemiparesis.

Bruit.

Dysphasia.

Investigations

CT: can identify large arteriovenous malformations (AVMs), especially when calcified.

MRI and MR angiography: can identify large (≥1.5 cm) aneurysms easily and is very useful for AVMs. Four-vessel cerebral angiography is most definitive diagnostically and helpful therapeutically.

- Make sure to evaluate for second aneurysm, present in 20%–30% of cases.

Lumbar puncture: for evaluation for subarachnoid hemorrhage if headache is present.

Complications

Intracerebral hemorrhage.

Progressive seizures, weakness, or neural compression.

Differential diagnosis

Cerebral neoplasm, especially vascular meningiomas.

Cerebral abscess.

CNS sarcoidosis.

Venous angioma or cavernous hemangioma.

Etiology

- Most AVMs are congenital.
- Aneurysms may be defects in the media of vessels at bifurcations or posttraumatic.
- Aneurysms can also be mycotic (subacute bacterial endocarditis), fungal, or neoplastic.

Epidemiology

- 7%–20% of patients with subarachnoid hemorrhage due to aneurysm rupture have a first-degree relative with an aneurysm.
- 20%–30% of patients with one aneurysm have multiple aneurysms.
- Rebleed rate is 3.5% per year for untreated aneurysms.
- Aneurysms found in association with polycystic kidney disease, Ehlers-Danlos syndrome, Marfan syndrome, and neurofibromatosis type 1.
- AVM incidence is one-seventh that of aneurysms.

Treatment

Diet and lifestyle

- Limit sports or activities that can cause head trauma.
- Pregnancy increases the likelihood of rupture.

Pharmacological treatment

Anticonvulsant agents for seizures as required.

Control hypertension aggressively.

Embolization, radiosurgery, and resection of accessible AVMs.

Treatment aims

To prevent cerebral hemorrhage.

To treat seizures.

Other treatments

Clipping and/or endovascular thrombosis of aneurysms (endovascular coil thrombosis especially effective in lesions with small necks).

Prognosis

Aneurysm rebleed rate, 3.5% per year.

AVM morbidity/mortality, 3%–4% per year.

- Posterior fossa AVMs have a particularly poor prognosis.
- Larger AVMs may be less likely to rupture.
- CNS steal syndromes may lead to ischemic deficits.

Follow-up and management

Follow-up seizures and neurological examination every 6–12 months and refer to neurosurgery for definitive management.

General references

Gobin YP, Laurent A, Merienne L, *et al.*: Treatment of brain arteriovenous malformations by embolization and radiosurgery. *J Neurosurg* 1996, **85**:19–28.

Scheinevink WI: Intracranial aneurysms. *N Engl J Med* 1997, **336**:28–40.

Sinson G, Phillips MF, Flamm ES: Intraoperative endovascular surgery for cerebral aneurysms. *J Neurosurg* 1996, **84**:63–70.

Angina pectoris, stable

Diagnosis

Symptoms

• Angina is a clinical syndrome characterized by discomfort in the chest, jaw, shoulder, back, or arm. Typical angina consists of 1) substernal chest discomfort with a characteristic quality and duration that is provoked by 2) exertion or emotional stress, and 3) relieved by rest or nitroglycerin. Probable angina meets two of these characteristics, and noncardiac chest pain meets fewer than one of the typical angina characteristics.

• The Canadian Cardiovascular Society Classification of Angina is as follows: class I: Angina occurs only with strenuous or rapid or prolonged exertion; b) class II: Ordinary activity (*e.g.*, climbing more than one flight of ordinary stairs or walking 2 blocks at a normal pace and in normal conditions) is slightly limited; c) class III: Ordinary activity is markedly limited; class IV: Inability to carry out any physical activity without discomfort—angina present at rest.

Signs

• Typically no signs are manifest, but patients should be examined for evidence of the following:

Hypertension.

Hyperlipidemia.

Diabetes.

Left ventricular outflow obstruction: *i.e.*, aortic stenosis, hypertrophic cardiomyopathy.

Previous myocardial damage.

Investigations

Hematocrit: anemia exacerbates angina.

Clinical biochemistry: 1) Serum lipids: LDL and HDL cholesterol, triglyceride level, 2) serum homocysteine level: particularly in young patients and patients with a strong family history, 3) fasting glucose: to rule out underlying diabetes mellitus, 4) thyroid function tests: to exclude hypothyroidism particularly, in the elderly.

Rest ECG: to detect left ventricular hypertrophy, previous Q-wave myocardial infarction or ST-T changes.

Rest echocardiography: done only when there is clinical suspicion of aortic stenosis or hypertrophic cardiomyopathy.

Exercise ECG: to precipitate symptoms, document workload at onset, and record any associated ECG abnormality (*e.g.*, 1 mm of horizontal or downsloping ST-segment depression or elevation for 60–80 ms after the end of the QRS complex) or arrhythmia.

Exercise myocardial perfusion imaging or exercise echocardiography: in patients who have one of the following baseline ECG abnormalities: left bundle-branch block, more than 1 mm of rest ST-segment depression, and 3) patients with electronically paced ventricular rhythm and those with previous revascularization (percutaneous transluminal angioplasty or coronary artery bypass grafting) or those in whom considerations of functional significance of lesions or myocardial viability are important.

Coronary angiography: gold standard: provides detailed anatomical information about site and severity of luminal narrowing due to coronary atherosclerosis and less common nonatherosclerotic causes, such as coronary artery spasm, coronary anomaly, Kawasaki disease, primary coronary artery dissection, and radiation-induced coronary vasculopathy. Coronary angiography should be considered if noninvasive testing reveals ST-segment or T-wave changes at low levels of exercise, blood pressure reduction during exercise, significant left ventricular dysfunction, or multiple or large transient perfusion defects.

Complications

Unstable angina.

Acute myocardial infarction.

Arrhythmias.

Death.

Differential diagnosis

Cardiac

Pericarditis.

Myocardial infarction.

Aortic dissection.

Noncardiac

Esophageal spasm.

Reflux esophagitis.

Peptic ulceration.

Musculoskeletal pain.

Cervical spondylosis.

Da Costa's syndrome.

Etiology

Causes

Coronary atherosclerosis in 99% of patients.

Aortic stenosis.

Hypertrophic cardiomyopathy.

Arteritis.

Risk factors

Family history.

Smoking.

Diabetes.

Hypertension.

Hyperlipidemia.

Obesity.

Post menopause

Epidemiology

• Coronary atherosclerosis is endemic in industrialized countries, but the incidence is decreasing.

• In the United States, >500 000 myocardial infarctions are reported per year.

• No accurate figures are available for the prevalence of angina pectoris, but, in people aged >30 years, it is >2.6%.

Treatment

Diet and lifestyle

Treatment of hypertension according to the Joint National Conference VI guidelines. (*See* Hypertension.)

Smoking cessation therapy; management of diabetes; exercise training program.

• Lipid-lowering therapy in patients with documented or suspected coronary artery disease and LDL cholesterol level of 130 mg/dL; target LDL cholesterol level <100 mg/dL.

• Weight reduction in obese patients who have hypertension, hyperlipidemia, or diabetes mellitus.

Pharmacological treatment

Pharmacotherapy to prevent myocardial infarction and death

• Antiplatelet agents

Aspirin: effective in preventing first myocardial infarction and 33% risk decrease in adverse cardiovascular events. *Clopidogrel:* when aspirin is contraindicated.

• Lipid-lowering agents

In the Scandinavian Simvastatin Survival Study, hydroxymethylglutaryl-coenzyme reductase inhibitors given to patients with a baseline total cholesterol level of 212–308 mg/dL was associated with a significant reduction in the risk for fatal and nonfatal myocardial infarction and the need for revascularization.

If triglyceride levels are elevated, fibrates should be considered.

Lipid-lowering therapy can expect to prevent 20–30 deaths or myocardial infarctions per 1000 patient-years.

Pharmacotherapy to reduce ischemia and relieve symptoms

• Nitrates

Nitrates improve exercise tolerance, increases the time to onset of angina, and decrease ST-segment depression during treadmill exercise. The main side effect is hypotension.

Sublingual glyceryl trinitrate (GTN) remains the mainstay of treatment. The major side effect is headache. It should be taken for pain and taken prophylactically before known precipitating events.

Long-acting nitrates (*e.g.*, isosorbide mononitrate) are particularly useful in patients who gain relief from sublingual GTN.

Special points: combined with β-blockers or calcium antagonists, nitrates produce greater anti-anginal and anti-ischemic effects in patients with stable angina.

• β-blockers

Preferred initial therapy (in the absence of contraindications), particularly in patients with previous myocardial infarction, for which this class of drugs has been shown to reduce mortality. **β-blockers may aggravate coronary spasm.**

Dosage: adjust dose to reduce rest heart rate 55 to 60 beats/min, or, in patients with more severe angina, to below 50 beats/min (provided there are no symptoms or heart block does not develop). Atenolol, 50–100 mg/d, is usually prescribed. Metoprolol, 25–50 mg/d, is often used when renal function is impaired.

• Calcium-channel antagonists

Appropriate initial therapy in patients with contraindications to β-blockers, as a substitute for β-blockers in patients who develop unacceptable side effects of β-blockers, or in combination with -blockers when initial β-blocker therapy is not successful.

Diltiazem and verapamil are usually prescribed, but in the setting of impaired left ventricular function, amlodipine is preferred

• Investigational drugs: Nicorandil, a potassium channel activator, can be useful in selected patients and is currently approved only in Europe.

Alternative medicine

Recommended use: carnitine; pantethine.

Common use: coenzyme Q_{10}; Hawthorn (*Crataegus* spp); khella (*Ammi visnaga*); Ethylenediaminetetraacetic acid chelation.; curcumin; acupuncture.

Caution: avoid garlic and high-dose vitamins before cardiac surgery; higher doses of pure khellin (120–150 mg/day) may cause anorexia, nausea, and dizziness.

Treatment aims

To control symptoms and restore normal exercise tolerance.

To prevent disease progression (myocardial infarction and death).

To improve prognosis.

Other treatments

Percutaneous transluminal coronary angioplasty (with or without coronary stent): complementary to drug treatment and surgery; no improvement in survival.

Coronary artery bypass grafting.

Prognosis

• 14% of patients with newly diagnosed angina pectoris progress to unstable angina, myocardial infarction, or death within 1 year.

• Mortality at coronary artery bypass grafting with normal ventricular function is 1%.

Follow-up and management

• Patients with successfully treated chronic stable angina pectoris should have a follow-up evaluation every 4–12 months. During the first year of therapy, evaluations every 4-6 months are recommended. After first year of therapy, annual evaluations are recommended if the patient is stable.

• During follow-up, 5 questions must be answered by the patient receiving treatment:

• Has patient decreased level of physical activity since last visit?

• Have the patient's symptoms increased in frequency and become more severe since last visit?

• How well is the patient tolerating therapy?

• How successful has the patient been in reducing modifiable risk factors and improving knowledge about ischemic heart disease?

• Has the patient developed any new comorbid illnesses or has the severity or treatment of known comorbid illnesses worsened the patient's angina?

General references

Aaberge L, *et al.*: Transmyocardial revascularization with CO_2 laser in patients with refractory angina pectoris. Clinical results from the Norwegian randomized trial. *J Am Coll Cardiol* 2000, **35**:1170–1177.

Murray S, Collins PD, James MA: Neurostimulation for angina pectoris. *Heart* 2000, **83**:217–220.

Angina pectoris, unstable

Diagnosis

Symptoms

Rest angina: angina occurring at rest and usually prolonged >20 minutes occurring within a week preceding presentation.

New-onset angina: angina of at least class III (Canadian Cardiovascular Society classification) severity with onset within 2 months before initial presentation.

Increasing angina: previously diagnosed angina that is distinctly more frequent, longer in duration, or occurring at a lower threshold.

Signs

•The objective of the physical examination is to:

1. Determine the likelihood of severe underlying coronary artery disease (*e.g.*, rales, S3 gallop, or acute mitral regurgitation). The presence of pulse deficits, bruits, or other signs of extracardiac vascular disease suggests a higher likelihood of significant coronary artery disease.

2. Assess the hemodynamic effects of the ischemic events and therefore vital signs (blood pressure in the arms, heart rate, temperature); a thorough cardiovascular and chest examination should be performed.

3. Identify potential precipitating causes of angina, *e.g.*, uncontrolled hypertension or thyrotoxicosis.

4. Identify comorbid conditions, *e.g.*, pulmonary disease.

Investigations

C-reactive protein: elevated levels during onset of symptoms are associated with increased mortality. Persistently high C-reactive protein levels 1on discharge is associated with higher risk for recurrent instability and myocardial infarction.

Cardiac troponin measurements: elevated troponin T level is associated with increased risk for cardiac events, whereas elevated troponin I level has shown to be associated with increased mortality.

ECG: a completely normal ECG in a patient with pain does not exclude the diagnosis. New or reversible ST-segment deviation of 0.5 mm or more from baseline or left bundle-branch block at time of admission is associated with increased mortality or risk of myocardial infarction at one year. Isolated T-wave inversion is not a marker of adverse prognosis.

Exercise testing and nuclear imaging: exercise or pharmacologic stress testing provides important information about a patient's risk, and the use of nuclear imaging improves the study's sensitivity and specificity. Both thallium-201 imaging and dipyridamole sestamibi tomography help distinguish between low-risk and high-risk patients with unstable angina in a population at intermediate clinical risk before testing. A normal result on nuclear imaging is associated with a lower rate of cardiac events during a 2-year follow-up period than an abnormal result is. The presence of a reversible or a fixed perfusion defect has an independent predictive value for future cardiac events.

Coronary angiography: approximately 50%–60% of patients with unstable angina require coronary angiography and revascularization because of the "failure" of medical therapy, defined as either recurrent ischemia at rest while the patient is in the hospital or ischemia that can be provoked during a test to assess risk before discharge.

Complications

Myocardial infarction.

Ventricular tachycardia, ventricular fibrillation.

Differential diagnosis

Cardiac

Myocardial infarction.

Aortic dissection.

Pericarditis.

Acute myocarditis.

Noncardiac

Pulmonary embolism.

Etiology

Plaque erosion and rupture.

Platelet adhesion and aggregation.

Thrombus formation.

Endothelial dysfunction: episodic vasospasm may contribute to vascular instability by altering pre-existing coronary plaques, a process that causes intimal disruption.

Epidemiology

• The estimated incidence is 2 per 1000 admissions annually; accounts for more than 1 million hospital admissions annually.

• 14% of patients with newly diagnosed stable angina progress to unstable angina, myocardial infarction, or death within 1 year.

Treatment

Diet and lifestyle

- Patients should be hospitalized, with strict bed rest, possibly with sedation.

Management

- Early triage is enhanced by thorough assessment.
- Low-risk patients do not have pain at evaluation, have an unchanged or normal ECG, have normal cardiac enzyme level, and are hemodynamically stable.
- Intermediate-risk patients have new-onset or accelerated angina or angina at rest ongoing for more than 20 minutes, with no changes in cardiac enzyme levels or ECG.
- High-risk patients have had angina at rest, prolonged angina, or persistent angina, with dynamic ST-segment changes or hemodynamic instability.
- Low- or intermediate-risk patients should be treated with aspirin and evaluated further. If they are asymptomatic for more than 24 hours, they may undergo evaluation on an outpatient basis if the evaluation can be completed within 72 hours after discharge.
- High-risk patients urgently require simultaneous evaluation and treatment.

Pain relief

- Sublingual nitroglycerine tablets, 0.4 mg, or spray taken 5 minutes apart.
- Morphine sulfate, 1 to 5 g i.v..
- Naloxone (0.4–2.0 mg) i.v. Meperidine hydrochloride can be substituted in patients allergic to morphine.
- Antiplatelet therapy should be initiated promptly.
- Aspirin blocks. Initial dose is 160–325 mg nonenteric formulation, followed by 80–160 mg of enteric or nonenteric formulation per day.
- Ticlopidine may be substituted for aspirin in patients with hypersensitivity to aspirin or gastrointestinal intolerance.
- Clopidogrel combined with aspirin is useful in preventing coronary-stent thrombosis. A loading dose of 300 mg is followed by 75 mg/d.
- Platelet glycoprotein IIb/IIIa receptor antagonists consist of 3 classes: *Murine-human chimeric antibody*, e.g., abciximab, 0.25 mg/kg bolus, followed by an infusion of 0.125 μg/kg/min (maximum, 10 μg/min) for 12–24 hours.

Synthetic peptide forms, e.g., eptifibatide 80 μg/kg bolus, followed by an infusion of 2.0 μg/kg/min for 72–96 hours. *Synthetic nonpeptide forms, e.g.*, tirofiban and lamifiban. Tirofiban, 0.4 μg/kg/min for 30 minutes, followed by an infusion of 0.1 μg/kg/min for 48–96 hours.

- A platelet glycoprotein IIb-IIIa receptor antagonist should be administered with aspirin and heparin to patients with unstable angina and continuing ischemia or with other high-risk features. Eptifibatide and tirofiban are approved for this use. Abciximab can be administered for patients who will undergo a percutaneous interventional procedure.
- These drugs can be used as primary medical therapy or as an adjunct to invasive coronary interventions.

Antithrombin therapy

- Unfractionated heparin: bolus, 60–70 U/kg i.v., followed by infusion of 12–15 U/kg/h titrated to a partial thromboplastin time of 1.5–2.5 times control.
- LMWH include dalteparin and enoxaparin.
- Direct antithrombins.
- Warfarin.

Thrombolytic therapy

- Avoid. *Aspirin:* possible unstable angina. *Aspirin plus i.v. heparin or s.c. LMWH:* likely/definite unstable angina. *Aspirin plus i.v. heparin or s.c. LMWH plus i.v. glycoprotein IIb/IIIa antagonist:* definite unstable angina with continuing ischemia.

Conventional anti-anginal therapy

- β-blockers are administered to reduce cardiac work and myocardial oxygen demand.
- Intravenous nitroglycerine is recommended for patients who do not respond to sublingual nitroglycerine and for nonhypotensive high-risk patients.
- Calcium antagonists are useful for controlling ongoing or recurring ischemia-related symptoms in patients already receiving adequate doses of nitrates and β-blockers, in patients unable to tolerate adequate doses of one or both of these agents, or in patients with variant angina.

Treatment aims

To prevent complications, while allowing healing of the ruptured plaque.

Other treatments

- Unstable angina is a medical emergency: patients whose symptoms do not resolve rapidly with medical treatment should be transferred to a cardiothoracic center for coronary angiography with a view to revascularization.
- Revascularization: The decision regarding the revascularization procedure (*e.g.*, coronary artery bypass grafting, percutaneous transluminal angioplasty, stent placement, or atherectomy) is based on coronary anatomy, left ventricular function, the experience of the medical and surgical personnel, presence or absence of coexisting illnesses, and preferences of the patient and the physician.

Prognosis

- The course of the disease varies widely. In some patients, an anginal attack progresses rapidly to myocardial infarction or death, whereas in others uneventful recovery occurs in 24 hours.
- High risk for myocardial infarction (15%–20%) and death (15%) in ensuing 3 months.
- In hospital, the mortality rate is 1%; rate of nonfatal myocardial infarction is 8%.

Alternative medicine

Recommended use: carnitine; pantethine.
Common use: coenzyme Q10; Hawthorn (Crataegus spp); khella (Ammi visnaga); Ethylenediaminetetraacetic acid chelation.; curcumin; acupuncture.
Caution: avoid garlic and high-dose vitamins before cardiac surgery; higher doses of pure khellin (120–150 mg/day) may cause anorexia, nausea, and dizziness.

General references

Goy JJ: Contemporary approach to management of unstable angina. *Lancet* 1999, **354:** 694–695.

Yeghizarians Y, Braunstein JB, Askari A, *et al.*: Unstable angina pectoris. *N Engl J Med* 2000, **342:**–101–114.

Ankylosing spondylitis

Diagnosis

Symptoms

• Symptoms usually begin during the third decade, although some patients present in their teens and a few in their 30s [1].

• Onset is insidious, not associated with trauma.

Back pain and stiffness: worse in morning, improving with exercise, deteriorating with rest.

Peripheral joint symptoms: in 40%; affecting particularly shoulders, hips, knees.

Fatigue.

Uveitis and other stigmata of the spondylarthropathies: *e.g.*, related to psoriatic spondylitis, reactive arthropathy, enteropathic arthritis.

Signs

• Signs may be nonexistent or minimal.

Decreased mobility of lumbar spine, reduced chest expansion, poor mobility of cervical spine.

Decreased mobility of hips and shoulders, knee synovitis, Achilles tendinitis, dactylitis, psoriasis, psoriatic nail change.

Evidence of uveitis: during active attack.

Increasing "stoop": with disease progression.

Anemia of chronic disease: particularly in patients with peripheral joint involvement.

Investigations

Radiography of pelvis: reveals sacroiliitis (sacroiliac change may be minimal, moderate, or severe), juxta-articular sclerosis and erosions, lumbar spine changes, calcification, cervical spine involvement.

ESR, plasma viscosity, CRP measurement: raised values in 50% of patients, but laboratory changes may be absent even in severely ill patients.

Complications

Hip deterioration: ~20% of patients who develop the disease in their teens or early 20s need one or two new hips within 15 years of disease onset.

Knee involvement: occasionally results in need for total knee replacement.

Deteriorating vision: resulting from persistent uveitis.

Spinal fracture: can occur as a result of osteoporotic changes associated with spinal fusion; resulting spinal-cord injury can be catastrophic.

Cauda equina syndrome: rare.

Pulmonary apical fibrosis: may be worse in smokers.

Differential diagnosis

Reactive arthropathy (Reiter's syndrome) [2], psoriatic arthropathy, inflammatory bowel disease.

Nonspecific back pain (much more common): radiography differentiates the two.

Other causes of peripheral joint disease with coincidental back pain [3].

Etiology [1]

• Ankylosing spondylitis is the result of interplay between HLA B27 and other genes and environmental triggers.

• Environmental triggers probably include agents recognized in other forms of reactive arthropathy (*e.g.*, *Chlamydia* spp.; ureaplasma; *Campylobacter*, *Shigella*, *Yersinia*, and *Salmonella* spp.; and other gram-negative organisms) [2].

Epidemiology

• Ankylosing spondylitis occurs in 0.5% of the population in communities where HLA B27 is prevalent (northern Europe, United States, Asia, Central America).

• The male:female ratio is 2.5:1 overall, 3:1 in teenagers, and 1.5:1 with onset in the late 20s.

Treatment

Diet and lifestyle

• Exercise is of paramount importance [4].

• Attention to posture throughout the day and night is essential.

• Hydrotherapy and physical therapy are needed as an initial introduction to a lifelong exercise program.

• Patients and family members must understand the concept of treatment, and literature should be available describing the precise exercise program needed.

• Patients should avoid smoking.

Pharmacological treatment

• NSAIDs are needed by 80% of patients [4].

Standard dosage	Indomethacin, 75 mg slow release once or twice daily; dose and frequency titrated against patient's needs.
Contraindications	Active peptic ulcer disease, indomethacin intolerance (alternative NSAID should be tried); caution in elderly patients, those on anticoagulants, and those with past history of gastrointestinal bleed or perforation.
Main drug interactions	Warfarin and other anticoagulants.
Main side effects	CNS disturbance, gastrointestinal problems.

• Sulfasalazine may be useful in patients with peripheral joint involvement but may have little effect on spinal disease [4–6].

Alternative medicine

Recommended use: none.

Common use: meadowsweet (*Filipendula ulmaria*); willowbark (*Salix* spp.); prickly ash (*Zanthoxylum clava-herculis*); nettles (*Urtica dioica*); black cohosh (*Cimicifuga racemosa*).

Caution: none.

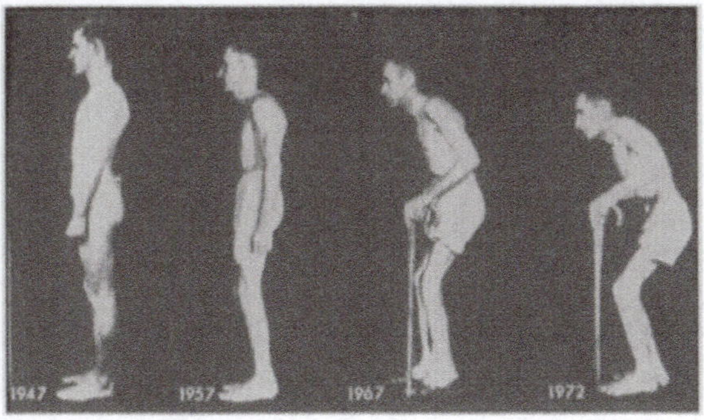

Sequence of progressive deformity.

Treatment aims

To allow a good night's sleep.

To decrease morning stiffness (pharmaco-logical treatment).

To enable patient to follow the important exercise program.

To maintain good function and posture.

Prognosis

• Outcome is determined by genetic and environmental factors.

• Although the disease does not burn out, most patients can follow a normal social, family, and professional life.

• Up to 10% of patients have relentless progression, with deteriorating posture and spinal fusion, perhaps requiring surgery.

• Patients with early age of onset and lower educational or social status may be at most risk of severe disease.

Follow-up and management

• After the patient has become stable, visits every 6–12 months to the rheumatologist suffice.

• For patients with severe disease, specialist inpatient management may be appropriate.

Patient support

Spondylitis Association of America
PO Box 5872
Sherman Oaks, CA 91413

Key references

1. Gran JT, Husby G: The epidemiology of ankylosing spondylitis. *Semin Arthritis Rheum* 1993, **22**:319–334.
2. Hughes RA, Keat AC: Reiter's syndrome and reactive arthritis: a current view. *Semin Arthritis Rheum* 1994, **24**:190–210.
3. Leirisalo-Repo M: Enteropathic arthritis, Whipple's disease juvenile spondyloarthropathy and uveitis. *Curr Opin Rheumatol* 1994, **6**:385–390.
4. Creemers MC, *et al.*: Treatment of seronegative spondyloarthropathies. *Semin Arthritis Rheum* 1994, **24**:71–81.
5. Dougados M, *et al.*: Sulfasalazine in the treatment of spondyloarthropathy. A randomized multi-center double-blind placebo controlled study. *Arthritis Rheum* 1995, **38**:618–627.
6. Cuellar ML, Espinoza LR: Management of spondyloarthropathies. *Curr Opin Rheumatol* 1996, **8**:288–295.

Anorexia & bulimia nervosa

Diagnosis [1]

Symptoms and signs

Anorexia nervosa

Body weight <85% of expected weight or body mass index < 17.5. Body mass index is approximately equal to weight (lbs) × 703/height $(in)^2$.

Intense fear of weight gain.

Inaccurate perception of own body size, weight, or shape.

Amenorrhea (in girls and women after menarche).

Dry skin, acrocyanosis, and breast atrophy.

Bulimia nervosa

Recurrent binge eating (at least two times per week for 3 months).

Recurrent purging, excessive exercise, or fasting (at least two times per week for 3 months).

Excessive concern about body weight or shape.

Absence of anorexia nervosa.

• Swelling of the parotid and submandibular glands, abnormal dentition, and abrasions on the dorsum of the hand (caused by scraping against the incisors during attempts at vomiting) may be seen in association with chronic self-induced vomiting.

• An undisclosed eating disorder should be suspected in any young to middle-aged adult who demonstrates difficulty eating in social contexts, social withdrawal, absence from school or work, substance abuse, or excessive exercise.

Investigations [2]

• In taking the history, a straightforward, empathic, and nonjudgmental approach should be taken.

• Careful history of weight changes, dietary patterns, and the frequency and severity of purging behavior and excessive exercise should be taken. Purging behavior may include emesis or use of laxatives, enemas, diuretics, anorexic drugs, or caffeine.

• Evaluation for suicidal behavior or ideation should be routine.

• Nutritional status should be assessed through basic chemistries, including serum albumin, and blood counts. Electrocardiography is essential to assess the QT interval, to monitor electrolyte abnormalities, and to guide therapy. Bone densitometry should be considered.

Complications

• The QT interval is sometimes prolonged in anorexia nervosa, even when serum electrolytes are normal. Left ventricular mass is often reduced in anorexia nervosa, although systolic function is typically preserved. Mitral valve prolapse may develop but is usually mild. Intestinal dilatation from chronic severe constipation and diminished intestinal motility as a result of long-term laxative abuse or withdrawal may be associated with anorexia or bulimia nervosa. Electrolyte disturbances can include hypokalemia, acid-base abnormalities, and hyponatremia.

• Osteoporosis is a serious, common clinical problem and can be established in young women after as little as 6 months. In 50% of women with anorexia nervosa, bone density is more than 2 standard deviations below normal.

• Suicidal behavior often accompanies anorexia and bulimia nervosa and is a chief contributor to the high mortality rate among patients with anorexia nervosa.

Differential diagnosis

Depression.

Diabetes mellitus.

Thyroid disease.

Inflammatory bowel disease.

Cancer.

Etiology

Etiology unknown, but these two conditions appear to be caused by a combination of genetic, neurochemical, psychodevelopmental, and sociocultural factors.

Epidemiology [1]

Most common among adolescent girls or young women, although 5%–15% of cases occur in males.

Approximately 3% of young women have some degree of eating disorder.

Onset usually during adolescence, but can occur after age 40.

Eating disorders affect all socioeconomic classes and major ethnic groups in the United States.

Treatment

• Most patients with clinically significant anorexia or bulimia nervosa are best managed in conjunction with a psychiatrist or behavioral management program with experience in eating disorders.

Diet and lifestyle

• Education and counseling about the importance of addressing symptoms and of monitoring weight, vital signs, and electrolytes (if purging or excessive water intake is ongoing) are a mainstay of therapy.

• Counseling about nutrition and limitations on exercise should be provided.

Pharmacological treatment

Anorexia nervosa

• Vitamin supplementation, calcium (1000–1500 mg/d), and vitamin D (400 IU/d).

• Role of bisphosphonates not established.

• Estrogen replacement (with progestin) may be offered if patient has symptoms of estrogen deficiency.

• Psychopharmacology is generally not effective in treating the primary symptoms.

Bulimia nervosa

• Antidepressants

Usual dosage	Fluoxetine, up to 60 mg/d; desipramine, up to 300 mg/d; and imipramine, up to 300 mg/d, have been shown to improve symptoms. Only fluoxetine is approved by the Food and Drug Administration for this indication.
Contraindications	Desipramine and imipramine: prolonged QT interval; tricyclic antidepressants: relatively contraindicated in patients with ischemic heart disease who have recently had myocardial infarction and in those with heart block; desipramine: pregnancy rating C.
Special points	Fluoxetine generally has fewer side effects than tricyclic antidepressants, but individual responses will vary.
Main drug interactions	Potentially fatal interactions with monoamine oxidase inhibitors (MAOIs) and antiarrhythmic agents. Serotonergic crisis (hypertension, hyperpyrexia, seizures) possible in patients receiving fluoxetine and other serotonergic medications (*e.g.*, MAOIs, lithium, carbamazepine). Fluoxetine inhibits hepatic cytochrome P450, yielding many potential drug interactions.
Main side effects	*Fluoxetine:* gastrointestinal upset, anorexia, vomiting, diarrhea, agitation, insomnia, sexual dysfunction.

Tricyclic antidepressants (desipramine and imipramine): cardiac dysrhythmias, anticholinergic side effects (dry mouth, orthostasis, constipation), lower seizure threshold.

Nonpharmacological treatment

• Psychotherapy, including a combination of individual, group, and family treatment, is often beneficial.

• For bulimia nervosa, the best-established approaches are cognitive-behavioral therapy—a structured, time-limited therapy that addresses the relationships among thoughts, affect, and behavior; and interpersonal psychotherapy—focused, time-limited therapy that addresses interpersonal sources of stress.

• Behavioral therapy is often helpful to control specific behaviors around eating and purging.

• Indications for inpatient treatment include:

Extremely low weight (e.g., <75% of ideal body weight).
Rapid weight loss.
Severe electrolyte imbalances, cardiac disturbances, or other acute medical problems.
Intractable purging.
Psychosis or high risk of suicide.

Treatment aims

Stabilization of medical and nutritional status.

Identification and resolution of psychosocial precipitants of the disorder.

Re-establishment of healthful patterns of eating.

Prognosis

About half of patients with anorexia or bulimia nervosa recover fully, 30% have a partial recovery, and 20% have no substantial improvement in symptoms.

Follow-up and management

Appropriate follow-up depends on severity of illness. After clinical recovery, follow-up and routine monitoring for symptoms should be continued for several years because residual symptoms can persist even in mild cases and relapses can occur spontaneously or with periods of increased stress.

Key references

1. *Diagnostic and Statistical Manual of Mental Disorders*, edn 4. Washington, D.C.: American Psychiatric Association; 1994:539–550, 729–731.

2. Becker AE, Grinspoon SK, Klibanski A, Herzog DB: Current concepts: eating disorders. *N Engl J Med* 1999, **340**:1092–1098.

Aortic dissection

Diagnosis

Symptoms

Abrupt and severe retrosternal chest or interscapular pain: sharp (in 90%) or tearing quality (in 50%); migration down the back occurs in 16% of patients [1]

Neck or jaw pain: suggests involvement of the aortic arch.

Nausea, vomiting, and sweating.

Syncope: in about 10% of patients [1].

Dyspnea: resulting from shortness of breath.

Paraplegia.

Abdominal pain.

Signs

General

Hypertension present in 70% of patients; mild pyrexia.

Proximal dissection

Loss of upper limb or differential limb blood pressure: pulse deficit occurs in 20% of patients with type A dissection [1].

Aortic regurgitation: in about one-third of the patients [1].

Cardiac tamponade.

Neurologic deficit.

Hypotension: often associated with cardiac tamponade.

Distal dissection

Lower-limb ischemia: occurs in 20% of patients [2].

Oliguria or anuria: kidneys are involved in 15% [2].

Distinction between proximal and distal dissection should not be based solely on clinical criteria.

Investigations

ECG: to detect acute myocardial infarction (in 3%) and hypertensive changes (in 26%); most frequently shows nonspecific abnormalities; in one study, results were normal in about one-third of patients [1].

Chest radiography: widened mediastinum (in 60%), pleural effusion (in 19%), pericardial effusion.

Echocardiography: to detect flap in ascending aorta, presence of aortic regurgitation, and pericardial effusion and to assess myocardial function.

Transesophageal echocardiography: to detect true and false channel, presence and extent of intimal flap in thoracic aorta, relationship to coronary ostia, pericardial effusion, presence of aortic regurgitation. Sensitivity, 95%–100%; specificity, 85%–90%. Advantages: rapid diagnosis, can be performed by bedside. *Disadvantages:* requires sedation, may precipitate hypertensive reaction, does not visualize proximal aortic arch, misses branch involvement and entry site.

Ultrafast CT or MRI: to detect presence and extent of intimal flap, true and false channel, pericardial effusion, extension of dissection to abdominal aorta. Sensitivity, 0%–100%; specificity, 95%–100%. *Advantages*: visualizes entire aorta, identifies visceral jeopardy, shows aortic branches, is noninvasive. *Disadvantages*: requires transfer of unstable patient to scanning area, is time-consuming.

Contrast angiography: Many centers prefer aortic and coronary angiography before surgery. Sensitivity, 80%–90%; specificity, 90%–95%. *Advantages:* shows entry site and aortic branches. *Disadvantages:* uses nephrotoxic dye load, misses intramural hematoma.

Complications

Death.
Aortic rupture.
Stroke.
Paraplegia.
Ischemic bowel.
Renal infarction.
Limb ischemia.
Acute myocardial infarction.

Differential diagnosis

Acute myocardial infarction.
Acute myocardial ischemia.
Acute aortic regurgitation.
Thoracic aortic aneurysm.
Musculoskeletal chest pain.
Pulmonary embolism.
Pericarditis.

Etiology

Factors increasing stress on arterial wall:
Hypertension.
Aortic dilatation and wall thinning.
Unicommissural or bicuspid aortic valve.
Aortic coarctation.
Aortic arch hypoplasia.
Iatrogenic: cardiac surgery, percutaneous catheters.

Factors reducing resistance of arterial wall
Aging.
Pregnancy.
Marfan syndrome.
Cystic medial necrosis of the aorta.

Epidemiology

- The annual incidence of acute aortic dissection is ~5–10 in one million population.
- 80%–90% of patients are aged >60 years.

Classification

DeBakey classification
Type I: tear in ascending aorta, with dissection extending into arch and descending aorta.
Type II: tear and dissection localized to ascending aorta.
Type III: originates in descending aorta, usually propagating distally for a variable distance.

Stanford classification
Type A: includes all proximal dissections and distal dissections that extend proximally to involve the arch and ascending aorta.
Type B: all other dissections without proximal extension.

Acute versus chronic
Acute: symptom onset within 2 weeks.
Chronic: symptom onset longer than 2 weeks.

Treatment

Diet and lifestyle

• After surgical repair, patients are generally advised to avoid circumstances that cause an acute rise in blood pressure, *e.g.*, lifting or carrying heavy objects or weights.

Pharmacological treatment

• Treatment for patients with acute type A dissections is primarily surgical.

• Pharmacological treatment is usually reserved for patients with type B dissections.

• Endovascular stents for type B dissections without proximal extension [3].

• All patients require chronic medical therapy to control hypertension, particularly beta-blocking drugs.

Emergency treatment

• Bed rest and intra-arterial blood pressure monitoring.

Blood pressure control to maintain systolic blood pressure at 100–120 mm Hg: β-blockers and sodium nitroprusside.

Subsequent treatment

• Long-term management of hypertension (*see* Hypertension *for details*).

Nonpharmacological treatment

Indications for surgery

Type A dissection.

Type B dissection: retrograde extension into the ascending aorta, progression of dissection, impending aortic rupture, refractory hypertension, localized false aneurysm, continued pain, or end-organ ischemia caused by compromise of the aortic branches.

Types of surgery

Excision of intimal tear.

Obliteration of proximal false lumen.

Resuturing of aorta, possibly with interposition graft.

Resuspension of aortic valve in patients with aortic regurgitation secondary to proximal extent of dissection.

Aortic valve replacement.

• Bentall-deBono operation: composite aortic graft (with attached mechanical aortic valve replacement) and reimplantation of coronary arteries; operation of choice in patients with Marfan syndrome.

• Interposition aortic graft to descending aorta (vital organ perfusion may arise from false lumen, which may need to be left open at its proximal or distal end).

Complications of surgery

Death.

Bleeding.

Infection.

Renal failure.

Spinal-cord ischemia with paraplegia.

Progressive aortic regurgitation.

Aneurysm formation.

Redissection.

Acute myocardial infarction.

Percutaneous catheter techniques

• Stent-graft placement requires state-of-the-art imaging technology and precise manipulation of catheters and positioning of the stent. Although long-term consequences of endovascular stents are not known, the stents may be beneficial in the following instances:

Dissections extending distally in patients whose condition is stable with medical therapy.

Evidence of visceral or lower-extremity ischemia.

Dissections extending in a retrograde direction, into the ascending aorta.

Chronic dissections that are being managed medically.

Treatment aims

To provide analgesia and sedation.

To stabilize dissection flap.

To treat underlying condition, usually systemic hypertension.

Prognosis

• If the condition is left untreated, 36%–72% of patients die within 48 hours of diagnosis, and 62%–91% die within 1 week.

• The current mortality rate among patients who receive medical therapy for type B dissection remains about 20%, whereas the mortality rates among patients who undergo surgical repair of acute type A and B dissections are about 29% and 35%, respectively. However, for acute disease complicated by end-organ ischemia, the surgical mortality rate exceeds 50%.

Follow-up and management

• Follow-up should be supervised by cardiologist.

• Regular MRI, spiral CT, or transesophageal echocardiography is advised to screen for aneurysm formation. These tests are usually performed twice yearly to identify aneurysm of the dissected false channel or to detect new aneurysm formation in previously unaffected segments.

Key references

1. Hagan PG, *et. al.*: The International Registry of Acute Aortic Dissection. *JAMA* 2000, **283**:897–203.
2. Pretre R, Von Segesser LK: Aortic dissection. *Lancet* 1997, **349**:1461–1464.
3. Vlahakes GJ: Catheter-based treatment of aortic dissection. *N Engl J Med* 1999, **340**.

General references

Cigarroa JE *et al.*: Diagnostic imaging in the evaluation of suspected aortic dissection. *N Engl J Med* 1993, **328**:35–43.

Nienbar CA, *et al.*: The diagnosis of thoracic aortic dissection by noninvasive imaging procedures. *N Engl J Med* 1993, **328**:1–9.

Aortic regurgitation

Diagnosis

Symptoms

- Many patients are asymptomatic and may have normal or depressed left ventricular function.

Dyspnea and fatigue: due to left ventricular impairment and low cardiac output initially on exertion.

Symptoms of left ventricular failure: later.

Angina: less common than in aortic stenosis; usually indicates coronary artery disease.

Signs

Pulse

Large volume, rapid fall with low diastolic pressure: "collapsing."

Head nodding in time with pulse: Musset's sign.

Visible pulsation in neck: Corrigan's sign.

Capillary pulsation in fingernails: Quincke's sign.

A booming sound heard over femorals: "pistol-shot" femorals or Traube's sign.

Systolic and diastolic murmur: produced by compression of femorals by stethoscope; Duroziez's sign.

Heart

- Heart sounds are usually normal.

Forceful, displaced, "heaving" apex: may be seen and felt.

Third heart sound: in early systole with bicuspid aortic valve.

Ejection click: suggests underlying bicuspid aortic valve.

High-frequency early diastolic murmur: maximal at left sternal edge in expiration.

Mid-diastolic murmur (Austin Flint): at apex, low-pitched, similar to murmur of mitral stenosis but without preceding opening snap.

Hypertension, loud pulmonary component of second heart sound: suggests pulmonary hypertension.

Investigations

Chest radiography: usually normal in mild aortic regurgitation; possibly valvular calcification; cardiomegaly almost always in severe aortic regurgitation— "cor bovinum" (bovine ox heart).

ECG: signs of left ventricular hypertrophy and strain (increased QRS amplitude and ST/T wave changes in precordial leads) and left atrial hypertrophy (wide P wave in lead II and biphasic P in lead V_1).

Echocardiography: indicated to confirm the diagnosis of aortic regurgitation; determine cause; assess valve structure; determine a semi-quantitative estimate of severity of regurgitation; assess left ventricular dimension and mass and systolic function; and assess aortic size.

Doppler echocardiography: best method of detecting aortic regurgitation.

Exercise testing: in severe aortic regurgitation when patient is sedentary or has equivocal symptoms; useful for assessing functional capacity, symptomatic responses, and hemodynamic effects of exercise.

Radionuclide angiography: useful in asymptomatic patients with echocardiographic images of insufficient quality.

Doppler ultrasonography: best method of detecting aortic regurgitation.

Cardiac catheterization: essential when coronary artery disease suspected (*e.g.*, in patients >40 years) and when severity of aortic regurgitation doubted; injection of contrast into aortic root gives information on degree of regurgitation and state of aortic root (presence of dilatation, dissection, root abscesses).

MRI or spiral CT: for assessment of aortic root.

Complications

Cardiac failure: most important cause of disability and death.

Infective endocarditis: should be considered in patients with unexplained illness; may lead to sudden and catastrophic aortic regurgitation.

Arrhythmias: ventricular tachycardia, usually indicating left ventricular failure.

Differential diagnosis

Pulmonary regurgitation: usually accompanying signs of pulmonary hypertension; echo-Doppler examination should resolve.

Patent ductus arteriosus: continuous murmur heard well to the left of sternum; echo-Doppler is definitive investigation.

Etiology

Chronic aortic regurgitation: common

Rheumatic fever.
Hypertension.
Atherosclerosis.
Infective endocarditis.
Idiopathic dilation of aortic root & annulus.
Calcific degeneration.
Marfan syndrome.
Bicuspid aortic valve.

Chronic aortic regurgitation: less common

Traumatic injuries to the aortic valve.
Cystic medial necrosis.
Rheumatoid arthritis.
Seronegative arthritis.
Osteogenesis imperfecta.
Ehlers-Danlos syndrome.
Discrete subaortic stenosis.
Ventricular septal defects with prolapse of an aortic cusp.
Syphilis.

Acute aortic regurgitation

Infective endocarditis.
Aortic dissection.
Trauma.

Epidemiology

- Aortic regurgitation is one of the most common valve lesions.
- In the Helsinki Aging study, 13% of persons aged 75–86 years had moderate to severe aortic regurgitation.

Natural history

- Symptomatic patients: annual mortality rate is >10%.
- Asymptomatic patients with left ventricular systolic dysfunction: >25% develop symptoms by the end of 1 year.
- Asymptomatic patients with normal left ventricular systolic function: 1) <6% progress to symptoms or left ventricular dysfunction every year; 2) <3.5% progress to asymptomatic left ventricular dysfunction every year; and 3) <0.2% have sudden death in 1 year.

Treatment

Diet and lifestyle

• Competitive sports should be discouraged.

• Asymptomatic patients with normal left ventricular systolic function may participate in all forms of normal daily physical activity, including mild forms of exercise and, in some cases, competitive athletics. Isometric exercise should be avoided.

Pharmacological treatment

Antibiotic prophylaxis

• Prophylaxis is needed against infective endocarditis in asymptomatic patients with known aortic regurgitation; it is particularly important before dental procedures. *See* Endocarditis *for specific details.*

• Vasodilators are useful in chronic severe aortic regurgitation; the uses include:

Long-term treatment of patients with severe aortic regurgitation who have symptoms or left ventricular dysfunction and are considered poor candidates for surgery because of other factors.

Improvement of hemodynamic profile before aortic valve replacement. In such patients, vasodilating agents with negative inotropic effects should be avoided.

Prolongation of the compensated phase of asymptomatic patients who have volume-loaded left ventricles but normal systolic function.

• The goal of vasodilator therapy is to reduce systolic blood pressure. However, it is rarely possible to reduce systolic blood pressure to normal because of increased left ventricular stroke volume; thus, drug dosage should not be increased excessively in an attempt to achieve this goal. The benefit of vasodilator therapy in patients with normal blood pressure and or normal left ventricular cavity size is not unknown and hence is not recommended in these patients.

• Angiotensin-converting enzyme (ACE) inhibitors have a role in reducing systemic vascular resistance and decreasing aortic regurgitation. For patients unable to take ACE inhibitors, nifedipine (a calcium-channel blocker) is a reasonable alternative.

Nonpharmacological treatment

• **Surgery** is the main form of treatment for aortic regurgitation. Indications for surgery include:

• Patients with normal systolic function (left ventricular ejection fraction ≥0.50 at rest) who have New York Heart Association (NYHA) functional class III or IV or Canadian Heart Association class III or IV angina.

Patients with NYHA functional class II, III, or IV symptoms and mild to moderate left ventricular systolic dysfunction (ejection fraction, 0.25—0.49).

NYHA functional class II and III in patients with severe left ventricular dysfunction (ejection fraction < 0.25 and/or end-systolic dimension > 60 mm).

In patients with NYHA functional class IV symptoms and ejection fraction < 0.25, the high risks associated with aortic valve replacement and subsequent medical management of left ventricular dysfunction are usually a better alternative than the higher risk of long-term medical management alone.

Asymptomatic patients with at least 2 consecutive measurements showing an ejection fraction < 0.50 or severe left ventricular dilatation (end-diastolic dimension > 75 mm or end-systolic dimension > 55 mm), even if the ejection fraction is normal.

• **Aortic valve with or without root replacement** is indicated for onset of symptoms, increased heart size, and change in ECG, all of which indicate onset of left ventricular dysfunction. By echocardiography, end-systolic left ventricular diameter >55 mm may be used to determine operative timing in patients with no or minimal symptoms.

Treatment aims

To prevent or delay deterioration of left ventricular systolic function and relieve symptoms of dyspnea and fatigue.

Prognosis

• Prognosis depends mainly on the etiology and left ventricular function.

• Rheumatic aortic regurgitation, if detected early, has an excellent prognosis.

• Acute aortic regurgitation due to a dissection or endocarditis is fatal unless treated promptly.

• Patients with an underlying collagen disorder have a poor prognosis.

Follow-up and management

• Asymptomatic patients with mild mitral regurgitation, little or no left ventricular dilation, and normal systolic function may be followed up annually with recommendation to alert the physician if symptoms develop in the interim.

• Asymptomatic patients with normal systolic function but severe atrial regurgitation and significant left ventricular dilation should be followed up every 6 months, preferably with echocardiography.

• Asymptomatic patients with normal systolic function but severe atrial regurgitation and with more severe left ventricular dilation (end-diastolic dimension >70 mm or end-systolic dimension >50 mm) have a 10%–20% risk for developing symptoms and hence should have serial echocardiography every 4 months.

• Patients who have had valve replacement should also be seen regularly and monitored for signs of failure of the aortic valve prosthesis and endocarditis.

General references

Bonow RO, *et al.*: ACC/AHA guidelines for the management of patients with valvular heart disease: executive summary. *Circulation* 1998, **98**:1949–1984.

Carabello BA: Valvular heart disease. *N Engl J Med* 1997, **337**:32–41.

Greenberg B, *et al.*: Long-term vasodilator therapy of chronic aortic insufficiency. A randomized double-blinded placebo-controlled clinical trial. *Circulation* 1988, **78**:92–103.

Lindroos M, *et al.*: Prevalence of aortic valve abnormalities in the elderly: an echocardiographic study of a random population sample. *J Am Coll Cardiol* 1993, **21**:1220–1125.

Aortic stenosis

Diagnosis

Symptoms

• Many patients are asymptomatic.

Angina: ~70% of adults.

Syncope: 25% of patients, during or immediately after exercise.

Dyspnea: common; severe dyspnea, paroxysmal nocturnal dyspnea, orthopnea indicate left ventricular dysfunction.

Signs

Pulse

• **Normal pulse** in mild aortic stenosis when the gradient is <50 mm Hg.

Slow increase with diminished "volume," sometimes with notch on the upstroke ("anacrotic"): double pulse may be felt ("bisferious").

Heart

"Thrusting" apex beat that is not displaced: thrill may be palpable at base of heart.

Delayed or absent aortic component of S2.

• Ejection click may be heard at apex in bicuspid valve.

• When present, S3 implies impaired left ventricular dysfunction.

• S4 may be heard in severe aortic stenosis.

• Mid-systolic murmur; rough; best heard at the base of the heart in second right intercostal space but often heard over the precordium, almost always radiating to neck and right clavicle in severe aortic stenosis, increase in expiration; may be very soft with poor left ventricular function and low cardiac output.

Investigations

ECG: usually shows left ventricular hypertrophy, possibly left axis deviation, later left atrial hypertrophy (negative P waves in V_1), conduction abnormalities due to calcification of conducting tissues (first-degree heart block, left bundle-branch block).

Chest radiography: may show cardiac enlargement, poststenotic dilatation of aorta, calcification of aortic valve (particularly in older patients).

Echocardiography: useful in diagnosing and assessing severity of aortic stenosis; normal valve appearance excludes significant aortic stenosis in adults; also helps to define the level of obstruction. Useful in assessment of left ventricular size, function, and hemodynamics. Useful in reevaluation of patients with known aortic stenosis with changing symptoms and signs. Useful in reevaluation in asymptomatic patients with severe aortic stenosis and assessment of patients with known aortic stenosis during pregnancy. *Note:* degree of aortic stenosis is graded as: mild (valve area > 1.5 cm^2), moderate (area > 1.0 to 1.5 cm^2), or severe (area ≤1.0 cm^2).

Exercise testing: in adults with aortic stenosis, discouraged because of safety; it should not be performed in symptomatic patients; in asymptomatic patients, an abnormal hemodynamic response is sufficient to consider atrial valve replacement. May be useful to provide a basis for advice about physical activity.

Cardiac catheterization: to assess coronary circulation and to confirm or clarify diagnosis. When echocardiography is inadequate, cardiac hemodynamic testing using left- and right-heart catheterization is indicated and requires: measurement of transvalvular flow, determination of transvalvular pressure gradient, and calculation of effective valve area.

Complications

Sudden death: in 10%–20% of adults and 1% of children. Rarely documented to occur without prior symptoms; uncommon.

Cardiac failure: indicates poor prognosis unless the valve is replaced.

Arrhythmias and conduction abnormalities: ventricular arrhythmias more common than supraventricular; heart block may occur.

Systemic embolization.

Infective endocarditis: consider in patients with aortic stenosis who have unexplained illness.

Hemolytic anemia.

Differential diagnosis

Aortic sclerosis: old age, normal pulse character, echocardiogram with mild thickening of leaflets without restricted motion or gradient.

Flow murmur (pregnancy, anemia, thyrotoxicosis): large-volume pulse, normal echocardiogram, no gradient.

Mitral regurgitation: holosystolic murmur, no radiation to neck, mitral valve abnormality on Doppler echocardiography.

Hypertrophic cardiomyopathy: late systolic murmur, jerky pulse, echocardiogram showing asymmetrical septal hypertrophy, systolic anterior motion of mitral valve.

Ventricular septal defect: pansystolic murmur at left sternal edge with thrill, jet detected on Doppler echocardiography.

Etiology

Valvular stenosis.

Degenerative-calcific process (most common cause in adults).

Rheumatic fever.

• Congenital stenosis often due to bicuspid valve. It may be associated with patent ductus arteriosus or coarctation of aorta.

• Subvalvar stenosis is more common in boys and accounts for 10% of congenital cases

• Supravalvar stenosis is rare, usually a component of Williams syndrome

Epidemiology

• Valvular aortic stenosis is the most common valve lesion in adults in industrialized nations.

• 70% of patients have calcific stenosis (60% bicuspid, 10% tricuspid), 15% rheumatic, and 15% other forms.

Natural history

• In adults with aortic stenosis, the obstruction develops gradually (usually over decades) and consists of a prolonged latent period during which morbidity and mortality are low. Progression in an individual patient cannot be predicted.

• Once symptoms appear, survival is limited: the median survival is only 5 years after angina develops, 3 years after syncope occurs, and 2 years after symptoms of heart failure appear.

Treatment

Diet and lifestyle

• Physical activity is not restricted in asymptomatic patients with mild aortic stenosis.

• Asymptomatic patients with moderate aortic stenosis should avoid competitive sports that involve high dynamic and static muscular demands; other forms of exercise can be performed safely, but it is advisable to evaluate such patients with an exercise test before they begin an exercise or athletic program.

• Asymptomatic patients with severe stenosis should limit their activity to relatively low levels.

Pharmacological treatment

• Drug treatment has no place in the treatment of patients with aortic stenosis who are fit for surgery, but patients should be given antibiotic prophylaxis against infective endocarditis (*see* Endocarditis).

In patients who cannot undergo surgery because of serious comorbid conditions, medical therapy is used to control symptoms.

Pulmonary congestion: patients may benefit from diuretics, digitalis, angiotensin-converting enzyme inhibitors. β-blockers and other drugs with negative inotropic effects should not be used in patients with heart failure caused by aortic stenosis.

Atrial fibrillation: cardioversion; if this is not successful, pharmacological control with digitalis or amiodarone

Angina: cautious use of nitrates and β-blockers can provide relief.

Nonpharmacological treatment

Surgery

• Surgery is mandatory for symptomatic patients and should be considered in asymptomatic patients objectively with severe aortic stenosis (peak-to-peak gradient > 50 mm Hg), particularly when any one or more of the following features is present: left ventricular systolic dysfunction, abnormal response to exercise (*e.g.*, hypotension), ventricular tachycardia, marked excessive left ventricular hypertrophy (≥15 mm), and valve area < 0.6 cm^2.

• Patients with severe aortic stenosis, with or without symptoms, who are undergoing coronary artery bypass surgery, surgery on the aorta, or surgery on other heart valves should undergo atrial valve replacement at the time of surgery. In asymptomatic patients with moderate aortic stenosis, it is generally acceptable to perform atrial valve replacement in those who are undergoing mitral valve or aortic root surgery or coronary artery bypass surgery.

• Age alone is not a contraindication.

• Patients with severe aortic stenosis should have valve replacement early to avoid deterioration.

• Absolute valve area (or transvalvular pressure gradient) is not usually the primary determinant of the need for aortic valve replacement.

Balloon valvuloplasty

• This is useful in infants (in whom the results of surgery are poor) and in children and young adults (in whom the valve apparatus is not calcified).

• In adults, it is recommended as a "bridge" to surgery in hemodynamically unstable patients who are at high risk for atrial valve replacement, as palliation in patients with serious comorbid conditions, and for patients who require urgent noncardiac surgery.

Treatment aims

To replace valve before left ventricular dysfunction occurs.

Prognosis

In adults, the 5-year survival rate is 40%.

• The prognosis after surgery depends on age and left ventricular function.

• Up to 20% of patients with severe congestive aortic stenosis die during childhood, mainly because of progressive heart failure.

Follow-up and management

• Patients with mild to moderate aortic stenosis should be monitored for increasing severity.

• Patients who have had valve replacement should be monitored for failure of the valve prosthesis (particularly biological valves) and endocarditis.

General references

Bonow RO, *et. al.*: ACC/AHA guidelines for the management of patients with valvular heart disease: executive summary: a report of the American College of Cardiology/ American Heart Association Task Force on Practice Guidelines (Committee on Management of Patients With Valvular Heart Disease). *Circulation* 1998, **98:** 1949–1984.

Carabello BA: Valvular heart disease. *N Engl J Med* 1997, **337:**32–41.

Carabello BA: Aortic sclerosis—a window to the coronary arteries? *N Engl J Med* 1999, **341:**193–195.

Arthritis, psoriatic

Diagnosis

Symptoms and signs

Hallmarks of psoriatic arthritis: cutaneous lesions of psoriasis, nail disease, and enthesopathy.

Psoriatic arthritis may present in several patterns:

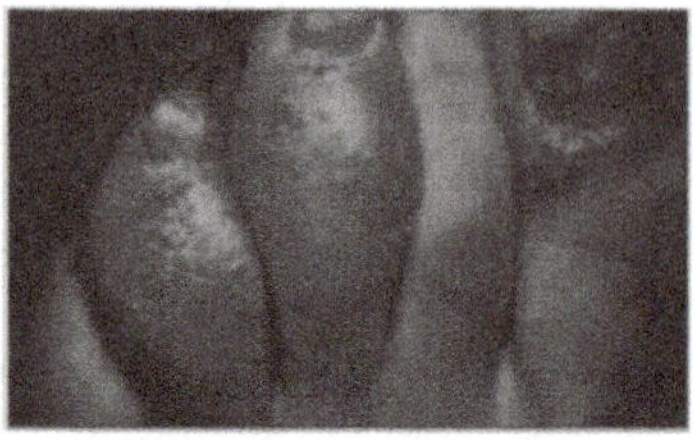

Psoriatic arthritis. (*See* Color Plate.)

• **Peripheral asymmetric oligoarthritis:** manifested in 80% of patients with psoriatic arthritis; involves small joints of hands and feet, large joints of legs, or both; hands may reveal dactylitis. Five percent of these patients have a highly distinctive, classic form of psoriatic arthritis involving predominantly distal interphalangeal joints of the hands and feet.

• **Peripheral symmetric oligoarthritis:** involves the same basic pattern of joints but is found in only 15% of patients with psoriatic arthritis.

• **Axial disease:** 5% of patients with psoriatic arthritis; involvement of the spine and sacroiliac joints (ankylosing spondylitis) is typical; peripheral joint disease may or may not be present.

Associated features:

• **Cutaneous psoriatic lesions:** possibly after years of arthritis.

• **Tenosynovitis.**

• **Enthesopathy:** clinically distinctive feature; inflammation involving the periarticular structures, particularly tendons and ligaments at their points of insertion.

• **Psoriatic nail changes:** may accompany involvement of distal interphalangeal joints.

• **Arthritis mutilans:** with telescoping of digits; usually only one or a few joints destroyed; occurs in approximately 5% of patients with psoriatic arthritis.

Investigations

Blood tests: rheumatoid factor absent; biochemical response to active disease similar to rheumatoid arthritis; erythrocyte sedimentation rate and acute-phase reactant level elevated; uric acid level may be elevated, reflecting increased cell turnover of psoriatic skin.

Radiography: shows asymmetrical small joint changes, tendency to ankylosis, osteolysis with pencil-in-cup deformity, whittling terminal phalanges (especially hallux); enthesitis; asymmetrical sacroiliitis and syndesmophytes.

Complications

Exfoliation of skin: rare.

Differential diagnosis

Rheumatoid arthritis.

Reactive (Reiter's syndrome).

Etiology

• Psoriatic arthritis has a genetic component: HLA B27 positive in 71% of patients with psoriatic spondylitis, 32% in distal joint group.

• It may be triggered by trauma.

• Immunologic and infectious factors have also been suggested.

Epidemiology

• 5%–8% of patients with all types of psoriasis have psoriatic arthritis; the incidence is greater with severe skin involvement.

• In one of seven cases of psoriatic arthritis, the arthritis precedes the development of psoriasis.

• The male:female ratio is equal, but more men have the distal-joint and spondylitic forms.

• Juvenile psoriatic arthritis is rare; monoarticular disease is more common.

Treatment

Diet and lifestyle

• Avoid repetitive injury.

• Maintain activity for function and range of joint motion per rheumatologist or physical therapist.

• No special diet is necessary, except when indicated for certain medications.

Pharmacological treatment

Principles

For psoriasis (localized involvement): topical steroids, coal tar (*see* Psoriasis *for further details*).

For arthritis (simple cases): NSAIDs, analgesics.

For severe cases: second-line treatment according to severity.

Second line for arthritis alone

Standard dosage	Sulfasalazine, 1 g twice daily.
Contraindications	Hypersensitivity to sulfonamides or salicylates.
Special points	Requires monitoring of complete blood count and liver function tests.
Main side effects	Nausea (dose must be reduced), reversible azoospermia, bone-marrow suppression.

Gold sodium thiomalate has been reported to improve symptoms in patients with moderately severe arthritic disease, but its efficacy is controversial. Caution should be used because it may exacerbate psoriatic skin lesions.

Antimalarial agents (*e.g.*, chloroquine, hydroxychloroquine) may also be of use.

Second line for arthritis and skin involvement

• Treatment should be given under specialist supervision.

Standard dosage	*Acitretin, methotrexate, cyclosporine:* dose should be determined by a specialist with experience in systemic therapy.
Contraindications	*Acitretin:* childbearing potential, preexisting hepatic disease, hypertriglyceridemia.
	Methotrexate: history of hypersensitivity to drug, hepatic disease, alcohol abuse, pregnancy.
	Cyclosporine: hypertension, renal insufficiency, underlying systemic infection.
Special points	*Acitretin:* teratogenic potential is present for up to 3 years after drug cessation (and possibly longer).
	Methotrexate: can be given orally or intramuscularly; medication should first be administered with a test dose; requires monitoring of complete blood count, liver function tests, and periodic liver biopsy, depending on total dosage ingested.
	Cyclosporine: best for short-term treatment of erythrodermic or pustular psoriasis; side effects limit long-term use; may be used for severe refractory psoriasis and psoriatic arthropathy; blood pressure, serum creatinine levels, and creatinine clearance should be monitored.
Main drug interactions	*Methotrexate:* trimethoprim–sulfamethoxazole, alcohol, NSAIDs, probenecid, retinoids.
	Cyclosporine: use caution with medications that affect renal function and drugs that inhibit the cytochrome P-450 system.
Main side effects	*Acitretin:* drying of skin and mucosa, elevated liver enzyme and triglyceride levels, myalgias, teratogenicity.
	Methotrexate: gastrointestinal effects, bone marrow suppression, immunosuppression, dose-dependent risk for hepatic fibrosis/cirrhosis, teratogenic effects, abortifacient.
	Cyclosporine: dose-dependent hypertension and nephrotoxicity, electrolyte imbalances, immunosuppression.

Treatment aims

To relieve pain and stiffness.

To achieve full functional capacity.

To prevent progression of arthritis.

To minimize skin lesions.

Prognosis

• Prognosis is usually good.

• A few patients are disabled.

Follow-up and management

• A few patients need regular review.

• Second-line drugs need blood monitoring.

Orthopedic guidelines

• Psoriatic arthritis has the same indications as other arthropathies.

• It has no more infective complications than other diseases.

• Physicians should consult with medical, physical therapy, and occupational therapy staff.

• Early postoperative mobilization is advised.

General references

Gladman DD: Psoriatic arthritis. *Rheum Dis Clin North Am* 1998, **24:**829–844.

Mahrle G, *et al.*: Anti-inflammatory efficacy of low-dose cyclosporin A in psoriatic arthritis. A prospective multicentre study. *Br J Dermatol* 1996, **135:**752–757.

McGonagle D, *et al.*: Psoriatic arthritis: a unified concept twenty years on. *Arthritis Rheum* 1999, **42:**1080–1086.

Pioro MH, Cash JM: Treatment of refractory psoriatic arthritis. *Rheum Dis Clin North Am* 1995, **21:**129–149.

Ross EL, *et al.*: Pathogenic mechanisms in psoriatic arthritis. *Hosp Med (Br)* 1998, **59:**534–538.

Arthritis, rheumatoid

Diagnosis

Symptoms

Painful, swollen, warm joints, with morning stiffness and impaired function: onset usually insidious, sometimes rapid; characteristically in hands or feet, occasionally monoarticular (most often in a knee); often accompanied by tiredness.

Signs

Articular

Warm, tender, swollen joints: decreased range of movement; peripheral joints most often affected; characteristic symmetry of involvement; proximal interphalangeal, metacarpophalangeal, wrist, and metatarsophalangeal joints usually affected.

Extra-articular

Bursitis: *e.g.*, olecranon.

Tenosynovitis.

Nodules: extensor surfaces.

Serositis: *e.g.*, pleurisy.

Keratoconjunctivitis sicca: secondary Sjögren's syndrome.

Vasculitis, scleritis.

Fibrosing alveolitis.

Investigations

• No single diagnostic test is available; the diagnosis relies on some or all of the following:

ESR, CRP, plasma viscosity measurement: for evidence of inflammation.

Immunology: rheumatoid factor positivity (not essential for diagnosis); present in up to 80%.

Radiography: initially shows periarticular osteoporosis, followed by erosions around affected joint.

Blood count: for anemia of chronic disease, thrombocytosis.

Serum immunoglobulin measurement: for polyclonal gammopathy.

• In addition, the duration of morning stiffness, level of functional impairment, and number of inflamed joints must be monitored in established disease.

Complications

• The following occur in patients with established disease and global decline in function or severe systemic malaise.

Widespread active synovitis.

Septic arthritis.

Systemic rheumatoid disease.

Iatrogenic problems: *e.g.*, NSAIDs and anemia, gold and renal impairment.

Atlantoaxial subluxation.

Non-Hodgkin's lymphoma: possible.

Amyloidosis.

Incapacitation: patient may become bedridden.

Differential diagnosis

Seronegative spondyloarthritis.

Reactive arthritis: gastrointestinal or sexually acquired.

Viral arthritis: *e.g.*, rubella, hepatitis B virus infection.

Septic polyarthritis: *e.g.*, staphylococcal or gonococcal infections.

Crystal polyarthritis: *e.g.*, gout.

Generalized nodal osteoarthritis: may have inflammatory component in 10%.

SLE.

Etiology

• The cause of rheumatoid arthritis is unknown, but the following have a role:

Genetic factors: subtypes of HLA DR4 and DR1.

Hormonal factors: remission during pregnancy; contraceptive pill protects from disease.

Epidemiology

• Rheumatoid arthritis is a significant disease that affects 1%–2% of the population.

• It is a chronic disease, with high prevalence and low incidence.

• It is a modern disease, with little evidence to indicate its presence >400 years ago.

• The female :male ratio is 3:1.

Treatment

Diet and lifestyle

- Activity should be encouraged, but heavy work intensifies joint inflammation.
- Physical therapy, taught exercise, and "joint protection" are helpful to maintain strength and function.
- Omega-3 fatty acids may reduce inflammation [1].

Pharmacological treatment

NSAIDs

- The response is variable and idiosyncratic; if one drug fails, another from a different group may be worth trying.
- The most commonly used drugs are diclofenac, ibuprofen, indomethacin, naproxen, and salicylate.

Standard dosage	Depends on drug used.
Contraindications	Caution in peptic ulceration, asthma, renal impairment, pregnancy, and elderly patients.
Special points	No influence on disease progression.
Main drug interactions	Diuretics, warfarin.
Main side effects	Dyspepsia, renal impairment, fluid retention.

Second-line agents

- These are increasingly started early in the disease process, particularly in patients who do not respond to NSAIDs or who respond partially but have evidence of active disease [2–4].

Standard dosage	Sulfasalazine, 2–3 g daily, with gradual build-up over 4 weeks. Methotrexate, 2.5–15 mg orally once weekly (not daily) [4,5].
Contraindications	*Sulfasalazine:* sulfonamide and salicylate hypersensitivity. *Methotrexate:* pregnancy, liver disease.
Special points	*Sulfasalazine:* complete blood count every 4 weeks for 2 months, monthly for 2–3 months, then 3-monthly; liver function test at onset, monthly for 3 months, then 3-monthly. *Methotrexate:* complete blood count monthly, liver function test 3-monthly; close monitoring in renal impairment; alcohol use should be avoided; NSAIDs must be used cautiously.
Main drug interactions	*Sulfasalazine:* warfarin, co-trimoxazole. *Methotrexate:* co-trimoxazole, trimethoprim, phenytoin.
Main side effects	*Sulfasalazine:* nausea, vomiting, rashes, reversible azoospermia. *Methotrexate:* nausea, diarrhea, rash, pulmonary hypersensitivity, blood dyscrasias.

Other options [2,4,6,7]

Gold (oral or i.m.) [4].
Hydroxychloroquine.
Penicillamine.
Local steroids.
Etanercept.
Leflunomide.

Systemic steroids: either induction before or adjunctive to second-line agents in poorly controlled disease [3].

Immunosuppressants: for severe articular or extra-articular disease.

Minocycline [6].

Nonpharmacological treatment

Physical therapy: during active disease.

Occupational therapy.

Surgery: synovectomies, arthroplasty, arthrodesis, tendon repair; for painful joints (particularly at night), functionally restricted joints, and joints that do not respond to other treatments.

Treatment aims

To decrease pain and symptoms and signs of inflammation.
To prevent progression of irreversible joint damage.
To monitor for and treat extra-articular manifestations.
To restrict disability and handicap.

Prognosis

- The prognosis is variable.
- Poor prognostic markers include female sex, insidious onset, high-titer rheumatoid factor, low educational achievement, persistently raised ESR or CRP, and extra-articular manifestations [8].

Follow-up and management

- Second-line treatment must be monitored regularly.
- Stable disease needs occasional assessment for progressive functional decline.
- Active disease needs regular follow-up so that modifying the various treatment options can be considered.
- Care should be shared between primary care and musculoskeletal specialists (rheumatologist, orthopedic surgeon, physiatrist).

Key references

1. Geusens P, *et al.*: Long term effect of omega 3 fatty acid supplementation in active rheumatoid arthritis; a 12 month double blind controlled study. *Arthritis Rheum* 1994, **37**:824–829.
2. Anonymous: Slow-acting antirheumatic drugs. *Drug Ther Bull* 1993, **31**:17–20.
3. Harris ED: Rheumatoid arthritis. Pathophysiology and implications for treatment. *N Engl J Med* 1990, **332**:1277–1289.
4. Wilke WS, *et al.*: Early aggressive therapy for rheumatoid arthritis concerns, descriptions and estimates of outcome. *Semin Arthritis Rheum* 1993, **23**:26–41.
5. Weinblatt ME, *et al.*: Methotrexate in rheumatoid arthritis. A five year prospective multi-center study. *Arthritis Rheum* 1994, **37**:1492–1498.
6. Kloppenburg M, *et al.*: Minocycline in active rheumatoid arthritis: a double blind placebo controlled trial. *Arthritis Rheum* 1994, **37**:629–636.
7. Jain R, Lipsky PE: Treatment of rheumatoid arthritis. *Med Clin North Am* 1997, **81**:57–84.
8. Tugwell P, *et al.*: End points in rheumatoid arthritis. *J Rheumatol* 1994, **42(suppl)**: 2-8; 20-24.

Diagnosis

Symptoms

• Symptoms and signs are more difficult to interpret in the presence of pre-existing joint disease and may be muted in immunosuppressed or elderly patients [1].

• Polyarticular infection occurs in 10%–15% of patients [1–3].

Pain: most consistent feature; typically progressive; may be worse at night; with pre-existing joint disease, change or exacerbation of pain is an important warning sign [3].

Loss of function, limp: possibly presenting feature in children [2].

Fever: possibly only manifestation, particularly in elderly patients [3].

Signs

Swelling and local tenderness, pain and restriction of movement: most marked in previously fit younger patients [2].

Local erythema: possibly but often less marked than in crystal synovitis.

Fever: although temperature normal in up to one-third of patients.

Confusion: possibly prominent feature in elderly patients [3].

Investigations

• Most investigations are nonspecific, and results may be normal; a high index of suspicion is necessary to make the diagnosis [4].

• Adequate specimens must be obtained for microbiological examination before antimicrobial treatment is started.

Synovial fluid analysis: Gram stain positive in 50% of patients; culture positive in 75%; presence of leukocytes not diagnostic; crystals may coexist with sepsis.

Blood cultures: positive in 50% (may be presenting feature of subacute bacterial endocarditis).

Urogenital swabs: should be obtained if gonococcal infection suspected.

Plain radiography: usually unhelpful in early stages of infection [4].

Complications

Death: in up to 15%, especially elderly, immunosuppressed, and rheumatoid arthritis patients.

Loss of function of joint.

Loss of prosthesis.

Osteomyelitis: from direct spread.

Bacterial endocarditis, disseminated intravascular coagulation.

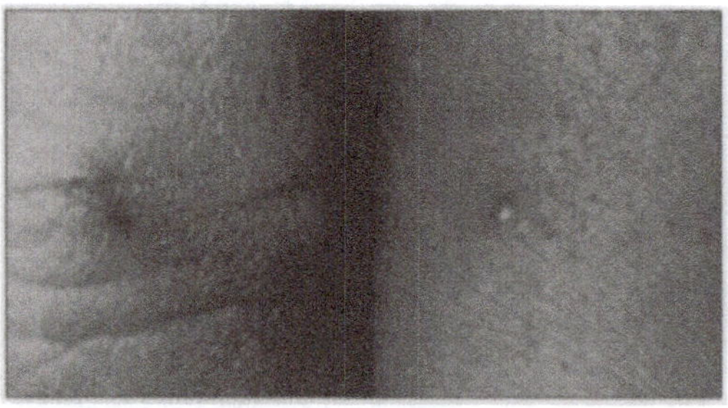

Septic arthritis. (*See* Color Plate.)

Differential diagnosis

Acute flare of inflammatory joint disease.

Crystal synovitis.

Hemarthrosis.

Bacterial endocarditis.

Etiology

• Pathogens depend on age and predisposing factors; most infections are due to *Staphylococcus aureus* and streptococci; in children aged <5 years, *Haemophilus influenzae* type b has been an important pathogen; gonococcal infection appears to be in decline but should be considered in sexually active patients.

• Spread is usually hematogenous; joint disease or blunt trauma may act to localize blood-borne pathogens.

• Direct inoculation during surgery, injection, or trauma occurs but is unusual.

• Risk factors include extremes of age, previous joint disease, diabetes mellitus, immunosuppression, prosthetic joint material, and corticosteroids.

Epidemiology

• The incidence of septic arthritis is unknown but is estimated to be 3–10 in 100 000 population.

Treatment

Diet and lifestyle

• No special precautions are necessary.

Pharmacological treatment

General principles

• A possible septic arthritis is a medical emergency and should be urgently referred to a specialist (rheumatologist or orthopedic surgeon).

• High-dose antibiotics are given i.v. for at least 2 weeks, then orally for at least a further 2–4 weeks, depending on the clinical response and presence of prosthesis.

• Antibiotics should be started only after appropriate specimens for culture have been obtained.

• Initially, a "best guess" choice of antibiotics is used, based on the most probable pathogen, patient's age, and sensitivities of pathogen; treatment is later tailored by the results of the Gram stain and culture.

Possible "best-guess" regimen

Child aged <5 years: cefotaxime and nafcillin [2].

Child aged >5 years: nafcillin (with penicillin G if gonococcal infection likely) [1–3,5,6].

Adult, immunosuppressed, prosthetic-joint patient: cefotaxime and floxacillin. Vancomycin i.v. for methicillin-resistant *S. aureus*.

Specific drugs

Standard dosage	Nafcillin, 2 g i.v. every 4 hours. Penicillin G, 4.8–9.6 g i.v. daily. Cefotaxime 3–6 g i.v. daily. Vancomycin, 1 g i.v. every 12 hours.
Contraindications	Hypersensitivity.
Special points	Complete blood count needed twice weekly. Aminopenicillin can be used instead of penicillin V for oral treatment.
Main drug interactions	None.
Main side effects	Rash, hypersensitivity reaction (rare), neutropenia (after prolonged treatment), diarrhea.

Other treatments

• Repeated medical aspiration with adequate drainage may be associated with better outcome than surgical drainage [7].

• Surgery is indicated for the following [8]:

Inability to drain medically.

Failure to improve on antibiotic or medical management.

Osteomyelitis.

Prosthetic joints (surgical drainage, debridement, or removal).

Treatment aims

To prevent septicemia or osteomyelitis.

To preserve joint function.

To resolve infection.

Prognosis

• The overall mortality is 15%.

• The prognosis is worse if treatment is delayed, in elderly patients with gram-positive infection, and in patients with predisposing joint or systemic disease.

• Infection of prosthetic material carries a particularly poor prognosis; revision or removal of the prosthesis is a common outcome.

Follow-up and management

• Patients with infected prostheses may need long-term suppressive antibiotic treatment, although, in most, revision surgery is delayed rather than prevented.

Key references

1. Goldenberg DL: Bacterial arthritis. *Curr Opin Rheumatol* 1994, **6**:394–400.
2. Shaw BA, Kasser JL: Acute septic arthritis in infancy and childhood. *Clin Orthop* 1990, **257**:212–225.
3. Esterhai JL Jr, Gelb I: Adult septic arthritis. *Orthop Clin North Am* 1991, **3**:503–514.
4. Hendrix RW, Fisher MR: Imaging of septic arthritis. *Clin Rheum Dis* 1986, **12**:459–487.
5. Norden C, *et al.*: Evaluation of new anti-infective drugs for the treatment of infectious arthritis in adults. *Clin Infect Dis* 1992, **15(suppl)**:S167–S171.
6. Steere AC: Diagnosis and treatment of Lyme arthritis. *Med Clin North Am* 1997, **81**:179–194.
7. Broy SB, Schmid FR: A comparison of medical drainage (needle aspiration) and surgical drainage (arthrotomy or arthroscopy) in the initial treatment of infected joints. *Clin Rheum Dis* 1986, **12**:501–522.
8. Parisien JS, Shaffer R: Arthroscopic management of pyarthrosis. *Clin Orthop* 1992, **275**:243–247.

Diagnosis

Symptoms

Uncomplicated ascites

Abdominal distension and discomfort.

Dyspnea: due to splinting of diaphragm.

Fatigue, encephalopathy, and other symptoms of chronic liver disease: present to variable degrees.

Spontaneous bacterial peritonitis

Pain, fever: in <50% of patients.

Deterioration in liver function, renal impairment, gastrointestinal hemorrhage, encephalopathy: present to variable degrees.

Signs

Uncomplicated ascites

Physical examination often insensitive.

Distension.

Shifting dullness on percussion of flanks, fluid wave.

Ballotable liver.

Spontaneous bacterial peritonitis

- Often no additional clinical signs are manifest.

Fever, encephalopathy: more common than tenderness, rebound, rigidity.

Investigations

In all cases

Measurement of serum and ascitic albumin levels: to allow calculation of concentration gradient (*i.e.*, serum albumin in g/dL–ascites albumin in g/dL) [1].

Cell count using ascites: >250 polymorphonuclear neutrophils/mL suggests peritonitis; lymphocyte predominance suggests tuberculosis or malignancy.

Cytological study: of fluid to evaluate for malignancy.

Gram stain and culture of ascites: blood culture bottle inoculation; polymicrobial infections suggest perforation of the gastrointestinal tract.

Urine electrolytes analysis.

Serum electrolytes, blood urea nitrogen, creatinine.

Specific tests for selected presentations

Amylase measurement: concentration raised in pancreatic ascites.

Cholesterol or triglyceride measurement: concentration raised in chylous ascites.

Total protein: high in malignancy, tuberculosis, cardiac ascites.

Laparoscopy and biopsy: for tuberculosis.

Abdominal ultrasonography or computed tomography: for malignant ascites.

Complications

Spontaneous bacterial peritonitis: most common in patients with high serum-ascites albumin gradients or low ascites protein.

Pleural effusion: may occur without ascites.

Inguinal, femoral, or umbilical hernias.

Mesenteric venous thrombosis.

Renal failure, hepatorenal syndrome.

Umbilical rupture.

Empyema.

Differential diagnosis

High serum-ascites albumin gradient (*i.e.*, ≥1.1 g/dL)

Portal hypertension.

Cirrhosis.

Cardiac ascites.

Fulminant hepatitis.

Budd-Chiari/veno-occlusive disease.

Myxedema.

Low serum-ascites albumin gradient (*i.e.*, <1.1 g/dL)

Peritoneal carcinomatosis.

Tuberculosis.

Pancreatic ascites.

Biliary ascites.

Nephrotic syndrome.

Chylous

Trauma and surgery, abdominal tuberculosis, lymphoma or other malignancy, filariasis.

Etiology

High serum-ascites albumin gradient

Overflow hypothesis: primary increase in renal sensitivity to aldosterone, causing sodium retention or volume expansion, ascites forming in abdomen because of portal hypertension and hypoalbuminemia.

Underfill hypothesis: fluid sequestration in abdomen, causing renal hypoperfusion and secondary hyperaldosteronism, renal retention of sodium to maintain circulating volume.

Vasodilatation hypothesis: overflow factors initiating and underfill factors perpetuating ascites.

Low serum-ascites albumin gradient

Increased capillary permeability.

Chylous

Lymphatic leakage.

Epidemiology

- 80% of patients with cirrhosis develop ascites during their course (spontaneous bacterial peritonitis in 10%).

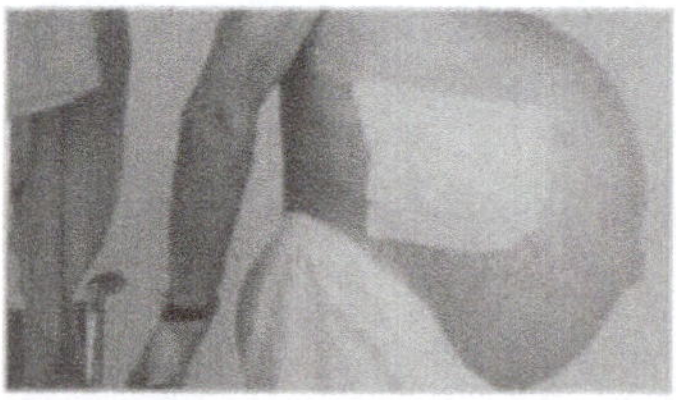

Distended abdomen with protuberant umbilicus in a patient with massive ascites. (*See* Color Plate.)

Treatment

Diet and lifestyle

• Patients should have a low-salt diet (<2 g daily) and maintain an adequate intake of calories.

• Bed rest during mobilization of ascites may be of benefit by lowering renin–angiotensin concentrations.

Pharmacological treatment

For uncomplicated ascites [2]

• Initially, treatment should involve spironolactone, with high-volume paracentesis reserved for patients with respiratory compromise or those with disease that is refractory to diuretic management.

• Furosemide can be added if no response is seen after 3 days and is more effective in patients with peripheral edema.

Standard dosage	Spironolactone, 100 mg daily, and furosemide, 40 mg daily, aiming for 1.0 kg of weight loss per day if pedal edema is present and 0.5 kg per day if there is no pedal edema; dosage is increased slowly depending on diuresis to maximum spironolactone, 400 mg, or furosemide, 160 mg daily.
Contraindications	Renal failure.
Special points	Renal function should be watched carefully and diuretics decreased or witheld for any increase in creatinine of 0.5 mg/dL over baseline. Hyponatremia with sodium level <122 mEq/L should be treated with fluid restriction. Hyperkalemia should be managed by a decrease in spironolactone or an increase in furosemide.
Main drug interactions	Diuretics and aminoglycosides may have increased nephrotoxicity in this context; NSAIDs should be avoided.
Main side effects	Hyponatremia, impaired renal function with raised creatinine level, hyperkalemia [3]. For patients with gynecomastia from spironolactone, amiloride is an alternative (5–10 mg daily).

Nonpharmacological treatment [3,4]

• High-volume paracentesis (removal of >6 L of ascites) should be done for tense ascites or in cases refractory to diuretic management. Caution should be exercised in patients with renal dysfunction (creatinine level >2.0 mg/dL). Intravenous albumin (10 g/L of ascites removed) administered to patients with elevated creatinine level or those without pedal edema may protect against progressive renal dysfunction [3].

For functional renal failure: renal failure is often precipitated by infection, hemorrhage, hypotension, or overaggressive diuretic treatment; it may reverse after orthotopic liver transplantation. Treatment involves central venous monitoring, volume expansion, and treatment of precipitating factors; renal vasodilators are of no proven benefit.

For resistant ascites: juguloperitoneal shunt, transhepatic intravascular portal systemic stent shunt, or orthotopic liver transplantation(s).

For spontaneous bacterial peritonitis [4]

• 80% of organisms are aerobic gram-negative bacilli; 20% are nonenteric organisms.

• Cefotaxime (2g intravenously every 8 hours) or ceftizoxime is effective in up to 85%; ciprofloxacin and amoxicillin may be as effective, but gentamicin is potentially more toxic.

• Treatment should last 5–7 days.

• Antibiotic treatment is influenced by hospital sensitivities.

• Clearance of ascitic leukocytes should be considered after 3 days in severely ill patients, and renal function should be monitored daily.

• Long-term antibiotic prophylaxis with antibiotics (*e.g.*, norfloxacin) may prevent recurrence; consider in patients with previous episodes of spontaneous bacterial peritonitis or patients with ascites fluid protein <1.0 g/dL.

Treatment aims

To reduce ascitic volume.

Prognosis

• 1-year and 5-year survival rates after development of ascites without renal impairment are 50% and 20%, respectively.

• 80% of patients respond to medical treatment.

• 30% develop functional renal failure within 24 months.

• When urine sodium level is <5 mmol/L or diuretic-resistant ascites has developed, 1-year survival is <50%.

• Spontaneous bacterial peritonitis has a hospital mortality of up to 50%.

• >50% of survivors have a recurrence in the following year.

Follow-up and management

• Patients with uncomplicated ascites must be monitored by using weight and daily fluid input and output charts.

• If no response is seen at maximum tolerated dose of diuretic, the development of hepatoma, portal-vein thrombosis, or spontaneous bacterial peritonitis must be excluded.

Key references

1. Runyon BA, Management of adult patients with ascites caused by cirrhosis. Hepatology 1998, **27**:264–272.
2. Strauss RM, Boyer TD: Diagnosis and management of cirrhotic ascites. In *Hepatology: A Textbook of Liver Disease*. Edited by Zakim D, Boyer TD. Philadelphia: WB Saunders; 1996:764–788.
3. Runyon BA: Patient selection is important in studying the impact of large-volume paracentesis on intravascular volume. *Am J Gastroenterol* 1997, **92**:371–373.
4. Runyon BA: Care of patients with ascites. *N Engl J Med* 1994, **330**:337–342.
5. Jalan R, Hayes PC: Hepatic encephalapathy and ascites. *Lancet* 1997, **350**:1309–1315.

Asthma

Diagnosis

Symptoms

Wheezing.

Breathlessness.

Chest tightness: not pain.

Cough: with or without sputum; may be the only symptom, especially in children.

Exercise-induced cough or wheezing.

• Symptom severity shows considerable temporal variation; they are often worse at night or in early morning.

Signs

Tachypnea.

Diffuse wheezing.

Use of accessory muscles of respiration: in severe attack, due to high negative intrapleural pressure or rapid respiratory rate.

Tachycardia: in severe attack.

Pulsus paradoxus: in severe attack.

Cyanosis or confusion: signs of impending respiratory arrest; wheezing may be absent.

Rhinitis, nasal polyps, atopic dermatitis: often associated with asthma.

Investigations

On presentation

Spirometry: forced expiratory volume in 1 second (FEV_1) and forced vital capacity; response to beta-2 agonist (>15% improvement in FEV_1 confirms reversible airflow obstruction; failure to improve does not exclude asthma).

Serial peak flow monitoring: early peak flow often low in asthma; >15% diurnal variation strongly suggests asthma, peak flow reduced after work or exposure to sensitizing agent.

Airways hyperresponsiveness test: increased sensitivity to methacholine, shown by 20% fall in FEV_1 to abnormally small doses of nebulized methacholine.

For acute episodes

Spirometry or peak flow rate measurement: to assess severity.

Arterial blood gas analysis: partial oxygen pressure reduced; partial carbon dioxide pressure usually low in acute episode; rising or raised partial carbon dioxide pressure suggests exhaustion and impending respiratory arrest; different patterns in acute exacerbations of chronic obstructive pulmonary disease (*see* Chronic obstructive pulmonary disease *for details*).

Chest radiography: to check for pneumothorax or pneumonia and to exclude heart failure.

ECG: if cause of breathlessness unclear.

Sputum culture: good samples often difficult to obtain; most exacerbations due to viral not bacterial infection.

Complications [1]

Respiratory arrest and death.

Pneumothorax.

Recurrent bronchial infection.

Irreversible airflow limitation.

Differential diagnosis

Acute or chronic bronchitis.

Irreversible airway obstruction (chronic obstructive pulmonary disease).

Rhinitis with postnasal drip.

Left ventricular failure.

Pulmonary embolism.

Etiology

• Asthma has an important genetic component, which is inherited separately from the genetic tendency to atopy.

• ~50% of patients have associated atopic allergy, especially children.

• All grades of asthma show airway inflammation, with eosinophils, mononuclear cells, and epithelial desquamation.

• Viral infections are clearly linked to exacerbations of asthma and may be responsible for initiating asthma in patients with adult-onset disease.

• Exposure to environmental chemicals and pollution is blamed for the current increase in prevalence: clear evidence of a causal relationship is awaited.

Epidemiology

• The prevalence of asthma appears to be increasing in the United States; an estimated 5%–10% of the population is asthmatic.

• Asthma is more common in children, and may remit as they grow.

Treatment

Diene and lifestyle

• Special diets are not usually needed; patients with salicylate or sulfite sensitivity should avoid foods containing salicylates or sulfites.
• Exercise is encouraged; swimming is often better tolerated than outdoor sports (exercise-induced asthma is triggered by cold dry air).
• Patients should be educated to develop a partnership in asthma management; this is a critical component.

Pharmacological treatment [2–8]

Corticosteroids [5,6]

Standard dosage	*Inhaled corticosteroids:* starting dose varies according to severity and corticosteroid formulation (*e.g.*, beclomethasone, 200–400 µg twice daily). *Oral corticosteroids:* prednisone, 30 mg daily for 5 days; longer courses may be needed if improvement is slow; dose need not be tapered if course lasts <14 days.
Contraindications	None.
Special points	Rinsing mouth after inhaling steroids reduces risk of oropharyngeal side effects. Spacer device should be used.
Main drug interactions	None.
Main side effects	*Inhaled steroids:* hoarse voice, oropharyngeal candidiasis. *Oral steroids:* cushingoid features, especially osteoporosis, bruising, weight gain.

Short-acting beta-2 agonists [3,5]

Standard dosage	Depends on agent and device, *e.g.*, albuterol, terbutaline, 1–2 puffs as needed.
Contraindications	None.
Special points	Frequent use of short-acting beta-2 agonists suggests suboptimal control.
Main drug interactions	Beta-blockers must be avoided.
Main side effects	Tremor.

Leukotriene inhibitors [2,5]

Standard dosage	Zafirlukast 20 mg twice daily. Zileutin 600 mg four times daily. Montelukast 10 mg at bedtime.
Main side effects	*Zileutin*: elevation of hepatic enzymes.

Xanthines [5,8]

Standard dosage	Theophylline, dose adjusted to give blood concentrations of 10–15 mg/L.
Contraindications	Liver disease, heart disease, epilepsy, porphyria.
Special points	Narrow therapeutic margin, so dose should be low initially and adjusted with aid of plasma drug concentrations.
Main drug interactions	Plasma concentration increased with many other drugs, *e.g.*, antibiotics (ciprofloxacin, erythromycin), cimetidine, antidepressants, diltiazem, verapamil, fluconazole.
Main side effects	Nausea, reflux esophagitis, tremor.

For severe attacks [1]

Hospital admission.
Severity assessment (especially spirometry and blood gases).
Oxygen administration as needed.
Maximal bronchodilatation (nebulizer).
Intravenous prednisone administration.
Ventilation if patient is tired or weakening or if blood gases show rising arterial blood pressure.

Alternative medicine

Recommended use: None.
Common use: nettles (*Urtica dioica*); garlic (*Allium sativa*); echinacea (*Echinacea purpura* and *E. angustifolia*); licorice (*Glycyrrhiza glabra*).
Caution: licorice at high dosages can cause hypertension and hypokalemia.

Treatment aims

To find minimum level of treatment to suppress symptoms.
To enable patients to take responsibility for day-to-day management of the condition.
To enable patients to avoid days off work or school.
To reduce the frequency of exacerbations and to avoid hospital admissions.

Prognosis

• Many children with asthma experience spontaneous remission in their second decade of life.
• Adult-onset asthma rarely remits.
• Most asthmatic patients cope well with their disease and have a normal life expectancy.
• A few severely ill or unstable asthmatic patients are at risk of respiratory arrest; often, these patients need large doses of oral corticosteroids to control the disease.

Follow-up and management

• Exacerbations should be treated by the following:
Increased dose of inhaled corticosteroid.
Oral prednisone, 30 mg daily for 5–7 days.
Antibiotics if patient is febrile or sputum discoloured.
Increased dose of bronchodilators.

Key references

1. Corbridge TC, Hall JB: The assessment and management of adults with status asthmaticus. *Am J Respir Crit Care Med* 1995, **151**:1292–1316.
2. Drazen JM, Israel E, O'Byrne PM: Treatment of asthma with drugs modifying the leukotriene pathway. *N Engl J Med* 1999, **340(3)**:197–206.
3. Nelson HS: Beta-adrenergic bronchodilators. *N Engl J Med* 1995, **333**:499–506.
4. National Asthma Education and Prevention Program—Expert Panel Report 2: *Guidelines for the Diagnosis and Management of Asthma*. Washington, D.C.: U.S. Department of Health and Human Services, Public Health Service, National Institutes of Health; 1997.
5. Lemanske RF Jr, Busse WW: Asthma. *JAMA* 1997, **278(22)**:1855–1873.
6. McFadden E Jr: Dosages of corticosteroids in asthma. *Am Rev Respir Dis* 1993, **147**:1306–1310.
7. Barnes PJ: Inhaled glucocorticoids for asthma. *N Engl J Med* 1995, **332**:868–875.
8. Weinberger M, Hendeles L: Theophylline in asthma. *N Engl J Med* 1996, **334**:1380–1388.

Asthma, occupational

Diagnosis

Symptoms

Breathlessness at rest or on exertion, wheezing, worsening after work, improvement at weekends or during holidays.

Signs

Diffuse wheezing.

Use of accessory muscles of respiration: due to high negative intrapleural pressure or rapid respiratory rate.

Tachycardia: in severe attack.

Pulsus paradoxus: in severe attack.

Rhinitis.

Cough.

Investigations [1,2]

Baseline spirometry: response to beta-2 agonist.

Bronchial hyper-responsiveness test: using methacholine PC_{20} (>20% fall in forced expiratory volume in 1 second, with no such change on control day).

Serial measure of airway responsiveness.

Detailed peak flow monitoring: at work and on days off or vacations.

Detailed list of materials encountered in the workplace.

Specific challenge tests: to confirm role of new agent in causing asthma or to determine responsible agent when several agents are present in the workplace (available only in very specialized centers).

Complications

Interstitial fibrosis.

Respiratory failure.

Chronic breathlessness.

Differential diagnosis

Asthma due to nonoccupational causes.

Other causes of breathlessness.

Irritant effect of chemical at work.

Etiology [3,4]

Animal hair.

Laboratory animals.

Chemicals: *e.g.*, formalin in hospital workers, urea formaldehyde in insulation workers.

Food processing.

Enzymes (detergents).

Hairdressing.

Metals: platinum and vanadium.

Materials used in plastics: especially toluene diisocyanate and trimetallic anhydride.

Epidemiology

- The incidence of occupational asthma is increasing and now accounts for >50% of industrial lung disease.

Treatment

Diet and lifestyle

• Exposure should be reduced (to zero if possible) by moving to low-exposure zone, provision of personal respirator, or leaving employment.

Pharmacological treatment [4–6]

• Treatment is the same as for other forms of asthma (*see* Asthma *for details*).

• All cases of occupational lung disease need specialist assessment to ensure that the correct diagnosis is reached and appropriate treatment instituted.

• Most patients need inhaled corticosteroids and bronchodilators.

Standard dosage	Beclomethasone, 400–800 µg daily.
Contraindications	None.
Special points	Rinsing of mouth after inhaling steroids reduces risk of oropharyngeal side effects. Spacer device should be used.
Main drug interactions	None.
Main side effects	Hoarse voice, oropharyngeal candidiasis.

Treatment aims

To control symptoms of asthma and restore normal levels of activity.

To reduce risk of developing chronic asthma.

Prognosis

• Most patients improve when withdrawn from exposure.

• >40% should have no residual signs or symptoms of asthma, but up to 30% have chronic persistent symptoms, despite full withdrawal from exposure.

• Persistent asthma is especially frequent with low molecular weight sensitizers but can also occur with high molecular weight (protein) antigens.

Follow-up and management

• Patients should be followed carefully to check whether asthma resolves with time.

• Regular radiographic monitoring is necessary for patients with interstitial fibrosis.

Key references

1. Chan-Yeung M, Malo JL: Occupational asthma. *N Engl J Med* 1995, **333**:107–112.
2. Bright P, Burge PS: Occupational lung disease: 8. The diagnosis of occupational asthma from serial measurements of lung function at and away from work. *Thorax* 1996, **51**:857–863.
3. Bernstein IL, *et al.* (eds.): *Asthma in the Workplace.* New York: Marcel Dekker; 1993.
4. Newman LS: Occupational asthma: diagnosis, management, and prevention. *Clin Chest Med* 1995, **16**:621–636.
5. Garshick E, Schenker MB, Dosman JA: Occupationally induced airway obstruction. *Med Clin North Am* 1996, **80**:851–878.
6. Schwartz DA, Peterson MW: Occupational lung disease. *Disease-A-Month* 1998, **44(2)**:41–84.

Ataxia & cerebellar disorders

Diagnosis

Symptoms

Gait imbalance: including the following:

Wide-based gait.

Tremor.

Difficulty with fine coordinated movements, clumsiness.

Falls.

Signs

Wide-based gait.

Titubation.

Dysmetria, dysdiadochokinesis.

Dysarthria.

Rotated or tilted head postures.

Hypotonia.

Investigations

Family history evaluation, genetic testing—SCA 1, 3, 7.

TSH, T_3, T_4.

Vitamin E levels.

MRI, PET.

CSF examination or angiography if relevant illness suspected.

Check for drug toxicity, heavy metal toxicity.

Ceruloplasmin.

Lipid and fatty acid and aryl sulfatase levels.

Complications

Inability to walk.

Falls, hip fracture.

Differential diagnosis

Acute intoxication.

Hysteria and malingering.

Miller-Fisher variant of Guillain–Barré syndrome.

Etiology

- Degenerative disorders are most common:

Alcoholic degeneration, olivopontocerebellar atrophy, Friedreich's ataxia, multiple system atrophy.

Vascular hemorrhage or infarction.

Multiple sclerosis.

Neoplastic or paraneoplastic syndrome.

Drug toxicity.

Inherited malformations (Dandy–Walker syndrome, Arnold–Chiari deformity).

Viral infections in children and young adults.

Myxedema.

Epidemiology

- Chronic alcoholism is probably the most common cause of chronic progressive ataxia in adults.

Treatment

Diet and lifestyle

- Patients should abstain from alcohol.
- Consider use of walker to prevent falls.

Pharmacological treatment

Clonazepan, 0.5–2 mg twice daily, may relieve symptoms.

Treatment of underlying disorder (*e.g.*, immunosuppression for multiple sclerosis, thyroid replacement, decoppering, or penicillamine for Wilson's disease).

Treatment aims

To maintain safety.

To treat tremor.

Other treatments

Physical therapy for gait retraining and adaptation.

Posterior fossa decompression for some malformations with progressive compression of cerebellar structures.

Address safety issues in patient's home.

Prognosis

- Depending on illness, degenerative disorders usually progress gradually over a decade.

Follow-up and management

Neurological examinations and discussion of function and safety every 6 months.

General references

Gilman S: Cerebellar disorders: clinical features and treatment. In *Movement Disorders: Neurologic Principles and Practice*. Edited by Watts RL, Koller WE. New York: McGraw Hill; 1997.

Harding S: Ataxic disorders. In *Neurology in Clinical Practice*, vol 1. Edited by Bradley WG, Daroff RB, Fenichel GM, Marsden CD. Boston: Butterworth Heinemann; 1991:337–346.

Atrial septal defect

Diagnosis

Symptoms

Ostium secundum defect: anatomically in the region of the fossa ovalis.

• Asymptomatic, particularly small defects with minimal left-to-right shunting. Moderate or large defects often have no symptoms until third or fourth decades, despite substantial left-to-right shunting (characterized by a ratio of pulmonary to systemic flow of 1.5 or more).

Fatigue.
Palpitation.
Dyspnea.
Productive cough.
Symptoms of paradoxical emboli.
Right heart failure.

Ostium primum defect: in the lower part of the atrial septum

• Patients may develop symptoms and heart failure in childhood.

Failure to thrive, chest infections, poor development.

• In adults, in addition to the same symptoms as for secundum defect, the following occur:

Syncope, symptoms of infective endocarditis.

Signs

Pulse

Normal or small-volume pulse.

Normal or raised venous pressure: raised pressure with pulmonary hypertension and right ventricular enlargement.

Heart

A right ventricular or pulmonary arterial impulse.

• S1 is normal.

• Wide and fixed splitting of S2.

• A systolic ejection murmur is audible in the second left intercostal space, peaks in mid-systole, ends before S2, and is usually so soft that it is mistaken for an "innocent" flow murmur.

• Mid-diastolic tricuspid flow murmur.

• Holosystolic murmur of mitral regurgitation heard only in ostium secundum defect.

Investigations

ECG: often shows right-axis deviation and incomplete right bundle-branch block. In ostium primum defects, left-axis deviation also occurs, whereas a junctional or low atrial rhythm occurs in sinus venosus defects.

Chest radiography: prominent pulmonary arteries and a peripheral pulmonary vascular pattern of "shunt vascularity."

Echocardiography: Transthoracic echocardiography visualizes ostium secundum and primum defects but usually does not identify sinus venosus defects. Sensitivity can be enhanced by injecting microbubbles in the peripheral vein, after which the movement across the defect can be seen. Transesophageal and Doppler color-flow echocardiography is useful in detecting and determining the location of atrial septal defects and in identifying anomalous venous drainage and sinus venosus defects.

Cardiac catheterization: often unnecessary in diagnosis but useful in determining the magnitude and direction of shunting and determining the severity and reversibility of pulmonary hypertension

Complications

Atrial arrhythmias: atrial fibrillation most common; often accompanied by tricuspid regurgitation; patient usually have normal sinus rhythm in the first 30 years of life, after which atrial arrhythmias, including atrial fibrillation and supraventricular tachycardia,may appear.

Pulmonary hypertension with the development of right ventricular disease.

Eisenmenger's syndrome with reversal of shunt.

Paradoxical embolus.

Infective endocarditis in patients with ostium primum defects only.

Recurrent pulmonary infections.

Differential diagnosis

Uncomplicated ostium secundum defect
Mild pulmonary stenosis.

Atrial septal defect with pulmonary hypertension
Rheumatic mitral and tricuspid valve disease.
Mitral valve prolapse.
Primary pulmonary hypertension.
Cor pulmonale.

Etiology

• The cause is unknown.

• Most result from spontaneous genetic mutations; some are inherited.

Epidemiology

• Atrial septal defect constitutes 7% of all congenital heart disease and 30% of congenital heart disease in adults.

• The female : male ratio is 2 : 1.

Types

Ostium secundum
Defect of fossa ovalis (most common; 70% of all defects). Associated mitral valve prolapse may occur.

Ostium primum
Defect in septum inferior to fossa ovalis; may occur in isolation or as atrial component of atrioventricular septal defect. Mitral regurgitation occurs due to a cleft in the anterior leaflet of mitral valve.

Sinus venosus
Defect at base of superior vena cava/upper part of interatrial septum; often associated with anomalous pulmonary venous drainage.

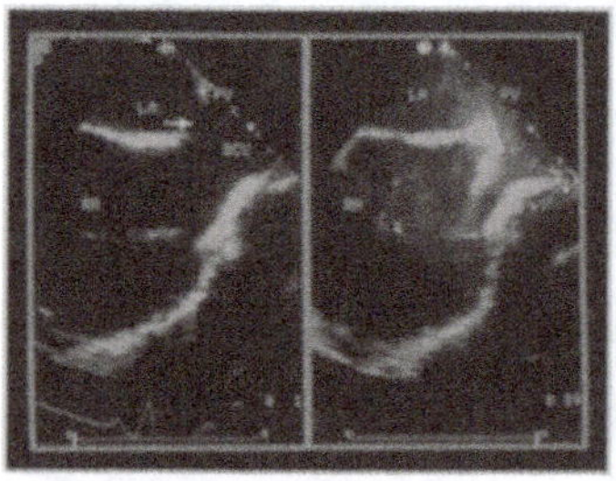

Sinus venosus atrial septal defect (*arrow*). (See Color Plate.)

Treatment

Diet and lifestyle

- No special precautions are necessary.

Pharmacological treatment

- Drug treatment has a role only in the management of complications of the defect such as atrial fibrillation (antiarrhythmic agents), right ventricular failure (diuretics).
- Prophylaxis against infective endocarditis is not recommended for patients with atrial septal defects (repaired or unrepaired) unlesss a concomitant valvular abnormality (*e.g.*, mitral-valve cleft or prolapse) is present.

Nonpharmacological treatment

- Treatment of the defect itself involves surgical closure or transcatheter delivery of an umbrella or clamshell device across the defect.

Ostium secundum defect

- Asymptomatic infants and children are usually followed, with closure advocated before the age of 10 years, if the pulmonary : systemic flow ratio is >1.5 : 1; the feasibility of device closure is determined on transthoracic and transesophageal echocardiography.
- If the child is unsuitable for transcatheter closure, surgical placement of pericardial or Dacron patch should be used.
- For adults, the debate continues on whether closure is worthwhile, but, if symptomatic with shunt >2 : 1, most experts advocate closure; transcatheter device closure may be feasible. In a recent study, surgical repair of atrial septal defects in middle-aged and elderly patients improved longevity and reduced functional limitation due to heart failure and was therefore considered superior to medical treatment. However, the risk of atrial arrhythmias (especially fibrillation and flutter) and the attendant risk of thromboembolic events are not reduced by closure of the defect.
- Contraindications to closure are pulmonary vascular resistance >6 Woods units, and age >65 years with small shunt.

Ostium primum defect

- All patients with significant shunt, unless complicated by severe pulmonary vascular disease, should have surgical closure, with repair of associated mitral valve abnormalities.

Treatment aims

To prevent late-onset pulmonary hypertension.

To avoid right ventricular failure.

To reduce or delay incidence of atrial arrhythmias.

Prognosis

- In patients with ostium secundum defect, mortality of repair in an uncomplicated case is <1%; in older patients with rise in pulmonary vascular resistance, mortality is higher.
- Most patients with unoperated ostium primum defect die by the age of 30 years; operative mortality varies with the complexity of the defect but is usually 5%–10%.

Follow-up and management

- Patients must be observed for symptoms of atrial arrhythmias, developing pulmonary hypertension, and right ventricular failure.
- After repair of an ostium primum defect, heart block is possible.

General references

Brickner ME, Hillis LD, Lange RA: Congenital heart disease in adults. *N Engl J Med* 2000, **342**:256–263.

Bacterial overgrowth of the small intestine

Diagnosis

Definition

• Normally, the microflora of the small intestine consists of a small number of aerobic, gram-positive organisms derived from the upper gastrointestinal tract. In bacterial overgrowth, these are replaced by anaerobic, facultative gram-negative organisms, especially *Escherichia, Bacteroides,* and *Clostridium* spp. at $>10^5$ colony-forming units/mL on culture [1]. Bacterial overgrowth may also occur in segments of the intestinal tract excluded surgically (*e.g.*, by a Billroth II procedure) or due to fistualizations (*e.g.*, Crohn's disease).

Symptoms

• Many patients are asymptomatic and have no adverse effects.

• Bacterial overgrowth of the proximal small intestine tends to produce more marked symptoms than overgrowth of the distal small bowel.

Diarrhea: watery, without blood.

Abdominal pain, weight loss, nausea, and vomiting.

Signs

Steatorrhea: bulky, oily stools.

Anemia: megaloblastic, secondary to vitamin B_{12} deficiency.

Ataxia, neuropathy: due to vitamin B_{12} deficiency.

Fevers, peritoneal signs, bleeding: suggest an alternative diagnosis.

Ecchymosis: vitamin K deficiency.

Investigations

• Diagnosis is often rendered solely on symptoms and signs in susceptible patients in whom other competing diagnoses have been eliminated.

Complete blood count: macrocytic anemia present in those with long-standing disease.

Vitamin B_{12} measurement: concentration low or normal in long-standing disease.

Serum or erythrocyte folate measurement: concentration high or normal; "inverted" profile (*i.e.*, elevated folate with low B_{12}), suggestive but nonspecific marker.

Schilling test with intrinsic factor: absorption not corrected; also found in terminal ileal disease.

Qualitative (*i.e.*, spot) fecal fat analysis with Sudan red: marker for neutral stool fat.

3-day fecal fat collection: useful but unpopular test to quantify steatorrhea.

Barium follow-through: for jejunal diverticulosis, strictures, and fistulas; delayed transit of barium through small intestine is indirect evidence of impaired motility.

Duodenal aspiration: gold standard for culture and species identification; presence of detectable concentrations of unconjugated bile acids and short-chain fatty acids can provide useful adjunct, although these tests are not widely available; false-negative results do not exclude bacterial overgrowth distal to ligament of Treitz.

Duodenal biopsy: to assess villous architecture and exclude parasitic infestation (*i.e.*, giardiasis, Whipple's disease, celiac sprue).

Breath tests: simple, noninvasive, and increasingly available; early rise of breath hydrogen after ingestion of 50 g glucose has a 60% sensitivity and 80% specificity for overgrowth.

Complications

• In patients with long-standing symptoms, complications result in chronic malnutrition and debility.

Secondary weight loss: if food exacerbates abdominal pain.

Neuropathy: after profound vitamin B_{12} deficiency (rare).

Dehydration.

Differential diagnosis

Celiac disease.

Chronic pancreatitis.

Crohn's disease

Infections: *Yersinia* or *Campylobacter* spp. (bacterial); *Giardia lamblia* (protozoan); *Ascaris* or *Strongyloides* spp. (helminthic); AIDS enteropathy (viral), Whipple's disease.

Lactose intolerance.

Etiology/risk factors

• Usually caused by stasis within the small intestine (*e.g.*, structural abnormality or motility disorder), reduced gastric clearance of ingested bacteria (*i.e.*, excessive bacterial load to the small intestine), or impaired immunity.

Structural abnormalities causing stasis

Jejunal diverticulosis.

Blind loops of the gastrointestinal tract.

Adhesions.

Motility disorders

Autonomic neuropathy (*e.g.*, diabetes mellitus).

Progressive systemic sclerosis, amyloidosis.

Postoperative ileus.

Excessive bacterial load

Diminished gastric acid production (gastric atrophy with achlorhydria, post-gastric surgery, acid reduction therapy with antisecretory medications) [2,3].

Incompetent ileocecal valve.

Incompetent pyloric valve.

Ileocolic fistula (Crohn's).

Impaired immunity

Primary immunodeficiencies (e.g., IgA deficiency).

Acquired immunodeficiencies (e.g., HIV, malignancies).

Malnutrition.

Epidemiology

• Prevalence studies are difficult because of the lack of a suitable screening test.

• The frequency of achlorhydria and other risk factors noted above make this a common and often overlooked cause of diarrhea in the elderly.

Treatment

Diet and lifestyle

• A high-protein, high-energy, high-fat diet is recommended.

• Vitamin supplementation, especially injections of vitamin B_{12} and fat-soluble vitamins (A, E, D, K), or oral iron may be beneficial.

• Total parenteral nutrition is rarely necessary.

• Lactose is poorly tolerated during periods of bacterial overgrowth.

Pharmacological treatment

• Treatment is often empirical, the diagnosis being made by observing improvement in symptoms and biochemical abnormalities after treatment.

• A single antibiotic with broad aerobic coverage is first line treatment (representative agents listed below). For refractory cases, two drugs and increased anaerobic coverage are required [4,5].

Antibiotics

Standard dosage	Amoxicillin-clavulanic acid, 500 mg 3 times daily. Trimethoprim, 160 mg/sulfamethoxazole, 800 mg twice daily (2-week course). Tetracycline, 250 mg 4 times daily (2-week course). Norfloxacin, 800 mg/day (1-week course). Maintenance with alternating courses may be needed.
Contraindications	*Amoxicillin-clavulanic acid:* penicillin allergy. *Trimethoprim/sulfamethoxazole:* sensitivity to sulfa. *Tetracycline:* renal insufficiency, children aged <12 years, lactation.
Special points	*Tetracycline:* permanent tooth discoloration if used during dental development.
Main drug interactions	*Trimethoprim/sulfamethoxazole:* potentiates anticoagulant effect of warfarin, prolongs half-life of phenytoin and sulfonylureas. *Tetracyclines:* calcium, magnesium, iron, and aluminum salts (*e.g.*, milk, antacids) impair absorption. *Norfloxacin:* magnesium, aluminium salts inhibit absorption; theophylline levels raised; anticoagulants potentiated.
Main side effects	*Tetracyclines:* gastrointestinal disturbances, photosensitive rash, hypersensitivity (rare). *Amoxicillin-clavulanic acid, norfloxacin:* gastrointestinal symptoms, rashes, restlessness, dizziness, pruritis, tremor, convulsions.

Treatment aims

To clear and prevent recurrence of bacterial overgrowth.

To reduce diarrhea.

To correct hematological abnormalities and secondary nutritional deficiencies.

Other treatments

Surgery to correct underlying anatomical abnormality; may cause prolonged postoperative ileus.

Prognosis

• The prognosis depends on the underlying disease: motility disorders have the worst prognosis.

Follow-up and management

• Relapses are frequent unless underlying cause is corrected.

• Regular infrequent outpatient follow-up may be needed to monitor for symptoms and to detect relapses early.

• Long-term maintenance antibiotic treatment is only rarely needed, and surgical treatment is a consideration for patients refractory to medical management.

Key references

1. Kirsch M: Bacterial overgrowth. *Am J Gastroenterol* 1990, **85**:231–237.

2. Larner AJ, Hamilton MIR: Infective complications of therapeutic gastric inhibition. *Aliment Pharmacol Ther* 1994, **8**:579–584.

3. Fried M, *et al.*: Duodenal bacterial overgrowth during treatment in outpatients with omeprazole. *Gut* 1994, **35**:23–26.

4. Attar A, *et al.*: Antibiotic efficacy in small intestinal bacterial overgrowth-related chronic diarrhea: a crossover, randomized trial. *Gastroenterology* 1999, **117**:794–797.

5. Banerjee S, LaMont JT: Treatment of gastrointestinal infectinos. *Gastroenterology* 2000, **118**:S48–S67.

Basal cell carcinoma

Diagnosis

Symptoms

New appearance or progression of skin lesion.

Bleeding with trauma.

Nonhealing sore or ulcer.

Pain or itching.

Signs

Skin findings

Papules: typically pink to flesh-colored with a translucent surface and overlying telangiectatic vessels; may have a rolled border and central ulceration; may bleed intermittently; occur on sun-exposed areas of the head, neck, and upper trunk; most common location is the face, especially the nose.

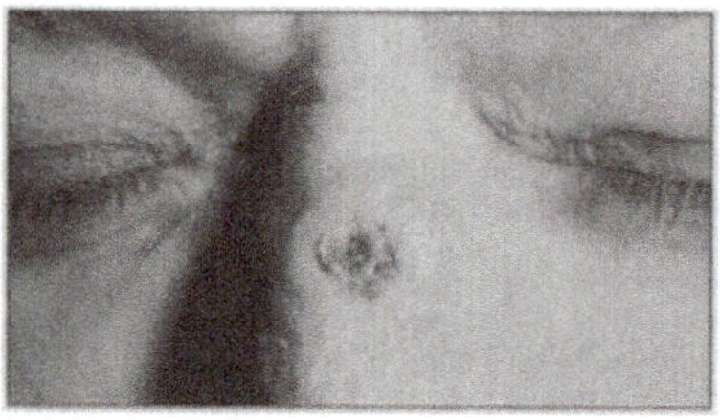

Classic basal cell carcinoma. (*See* Color Plate.)

Clinical variants

Superficial basal cell carcinoma (BCC): frequently occurs as a dry, scaly psoriasis-like lesion on the covered portions of the trunk; edge of lesion shows a thread-like raised border.

Pigmented BCC: shows brown or black, often variegate, pigmentation in addition to typical features; seen more frequently in Latin Americans, Asians.

Morpheaform (sclerosing) BCC: waxy white plaque most commonly found on the head and neck; characteristically lacks a rolled border, so edges are ill-defined; resembles a small scar.

Basal cell nevus syndrome (BCNS): rare, autosomal dominant disorder of the skin and internal organs; patients develop multiple BCCs, sometimes hundreds (the BCCs may have typical appearance or appear nonspecific); usually develops before 20 years of age; associated signs are "pitting" of the palms and soles, mandibular cysts, bifid ribs, and frontal bossing. Patients are also predisposed to other neoplasms, including ovarian fibroma and medulloblastoma.

Investigations

The physician should obtain an accurate history of the duration and behavior of the lesion; predisposing etiologic factors.

- Biopsy is required for diagnosis and accurate histological classification, which may be important in choosing the method of treatment.

Complications

- A neglected BCC that slowly progresses over many years may become a large, gnawed-out mutilating lesion known as a "rodent ulcer."
- The incidence of metastases for BCC has been reported to be slightly <0.1%.
- An increased incidence of metastatic BCC has been noted in AIDS patients.

Differential diagnosis

Typical BCC
Nevus, fibrous papule, seborrheic keratosis, amelanotic melanoma, squamous cell carcinoma, keratonacanthoma.

Superficial BCC
Psoriasis, nummular eczema, Bowen's disease, extramammary Paget's disease.

Pigmented BCC
Pigmented seborrheic keratosis, malignant melanoma.

Morpheaform BCC
Scar.

Etiology

UV radiation (sunshine) most common.

Trauma.

Long-term arsenic exposure.

Genodermatoses (BCNS, albinism, xeroderma pigmentosum).

Radiation therapy (used in the treatment of acne vulgaris until 1950).

Immunosuppression (secondary to organ transplantation, chemotherapy, or AIDS).

Certain long-standing lesions (linear epidermal nevi, nevus sebaceous, and porokeratosis of Mibelli).

Chronic venous stasis dermatitis and stasis ulcers.

- BCNS the gene responsible for BCNS is the *PATCHED* gene, located on chromosome 9. In normal embryonic development, the *PATCHED* gene, which represses growth, works in counterbalance with the *HEDGEHOG* gene, which stimulates growth. It appears that a mutation in the *PATCHED* gene allows for the cutaneous and extracutaneous overgrowth found in BCNS.

Epidemiology

- BCC is the most common of all human cancers.
- It affects 750 000 people yearly in the United States.
- It is most common in light-skinned people aged >40 years with a history of UV exposure.
- BCNS affects 1 in 56 000 individuals.

Treatment

Diet and lifestyle
• No special diet is necessary.
• Emphasize the importance of sun avoidance and sun protection. Sun protection includes the use of protective clothing (hats, long-sleeved shirts) and daily sunscreens, preferably of broad-spectrum UVA plus UVB with SPF of 15 or higher.

Surgical treatment
For high-risk BCCs
• Mohs' microscopic surgery (a very precise staged method of excision) is the treatment of choice. Indications for Mohs' surgery include: location in the canthi, nasolabial folds, or postauricular folds; size >2 cm; aggressive histological growth pattern including morpheaform and keratinizing BCCs; recurrent tumors after any treatment modality; tumors arising in areas of previous radiation exposure; incompletely excised tumors; tumors with clinically ill-defined borders; tumors with perineural invasion.
Advantages: achieves the highest cure rate available (99% for primary BCCs, 94% for recurrent BCCs).
Disadvantages: cost, availability.

For low-risk BCCs
Treatment of choice:
For lesions 5 mm–2 cm in diameter, simple elliptical excision with 2–5-mm margins.
For lesions <5 mm: punch biopsy or tangential (shave) excision with curettage and electrodessication of the lesion base.
Advantages: electrodessication and curettage had a cure rate of 90%–93% for primary BCCs; less expensive than Mohs' surgery.
Disadvantages: recurrence rate up to 40% for high-risk BCCs.

For prophylaxis
• For patients with severely sun-damaged skin who are experiencing frequent precancerous and cancerous lesions, prophylaxis may be obtained with 5% 5-fluorouracil cream and low-dose isotretinoin.

Standard dosage	5-fluorouracil, 5% cream topically to affected area twice daily for 2–4 weeks; may be repeated twice yearly. Low-dose isotretinoin, 10 mg/day.
Contraindications	*5-fluorouracil:* unavoidable sun exposure. *Low-dose isotretinoin:* pregnancy; pre-existing hepatic disease, hypertriglyceridemia.
Special points	*Low-dose isotretinoin:* liver function tests and serum lipoprotein levels should be monitored monthly.
Main drug interactions	*5-fluorouracil:* none. *Low-dose isotretinoin:* concomitant use with tetracycline, minocycline, or doxycycline may increase risk of pseudotumor cerebri.
Main side effects	*5-fluorouracil:* extensive swelling, erosions, and pain 3–5 days after the start of treatment; may require analgesics, topical steroids, oral and/or topical antibiotics; ideally treatment should be carried out in the winter; patients usually cannot tolerate the use of sunscreen on areas undergoing 5-fluorouracil therapy until they heal; contact dermatitis may develop with repeated courses of 5-fluorouracil; diagnostic clues include development of pruritus and extension of the erythema and crusts beyond the treated areas. *Low-dose isotretinoin:* drying of skin and mucosa, elevated liver enzymes and triglyceride levels, myalgias teratogenicity side effects are significantly less common with lower dosages.

For patients with BCNS
• A team approach is required.
• Current management recommendations include regular visits to a dermatologist every 2–3 months beginning in adolescence or earlier as necessary, with simple excision or Mohs' microscopic surgery for developing BCCs.
• Patients should have yearly panoramic radiographs of the jaws with referral to an oral surgeon for excision if odontogenic cysts are found.
• Infants at risk should have an annual MRI to exclude medulloblastoma and periodic radiographs to rule out skeletal anomalies and cardiac fibromas.
• Photodynamic therapy is a relatively new form of cancer treatment that may be effective in adults with BCNS. Radiation therapy should be used with caution.
• Management should always include appropriate genetic counseling because each affected individual carries a 50% risk of transmitting the disease to his/her children.

Treatment aims
To achieve a cure with the best cosmetic result.

Other treatments
For patients unable or unwilling to tolerate surgical intervention:
Ionizing radiation therapy, intralesional alpha-interferon treatment, cryotherapy, imiquimod 5% cream.

Prognosis
• BCC growth is usually slow but relentless; recurrences are usually seen during the first 4–12 months after treatment.
• The risk of development of a second BCC is approximately 40%.

Follow-up and management
• All patients should be evaluated 3 months after treatment and a minimum of every 6 months owing to the risk of recurrence and development of additional primary tumors.
• Follow-up must be continued over the patient's lifetime.

General references

Beutner KR, *et al.*: Therapeutic response of basal cell carcinoma to the immune response modified imiquimod 5% cream. *J Am Acad Dermatol* 1999, **41**:1002–1007.

Johnson TM, *et al.*: Unusual basal cell carcinomas. *Cutis* 1994, **54**:85–92.

Nelson B: Malignant cutaneous tumors. *Dermatol Focus* 1996, 15:1–7.

Telfer NR, *et al.*: Guidelines for the management of basal cell carcinoma. *Br J Dermatol* 1999, **141**:415–423.

Thissen MR, *et al.*: A systematic review of treatment modalities for primary basal cell carcinomas. *Arch Dermatol* 1999, **135**:1177–1183.

Walker DC, Tschen JA: Basal cell carcinoma: predisposing genetic syndromes and clinical settings. In: *Cutaneous Oncology: Pathophysiology, Diagnosis and Management.* Edited by Miller SJ, Maloney ME. Malden, MA: Blackwell Science; **1998**:619–624.

Benign prostatic hyperplasia

Diagnosis

Symptoms [1]

Obstructive

Sensation of incomplete bladder emptying, decreased force of urine stream, straining to urinate, dribbling.

Irritative

Urgency, frequency, nocturia, dysuria.

• Self-administered questionnaire to evaluate symptom severity and response to therapy is shown in the table [2].

American Urological Association Symptom Index

Over the past month or so, how often have you:	Possible answers for questions 1–6:
1. Had the sensation of not emptying your bladder completely after you finished urinating? 2. Had to urinate again less than 2 hours after you finished urinating? 3. Found you stopped and started again several times when you urinated? 4. Found it difficult to postpone urination? 5. Had a weak urinary stream? 6. Had to push or strain to begin urination?	0=Not at all. 1=Less than one time in 5. 2=Less than half the time. 3=About half the time. 4=More than half the time. 5=Almost always.
7. Over the past month, how many times did you typically get up to urinate from the time you went to bed at night to the time you got up in the morning?	Possible answers: 0,1,2,3,4, ≥5 times

Symptom score (sum of all the answers): Mild symptoms: 0–7 points; Moderate symptoms: 8–19 points; Severe symptoms: 20–35 points

Signs

• None; size of prostate on physical examination does not correlate with symptoms.

Investigations [1]

For all patients

Comprehensive history and physical examination.

Detailed urinary history: with focus on symptom severity using American Urological Association (AUA) symptom index.

Digital rectal examination and focused neurological examination: perineal sensation, rectal tone, presence of diabetic neuropathy.

Urinalysis and sediment examination: to rule out infection or hematuria.

Serum creatinine: to assess renal function

Additional studies if clinically indicated

Postvoid residual (PVR) urine volume if concern for large retained urine volumes: palpable bladder, overflow incontinence.

Pressure-flow studies: if there is concern for primary bladder dysfunction from neurological disease.

Urethrocystoscopy: if surgical therapy is planned.

• Prostate-specific antigen (PSA) testing is optional, because benign prostatic hypertrophy (BPH) may raise PSA levels; therefore PSA does not discriminate well between BPH and early prostate cancer.

Complications

Acute urinary obstruction: may be precipitated by alcohol, sedatives, sympathomimetics, or anticholinergics.

Obstructive uropathy with chronic renal insufficiency: rare.

Urinary tract infections and bladder decompensation: rare.

Bladder stones: 1%–2% found at time of prostate surgery.

Differential diagnosis

Dysuria: urinary tract infection.

Urgency, frequency: infection, excessive caffeine intake.

Polyuria: diabetes mellitus, diabetes insipidus, hypercalcemia.

Bladder tumor.

Detrusor muscle instability.

Neurological bladder dysfunction, such as neurogenic bladder with diabetes or spasticity with prior cerebrovascular accident.

Etiology

Hyperplasia of prostatic tissue, both stromal and epithelial components.

Risk factors are advancing age and presence of androgens.

Epidemiology

• Histologic evidence of BPH is evident in 10% of men at age 30 years, >50% at age 60, >90% at age 85.

• Only 50% of patients with histological evidence of BPH have clinical symptoms.

• 10% of men with BPH will require transurethral resection of prostate (TURP) for urinary obstruction.

• 400 000 surgical procedures are performed per year in the United States.

Treatment

Diet and lifestyle

• Avoidance of caffeine may improve frequency, urgency.

• Avoid fluid intake after dinner to decrease nocturia.

Decision making

• For mild symptoms (AUA scores 0–7) watchful waiting is appropriate.

• For moderate to severe symptoms (AUA scores 8–35), risks and benefits of surgery vs. watchful waiting vs. medical therapy should be discussed.

Pharmacological treatment [1]

Alpha-blockers

Standard dosage	Prazosin, doxazosin, terazosin, or tamsulosin decrease symptoms; terazosin doses titrated from 1 to 5–10 mg every night.
Contraindications	Known hypersensitivity, hypotension, or postural hypotension.
Special points	First-dose hypotension (1%–2%), orthostasis best prevented by nightly dosing, caution in the elderly.
Main drug interactions	Caution with other antihypertensive medications.
Main side effects	Aesthenia (6%–10%), postural hypotension (6%–8%), dizziness (5%–10%), rhinitis (6%–8%).

Finasteride

Standard dosage	5–10 mg daily.
Contraindications	Known hypersensitivity.
Special points	Beneficial only in patients with enlarged prostates and moderate to severe symptoms.
Main drug interactions	None.
Main side effects	Sexual dysfunction, loss of libido (1%–3%)

Intermittent straight-catheterization

Treatment of choice for patient with high PVR on maximal medical therapy who declines surgery or is not a surgical candidate.

Indications for referral to urologist

Uncertain diagnosis, especially if neurological bladder dysfunction is suspected secondary to CVA or diabetes.

Refractory urinary retention on maximal medical therapy.

Recurrent urinary tract infections.

Recurrent gross hematuria.

Bladder stones.

Renal insufficiency secondary to BPH.

Refractory symptoms despite maximal medical therapy.

Alternative medicine

Recommended use: saw palmetto (*Serenoa repens*); stinging nettles (*Urtica dioica*).

Common use: cernilton; pygeum (*Pygeum africanum*).

Caution: saw palmetto may cause headache or gastrointestinal disturbance.

Treatment aims

To relieve symptoms.

To improve quality of life.

To prevent infections and renal insufficiency.

Surgical therapy with TURP

Effective for symptoms in 80%–90%.

Postoperative mortality 0.2%–1.5%.

Retrograde ejaculation (75%).

Impotence (13%).

Urethral stricture (3%–5%).

Partial to complete incontinence (2%–5%).

Prognosis

• Disease progresses slowly and is quite variable among patients.

• Spontaneous improvement in symptoms common (30%–50%).

Follow-up and management

Regular review of symptoms and response to therapy.

Key references

1. McConnell JD, *et al.*: Benign prostatic hyperplasia: diagnosis and treatment. In *Clinical Practice Guideline*, no 8. Rockville, MD: Agency for Health Care Policy and Research (AHCPR), Public Health Service, U.S. Department of Health and Human Services. [AHCPR publication no 94-0582.]
2. Barry MJ, *et al.*: The American Urologic Association Symptom Index for benign prostatic hyperplasia. *J Urol* 1992, **148**:1549–1557.

Breast cancer

Diagnosis

Symptoms

•Symptoms of breast cancer are few. Some patients may note a mildly tender lump under the arm or in the breast.

Signs

•Signs are not always manifest.

Breast lump.

Abnormal skin over breast: dimpling, ulceration, edema, erythema.

Fixation of mass to chest wall.

Nipple changes: retraction, discoloration, erosion, discharge.

Adenopathy: axillary, cervical, supraclavicular, infraclavicular.

Investigations

For diagnosis

Bilateral mammography.

Needle aspiration of breast mass with cytological examination: 95% sensitivity; rapid, inexpensive, and painless; will not distinguish carcinoma in situ from invasive carcinoma.

Stereotactic core biopsy: more painful, but has lower false-negative rate than needle aspiration.

Excisional biopsy: provides optimum pathological specimen, but is more painful and has cosmetic effects.

For staging

Axillary node dissection with pathological examination of 10–20 nodes.

Chest radiography.

Complete blood, differential, and platelet counts: persistently abnormal complete blood count may be an indicator of bone-marrow involvement; bone-marrow biopsy should be performed.

Liver function tests: may indicate liver metastasis.

Bone scan for suspected stage III disease.

Head CT or MRI: if neurological symptoms are present.

Special investigations

Tumor estrogen and progesterone receptor status: useful in determining response to hormonal therapy with tamoxifen or toremifene.

Breast cancer antigen (CA 15-3) tumor marker level: useful more as a marker during follow-up examination of disease progression in patients with breast cancer.

***BRCA1* and *BRCA2* mutation analysis:** useful in familial breast cancer analysis and genetic counseling.

HER2 (c-erb B2) receptor status: usefull in determining response to Trastuzumab monoclonal antibody therapy.

Complications

Pain.

Pleural or pericardial effusion.

Metastases to bone, brain, liver.

Recurrent venous thrombosis.

Pathological fracture.

Differential diagnosis

Fibrocystic disease.

Mastitis.

Other tumors: lymphoma, sarcoma, melanoma, phyllodes tumors.

Etiology

• The cause of breast cancer is unknown but is presumed to be due to genetic mutations, the risk of which is increased by DNA damage.

• Patients who carry the *BRCA1* mutation have a 50% risk of developing breast cancer by age 45 years and an 85% lifetime risk of breast cancer. Increased risk is also conferred by the presence of the *BRCA2* mutation.

Epidemiology

• Breast cancer tumors are the most common tumors in women in the United States and account for 25% of all cancers in women.

• An association exists between breast cancer and a high-fat diet, long-term alcohol ingestion, age of menarche and menopause, and age at birth of first full-term child. There is a more controversial association with estrogen supplementation and high-fat diet.

• Women with a first-degree relative with breast cancer have a 2–3-fold increased risk for breast cancer.

Treatment

Diet and lifestyle

• Weight loss is not generally significant unless it is related to complications of chemotherapy.

• Patients should be encouraged to be active.

Treatment

• Treatment depends on disease stage, age, and tumor histology.

• Treatment should be given under specialist supervision.

Surgery

• Surgery is the mainstay of therapy, with procedures ranging from partial mastectomy to modified radical mastectomy available.

• Breast-conserving surgeries with or without radiation are possible when the tumor is small, but are contraindicated when the disease is multifocal or associated with diffuse indeterminate calcifications on mammogram.

• Axillary lymph node resection with removal of 10–20 nodes is performed at the time of definitive surgery, but may not be done in patients who are aged >65 years with no palpable nodes.

Radiation therapy

• Radiation therapy is used to prevent local recurrence after surgery.

• Some studies suggest radiation therapy can be omitted in postmenopausal women if the tumor is <2.5 cm and a quadrantectomy is performed.

Chemotherapy

• Complex decision making is based on disease stage, but chemotherapy may be administered in node-negative patients who are considered high risk.

• Adjuvant chemotherapy generally consists of a combination of two or more of the following agents: cyclophosphamide, methotrexate, vincristine, doxorubicin, 5-fluorouracil, or prednisone.

• Chemotherapy is the mainstay of stage IV disease and may include paclitaxel or mitomycin C.

Hormonal therapy

• Adjuvant tamoxifen or toremifene hormonal therapy is used in postmenopausal women of all stages and may also be used in premenopausal patients with breast cancer that is estrogen receptor–positive.

• Luteinizing hormone–releasing analogs, aminoglutethimide, and progestins are additional agents used in stage IV disease.

Monoclonal antibody (immunologic) therapy

• Useful alone or in combination with chemotherapeutic agents for patients with metastatic breast cancer whose tumors overexpress the HER2 protein.

Complications of therapy

Lymphedema after axillary node dissection, accelerated coronary artery disease after radiation to chest, osteoporosis, bladder dysfunction, hot flashes, vaginal dryness, emotional lability during antiestrogen therapy.

• Hypercalcemia and accelerated bone pain are sometimes seen with tamoxifen therapy.

Treatment aims

To identify patients with surgically resectable disease at the earliest stage.

To identify patients with more indolent disease histologies who do not require aggressive surgical management or adjuvant chemotherapy.

To prevent distant metastasis through adjuvant therapy.

To provide emotional support.

Prognosis

• Prognosis is directly related to the number of positive axillary nodes, tumor size, tumor histology and nuclear grade, and estrogen receptor status.

• Ductal carcinoma in situ has a 98% cure rate with local and regional therapy alone.

• Five-year survival for stages I–IIIB are 90%, 80%, 65%, 50%, and 40%, respectively.

Follow-up and management

Patients must be followed up regularly for local and distant recurrence and side effects of therapy.

Relapsed disease

• Chemotherapy is palliative in stage IV disease, with a median duration of response of 9–12 months.

•The advantage of high-dose chemotherapy with autologous bone marrow transplantation over standard therapies is unclear. Bone marrow transplantation may be appropriate for some patients and is best administered as part of a clinical study.

General references

American Joint Committee on Cancer: Breast. In *AJCC Cancer Staging Handbook*, edn 5. Edited by Fleming ID, Cooper JS, Henson DE, *et al*. Philadelphia: Lippincott-Raven; 1998:159–170.

Donegan WL: Tumor-related prognostic factors for breast cancer. *Cancer* 1997, **47**:28–51.

Ford K, Marcus E, Lum B: Breast cancer screening, diagnosis, and treatment. *Disease-A-Month* **45**:337–405.1

Hortobagyi GN: Treatment of breast cancer. *N Engl J Med* 1998, **339**:974–984.

Veronesi U, Luini A, Del Vecchio M, *et al.*: Radiotherapy after breast preserving surgery in women with localized cancer of the breast. *N Engl J Med* 1993, **328**:1587–1591.

Diagnosis

Symptoms

Cough, purulent, large-volume sputum, episodic fever or malaise, night sweats, nasal discharge, possibly with purulent sinusitis, dyspnea, wheezing, recurrent hemoptysis, pleuritic chest pain, recurrent pneumonia.

Weight loss, anemia: frequent.

Signs

Rhonchi, coarse crackles, tachypnea, hyperinflation, signs of weight loss.

Clubbing

Foul-smelling phlegm: classically separates into three layers.

Investigations [1]

Pulmonary function tests: to assess impairment.

Sputum culture: for *Staphylococcus aureus*, *Haemophilus influenzae*, *Pseudomonas* spp., and fungi, and to exclude active tuberculosis.

Sputum cytology: to exclude malignancy.

Serum immunoglobulin quantitaion.

Chest radiography: shows hyperinflation, crowded lung markings, and ring shadows.

High-resolution CT: shows airway dilatation ring and cystic lesions, and bronchial wall thickening.

Respiratory function tests: for obstructive or mixed ventilatory defect.

Aspergillus skin and precipitin tests.

Complications

Infective exacerbations: bacterial or viral.

Hemoptysis.

Pneumothorax.

Respiratory failure.

Cor pulmonale.

Empyema.

Chest pain: usually pleuritic, associated with an area of bronchiectasis.

Metastatic spread of infection: now rare; brain abscess was classic complication.

Arthropathy: rheumatoid arthritis and nonspecific seronegative arthritis related to activity of disease.

Amyloidosis.

Differential diagnosis

Asthma.
Interstitial fibrosis.
Chronic bronchitis.
Lung carcinoma.
Sinusitis with chronic cough.

Etiology [2,3]

- Bronchiectasis is caused by recurrent inflammation or infection. Congenital causes include cystic fibrosis, immunodeficiency states and alpha, antitrypsin deficiency.
- Acquired causes include defective mucociliary clearance, bronchial obstruction, inflammatory pneumonitis, fibrotic or granulomatous lung disease, previous severe infection, allergic aspergillosis, and acquired immunodeficiency (*e.g.*, AIDS, chemotherapy).

Epidemiology

- The estimated prevalence of bronchiectasis is declining with the advent of modern antibiotics.

Associated diseases

Rheumatoid arthritis.
Purulent sinusitis.
Allergic bronchopulmonary aspergillosis.
Malignancy.
Connective tissue disorders.
Vasculitis.
Infertility.
Primary ciliary dyskinesia.
Immune deficiency syndromes.
Sjögren's syndrome.

Treatment

Diet and lifestyle

• Adequate nutrition is important.

Pharmacological treatment [3,4]

General guidelines

• Treatment specific to the underlying cause includes the following:

Removal of foreign body or inspissated mucus.

Replacement of immunoglobulins: for panhypogammaglobulinemia, selective IgM and IgG, and possibly IgG_2 deficiency, but not for selective IgA deficiency (risk of anaphylaxis).

Treatment of associated conditions, *e.g.*, rheumatoid arthritis.

Antibiotics: drug choice based on sputum culture; given either for exacerbations or at regular intervals; courses should last 2–3 weeks, and antimicrobial agents should be given in high doses; for patients colonized with *Pseudomonas* spp., specific antipseudomonal antibiotics should be given, including nebulized antibiotics, *e.g.*, tobromycin, for maintenance treatment between courses.

Bronchodilators: for patients with demonstrable airflow obstruction.

Steroids: improved morbidity in short term, but effects on prognosis not known; inhaled steroids recommended for patients with prominent or reversible airflow obstruction.

DNase: has been shown to be effective in patients with cystic fibrosis, but not for those with idiopathic bronchiectosis.

Nonpharmacological treatment

Physical therapy

• Physical therapy is the main form of nonpharmacological treatment.

• Methods include chest percussion, postural drainage, deep cough, and forced expiratory maneuvers twice daily.

Other options

For hemoptysis: bed rest and antibiotics, selective embolization, intubation and balloon tamponade, or local resection.

For pneumothorax: aspiration, intercostal drainage, pleurodesis or partial pleurectomy (if recurrent or unresponsive).

For respiratory failure: supplemental oxygen therapy, nasal ventilation.

For severe localized disease: surgery.

Lung transplantation.

Treatment aims

To minimize lung damage by limiting pulmonary infection and increasing clearance of pulmonary secretion.

Prognosis

• The prognosis of bronchiectasis depends on the severity of the disease.

Follow-up and management

• All patients with moderate to severe bronchiectasis need regular care from a respiratory physician.

Patient support

Counselling regarding lung transplantation, fears of dying, reproduction, etc.

Key references

1. Smith IE, Flower CD: Review article: imaging in bronchiectasis. *Br J Radiol* 1996, **69**:589–593.
2. Cohen M, Sahn SA: Bronchiectasis in systemic diseases. *Chest* 1999, **116**: 1063.
3. O'Donnell A, Barker A, Ilowite J, *et. al.*: Treatment of idiopathic bronchiectasis with aerosolized recombinant human Dnase I. *Chest* 1998, **113**:1329.
4. Weg J: Bronchiectasis. *Semin Respir Med* 1992, **13**:177–189.

Bullous disorders

Diagnosis

Symptoms

Pemphigus vulgaris: pain, difficulty eating.

Bullous pemphigoid: pruritus, pain.

Dermatitis herpetiformis: intense, severe, pruritus (seemingly out of proportion to the sparse clinical signs).

Signs

Pemphigus vulgaris

Oral ulcerations: most patients present with oral erosions only; skin lesions develop on average 5 months later.
Flaccid blisters: rupture easily; only erosions may be visible on examination; Nikolsky sign is positive (gentle pressure on a bulla causes fluid to expand laterally into the normal skin, extending the lesion).

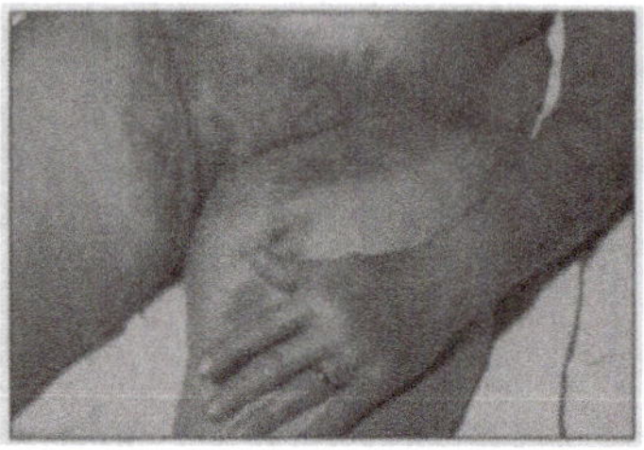

Bullous pemphigoid. (*See* Color Plate.)

Bullous pemphigoid

Large, tense blisters: often on urticarial or erythematous bases in elderly patients. Bullae may be preceded by a prodrome of pruritus or an urticarial rash lasting several weeks to months.
Oral involvement: only in up to one-third of patients; usually not extensive.

Dermatitis herpetiformis

Groups of papules and vesicles: often excoriated with a predilection for the extensor surfaces of the extremities and buttocks; symmetrical.

Investigations

Pemphigus vulgaris

Biopsy: of perilesional skin to detect intraepidermal blister.
Direct immunofluorescence: to detect IgG and C3 directed at keratinocyte cell membranes.
Indirect immunofluorescence: to detect circulating autoantibodies. Titers may be monitored to detect response to therapy because they parallel disease activity.

Bullous pemphigoid

Biopsy: of perilesional skin to detect subepidermal blister; many eosinophils.
Direct immunofluorescence: IgG and C3 directed at the dermoepidermal junction.
Indirect immunofluorescence: autoantibodies may be present, but titer does not correlate with severity of disease.

Dermatitis herpetiformis

Biopsy: of erilesional skin to detect papillary dermal neutrophilic abscesses (subepidermal).
Direct immunofluorescence: to detect granular deposits of IgA and C3 in the dermal papillary tips.

Complications

Pemphigus vulgaris

Malnutrition and dehydration: with severe oral involvement.
Secondary bacterial infection.
Sepsis: in severe cases (especially immunosuppressed patients).
Fluid and electrolyte imbalance: in severe cases.
Thymoma and myasthenia gravis (unusual).

Bullous pemphigoid

Secondary bacterial infection.
Underlying occult malignancy: controversial association.

Dermatitis herpetiformis

Gluten-sensitive enteropathy: in approximately 90% of cases.
Gastrointestinal lymphoma: increased incidence, especially in jejunum.

Differential diagnosis

Infections: *e.g.*, varicella zoster, herpes simplex, bullous impetigo, cellulitis.
Bullous bite reaction (insect bites).
Drug-induced pemphigus.
Epidermolysis bullosa.
Porphyria cutanea tarda.
Pseudo–porphyria cutanea tarda.
Diabetic bullosis.
Cicatricial pemphigoid.

Etiology

Pemphigus vulgaris

Autoantibody against keratinocyte surface glycoproteins (desmoglein), causing separation just above the basal cell layer. Associated with HLA-DR4/DR6 phenotype.

Bullous pemphigoid

Autoantibody against proteins in the hemidesmosomes that anchor keratinocytes to the basement membrane, causing separation at the dermoepidermal junction. Associated with HLA-B8/DR3 phenotype.

Dermatitis herpetiformis

Molecular immunopathogenesis plus HLA-B8- and DW3-associated autoimmune disorder; also associated with gluten-sensitive enteropathy.

Epidemiology

Pemphigus vulgaris

More common in patients with Jewish or Mediterranean heritage.

Bullous pemphigoid

Most common in patients 60–70 years of age (less common variant can occur in children).

Dermatitis herpetiformis

Onset between 2–4 decades of life.

Annual incidence of 1:100 000 in Scandinavian patients.

Treatment

Diet and lifestyle

• A gluten-free diet may be curative in dermatitis herpetiformis.

• Wound care of open erosions is essential to prevent secondary infection in all bullous diseases.

Pharmacological treatment

• Only those physicians with experience and training to monitor these diseases and the drugs used to treat them should follow these patients.

Potent topical steroids may be used for mild bullous pemphigoid: clobetasol ointment applied twice daily to erythematous or urticarial plaques and early blisters.

Tetracycline, 500 mg four times daily, may be used as maintenance therapy for mild to moderate bullous pemphigoid.

• Systemic steroids are the mainstay of therapy for moderate to severe pemphigus vulgaris and bullous pemphigoid.

• Other drugs listed may be used as steroid-sparing agents, adjunctive or maintenance therapy.

Standard dosage
Prednisone, 60–120 mg orally once daily to control, then 40–60 mg once daily followed by slow taper as tolerated.

Azathioprine, 50–150 mg daily.

Dapsone, 50–200 mg daily.

Contraindications
Prednisone: underlying systemic infection (*e.g.*, tuberculosis); use caution in patients with a history of osteoporosis, diabetes mellitus, hypertension, glaucoma, or peptic ulcer disease.

Azathioprine: underlying systemic infection, neutropenia.

Dapsone: glucose-6-phosphate dehydrogenase deficiency, severe anemia, poorly compensated congestive heart failure.

Special points
Dapsone: treatment of choice for dermatitis herpetiformis.

Main drug interactions
Azathioprine: allopurinol enhances effect and increases risk for bone marrow suppression.

Main side effects
Prednisone: osteoporosis, increased blood glucose level, hypertension, peptic ulceration, weight gain, psychiatric disturbances.

Azathioprine: bone marrow suppression (primarily leukopenia), increased liver enzyme levels, increased risk for secondary malignancies.

Dapsone: gastrointestinal effects, peripheral motor neuropathy, dose-related hemolysis and methemoglobinemia, idiosyncratic agranulocytosis and hepatotoxicity.

Treatment aims

To relieve pain and heal wounds.
To prevent secondary infection.
To suppress disease activity with lowest possible dose of drug.
To minimize complications of therapy.

Other treatments

Gold sodium thiomalate.
Plasmapheresis.
Cyclophosphamide.
Mycophenolate mofetil.

Prognosis

Pemphigus vulgaris

• Mortality rate is <10% and is often due to complications of therapy.

• Patients do very well with close control and monitoring of this chronic disease.

Bullous pemphigoid

• It is usually self-limited, with remission in 75% of patients in 3–6 years.

• Mortality rate of 10%–20% is related to systemic steroid treatment.

Dermatitis herpetiformis

• Has a chronic course when untreated.

• Response to dapsone is dramatic; pruritus and skin lesions resolve within the first week of therapy.

Follow-up and management

• Long-term follow-up by a specialist is advised.

General references

Fine T: Management of acquired bullous diseases. *N Engl J Med* 1995, **333**:1475–1484.

Guidice GJ, Diaz LA: New laboratory methods in the investigation of bullous diseases. *Dermatol Clin* 1993, **2**:419–427.

Korman NJ: Bullous pemphigoid. The latest in diagnosis, prognosis and therapy. *Arch Dermatol* 1998, **134**:1137–1141.

Nousari HC, Anhalt GJ: Pemphigus and bullous pemphigoid. *Lancet* 1999, **354**:667–672.

Nousari HC, *et al.*: Mycophenolate mofetil in autoimmune and inflammatory skin disorders. *J Am Acad Dermatol* 1999, **40**: 265–268.

Rye B, Webb JM: Autoimmune bullous diseases. *Am Fam Physician* 1997, **55**:2709–2718.

Candidiasis, buccal & esophageal in AIDS

Diagnosis

Symptoms

• 30% of patients are asymptomatic.

Altered taste sensation.

Oral discomfort or pain.

Coated mouth or tongue.

Dysphagia.

Odynophagia.

Loss of appetite.

Signs

Angular cheilitis.

Intraoral removable white plaques, with erythematous underlying mucosa.

Intraoral mucosal ulceration or erythema with or without whitish plaques.

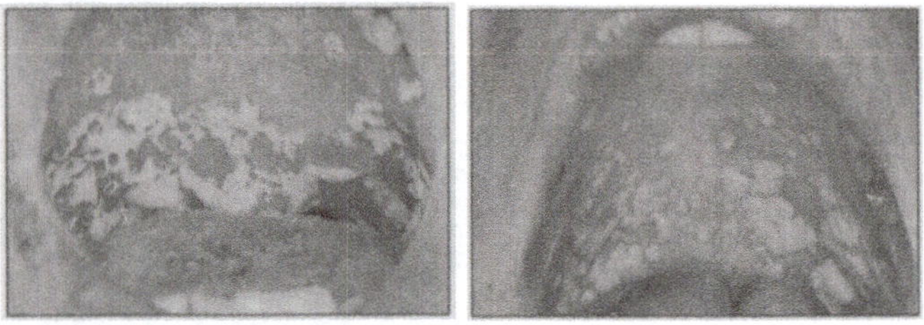

Curdish white plaques of pseudomembranous candidiasis. (*See* Color Plates.)

Investigations

Buccal candidiasis

• The diagnosis is usually obvious without further investigation.

Direct microscopy: direct staining of mouth scraping with hydrogen peroxide or Gram stain rapidly confirms presence of fungal hyphae — most often not necessary.

Esophageal candidiasis

Fiberoptic endoscopy: allows direct visualization of esophageal involvement, with biopsy confirming diagnosis; should be considered gold standard.

Barium-swallow radiography: can highlight linear filling defects.

Complications

Oral ulceration.

Weight loss: secondary to depressed appetite.

Esophageal obstruction: rarely, secondary to overgrowth of *Candida* spp. (systemic dissemination unusual).

Differential diagnosis

Oral hairy leukoplakia.

HIV-related gingivitis, periodontitis, herpes simplex, or giant aphthous ulcers.

Cytomegalovirus ulceration, Kaposi's sarcoma, or lymphoma.

Etiology

• In HIV infection, buccal candidiasis is often seen when the number of circulating CD4 lymphocytes is $<350 \times 10^6$/L, and esophageal candidiasis is seen when CD4 cells are $<250 \times 10^6$/L.

Epidemiology

• Previously, 90% of HIV-infected patients develop candidiasis at some stage of their illness.

• In the era of highly active antiretroviral therapy (HAART), the incidence of oral and esophageal candidiasis had declined.

Treatment

Diet and lifestyle

No special precautions are necessary.

Pharmacological treatment

Topical antifungals

• Nystatin and clotrimazole are of benefit in cases of buccal candidiasis; however, they do not treat any esophageal involvement.

• Some patients receiving HAART have improvement without specific antifungal treatment.

Fluconazole

• Fluconazole is effective for all esophageal candidiasis and oral candidiasis unresponsive to topical agents. Improvement results in 3–5 days. It is predominantly renally excreted so the patient does not suffer from hepatic metabolism problems.

Standard dosage	Fluconazole, 100 mg daily for 1 week for oral candidiasis, 3 weeks for esophageal candidiasis.
Contraindications	Azole hypersensitivity.
Special points	Reduced dose in patients with renal impairment.
Main drug interactions	Pentamidine, amphotericin-induced nephrotoxicity may impair renal excretion.
Main side effects	Abnormalities in liver function (higher doses), rashes.

Itraconazole

• Itraconazole is used in patients who cannot tolerate fluconazole (70% response rates at 1 week and 90% at 1 month) and is less hepatotoxic than ketoconazole.

Standard dosage	Itraconazole, 200 mg daily for 1–4 weeks.
Contraindications	Azole hypersensitivity.
Special points	An oral suspension is available with better absorption features.
Main drug interactions	Decreased absorption with antacids, cimetidine, or omeprazole; increased metabolism with rifampicin, rifabutin, or phenytoin.
Main side effects	Rash, nausea.

Suppression is not necessary.

Alternative medicine

Recommended use: None.

Common use: garlic (*Allium sativa*); aloe vera; probiotics (*Acidophilus* spp.); thyme (*Thymus vulgera*).

Caution: None.

Treatment aims

To suppress *C. albicans* overgrowth.

Prognosis

• 59% of patients with oral candidiasis are diagnosed with AIDS within 3 months.

• Many patients with acute *Pneumocystis carinii* pneumonia also have oral candidiasis.

• Patients with a successfully treated episode of oral or esophageal candidiasis may relapse within 3 months. Relapse rate is reduced in those receiving HAART.

Causes of treatment failure

Poor drug absorption.

Increased metabolism or excretion from other drugs.

C. albicans developing drug resistance.

Nonalbicans species or dual infection.

Immunodeficiency too severe for drug treatment alone to work.

No response to HAART.

General references

Barbara G, Barbiremi G, Di Lorenzo G: Fluconazole vs. itraconazole-flucytosine association in the treatment of esophageal candidiasis in AIDS patients: a double-blind multicenter, placebo-controlled study. *Chest* 1996, **110**:1507–1514.

Greenspan D, Greenspan JS: HIV-related oral disease. *Lancet* 1996, **348**:729–733.

Klein RS, et al.: Oral candidiasis in high risk patients as the initial manifestation of the acquired immunodeficiency syndrome. *N Engl J Med* 1984, **311**:354-358.

Cardiac failure & dilated cardiomyopathy

Diagnosis

Symptoms

- Dilated cardiomyopathy starts as asymptomatic left ventricular dysfunction.
- Cardiac failure is defined as symptomatic left ventricular dysfunction.

Major symptoms: exertional fatigue, dyspnea, ankle edema. New York Heart Association classification of functional capacity to estimate prognosis: Class I—asymptomatic; class II—dyspnea on accustomed exertion; class III—dyspnea on activities of daily living, such as having a shower and dressing; and class IV—dyspnea at rest. However it is often difficult to assign patients to one NYHA class; frequently, patients belong to two classes (*e.g.*, II/III or III/IV).

Less common symptoms: nocturia, urinary frequency, chest discomfort.

Signs

Cardiac failure

- Cardiac failure can be free of objective signs.

Signs of fluid retention: edema, raised jugular venous pressure, lung crepitations.

Signs of impaired perfusion: cold clammy skin, low blood pressure.

Signs of ventricular dysfunction: displaced left ventricular apex, right ventricular heave, S3 or S4, functional mitral or tricuspid regurgitation, tachycardia.

Underlying disorder

Valvular disease.
Atherosclerotic vascular disease.
Severe hypertension.
Severe anemia or volume overload: *e.g.*, arteriovenous shunt.
Pathological arrhythmia.
Evidence of generalized myopathy or poisoning.

Investigations

Chest radiography, echocardiography, cardiopulmonary exercise testing: to confirm diagnosis. Exercise testing is useful to identify ischemic heart disease. Cardiopulmonary exercise testing is useful to determine functional capacity before cardiac rehabilitation and to determine eligibility for cardiac transplantation.

ECG: to look for underlying cause, *e.g.*, ischemia or infarction, left ventricular hypertrophy, arrhythmia, other causes of pathological Q waves.

Echocardiography: to look for valvular disease; differentiates globally impaired left ventricle (*e.g.*, dilated cardiomyopathy) from segmental dysfunction (*e.g.*, ischemic heart disease). It provides an estimate of the ejection fraction; usually treatment is initiated when ejection fraction is ≥ 40%.

Blood tests: for rare causes, *e.g.*, hypocalcemic cardiomyopathy, thyroid heart disease, iron storage diseases, anemia, heavy metal poisons, amyloid (serum electrophoresis, rectal biopsy), sarcoid (serum angiotensin-converting enzyme [ACE]); for associated disease; renal, liver, and electrolyte disturbances common.

Coronary angiography: occasionally, to identify ischemic heart failure.

Ventricular biopsy: rarely, for specific myocarditis, especially viral.

Radionuclide ventriculography or echocardiography: for ejection fraction, to quantitate severity of systolic dysfunction.

24-hour Holter ECG monitoring: for ventricular arrhythmias.

Complications

Atrial and ventricular bradyarrhythmias and tachyarrhythmias: especially atrial fibrillation and ventricular tachycardia.

Peripheral emboli, postural hypotension.

Renal failure.

Hepatic congestion and dysfunction.

Poor gastrointestinal absorption.

Muscle wasting, tissue abnormalities, oxidative enzyme depletion, early fatigue.

Pulmonary congestion, nonasthmatic bronchial constriction, respiratory muscle weakness.

Pulmonary hypertension and right ventricular failure.

Differential diagnosis

Chronic lung disease.

Psychogenic dyspnea.

Etiology

- Ischemic heart disease: in 40%–70% of patients.
- Hypertension: in 10%–30%.
- Idiopathic, alcoholic, puerperal, or familial dilated cardiomyopathy: in 10%–20%.
- Valvular heart disease: in 5%–10%.
- Postviral myocarditis: possibly in 1%–10% (but presumed cause for many idiopathic cases).

HIV-related.

Epidemiology

- 1% of the general adult population has cardiac failure or dilated cardiomyopathy. Approximately 3 million Americans have heart failure. An additional 400,000 develop heart failure annually. Each year, 750,000 patients with heart failure are hospitalized and 250,000 die.
- The incidence increases with age (>10% in people aged ≥ 80 years).
- Heart failure is the most common cause of hospitalization in the elderly. Because the U.S. population is aging, the incidence of heart failure and its associated morbidity and mortality are expected to increase in the future.

Treatment

Diet and lifestyle

• Dietary sodium restriction may reduce the diuretic dose or the need for diuretics in patients with congestion. Restriction of fluid intake is 2 L or less, particularly in patients with hyponatremia.

• Avoid alcohol.

• On the basis of studies indicating that exercise can be safe under steady conditions, patients with stable cardiac failure should be encouraged to participate in exercise training.

• Patients should be encouraged to contact their doctor if the following occur: weight gain of more than 3 pounds in 1 week, or progressive weight gain over weeks or months; shortness of breath; swollen ankles or feet or generalized swelling of limbs, face, and neck; fatigue; palpitations or irregular heart beat; dizziness or coughing; loss of appetite; persistent cough.

Pharmacological treatment

Diuretics

• Patients with fluid retention should be given thiazides for mild disease, loop diuretics for moderate disease, and combinations of loop, thiazide, or potassium-sparing agents for severe cardiac failure; metolazone is particularly effective with loop diuretics.

Diuretic dosages

Drug	Starting dosage	Target or common dosage
Hydrochlorothiazide	25 mg qd	25–100 mg qd
Metolazone	2.5 mg qd	2.5–10 mg qd
Bumetanide	1 mg qd	1–10 mg qd–tid
Ethacrynic acid	25 mg qd	25–200 mg qd–bid
Furosemide	40 mg qd	40–400 mg qd–tid
Torsemide	20 mg qd	20–200 mg qd–bid

ACE inhibitors

• Indicated in the treatment of all patients with systolic heart failure.

ACE inhibitor dosages

Drug	Starting dosage	Target or common dosage
Captopril	6.25 mg tid	12.5–50 mg tid
Enalapril	2.5 mg bid	10 mg bid
Lisinopril	5 mg qd	10–20 mg qd
Ramipril	1.25 mg bid	5 mg bid
Trandolapril	1 mg qd	4 mg qd

Blockers

• β-blockers are indicated in all patients except those who are having rest dyspnea, are hemodynamically unstable, and are intolerant of this therapy (such as bradycardia or heart block).

Blocker dosages

Drug	Starting dosage	Target or common dosage
Bisoprolol	1.25 mg qd	10 mg qd
Carvedilol	3.125 mg bid	25–50 mg bid
Metoprolol	12.5 mg bid	50–75 mg bid
Metoprolol extended release	12.5 mg qd	200 mg qd

Digoxin: indicated in patients with heart failure or symptoms of heart failure; usual dosage is 0.25 mg/d.

Spironolactone: indicated in patients with heart failure who have dyspnea at rest (current or recent history) and lack significant renal impairment.

Direct-acting vasodilators: combination of hydralazine-isosorbide denitrate has shown to improve survival in heart failure; can be considered a potential alternative in patients with heart failure if the ACE inhibitors are poorly tolerated.

Calcium-channel blockers: have a limited role in the treatment of heart failure. First-generation agents were shown to have adverse outcomes in post-myocardial infarction patients with systolic dysfunction. Amlodipine has been shown to improve survival in nonischemic heart failure.

Inotropes: intravenous inotropes, indicated for patients hospitalized for acutely decompensated heart failure who do not respond adequately or in a timely manner for diuretic therapy. Phosphodiesterase inhibitors appear to have greater effects on pulmonary vasculature than dobutamine or dopamine do.

Treatment aims

To alleviate symptoms.

To delay disease progression.

To reduce mortality.

Other treatments

Coronary artery bypass grafting: in selected patients with severe coronary disease.

Heart transplantation: for younger patients with severe left ventricular disease; organ supply remains inadequate for demand.

Left ventricular assist devices are undergoing evaluation.

Prognosis

• Adverse prognostic features include the following: old age, low ejection fraction, poor exercise tolerance, ischemic origin, ventricular arrhythmias, reduced heart rate variability, high plasma noradrenaline concentration, low serum sodium concentration.

• The annual mortality rate is 50% in patients with severe heart failure and 10%–20% in patients with mild to moderate heart failure.

• Overall, nearly 50% of patients die within 5 years of symptom onset.

•Nonischemic cardiomyopathies may resolve within 12 months of symptom onset in approximately 30% of cases.

Follow-up

Follow-up is lifelong.

General references

Packer M, *et al.*: Consensus recommendations for management of chronic heart failure. *Am J Cardiol* 1999, **83**:1A–38A.

Cardiopulmonary resuscitation

Basic life support

Definition

• The term "basic life support" refers to maintaining an airway and supporting breathing and the circulation without equipment.

• This is a practical skill, and training must be sought.

• Health care professionals should also have more complex skills, including the use of airway adjuncts, *e.g.*, Guedel airway place face mask (with or without a nonreturn valve) or bag-mask ventilation and two rescuer resuscitation.

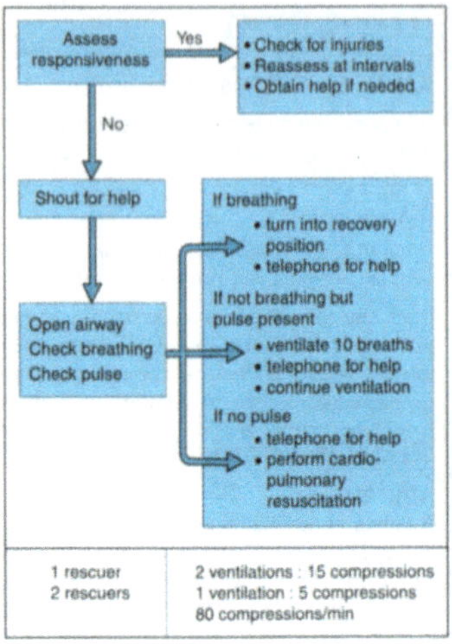

Basic life support.

Assessment

Approach

• Safety for the rescuer and the patient must be assessed.

Responsiveness

• The rescuer should gently shake the patient's shoulders and ask loudly, "Are you all right?"

• If the patient is unresponsive, the rescuer should call for help.

• The rescuer opens the airway by the combined maneuver of head tilt and chin lift; in most cases, this alone lifts the tongue from the back of the throat.

• If neck injury is likely, a chin lift or jaw thrust must be performed without moving the head or neck to open the airway.

• Any obvious obstruction should be removed from the mouth.

• Well-fitting dentures should be left in place because these help to maintain a mouth seal during ventilation.

Breathing

• After opening the airway, the rescuer should look for chest movements, listen for breath sounds at the mouth, and feel for exhaled air with the cheek.

• These steps must be done for 5 seconds before the rescuer decides that breathing is absent.

Pulse

• The best pulse to feel in any emergency is the carotid.

• The carotid should be palpated for 5 seconds to ensure that circulation is absent.

Action

For respiratory arrest

• If the patient is not breathing but a pulse is present, 10 breaths/min expired air ventilation must be given.

• The pulse must be checked after every 10 breaths, and full cardiopulmonary resuscitation (CPR) instituted if the pulse disappears.

For cardiorespiratory arrest

• If the patient is unconscious and not breathing and the pulse is absent, ventilation and initiation of chest compression are needed at a rate of two breaths: 15 compressions, with 80 compression/min (single rescuer).

• Chances are remote that effective spontaneous cardiac action will be restored without other techniques of advanced life support (including defibrillation), so time should not be wasted by further checks for the presence of a pulse.

• If, however, the patient makes a movement or takes a spontaneous breath, the carotid pulse should be checked to establish whether the heart is beating, taking no more than 5 seconds, and breathing should be checked.

• Otherwise, resuscitation must not be interrupted.

• The outcome after CPR with chest compression alone is similar to that after chest compression with mouth-to-mouth ventilation, and chest compression alone may be the preferred approach for bystanders inexperienced in CPR.

Advanced life support

• Cardiac arrest rhythms can be divided into two subsets: ventricular fibrillation/pulseless ventricular tachycardia (VF/VT) and non-VF/VT. Non-VF/VT incorporates both asystole and pulseless electrical activity. VF is defined as pulseless, chaotic, disorganized rhythm characterized by an undulating irregular pattern that varies in size and shape with a ventricular waveform of >150 beats/minute. The only difference in management between the two arrest rhythms is the need for rescuers to perform defibrillation for patients in VF/VT. Otherwise, the actions and interventions are essentially the same: basic CPR, tracheal intubation, epinephrine administration, and correction of reversible causes.

Components

Basic CPR at all times for pulseless patients (with the obvious exception of rhythm analysis and defibrillation shocks): in the event of a monitored arrest, a precordial thump should be considered.

Defibrillation: if the rhythm is VF/VT. Defibrillate until VT/VF is not present. Defibrillation should be performed as soon as VF/VT is recognized. Defibrillation energy levels should initially be 200 J for the first shock, 200 to 300 J for the second shock, and 360 J for the third and subsequent shocks.

Oxygenation and ventilation of the lungs through a patent secure airway, such as a tracheal tube: if tracheal intubation is impossible, the laryngeal mask airway or Combitube are acceptable initial alternatives in adults.

Intravascular access obtained immediately: if intravascular access is unattainable, epinephrine may be administered via the tracheal tube using at least double the intravascular dosage.

Epinephrine: administered using a dosage of at least 1 mg every 3 minutes.

Correction of reversible causes

• The use of buffers, antiarrhythmics, atropine, and pacing can be considered in certain special situations.

Treatment aims

To resuscitate the patient

To enhance basic life support (adrenaline).

Prognosis

• Survival from cardiac arrest is greatest when the event is witnessed, when a bystander starts resuscitation, when the heart arrests in ventricular fibrillation, or when defibrillation is done at an early stage.

Follow-up and management

• After resuscitation, patients should be observed, monitored, and treated in an intensive care unit.

• Patients must be checked by assessment of responsiveness, airway, breathing, circulation, and blood pressure; arterial blood gas and electrolyte measurements should be taken; chest radiography is advised.

Training

• Doctors need regular formal practical training in resuscitation.

• Advanced life support courses are available through local American Heart Association affiliates and most large emergency departments.

General references

Ewy G: Cardiopulmonary resuscitation: strengthening the links in the chain of survival. *N Engl J Med* 2000, **342**:1599–1601.

Ewy G, *et al.*: 31st Bethesda Conference: emergency cardiac care: Task Force 1: Cardiac arrest. *J Am Coll Cardiol* 2000, **35**:832–834.

Hallstrom A, *et al.*: Cardiopulmonary resuscitation by chest compression alone or with mouth-to-mouth ventilation. *N Engl J Med* 2000, **342**:1546–1553.

Kloeck W, *et al.*: The universal advanced life support algorithm. *Circulation* 1997, **95**:2180–2182.

Carpal tunnel syndrome

Diagnosis

Symptoms

Numbness, tingling, pain, burning in distribution of median nerve.

Weakness, loss of grip strength.

Incoordination: dropping objects.

Awakening from sleep, shaking hand and wrist to relieve tingling sensation: cardinal symptom.

Proximal upper extremity pain: uncommon.

Signs

Numbness.

Diminished pin-prick sensation.

Diminished grip strength.

Muscular atrophy of thenar eminence.

Phalen's test and reverse Phanlen's test: "praying hands" position recreates neuropathic symptoms.

Tinel's sign: percussion over median nerve at volar aspect of wrist with reflex hammer reproduces symptoms; nonspecific.

Investigations

Electromyography.

Complications

Numbness.

Decrease in grip strength.

Work impairment.

Atrophy of thenar eminence.

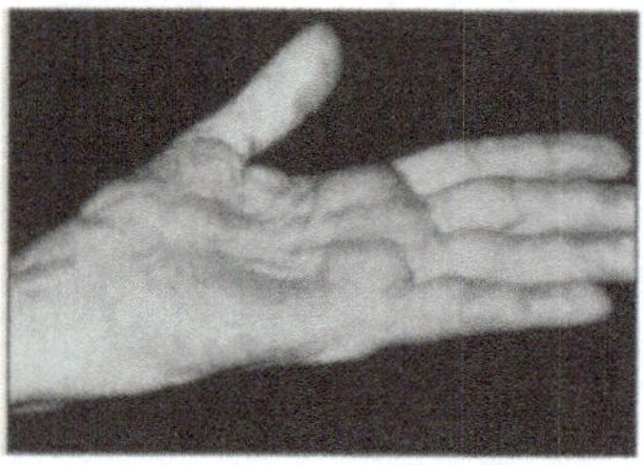

Carpal tunnel syndrome.

Differential diagnosis

Cervical radiculopathy.

• Other causes of localized wrist pain include:

Osteoarthritis.

Rheumatoid arthritis.

Etiology

Osteoarthritis.

Diabetes mellitus.

Pregnancy.

Hypothyroidism.

Rheumatoid arthritis.

Acromegaly.

Dysproteinemia (*e.g.*, multiple myeloma).

Amyloidosis.

Epidemiology

• Carpal tunnel syndrome has become the second most common cause of work impairment (after back pain).

Pathophysiology

Repetitive trauma (*e.g.*, jack hammer operators, meat cutters).

Infiltration (amyloidosis, hypothyroidism, diabetes).

Edema: osteoarthritis, pregnancy.

Idiopathic: 20% of cases are of unknown cause.

Treatment

Diet and lifestyle

- Patients should implement dietary changes such as those used to control diabetes.
- Wrists should be splinted.

Pharmacological treatment

- NSAIDs are of limited value.
- Corticosteroid injection into carpal tunnel volar sheath has a very limited role. It should be performed by an orthopedic surgeon or rheumatologist (if at all).

Nonpharmacological treatment

Splinting: symptomatic improvement may occur with inexpensive cock-up wrist splints. Custom-molded fabricated splints offer no additional advantage.

Rehabilitation.

Surgery: controversial, variable results.

Treatment aims

To eliminate symptoms of pain and numbness.

To improve function.

To improve sleep.

To restore grip strength.

Prognosis

- Carpal tunnel release surgery has variable results.
- Traditionally, cure rates exceeding 90% were routinely reported, however, postsurgical recurrences of carpal tunnel syndrome after return to repetitive stress work environments may approach 80%.
- Careful patient selection prior to surgery is crucial, along with rehabilitation for possible job modifications prior to return to work.

General reference

von Schroeder HP, Botte MI: Carpal tunnel syndrome. *Hand Clin* 1996, **12**:643–655.

Raudino F: Tethered median nerve stress test in the diagnosis of carpal tunnel syndrome. *Electromyogr Clin Neurophysiol* 2000, **40(1)**:57–60.

Diagnosis

Symptoms

• Only 50% of patients present with the classic symptoms of diarrhea associated with malabsorption. Many are diagnosed because of anemia (especially iron or folate deficiency).

Symptoms of steatorrhea: foul-smelling stools, oil residue, or undigested food particles in toilet bowl.

Weight loss and amenorrhea: common.

Skin rashes, easy bruising.

Signs

Evidence of weight loss [1].

Pallor: anemia due to iron or folic acid deficiency.

Ecchymosis: Malabsorption of vitamin K, other fat-soluble vitamins.

Calcium deficiency: with possible tetany.

Chelosis.

Papulovesicular rash of dermatitis herpetiformis on extensor surfaces.

Investigations [2]

Initial

Complete blood count; serum iron, ferritin, folate, and vitamin B_{12} measurement: to identify microcytic (iron deficiency) or macrocytic (folic acid, vitamin B_{12} deficiency) anemia, or a dimorphic pattern of anemia due to both.

Serum calcium and magnesium measurement: concentration possibly depressed.

Protime: prolonged in patients with vitamin K deficiency.

Fecal fat estimation: 3-day fecal fat excretion >7 g/day in patients ingesting at least 100 g fat daily (sensitive for malabsorption but not specific for celiac disease).

Contrast radiography: small bowel follow-through to assess small intestine; poor sensitivity, luminal dilation, and altered mucosal folds often observed.

Specific

Autoantibodies: serum IgA antiendomysium has a sensitivity and specificity that exceeds 90% in untreated patients; IgA antigliadin used for some for screening but is less specific [3].

Upper gastrointestinal endoscopy with biopsy of duodenum or proximal jejunum: reveals short (or absent) villi, intraepithelial lymphocytes, and crypt hyperplasia; for unequivocal diagnosis, at least six biopsy specimens should be obtained; celiac disease is confirmed when subsequent biopsy results are normal on a gluten-free diet.

Complications

Anemia: due to iron or folic acid deficiency.

Osteomalacia, osteoporosis: due to hypocalcemia and vitamin D malabsorption.

Ulcerative jejunitis: rare, possibly early manifestation of malignancy.

Small-intestinal lymphoma: T-cell lymphoma complicating 5%–10% of cases; may be manifest as unexplained small intestinal perforation.

Neuropathy: vitamin B_{12} deficiency.

Wernicke's encephalopathy or Korsakoff's psychosis: due to acute or prolonged vitamin B_1 (thiamine) deficiency.

Differential diagnosis

Infectious diarrhea.

Chronic pancreatitis.

Inflammatory bowel disease.

Giardiasis.

Tropical sprue.

Lactose intolerance.

Small bowel bacterial overgrowth.

Laxative abuse.

Whipple's disease.

Irritable bowel syndrome.

Etiology [3]

• In northern Europeans, 98% of cases of celiac disease are associated with the extended haplotype HLA B8, DR3, DQ2; in southern Europeans, HLA DR5/7, DQ2 accounts for one-third of cases.

• 10%–20% of first-degree relatives of probands are similarly affected.

• Family history often reveals a Celtic ancestry [3].

• Increased prevalence of autoimmune disorders [4].

Epidemiology

• Prevalence in the United States is approximately 1 in 2500 people.

• The prevalence of celiac disease in the United Kingdom is particularly high (1 in 1200 people, rising to 1 in 300 around Galway Bay in Ireland).

• Slightly more women than men have celiac disease.

• The incidence of presentation has three peaks:

Infancy (9–36 months), on introduction of foods containing gluten.

Third decade, frequently manifest as severe anemia of pregnancy.

Fifth decade, normally manifest with a specific nutritional deficiency, *e.g.*, iron, folic acid, or calcium.

Treatment

Diet and lifestyle

• A gluten-free diet is the mainstay of treatment and involves avoiding products containing wheat, rye, barley, or oats. Care should be taken to avoid any food contaminated by these cereals or their partial hydrolysates, including beer. Women of childbearing age who experienced amenorrhea due to nutritional deficiencies will probably have a return of regular menstruation. Men who have had long-standing disease may report impotence and infertility. These problems normally resolve within 2 years of starting a gluten-free diet.

• Specific nutritional deficiencies should be treated by replacement: iron, calcium, vitamin B_{12}, folic acid, or magnesium.

Pharmacological treatment

• For most patients, a gluten-free diet is sufficient; patients with refractory disease or severe malnutrition may benefit from steroid therapy.

Standard dosage	Prednisone, 20–40 mg daily initially, usually rapidly reduced to 5–10 mg daily. Hydrocortisone, 50–100 mg i.v. every 6 hours in patients who need i.v. fluid replacement.
Contraindications	Caution in diabetes mellitus, or pregnancy.
Special points	Care should be taken to avoid high-dose (prednisone >10 mg/day), long-term steroid treatment because of side effects.
Main drug interactions	Mild antagonism to thiazide diuretics.
Main side effects	Weight gain, fluid retention, osteoporosis, cushingoid facies, diabetes mellitus.

Treatment aims

To improve general well-being, small intestinal mucosal structure, and associated nutritional deficiencies.

To reduce the risk of development of small intestinal lymphoma.

Prognosis

• With a gluten-free diet, general health is improved within a few weeks.

• Untreated patients are at a 5%–10% risk of developing a small intestinal T-cell lymphoma, the incidence of which probably falls if they maintain a strict diet.

• Failure to improve suggests incorrect initial diagnosis, failure to adhere strictly to a gluten-free diet, or concurrent disorder (*i.e.*, malignancy) [4].

Follow-up and management

• Outpatients must be reassessed 6–8 weeks and 3–4 months after starting a gluten-free diet, when repeat biopsy should be done.

• A further biopsy should be done 1 year after starting treatment, when continued improvement in the structure of the small-intestinal mucosa should be expected.

• Annual hematological screening is recommended to exclude development of specific nutritional deficiencies.

• When the diagnosis is doubtful, a gluten challenge, with 40 g gluten or 4 slices of normal bread daily for 2 weeks (adults) or 6 weeks (children), may be followed by a repeat jejunal biopsy.

Key references

1. Godkin A, Jewell D: The pathogenesis of celiac disease. *Gastroenterology* 1998, 115:206–210.
2. Trier JS. Diagnosis of celiac sprue. *Gastroenterology* 1998, 115:211–216.
3. Valdimarsson T, *et al.*: Is small bowel biopsy necsesary in adults with suspected celiac disease and IgA antiendomysium antibodies? 100% predictive value for celiac disease in adults. *Dig Dis Sci* 1996, 41:83–87.
4. Ventura, *et al.*: Duration of exposure to gluten and risk for autoimmune disorders in patients with celiac disease. *Gastroenterology* 1999, 117:297–303.

Diagnosis

Symptoms

• Symptoms generally include the following, alone or in combination:

Epilepsy: in >50% of patients by presentation; associated focal features may suggest localization of brain tumor; simple partial seizures particularly common.

Dysphasia, hemiparesis, intellectual failure, personality change, cranial nerve abnormalities.

Headache, papilledema, visual failure, vomiting: alone or in combination indicate raised intracranial pressure due to intracranial mass lesions.

Signs

Papilledema, impaired visual acuity, visual field defects.

Diplopia: with or without clear III or VI nerve palsy.

Facial weakness.

Dysphasia.

Hemiparesis, hyperreflexia, extensor plantar response, hemisensory loss.

Signs of primary malignancy in secondary brain tumors: *e.g.*, site of previous melanoma excision visible in skin.

Investigations

Neuroradiography: primarily CT and MRI of brain; more invasive procedures (*e.g.*, angiography or PET) sometimes needed for management.

Chest radiography: important as part of general screening for extracerebral primary or metastatic tumor in lungs.

EEG: possibly needed as secondary investigation to elucidate epileptic manifestations.

Blood tests: possibly needed to clarify differential diagnosis, *e.g.*, blood cultures when metastatic brain abscess suspected.

Lumbar puncture: to identify meningeal spread of malignancy.

Complications

Blindness: papilledema due to progressive raised intracranial pressure leads to blindness if unrelieved.

Herniation: brain shift due to increasing mass of cerebral tumor can lead to central or transtentorial brain herniation, with irreversible ischemic brain damage and fatal apnea due to failure of brain stem function.

Differential diagnosis

Cerebrovascular disease.

Other organic brain disease (*e.g.*, encephalitis or demyelination).

Other extradural intracranial tumors (*e.g.*, meningioma).

Cerebral abscess: an important differential diagnosis; often no signs of acute infection in patients, despite relevant history of middle ear disease, bronchiectasis, or valvular heart disease.

Etiology

• The cause of most cerebral tumors remains unknown, although the incidence is increased after exposure to radiation, in patients with neurofibromatosis, and in some rare inherited immunodeficiency diseases.

• Increasing evidence indicates that cerebral astrocytomas are associated with loss of tumor suppressor gene function from chromosomes 17 and 10 and with amplification of epidermal growth factor receptor.

Epidemiology

• Primary cerebral tumors account for ~55% of intracranial tumors in adults and are the tenth most common tumors in men.

• The annual incidence of cerebral tumor is ~10 in 100 000 population.

• The peak incidence is in the fifth decade, with a small male preponderance (55%).

• Secondary brain tumors are common and account for 15%–20% of intracranial tumors in neurological series.

Treatment

Diet and lifestyle

- No special diet is necessary for patients with primary brain tumors.
- Impaired cognitive function, epilepsy.

Pharmacological treatment

For epilepsy

- Anticonvulsant drug treatment is usually started for supratentorial tumors in both epileptic and nonepileptic patients.

Standard dosage	Phenytoin, 300–400 mg daily, or carbamazepine, 600–1000 mg daily.
Contraindications	Hepatic impairment, severe cytopenia.
Main drug interactions	Analgesics, antibiotics, antidepressants.
Main side effects	Confusion, skin eruptions, gum swelling, diplopia, ataxia.

For raised intracranial pressure and stabilization of brain function

Standard dosage	Dexamethasone, 4 mg every 6 hours (adult) initially; up to 20 mg every 6 hours may be useful for a few weeks as palliative terminal treatment.
Contraindications	Peptic ulcers.
Special points	When surgical decompression and adjuvant radiation therapy have been completed, steroids may be gradually withdrawn or reduced to a minimum level that keeps the patient asymptomatic. While the patient is taking dexamethasone, the risk of peptic ulcers is increased; H_2 antagonists (such as ranitidine, 150 mg twice daily) or protien pump inhibitors (such as omepazole 20 mg once daily) are usually also prescribed.
Main drug interactions	Hypoglycemia agents, diuretics.
Main side effects	Peptic ulcers, weight gain, demineralization.

For acutely raised intracranial pressure

- In patients who are unconscious as a result of raised intracranial pressure from cerebral tumor or in those who have herniated, with respiratory arrest, artificial ventilation, mannitol as an osmotic diuretic, and i.v. dexamethasone may be needed in an emergency department or intensive care unit setting.

Chemotherapy

- After surgery and adjuvant radiation therapy, antitumor chemotherapy may be indicated for malignant glioma, either as an adjuvant or at the time of relapse.
- Nitrosoureas and procarbazine are the agents chiefly used.

Treatment aims

To relieve symptoms; curing malignant primary or secondary brain tumors is generally not possible.

Other treatments

Surgery: almost always indicated to establish histological diagnosis and grading and, where possible, to reduce tumor bulk.

Radiation therapy: localized to tumor and surrounding area, usually given for malignant primary cerebral tumors; secondary metastatic cerebral tumors treated by whole-brain radiation.

Prognosis

- Prognosis is related to tumor type and histological grade, patient age, and functional performance at the time of treatment.
- The median survival with grade 4 astrocytomas is ~9 months and with grade 2 astrocytomas ~6 years. Aggressive treatment improves the prognosis to 1–2 years.

Follow-up and management

- Clinical assessment of neurological and performance status, with follow-up brain scanning at intervals of 3–6 months, is used to monitor progress.
- At disease progression, further surgery is considered in 10%–15% of patients, as are novel treatments, *e.g.*, focused radiation or immunotherapy.
- The terminal phase is usually short, from a few days to 6 weeks, and patients may often be managed in the home, although hospice care may sometimes be preferable.

General references

Fernandez PM, Brem S: Malignant brain tumors in the elderly. *Clin Geriatr Med* 1997, **13**:327–338.

Mahaley MS: Neuro-oncology index and review (adult primary brain tumors). *J Neurooncol* 1991, **11**:85–147.

Newton HB, Turowski RC, Stroup TJ, McCoy LK: Clinical presentation, diagnosis, and pharmacotherapy of patients with primary brain tumors. *Ann Pharmacother* 1999, **33**:816–832.

Neuro-Oncology. Edited by Thomas DGT. London: Arnold; 1990.

Cholangitis, primary sclerosing

Diagnosis

Symptoms

• 25% of patients are asymptomatic; diagnosis is made after discovery of abnormal results on liver function tests, particularly in patients with ulcerative colitis.

Pruritis, fatigue: >50% of patients.

Right upper quadrant pain: intermittent.

Jaundice: intermittent.

Weight loss.

Fever:

Bleeding esophageal varices, edema, ascites: late features; however, this may be the initial clinical presentation in a subset of patients with occult disese.

Signs

• Signs are not always manifest [1,2].

Right-upper quadrant tenderness, fevers: during episodes of cholangitis.

Hepatomegaly: >50%.

Splenomegaly: ~30%.

Jaundice: in more advanced cases.

Spider nevi, palmar erythema, ascites: in patients with long-standing disease.

Investigations

Liver chemistries: cholestatic pattern with raised alkaline phosphatase (3- 5-fold elevations most common), gamma-glutamyl transpeptidase, bilirubin (late); low albumin, prolonged prothrombin time (late).

Laboratory abnormalities: immunoglobulins, particularly IgM, typically elevated; antimitochondrial antibody usually negative, antinuclear antibodies often positive for low titer; a serum CA 19-9 level > 100 U/mol has a 75% sensitivity and 80% specificity in identifying cholangiocarcinoma in patients with primary sclerosing cholangitis [4].

Cholangiography: the diagnostic test; endoscopic retrograde cholangiography first choice, percutaneous route only if endoscopic route fails; bile-duct stricturing interspersed with dilatation (beading); intra- and extrahepatic duct changes in most patients.

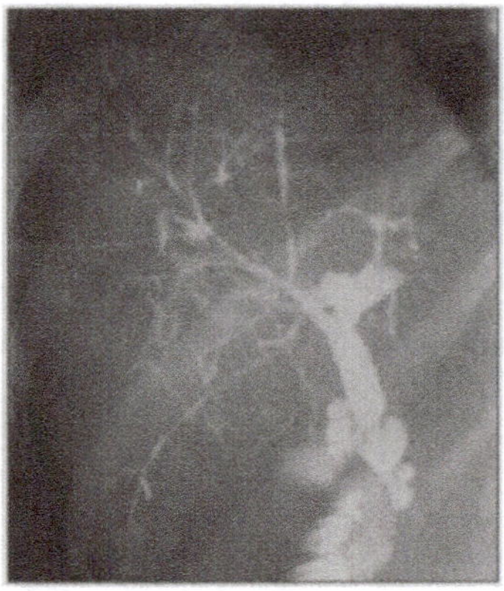

Classic intrahepatic changes of primary sclerosing cholangitis (bleeding and stricturing) on percutaneous cholangiography. The common bile duct is dilated because of involvement of the lower end by primary sclerosing cholangitis. Endoscopic cholangiography was unsuccessful.

• Distinction of benign primary sclerosing cholangitis stricture from cholangiocarcinoma is very difficult; brush or bile cytology is only 50%–60% sensitive.

Liver biopsy: changes suggestive (portal edema, fibrosis, duct proliferation) rather than diagnostic; biopsy staging: 1, portal changes; 2, periportal extension; 3, septum formation; 4, cirrhosis.

Complications

Recurrent cholangitis.

Cholangiocarcinoma: in 10%–15% of patients.

Metabolic bone disease.

Cirrhosis: portal hypertension, bleeding, ascites, enephalopathy in advanced disease.

Differential diagnosis

Bile duct stones.

Cholangiocarcinoma.

Drug-induced cholestasis.

Primary biliary cirrhosis.

Surgical stricture.

Secondary sclerosing cholangitis.

Metastatic tumor. (e.g. colon)

Granulomatous liver disease (e.g., sarcoid).

AIDS cholangiopathy.

Etiology

• Primary sclerosing cholangitis has a known strong association with inflammatory bowel disease (ulcerative colitis) and HLA B8 and DR3.

• The pathogenetic mechanism is unknown.

• The current hypothesis is that infection, absorption of bacterial products, or both occur in predisposed (HLA DR) individuals.

Epidemiology

• 70% of patients with primary sclerosing cholangitis have ulcerative colitis; 4% of patients with ulcerative colitis have primary sclerosing cholangitis.

• The prevalence of primary sclerosing cholangitis is 2–7 in 100 000.

• The male : female ratio is 2 : 1.

• The most common age of presentation is 25–45 years.

Treatment

Diet and lifestyle

- Careful attention to adequate nutrition is recommended.
- If steatorrhea is problematic, fat intake may be reduced.
- Maintain adequate fat soluble vitamin stores (vitamins A, D, E, and K).

Pharmacological treatment

Symptomatic

- Drugs are indicated to relieve pruritus.

Standard dosage	Cholestyramine, 4–8 g three times daily (before meals).
Contraindications	Complete biliary obstruction.
Special points	May interfere with absorption of fat-soluble vitamins, so supplementation may be needed.
Main drug interactions	Delayed or reduced absorption of digitalis, tetracycline, chlorothiazide, warfarin, thyroxine.
Main side effects	Increased bleeding tendency, constipation, diarrhea.

- Antihistamines of occassional benefit; phenobarbital (30–60 mg at bed time) or rifampin 10 mg/kg/day also of benefit in select patients. However, both induce P450 enzymes, which may result in altered metabolism of other medications.

Prophylactic

- For proven fat-soluble vitamin deficiency or jaundice, the following are indicated:

Vitamin K, 10 mg i.m. monthly.

Vitamin D, 100 000 U i.m. monthly.

Vitamin A, 100 000 U i.m. 3-monthly.

- Adequate calcium intake must be ensured.

Therapeutic

- No medical treatment has been definitively shown to delay progression or reverse changes of primary sclerosing cholangitis [3].
- Ursodeoxycholic acid, 10–15 mg/kg orally daily, improves liver function tests, but benefit for liver histology, cholangiography, or survival has not been established.
- The choice of antibiotics for cholangitis (when no remediable dominant stricture) depends on bile or blood culture; empiric considerations include ciprofloxacin, ampicillin, or a cephalosporin.

Treatment aims

To relieve symptoms.

To prevent recurrence of cholangitis.

Other treatments

Endoscopic or radiographical balloon dilation/stent placement: for symptomatic dominant strictures (cholangitis, itching).

Surgical palliation: appropriate for dominant stricture only if transplantation is not an option and an endoscopic or a percutaneous approach has failed.

Orthotopic liver transplantation: for refractory cases; ~70% 1-year survival; unexpected cholangiocarcinoma often found [5].

Colectomy in patients with ulcerative colitis does not influence the course of primary sclerosing cholangitis.

Prognosis

- Prognosis varies greatly.
- Factors at presentation related to prognosis (Mayo model) include serum bilirubin concentration, histological stage on liver biopsy, age, and presence of splenomegaly [3,6–8].

Follow-up and management

- Patients should be monitored clinically for signs and symptoms of cholangitis.
- Patients should be reviewed monthly if they have symptomatic or biochemical deterioration and are approaching transplantation.

Key references

1. Broome U, Olsson R, Loof L, *et al.*: Natural history and prognostic factors in 305 Swedish patients with primary sclerosing cholangitis. *Gut* 1996, **38**:610–615.
2. Chalasani N, *et al.*: Cholangiocarcinoma in patients with primary sclerosing cholangitis: a multicenter case-control study. *Hepatology* 2000, 31:7–11.
3. Dickerson ER, *et al.*: Primary sclerosing cholangitis: refinement and validation of survival models. *Gastroenterology* 1992, **103**:1893–1901.
4. Lindor KD: Ursodiol for primary sclerosing cholangitis. *N Engl J Med* 1997, **336**:691–695.
6. Narumi S, Roberts JP, Emond JC, *et al.*: Liver transplantation for sclerosing cholangitis. *Hepatology* 1995, **22**:451–457.
7. Shetty K, Rybicki L, Carey WD: The Child-Pugh classification as a prognostic indicator for survival in primary sclerosing cholangitis. *Hepatology* 1997, **25**:1049–1053.
8. Wiesner RH: Current concepts in primary sclerosing cholangitis. *Mayo Clin Proc* 1994, **69**:969–982.

Chronic fatigue syndrome

Diagnosis

Symptoms

Major

Fatigue: lasting >3–6 months, with 50% reduction in activity; worsened by physical or mental stress; relapsing, with good and bad days.

Prominent disturbance of concentration or short-term memory.

Minor

Initiating viral-like illness, with pyrexia and malaise, common.

Myalgia: especially limb and chest pain; worse after activity.

Joint pain: especially in large joints.

Abdominal pain or bloatedness, nausea, alternating constipation and diarrhea.

Headaches, dizziness, tinnitus, paresthesias.

Sleep disturbance: initially more sleep, followed by disturbed sleep or vivid dreams.

Sensitivity to heat or cold, inappropriate sweating.

Adverse effects of alcohol.

Signs

• Most patients have been previously well; few clinical signs are manifest.

Localized areas of tender muscle: about 1 cm diameter in affected muscle groups.

Enlarged lymph nodes, glands, or inflamed throat: in periods of relapse.

Muscle weakness: in patients who have been ill for many years.

Investigations

• Diagnosis must not be made on the presence of fatigue alone; the two major symptoms and at least four minor items from symptoms, clinical signs, or positive laboratory investigations must be present.

• No diagnostic test exists; investigations are designed to exclude other causes of a similar clinical syndrome.

Initial investigations

• All of the results should be normal, if other illnesses are to be excluded.

Hemoglobin measurement: to exclude anemia.

Leukocyte count: to identify infection or a hematological condition.

Thyroid function tests: to exclude thyroid disease.

Plasma viscosity or ESR and CRP measurement: nonspecific indicator of an underlying disorder.

Further investigations

• Other conditions suggested by the patient's history or examination must be excluded, especially infection, *e.g.*, tick bites (Lyme disease) or consumption of raw meat (toxoplasmosis).

Complications

Psychiatric disorder: especially depression and anxiety.

Irritable bowel syndrome.

Severe disability: patient may become bedridden.

Differential diagnosis

Infections, especially Epstein–Barr virus infection, Lyme disease, toxoplasmosis, hepatitis A, brucellosis.

Endocrine disease, especially hypothyroidism.

Psychiatric disease, especially if patient has been ill for many years.

Malignancy.

Autoimmune disease, sarcoidosis.

Drugs or toxins.

Etiology

• The cause is unknown; probably several conditions are involved, including continuing infection and immune response to infection.

Epidemiology

• Chronic fatigue syndrome occurs throughout the world.

• ~1.3 in 1000 population are affected.

• Both sexes and all ages are affected; women are more likely to have prolonged illness.

Nomenclature

• Chronic fatigue syndrome is also known as the following:

Postviral fatigue syndrome.

Myalgic encephalomyelitis.

Effort syndrome.

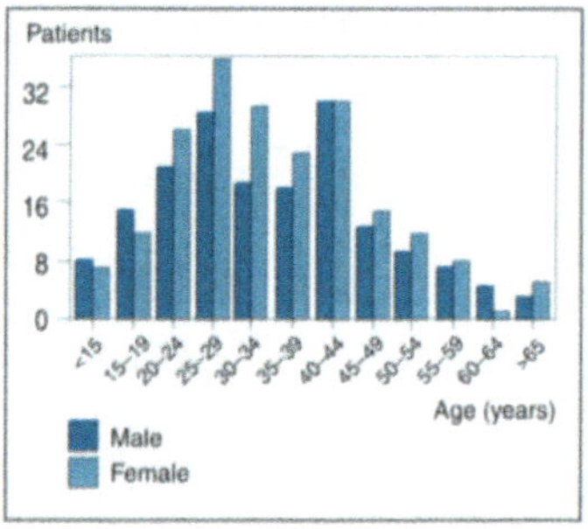

Patients affected by chronic fatigue syndrome, according to age and sex (204 females, 177 males; ratio, 1.2:1).

Treatment

Diet and lifestyle

• If patients have a normal diet, vitamins or mineral supplements are unnecessary.

• Patients should remain within their energy limits; sleep should not be resisted (at least 10 h/day); sleep and relaxation techniques increase energy levels; energy is lost through physical activities and mental exertion (such as concern about jobs, finances, and relationships).

Pharmacological treatment

• Although moderating activity is the best method of controlling symptoms, many patients need additional supportive treatment.

• Several drugs may have to be tried before the most appropriate is found.

Analgesics

• Mild analgesics, *e.g.*, acetaminophen or aspirin, should be tried initially; if they are unsuccessful, dihydrocodeine or ibuprofen may help.

Benzodiazepines

• Because of their hypnotic, sedative, anxiolytic, and muscle-relaxant actions, these drugs are useful in patients who have difficulty sleeping.

• Intermediate-acting compounds are best (temazepam, lormetazepam).

Standard dosage	Temazepam, 10 mg orally at night for 3–4 weeks.
Contraindications	Respiratory depression, phobic or obsessional states.
Main drug interactions	Alcohol.
Main side effects	Drowsiness, dizziness.

Antidepressants

• The most useful agents are amitriptyline, doxepin, dothiepin, and fluoxetine.

Standard dosage	Amitriptyline, 10 mg orally at night.
Contraindications	Heart disease.
Special points	Patients should be given low doses initially, with gradual increase if necessary.
Main drug interactions	Alcohol.
Main side effects	Dry mouth, blurred vision, nausea, constipation.

Alternative medicine

Recommended use: none.

Common use: echinacea (*Echinacea angustifolia*); milk thistle (*Silybum marianum*); burdock (*Arctium* spp.); Siberian ginseng (*Panax ginseng*).

Caution: none.

Treatment aims

To reduce fatigue and prevent relapses.

To relieve other symptoms.

To allow patient to resume normal activity, *e.g.*, to return to work or school.

Prognosis

• Patients may recover after a fluctuating illness, usually in the first 4 years, achieve stability at a lower energy level, or deteriorate and become chronically disabled.

Follow-up and management

• Patients should keep a daily diary, monitoring activities and energy levels.

• Activities may be increased and a return to work or school encouraged when energy levels are 70%–80% of normal.

Causes of treatment failure

Overoptimistic reassurance of recovery.

Patient's inability to change lifestyle.

Too much energy being spent pursuing alternative cures.

General references

Buchwald D: Fibromyalgia and chronic fatigue syndrome: similarities and differences. *Rheum Dis Clin North Am* 1996, **22**:219–243.

Thomas PK: The chronic fatigue syndrome: what do we know? *BMJ* 1993, **306**:1557–1558.

Tirelli U, *et al.*: Clinical and immunologic study of 205 patients with chronic fatigue syndrome. *Arch Intern Med* 1993, **153**:116–120.

Wallace DJ: The fibromyalgia syndrome. *Ann Med* 1997, **29**:9–21.

Chronic obstructive pulmonary disease

Diagnosis [1]

Symptoms

Cough: chronic bronchitis is defined as a cough productive of sputum on most days for at least 3 consecutive months in 2 successive years.

Productive sputum.

Increasing dyspnea: especially with exertion.

Weight loss.

History of smoking: present in most cases.

Signs

Onset usually in the 5th or 6th decade.

Barrel-shaped chest, decreased cardiac dullness and reduced breath sounds, palpable liver due to hepatic displacement, signs of hyperexpansion.

Increased respiratory rate, use of accessory muscles of respiration, "pursed lip" breathing, reduced breath sounds: signs of airflow obstruction.

Cyanosis.

Right ventricular heave, raised jugular venous pressure, peripheral edema: signs of pulmonary hypertension.

Fine inspiratory crackles: frequently found in chronic obstructive airway disease and do not necessarily imply coexistent heart failure.

Hyperresonance with percussion.

Investigations [3]

Complete blood count: polycythemia found in some patients.

ECG: to detect right axis deviation or signs of right-sided strain.

Chest radiography: to detect signs of chronic obstructive pulmonary disease (low flat diaphragms, long thin heart), emphysema (hypodense bullae, large retrosternal airspace on lateral radiography), or pulmonary hypertension (prominent hilum, with reduced peripheral vascular shadows).

Pulmonary function testing: to confirm obstructive picture and to show degree of reversibility to therapeutic agents; diffusing capacity estimates gas transfer.

Arterial blood gas measurement: to check for hypoxia and carbon dioxide retention; high bicarbonate concentration suggests more chronic carbon dioxide retention.

Chest CT scan: may confirm emphysema.

Complications

Infective exacerbations: acute bronchitis, pneumonia.

Pulmonary hypertension, cor pulmonale.

Pulmonary embolism.

Respiratory failure, death.

Pneumothorax.

Lung cancer: when smoking is cause of chronic obstructive pulmonary disease (COPD).

Hemoptysis.

Differential diagnosis

Asthma.

Left ventricular failure.

Large airway obstruction, *e.g.*, proximal tumor.

Allergic bronchopulmonary aspergillosis.

Aspiration.

Bronchiectasis.

Cystic fibrosis.

Etiology

Cigarette smoking: most important cause.

Atmospheric pollution: much less important than smoking.

Airway infections/inflammation.

Alpha$_1$ antitrypsin deficiency: rare; homozygous form present in 1 in 5000 people, and not all of these develop chest disease; causes basal emphysema [2].

Intravenous drug abuse.

Epidemiology

- Estimates indicate that ~15 million Americans have COPD.
- Chronic obstructive airway disease is estimated to cause >90 000 deaths per year.

Treatment

Diet and lifestyle

- Stopping smoking reduces the rate of deterioration of lung function to that of non-smokers and, at an early stage, may improve symptoms.
- Loss of weight improves functional capacity.
- Patients' homes can be assessed for the need for aids to daily living.

Pharmacological treatment [1,3–5]

- Inadequate inhaler technique is one of the main reasons for treatment failure; inhaler technique must always be checked before treatment is initiated or changed.

Inhaled anticholinergics

Standard dosage	Ipratropium bromide inhaler, 20–40 µg 4 times daily.
Contraindications	Hypersensitivity; caution in glaucoma (nebulized solutions).
Main drug interactions	None.
Main side effects	Dry mouth (rare).

Inhaled beta-2 agonists (*e.g.*, albuterol, metaproterenol, terbutaline)

Standard dosage	Two puffs up to 4 times daily (dosage varies with formulation).
Contraindications	Hypersensitivity.
Special points	Patient responses vary; clinical improvement may occur but may not be detected on spirometric assessment.
Main drug interactions	None.
Main side effects	Tremor, palpitations.

Inhaled steroids

- Inhaled steroids are indicated for patients who have shown an objective response.

Standard dosage	Dosage varies with formulation.
Contraindications	Hypersensitivity.
Special points	Systemic absorption can be reduced with a spacer device.
Main drug interactions	None.
Main side effects	Oral candidiasis.

Oral steroids

- Oral steroids are indicated for exacerbations of COPD and for maintenance treatment in severely ill steroid-responsive patients.

Standard dosage	Prednisone, 30–60 mg in the morning for exacerbations; lowest possible dose for maintenance treatment.
Contraindications	None.
Special points	After 3 weeks of prednisone, steroid responsiveness should be shown by >10% improvement in forced expiratory volume in 1 second.
Main drug interactions	None.
Main side effects	Osteoporosis, diabetes, steroid psychosis.

Theophyllines

- Use is controversial.

Standard dosage	Theophylline, 300–900 mg daily.
Contraindications	None.
Special points	Plasma concentrations must be monitored; they should be maintained at 10–20 µg/L.
Main drug interactions	Cimetidine, erythromycin, ciprofloxacin, and oral contraceptives reduce metabolism; cigarettes, alcohol, phenytoin, and rifampin increase metabolism.
Main side effects	Tachycardia, arrythmias.

Alternative medicine

Recommended use: none.

Common use: coltsfoot (*Tussilago farfara*); mallow (*Malva sylvestris*); thyme (*Thymus vulgaris*); mullein (*Verbascum thapsus*); ephedra/ma huang (*Ephedra sinica*); comfrey (*Symphytum officinale*).

Caution: avoid ephedra/ma huang if heart disease, hypertension, or thyroid disease is present; large doses of comfrey may be hepatotoxic; do not use coltsfoot for more than 6 weeks/year.

Treatment aims

To maximize functional capacity.
To reduce decline in lung function.

Other treatments [3,6]

Long-term oxygen therapy (>16 hours daily): indications include the following:
Partial pressure of oxygen <55 mm Hg on two successive occasions when patient is stable.
Increasing hypoxemia with sleep or exercise.
Nonsmoking patient.
Failure to show carbon dioxide retention after a trial of oxygen.
At least one episode of peripheral edema.
Lung volume reduction surgery: an experimental procedure with promising results.
Lung transplantation: an option in selected patients, particularly younger patients with alpha$_1$ antitrypsin.
Nasal intermittent positive pressure ventilation: may be suitable in patients who retain carbon dioxide with oxygen therapy.
Smoking cessation.
Chest percussion and postural drainage.
Aerobic exercise programs.

Prognosis

- The 5-year survival rate after the initial episode of respiratory failure averages 15%–20%.

Follow-up and management

- Forced expiratory volume in 1 second must be monitored.
- Response to treatment must be assessed.

Key references

1. American Thoracic Society: Standards for the diagnosis and care of patients with chronic obstructive pulmonary disease. *Am J Respir Crit Care Med* 1995, **152(52 Pt 2)**:S77–S121.
2. American Thoracic Society: Guidelines for the approach to the patient with severe hereditary alpha 1-antitrypsin deficiency. *Am Rev Respir Dis* 1989, **140**:1494–1497.
3. Ferguson GT: Recommendations for the management of COPD. *Chest* 2000, **117(2)**:23S–28S.
4. McEvoy CE, Niewoehner DE: Adverse effects of corticosteroid therapy for COPD: a critical review. *Chest* 1997, **111**:732–743.
5. Celli BR: Current thoughts regarding treatment of chronic obstructive pulmonary disease. *Med Clin North Am* 1996, **80**:589–609.
6. Tarpy SP, Celli BR: Long-term oxygen therapy. *N Engl J Med* 1995, **333**:710–714.

Cirrhosis, primary biliary

Diagnosis

Symptoms

• Often asymptomatic; may be an incidental finding (abnormal liver test results on routine screening for other conditions):

Lethargy and pruritus: >60%.

Right-sided abdominal pain: rare.

Signs

Jaundice: 10%; indicates advanced disease.

Xanthoma and xanthelasma: 10%.

Hepatomegaly: 25%.

Splenomegaly: 15%.

Spider nevi stigmata of chronic liver disease: often absent.

Ascites or variceal hemorrhage: indicating advanced disease with portal hypertension.

Investigations

Complete blood count: usually normal.

Liver chemistries:

• Cholestatic pattern with elevated alkaline phosphatase (> 3- to 4-fold) most common; the magnitude of alkaline phosphatase elevations does not have prognostic significance; hyperbilirubinemia usually found only in advanced disease.

• Transaminases typically normal or mildly elevated. AST or ALT > 200 U/L warrants consideration of alternative diagnoses.

• Prolonged PT or INR may signify reduced vitamin K stores (from malabsorption secondary to cholestasis) or advanced cirrhosis.

• Elevated cholesterol common.

Immunological tests:

• Elevated antimitochondrial antibody (>1:30 titer) most classic (relatively sensitive for primary sclerosing cholangitis with >95% of patients testing positive; however, not specific in that patients with other autoimmune hepatitis, may also test positive).

• Patients may have nonspecific elevations in immunoglobulins (IgM, IgG) and antinuclear antigens.

Liver histology: shows nonsuppurative destructive cholangitis or hepatitis involving portal tracts, which may also contain granulomas.

Hepatobiliary imaging:

•An ultrasound (and in select cases, ERCP, CT, or MRI) is typically required to exclude other competing diagnoses (*See* Differential Diagnosis).

•Ultrasound, ERCP, CT, and MRI are all normal except in advanced disease when findings suggestive of cirrhosis may be present.

Complications

Arthralgias, osteoporosis: hepatic osteopenia (35–50%).

Hypercholesterolemia (85%).

Gall stones: 30%.

End-stage liver disease: asciles, vanceal bleeding, encephalopathy in advanced disease.

Differential diagnosis [1]

Primary sclerosing cholangitis.

Autoimmune hepatitis.

Drug-induced jaundice.

Sarcoidosis.

Chronic viral hepatitis.

Gall stone disease.

Alcoholic liver disease.

Etiology

• The cause is unknown, although the following may have a role:

Infectious agents: bacterial or viral.

Autoimmune disorders.

Epidemiology

• In the United Kingdom, estimates of point prevalence of primary biliary cirrhosis are 2.3–14.4 in 100 000 people.

• The disease is less common in Africa and India.

Associated syndromes

Thyroid disease (15%).

Sicca syndrome (>50%).

Renal tubular andosis (50%).

Pulmonary fibrosis: rare.

Scleroderma (15%).

Histology [2]

Stage 1

Florid duct lesions, septal duct damage surrounded by dense inflammatory infiltrate, lymphoid aggregates; granulomas.

Stage 2

Ductular proliferation, fibrosis, fewer ducts.

Stage 3

Scarring (less inflammation), fibrous septa expanding from portal tracts; periportal cholestasis.

Stage 4

True cirrhosis; few or no bile ducts.

Treatment

Diet and lifestyle

• Patients must avoid regular alcohol intake.
• Careful attention must be paid to adequate nutrition, particularly adequate fat-soluble vitamin (*i.e.*, A, D, E, K) stores.
• Prolonged cholestasis may result in vitamin K deficiency as manifest by a prolonged prothrombin time.
• Calcium and vitamin D supplementation should be considered early.

Pharmacological treatment

Symptomatic

• Drugs are indicated to relieve pruritus.

Standard dosage	Cholestyramine, 4–16 g daily, or colestipol.
Contraindications	Complete biliary obstruction.
Special points	May interfere with absorption of fat-soluble vitamins, so supplementation may be needed.
Main drug interactions	Delayed or reduced absorption of digitalis, tetracycline, chlorothiazide, warfarin, thyroxine.
Main side effects	Increased bleeding tendency, constipation, diarrhea.

• Antihistamines of occasional benefit; phenobarbital (30–60 mg at bedtime) or rifampin 10 mg/kg/day also of benefit in select patients. However, both induce P450 enzymes that may result in altered metabolism of other medications.

• Treatment to prevent osteoporosis and supportive treatment for associated symptoms should also be provided.

Definitive

• Ursodeoxycholic acid (UDCA): demonstrated improvement in liver chemistries, clinical parameters, and survival [4].

Dosage	UDCA 10 to 15 mg/day orally in three to four divided doses.
Contraindications	Hypersensitivity to bile acids.
Special points	A number of trials are examining combined benefit of UDCA with colchicine, steroids, and immunosuppressants; data are not compelling regarding additional benefit from these agents.
Main interactions	Cholestyramine may interfere with absorption of UDCA
Main side effects	Not significantly different from placebo; much better tolerated than previous bile acid therapies (*i.e.*, chenodeoxycholic acid).

Alternative medicine

Recommended use: none.

Common use: milk thistle (*Silybum marianum*); ginseng (*Panax ginseng*); licorice (*Glycyrrhiza* spp.).

Caution: avoid comfrey, borage, coltsfoot, chapperel, and germander—these contain pyrrolizidine alkaloids, which are harmful to the liver. Licorice at high doses can cause hypertension and hypokalemia.

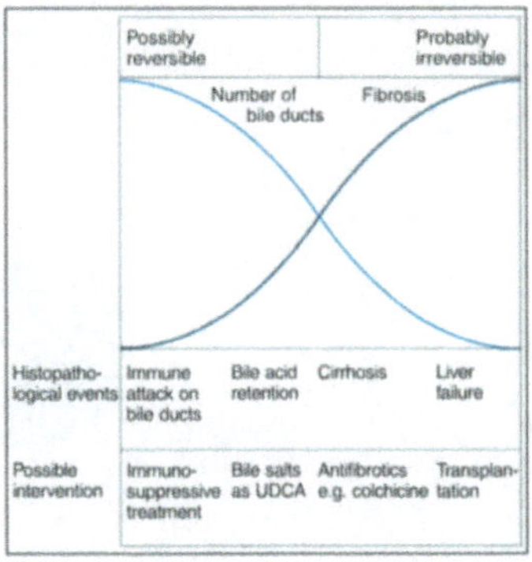

Progression of primary biliary cirrhosis and possible interventions. UDCA, ursodeoxycholic acid.

Treatment aims

To prevent progression.

To reverse symptoms.

Other treatments

Liver transplantation:
• Should be considered in patients with a serum bilirubin >8.2 mg/L (or earlier in patients with complications from advanced liver disease).
• Five-year survival after liver transplantation is >70% at most centers.
• Recurrence of primary biliary cirrhosis >15% and rarely of clinical consequence.

Prognosis [6]

• Prognosis depends on serum bilirubin concentration: >10 mg/dL implies an 18-month survival.
• The median time from diagnosis to death is 10 years.

Follow-up and management

• Follow-up with serial liver chemistries and monitoring for complications (particularly bone disease) is dicated by rate of progression.
• Consultation with a hepatologist should be sought early in disease course.

Key references

1. Laurin JM, Lindor KD: Primary biliary cirrhosis. *Dig Dis Sci* 1994, **12**:331–350.
2. Locke GR III, Therneau TM, Ludwig J, *et al.*: Time course of histological progression in primary biliary cirrhosis. *Hepatology* 1996, **23**:52–56.
3. Lindor KD: Primary biliary cirrhosis: questions and promises. *Ann Intern Med* 1997, **126**:733–735.
4. Lindor KD, Therneau TM, Jorgensen RA, *et al.*: Effects of ursodeoxycholic acid on survival in patients with primary biliary cirrhosis. *Gastroenterology* 1996, **110**:1515–1518.
5. Ricci P, Therneau TM, Malinchoc M, *et al.*: A prognostic model for the outcome of liver transplantation in patients with cholestatic liver disease. *Hepatology* 1997, **25**:672–677.
6. Metcalf JV, Mitchison HC, Palmer JM, *et al.*: Natural history of early primary biliary cirrhosis. *Lancet* 1996, **348**:1399–1402.

Colorectal cancer

Diagnosis

Symptoms

Change of bowel habit.

Blood in stools: often occult.

Weight loss.

Tenesmus: rectal lesions.

Abdominal pain or swelling: not a common presentation for colorectal cancer.

Signs

Pallor: in patients with anemia.

Mass or blood on digital rectal examination.

Mechanical bowel obstruction, abdominal mass, peitonitis: more common in patients who have ignored above symptoms.

Hepatomegaly: metastatic disease.

Cachexia, clinical evidence of weight loss.

Hematochezia: melena occasionally occurs with right-sided lesions.

Investigations

Screening [1–4]

Assessment of primary tumor

Colonoscopy: of patients with symptoms or signs of colorectal cancer; any polyps in these patients should be removed for histological examination; malignancy confined to the mucosa or Dukes' stage A (*see* Pathology) do not require surgery or chemotherapy if the lesion can be completely resected via the colonoscope (*i.e.*, the resection margins are free of disease [1].

Air contrast barium enema: highly competent radiologists can detect significant lesions at a sensitivity that approximates colonoscopy at a lower cost. However, the frequency of colonic lesions in older patients and inability to assess histology by this technique commonly favors colonoscopy.

Assessment of disseminated disease

Liver chemistry tests: metastatic disease often presents with an elevated alkaline phosphatase level.

Chest radiography: may detect solitary or multiple peripheral lung nodules.

Abdominal CT: to assess tumor burden in pelvis and to look for evidence of adenopathy or hepatic disease.

Liver ultrasonography: in absence of CT; inexpensive but lower sensitivity than CT.

Complications

Obstruction: usually left-sided lesions.

Perforation, sepsis.

Acute hemorrhage or iron-deficiency anemia.

Fistula formation.

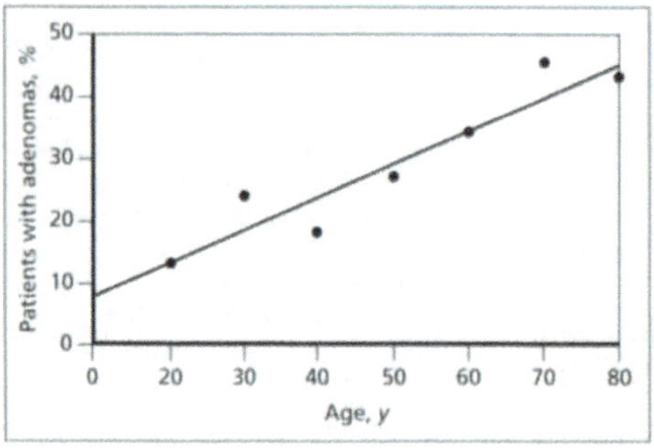

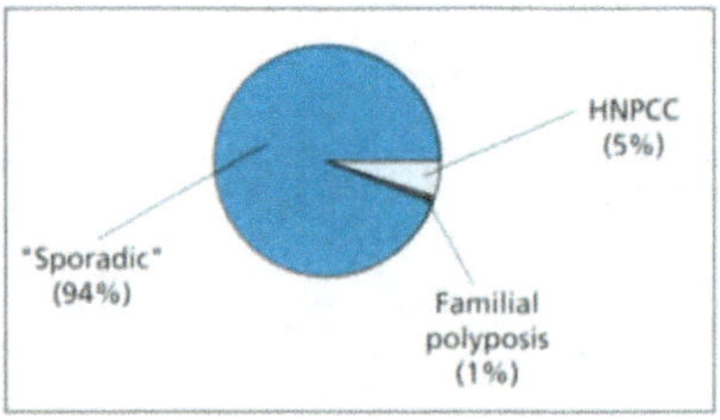

Differential diagnosis

Diverticular disease.
Inflammatory bowel disease.
Irritable bowel syndrome.
Adhesions.
Arteriovenous malformations.
Solitary rectal ulcer.
Mesenteric ischemia.
Nonsteoirdal antiinflammatory drug eneropathy.

Risk factors

High-fat, low-fiber diet.
Chronic ulcerative colitis (>10 years).
Genetic: hereditary nonpolyposis colorectal cancer, familial polyposis coli.
Colorectal adenomas.
Crohn's disease.

Epidemiology

- In an asymptomatic average adult in the United States, the lifetime risk of developing colorectal cancer is 6%.
- The peak incidence is at 60–69 years of age.
- Colon cancer is the second most frequent cause of death due to malignancy in developed countries.

Pathology

Microscopic: adenocarcinoma.
Macroscopic: polypoidal, ulcerative, annular, diffuse or colloidal lesions.

Site

Rectum: 30%.
Cecum and ascending colon: 25%.
Sigmoid colon: 20%.
Descending colon: 15%.
Transverse colon: 10%.

Spread

Direct, lymphatic, venous.

Treatment

Diet and lifestyle

• For primary prevention, fat intake should be reduced to 30% of energy intake. Unrefined fiber, fruit, and vegetable consumption should be increased. Regular aspirin intake has also been associated with a lower risk of colonic adenocarcinoma.

Pharmacological treatment [5]

• Postoperative chemotherapy is of benefit in patients with Dukes' stage C disease. 5-Fluorouracil appears to be the most important component coupled with either leucovorin (6 months) or levamisole (12 months). There is no evidence of benefit in disseminated disease [4–6].

Nonpharmacological treatment

Elective surgery

Curative resection: right hemicolectomy, left hemicolectomy, anterior resection, or abdominoperineal excision, depending on site and extent of lesion.

Palliative resection or bypass.

Local treatment for rectal lesions: local transanal resection (open or endoscopic), laser therapy, or intracavity radiation.

Emergency surgery

• 20% of patients present with obstruction, possibly with perforation.

Adjuvant radiation therapy

• For rectal carcinoma, preoperative or postoperative radiation therapy with 5-fluorouracil provides survival benefit.

Management of recurrence [5]

• Management depends on the site, size, and number of metastases.

• Serial carcinoembryonic antigen estimation can predict recurrence and may be followed if the patient is a candidate for aggressive surgical management of extracolonic lesions (*e.g.*, solitary hepatic mestastases).

• Fewer than 20% of patients with recurrence after a "curative" resection are suitable for another resection.

Site of recurrence: local (20%; related to stage), hepatic (30%), abdominal (20%), pulmonary (20%), retroperitoneal (10%).

For local disease: 50% amenable to further ablative surgery, with potential cure in 25%; radiation therapy effective palliation for rectal recurrence but limited by myelotoxicity.

For hepatic metastases: <20% (solitary or unilobar) amenable to curative resection; possible short-term benefit from hepatic artery infusion of 5-fluorodeoxyuridine; possible symptomatic relief for capsular distension with fractionated radiation therapy.

Treatment aims

To remove primary tumor and regional nodes, including mesorectum for rectal lesions (curative resection).

To remove or bypass the primary lesion with advanced local or metastatic disease, in order to ameliorate symptoms (palliative resection or bypass).

To control local disease in patients unfit for resection.

Prognosis

• 25% of patients have metastases at the time of presentation.

• In-hospital postoperative mortality (5%–7%) is related to intra-abdominal sepsis, obstruction, age, or cardiopulmonary complications.

• Overall 5-year survival rates are 80%–90% for Dukes' stage A, 50%–60% for stage B, 30% for stage C, and 5% for stage D.

Follow-up and management

• Patients resected for cure should undergo surveillance colonscopy within 6–12 months of resection to exclude missed lesions, and every 3–5 years in the absence of symptoms.

Key references

1. Winawer SJ, *et al.*: Colorectal cancer screening: clinical guidelines and rationale. *Gastroenterology* 1997, 112:594–642.
2. Goldberg ES: Colorectal polyps and polyposis syndromes. *Curr Pract Med* 1998, **1**:837–843.
3. Simon JB, Fletcher RH: Clinical debate: should all people over the age of 50 have regular fecal occult blood tests? *N Engl J Med* 1998, **338**:1151–1156.
4. Ransohoff DF, Lang CA: Screening for colorectal cancer with the fecal occult blood test: a background paper. *Ann Intern Med* 1997, **126**:811–822.
5. Boland CR, *et al.*: Colorectal cancer prevention and treatment. *Gastroenterology* 2000, **118**:S115–S128.

Diagnosis

Definition

• Coma is a state of unresponsiveness to external stimuli in which the patient lies with eyes closed.

• In practice, the condition may usefully be defined as a patient with a Glasgow coma scale of 8 (2:4:2) or less.

Symptoms

• Coma is a symptom.

Signs

Fever: indicating infection (meningitis, encephalitis, systemic).

Hypothermia: may be cause or effect.

Neck stiffness, Kernig's sign, papilledema.

Cardiac abnormalities: can indicate subacute bacterial endocarditis or emboli.

Hypertension or hypotension.

Slow, shallow respiration: may suggest drug intoxication.

Rapid respiration: suggesting infection or acidosis.

Anemia, jaundice, rash.

Intoxication, diabetes, hepatic failure.

Organomegaly.

Investigations

History from a witness: for evolution of coma, circumstances of patient's discovery, trauma, seizure, drugs, medical history.

Glasgow coma scale: for level of consciousness [1].

Brain stem function tests: pupillary response, spontaneous eye movements, oculovestibular responses.

Motor function tests: for lateralizing features.

Fundus examination: for papilledema, hemorrhage, emboli.

Blood analysis: for biochemistry, *e.g.*, glucose, electrolytes; hepatic, renal, and thyroid function; toxin exposure; etc.

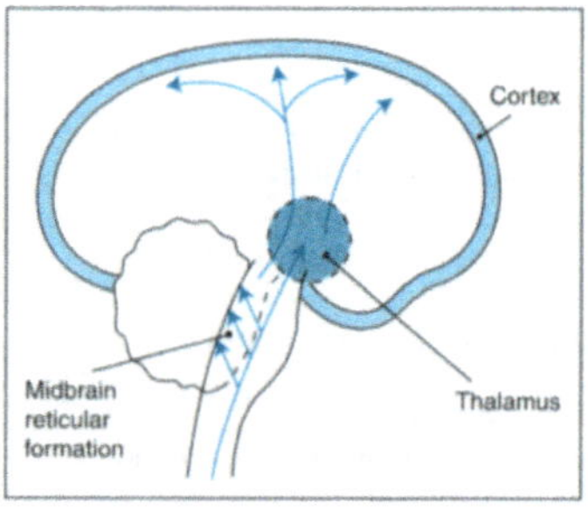

The anatomy of consciousness.

CT or MRI: for coma with focal signs or if the diagnosis is uncertain.

Lumbar puncture: for coma without focal signs but with stiff neck.

Hematological assays, chest radiography, EEG: for coma without focal signs or stiff neck (raised intracranial pressure must be excluded first).

Complications

Infections: particularly respiratory or renal, *e.g.*, aspiration pneumonia.

Metabolic abnormalities.

Disseminated intravascular coagulation.

Decubitus ulcers.

Contractures.

Deep venous thromboses.

Corneal abrasion.

Death.

Differential diagnosis [2]

Locked-in syndrome: voluntary response of eye opening and eye closure to command.

Vegetative state: spontaneous eye opening and sleep-wake cycles, but no evidence of cognition.

Psychogenic coma: intact oculovestibular responses and nystagmus to cold water caloric, blepharospasm, intact cranial nerve reflexes.

Etiology

Drug or alcohol overdose.

Trauma.

Space-occupying intracranial lesions.

Infections: encephalitis, meningitis, septicemia.

Intracranial hemorrhage or thrombosis.

Metabolic abnormalities.

Toxins.

Status epilepticus

Epidemiology

• 3% of emergency admissions to hospital are patients in coma.

• 40% of these patients have taken an overdose of sedative drugs.

Glasgow coma scale

Eye opening

1. Nil.
2. To pain.
3. *To speech.*
4. *Spontaneously.*

Motor response

1. Nil.
2. Extensor.
3. Flexor.
4. Withdrawal.
5. *Localizing.*
6. *Voluntary.*

Verbal response

1. Nil.
2. Groans.
3. *Inappropriate.*
4. *Confused.*
5. *Orientated.*

• Italics indicate no coma.

Treatment

Diet and lifestyle

• No special precautions are possible.

Avoid sedating medications in elderly patients.

Pharmacological treatment [3]

• Thiamine, glucose, Narcan, and flumacemil may be diagnostically and therapeutically useful in patients without available history.

• Patients may need treatment for causative or concurrent disorders: antibiotics and antiviral agents, antifungal agents, correction of metabolic abnormalities, removal of toxic substances, treatment of mass lesions, s.c. heparin to prevent thrombotic complications.

• Steroids or mannitol should not be given routinely in comatose patients but may help in specific instances when raised intracranial pressure, due to edema, can be corrected.

Treatment aims

To correct cause.

To maintain hydration and nutrition.

To reverse coma and return normal physiological and psychological function.

Prognosis

• Sedative drugs or alcohol overdoses are not usually lethal, and the prognosis is good if the circulation and respiration are protected.

• The prognosis of other causes of non-traumatic coma depends on the cause (metabolic coma has better prognosis than hypoxic ischemic coma), the depth (the deeper the coma, the worse the prognosis), the duration (the longer the coma, the worse the prognosis), and clinical signs, e.g., brain stem reflexes.

• Overall, only 15% of patients in non-traumatic coma for >6 hours make a good or moderate recovery.

Follow-up and management

• The airway must be maintained.

• The patient must be given adequate nutrition.

• Skin, chest, bladder, and bowel must be protected.

• Progress must be monitored.

Key references

1. Plumer F, Posner JB: *Stupor and Coma*, edn 3. Philadelphia: FA Davis; 1982.
2. Giacino JT: Disorders of consciousness: differential diagnosis and neuropathologic features. *Semin Neurol* 1997, **17**:105–111.
3. Bates D: The management of medical coma. *J Neurol Neurosurg Psychiatry* 1993, **56**:589–598.

Cor pulmonale

Diagnosis

Symptoms

• Cor pulmonale is the enlargement of the right ventricle, due to pulmonary hypertension, that occurs in diseases of the lung, the chest wall, or the pulmonary circulation. By definition, primary diseases of the left side of the heart and congenital heart diseases are excluded.

• Although overt right ventricular failure is often present, right ventricular failure is not necessary for cor pulmonale.

Pedal edema, chest pain, syncope with exertion, distended neck veins: symptoms related to right ventricular failure.

Exertional dyspnea, easy fatiguability, rough hemoptysis, weakness: nonspecific findings.

Hoarseness (due to left recurrent larygeal compression); right upper quadrant discomfort (due to hepatic congestion).

Symptoms of chronic obstructive pulmonary disease (COPD), arthritic symptoms of connective tissue diseases: symptoms of the underlying pulmonary disorder may often predominate.

Signs

Right ventricular heave, right ventricular gallop, increased P_2 distended neck veins, tender and enlarged liver, pedal edema, severe limitation to exercise, cyanosis, clubbing, and orthostatic syncope: signs of right-sided cardiac failure.

Polycythemia, arterial hypoxemia: oxygen saturation is often <85%.

COPD, cystic fibrosis, severe restrictive lung disease: signs of the underlying disorder may predominate.

Investigations

Arterial blood gases: should be done to assess the degree of arterial oxygen desaturation as well as the level of Pco_2 because COPD is the major cause of cor pulmonale.

Chest radiography: needed to assess the degree of pulmonary interstitial or parenchymal disease, to assess the size of the pulmonary arteries, and to document the enlarged right ventricle. Often the central pulmonary artery is enlarged, but distal pulmonary vessels are severely reduced, yielding "pruned tree" appearance.

Pulmonary function tests: needed to assess the degree of underlying lung disease; will distinguish between obstructive and restrictive causes of pulmonary impairment.

ECG: may show a right axis deviation with right ventricular hypertrophy and right atrial enlargement (*i.e.*, P pulmonale). Deep S-waves are often present in lead V-6; low voltage is often seen in the presence of COPD. Arrhythmias, especially atrial tachyarrhythmias, are common.

Echocardiography: helpful in ruling out left ventricular disease; it is less helpful in pure right ventricular failure because air in the distended lungs makes it technically difficult to assess the right ventricle. Doppler echocardiography may permit noninvasive estimation of pulmonary artery pressure

Ventilation perfusion scans: in the presence of right ventricular failure, these are not as helpful to assess vascular disease. Pulmonary angiography is the preferred method for diagnosis and assessment of pulmonary embolization.

Catheterization of the right side of the heart: will establish the ventricular and pulmonary artery pressures as well as determine cardiac output. Catheterization is often useful to exclude left ventricular failure.

Complications

Atrial tachyarrhythmias, particularly atrial fibrillation and supraventricular tachycardia: common.

Acute or chronic respiratory failure: often present because of the underlying lung disease in combination with the right ventricular failure. Emergency hospital admissions are often necessary as a result of respiratory infection.

• Complications of the underlying lung disease will often predominate (*e.g.*, in COPD, these would include infective exacerbations, respiratory failure and death, pneumothorax, and lung cancer).

Differential diagnosis

Left-sided congestive heart failure and chronic lung disease without right ventricular enlargement.

Etiology

• COPD is the most common cause of cor pulmonale. Diseases that primarily affect the pulmonary vasculature leading to cor pulmonale include large or multiple central emboli, small chronic embolization, and acute respiratory distress syndrome.

• Rarer causes include idiopathic pulmonary fibrosis, end-stage pneumoconiosis, primary pulmonary hypertension, sleep apnea syndrome, schistosomiasis, lymphangiatic spread of cancer, and obliterative pulmonary vascular disease as seen in connective tissue diseases.

• Cor pulmonale can also been seen in severe obesity, severe hypothyroidism with myxedema, severe muscle weakness, and severe kyphoscoliosis and at high altitude.

Epidemiology

• The most common cause of chronic cor pulmonale is severe COPD, both chronic bronchitis and emphysema. The most common cause of acute cor pulmonale is acute pulmonary embolism due to many large emboli, which causes a dramatic elevation in pulmonary artery pressure.

Treatment

Diet and lifestyle

• Patients should be encouraged to restrict sodium intake and maintain ideal weight.

• The use of alcohol and sedatives should be minimized to prevent episodes of respiratory failure.

Pharmacological treatment

Oxygen

• The mainstay of therapy is treatment of hypoxia by the administration of oxygen. The oxygen is most often given via nasal cannula but in chronic situations may also be given through a transtracheal catheter.

Diuretics

• Patients with cor pulmonale generally will need diuretics to minimize fluid retention. The smallest amount of diuretic necessary to achieve the desired effect should be used. Over-aggressive use of a loop diuretic may precipitously decrease cardiac output, causing orthostatic hypotension and syncope.

Standard dosage	Depends on the degree of fluid retention. Patients with mild fluid retention may be managed with thiazide diuretics. Progression to loop diuretics is needed for most moderate to severe disease; combination of loop and thiazide diuretics or calcium-channel blocker may be needed in the very severe cases. Fluid restriction may be needed in advanced disease.
Contraindications	Severe hypotension, renal failure, and hypokalemia (relative).
Main drug interactions	Potent diuresis seen occasionally with combination diuretic therapy.
Main side effects	Hypokalemia, renal impairment, orthostatic hypotension.

Vasodilators

• These agents are avoided in most cases because of significant adverse effects and only mild short-term improvement.

For underlying lung disorders

• Aggressive treatment of the underlying lung disorders is necessary. In most patients, this will be treatment of COPD, which would include bronchodilators, inhaled β_2 agonists and inhaled cholinergics, and inhaled steroids. Oral steroids would be indicated for acute exacerbations. (*See* Chronic obstructive pulmonary disease.)

• Antibiotics are appropriate for managing infective exacerbations of the pulmonary disorder, which often can contribute to worsening cor pulmonale.

• Digoxin is not used for right-sided failure unless the patient is in atrial fibrillation.

Treatment aims

To minimize alveolar hypoxia.

To minimize pedal edema.

To maximize respiratory function.

Other treatments

• Heart/lung transplantation should be considered, especially in younger patients with cor pulmonale.

Prognosis

• Prognosis in patients with cor pulmonale usually depends on the underlying pulmonary disease.

• The underlying pulmonary disease is a better predictor of survival than the severity of right ventricular failure.

• An average life expectancy in a patient after the development of cor pulmonale may be 2–5 years; however, this can vary widely.

General references

Klinger JR, Hill NS: Right ventricular dysfunction in chronic obstructive pulmonary disease: evaluation and management. *Chest* 1991, **99**:715.

MacNee W: Pathophysiology of cor pulmonale in chronic obstructive pulmonary disease. *Am J Respir Crit Care Med* 1994, **150**:833–1158.

Cranial arteritis

Diagnosis

Symptoms [1–3]

Headache: present in 75% of patients; at any site, often throbbing, unilateral or asymmetrical, worse at night; scalp soreness and tenderness frequent.

Polymyalgia: proximal limb pain and stiffness in 58%.

Malaise, fatigue, weight loss: in 56%.

Jaw pain and fatigue: masticatory "claudication" in 40%.

Fever: in 35%.

Cough: in 17%.

Amaurosis fugax: in 10%.

Permanent visual loss: in 8%.

Limb claudication: in 8%.

Transient ischemic attack or stroke: in 7%.

Depression or confusional state: in 3%.

Diplopia: in 2%.

Signs

Abnormal temporal artery: tenderness, nodularity, thickening or reduced pulsation in 49% of patients.

Scalp tenderness elsewhere.

Tenderness of common carotid arteries.

Diminished carotid or limb pulses.

Ischemic optic neuropathy: pale, swollen disc in a recently blinded eye.

Ophthalmoplegia: due to cranial nerve or brain stem lesion.

Confusional state or encephalopathy.

Investigations

ESR measurement: substantially raised in most patients; mean, 85 ± 32 mm/h (<30 mm/h in 3% of patients).

Complete blood count: mild anemia, thrombocytosis, and raised leukocyte count common.

Liver function tests: raised gamma glutamyltransferase, alkaline phosphatase, or aspartate transaminase in 15% of patients.

Lumbar puncture: necessary only if low-grade meningitis or cortical thrombophlebitis considered in differential diagnosis.

Temporal artery biopsy: essential when diagnosis not absolutely clear cut on clinical grounds; at least 2–3 cm length biopsy (longer segment more likely to yield positive result); occipital artery biopsy alternative in selected patients. Longitudinal sections helpfull.

Angiography: necessary only to exclude arterial dissection or other arteritides in selected patients; may show abnormalities in all major branches of aortic arch in cranial arteritis; lacks sensitivity and specificity as diagnostic test.

Complications

Permanent blindness: in 8% of patients.

Brain stem or carotid territory infarction: in <5%.

Myocardial infarction.

Scalp necrosis.

Limb ischemia.

Aortic rupture.

Differential diagnosis

Raised ESR

Other arteritides (rare in patients aged >70 years).
Myeloma.
Other skull metastases.
Subacute meningitis.
Infection with venous sinus thrombosis.

Normal ESR

Migraine.
Tension headache.
"Occipital neuralgia."
Cervical spine disease.
Paget's disease of the skull.
Vertebral or carotid dissection.
Temporomandibular joint disease.
Meningioma.

Etiology

- Cranial arteritis is presumed to be an autoimmune disorder, but the antigen is not known (perhaps component of internal elastic lamina).
- Immunoglobulin and complement deposits have been shown at the internal elastic lamina; other histological features suggest that cell-mediated mechanisms are also involved.

Epidemiology [4]

- The incidence is 9.3 in 100 000 population overall and 15–30 in 100 000 aged >50 years.
- The prevalence is 130 in 100 000 aged >50 years.
- Cranial arteritis rarely occurs in people aged <50 years.
- The median age of onset is 75 years (range, 56–92 years in published series).
- The female:male ratio is 3.7:1.

Pathology

- Cranial arteritis is an occlusive disease, involving large and medium-sized arteries arising from the aortic arch and sometimes the femoral arteries and aorta itself.
- Biopsy shows arterial luminal stenosis due to intimal proliferation, with disruption of the internal elastic lamina, mononuclear cell infiltration, necrosis of the media, giant cells, and granuloma formation; secondary thrombosis may be present. Involvement is patchy and may be missed by too small a biopsy.

Treatment

Diet and lifestyle

• No special precautions are necessary.

Pharmacological treatment [5]

General principles

• Cranial arteritis requires prompt treatment by corticosteroids to prevent the rare but serious complications, particularly blindness.

• Presenting symptoms are often nonspecific and "atypical" (*e.g.*, pyrexia of unknown origin, weight loss, anemia), so suspicion must be high and treatment initiated as soon as the diagnosis is seriously considered.

• Arterial biopsy is often taken after steroid treatment is started, but it should not be delayed by more than 2–3 days; the yield of positive histology in clinically probable cases falls from 60%–80% with early biopsy to only 10% in patients undergoing biopsy 1 week after starting steroid treatment.

• Traditional high doses of prednisolone are justifiable in all patients with visual symptoms or signs and in those with features of cerebral or myocardial ischemia.

• In critical cases (*e.g.*, visual loss in one eye and early symptoms in the other), infusion of high-dose methylprednisolone probably reduces the risk of complete blindness.

• In patients without visual symptoms, prospective trials suggest that most respond to much lower doses (even less needed for polymyalgia without symptomatic arteritis).

• The rate of reduction depends on clinical severity at presentation, starting dose, symptom control, and ESR.

• A maintenance dose of 5–10 mg daily is usually needed for 2–3 years.

• An alternate-day regimen is sometimes possible, when the dose is very low.

• 30%–50% of patients can discontinue treatment after 2 years.

• Some need treatment for several years, and a few apparently need long-term maintenance doses of 2–5 mg daily.

Steroid regimen [6]

Initial dose: prednisolone, 40–80 mg daily;
methylprednisolone, 1 g i.v. daily for 2–5 days in critical cases.

Months 1–2: reduced slowly to 20–40 mg daily.

Months 2–4: reduced slowly to 10–20 mg daily.

Months 4–24: reduced to maintenance dose 5–10 mg daily.

Months 24–36: withdrawal possible in ~50% of patients.

Complications of treatment

Vertebral compression fractures in 26%.

Other symptoms of osteoporosis.

Steroid myopathy in 11%.

Cataracts.

Gastrointestinal symptoms.

Other steroid side effects.

Other drugs

Methotrexate.

• Azathioprine has a modest steroid-sparing effect but is not of proven efficacy used alone.

• Cyclophosphamide is a possible fourth option but rarely used.

Treatment aims

To relieve symptoms.

To prevent complications.

To prevent and control steroid side effects.

Prognosis

• Prognosis is excellent with early and adequate steroid treatment, which is usually needed for at least 2–3 years.

• Subsequent morbidity is determined as much by steroid side effects as by the disease itself.

Follow-up and management

• Patients need regular monitoring of clinical symptoms, ESR, and potential steroid effects for at least 2 years, preferably in a specialist clinic (neurology or rheumatology).

Key references

1. Caselli RJ, Hunder GG, Whisnant JP: Neurologic disease in biopsy-proven giant cell (temporal) arteritis. *Neurology* 1988, **38**:352–359.
2. Hunder GG: Giant cell arteritis and polymyalgia rheumatica. *Med Clin North Am* 1997, **81**:195–219.
3. Turnbull J: Temporal arteritis and polymyalgia rheumatica: nosographic and nosologic considerations. *Neurology* 1996, **46**:901–906.
4. Nordborg E, Bengtsson BA: Epidemiology of proven giant cell arteritis (GCA). *Intern Med* 1990, **227**:233–236.
5. Evans J, Hunder GG: The implications of recognizing large-vessel involvement in elderly patients with giant cell arteritis. *Curr Opin Rheumatol* 1997, **9**:37–40.
6. Kyle V, Hazleman BL: Treatment of polymyalgia rheumatica and giant cell arteritis. Steroid regimens in the first two months. *Ann Rheum Dis* 1989, **48**:658–661.

Crohn's disease

Diagnosis

Symptoms

Diarrhea: nonbloody most common.

Abdominal pain.

Weight loss.

Recurrent perianal pain and inflammation.

Arthropathy, skin, eye symptoms in 10%–20%.

Signs

• Patients with mild to moderate disease most typically have a relatively normal examination.

Abdominal tenderness with occasional right lower quadrant mass or fullness: patients may present with signs of obstruction or peritonitis, in which case surgical consultation should be sought early.

Perianal disease: present in 50% of patients (abscess, fistula, atypical fissures).

Muscle wasting, easy bruising, glossitis: prolonged malabsorption indicating severe disease.

Aphthous stomatitis.

Skin findings (<4% of patients): tender red nodules of erythema nodosum, ulcerated lesions of pyoderma gangrenosum.

Arthropathy: large joint involvement (10%–20% of patients); sacroiliitis/ankylosing spondylitis (5% of patients).

Investigations

• Crohn's disease can be diagnosed only after interpretation of diagnostic studies in the context of the patient's clinical presentation (*i.e.*, radiographs, fiberoptic studies, or biopsies alone rarely in and of themselves make the diagnosis of Crohn's disease) [1].

Stool studies: infection must be excluded in all patients by sending samples for *Clostridium difficile* toxin, cultures, and ova/parasites.

Complete blood count: evaluate for anemia; elevated leukocyte count secondary to inflammation or infection.

ESR or CRP measurement: inflammatory markers of disease activity.

Electrolytes, blood urea nitrogen, creatine: abnormal in patients with dehydration.

Serum albumin: decreased in patients with malnutrition.

Colonoscopy: allows assessment of colonic disease and usually visualization of the terminal ileum and appropriate biopsy; Crohn's disease is characterized by intermittent disease (*e.g.*, aphthous or serpiginous ulcers) separated by areas of normal mucosa. Although perianal involvement is common, the rectum is often normal; strictures may be evidence of prior inflammation.

Mucosal biopsies: perform during fiberoptic endoscopy from areas of inflammation; considerable overlap in histologic features prevents distinguishing Crohn's disease from other inflammatory conditions, such as ulcerative colitis, solely on the basis of biopsy findings.

Upper gastrointestinal endoscopy: if relevant symptoms; lesions must undergo biopsy to confirm that they are due to Crohn's disease.

Barium contrast radiography: small bowel follow-through allows assessment of mucosa; used in part to distinguish active mucosal inflammation (*e.g.*, ulcerations) from the sequelae of chronic inflammation (*e.g.*, stricture, fistula).

Abdominal CT scan: useful when checking for extraintestinal inflammation (*e.g.*, abscesses).

Radioisotope-labeled leukocyte scans: may be of use in localizing inflammation not detected by studies above or in defining extent of disease prior to surgical management.

Complications

Intestinal obstruction or perforation.

Abscess or fistula formation: to bowel, bladder, vagina, or skin.

Malnutrition: vitamin B_{12} deficiency common (macrocytic anemia); short gut syndrome in severe cases.

Gastrointestinal bleeding: occult more common than visible blood loss, resulting in iron deficiency anemia.

Uveitis, episcleritis.

Cholestatic liver disease: *e.g.*, sclerosing cholangitis and rarely cholangiocarcinoma.

Renal oxalate stones: uncommon.

Deep venous thrombosis.

Infections: patients are often immunocompromised because of medications, chronic disease.

Differential diagnosis

Bacterial infections (*Salmonella, Shigella, Campylobacter* spp., *Escherichia coli, Yersinia*, tuberculosis, *Clostridium difficile*).

Viral gastroenteritis, cytomegalovirus.

Nonsteroidal anti-inflammatory drugs enteropathy.

Amebic infection, *Giardia* spp.

Ulcerative colitis.

Ischemia.

Colonic carcinoma.

Lymphoma.

Etiology

Unknown; environmental triggers such as smoking and unidentified infections in genetically susceptible individuals is the most popular opinion at this time. No specific dietary triggers have been identified [2].

Overall risk in first-degree relatives 5%–15%; higher with onset of disease in proband at a young age.

Epidemiology

• The prevalence of Crohn's disease is 1 in 1000.

• Ethnic clustering has been found.

• Onset may be in childhood.

• The disease most commonly presents in the third decade.

• The male : female ratio is equal.

Histology

Macroscopic

Patchy areas of disease with intervening areas of normal mucosa.

Terminal ileum involvement most common but disease can be found anywhere along the gastrointestinal tract.

Transmural inflammation.

Microscopic

Crypt distortion with inflammation.

Noncaseating granulomas: classic, but often not seen.

Lymphocytic infiltration.

Treatment

Diet and lifestyle

- Nutritional supplementats are needed in patients with severe illness, including parenteral nutrition in advanced disease. Elemental diets may be effective but are poorly tolerated due to unpalatability; remission induced by elemental diets does not continue after diets are stopped.
- Patients should be urged to quit smoking and to avoid nonsteroidal antiinflammatory drugs.
- Patients with extensive small-bowel disease tolerate lactose poorly.

Pharmacological treatment [3]

Corticosteroids

- The most efficacious medication in treatment of patients with moderate to severe disease.

Standard dose: Prednisone, 1 mg/kg up to a daily maximum of 60 mg/day; consider i.v. administration (*e.g.*, solumedrol 15mg i.v. every 6 hours) in patients with poor motility and absorptive function; topical steroids for rectal or perianal disease.

Contraindications: Overt sepsis; caution in hypertension and diabetes.

Special points: Does not prevent disease flair in patients in remission. Long-term use should be avoided, and tapering should be initiated when disease is in remission.

Main drug interactions: Significant immunosuppression with azathioprine or 6mP.

Main side effects: Fluid retention and hypertension, hyperglycemia, osteoporosis, cushingoid features, mood lability, aseptic necrosis, hyperphagia, increased energy.

5-aminosalicylic acid preparations (*e.g.*, mesalamine, olsalazine)

Standard dosage: 2.4–4.8 g orally each day.

Contraindications: Salicylate hypersensitivity.

Special points: Requires several weeks to realize beneficial effect; better at maintaining remission than in treating acute symptoms; preparations vary in site of action.

Main drug interactions: May increase warfarin requirements.

Main side effects: Nausea.

Other medications

Some patients with mild disease can be treated with antibiotics (*e.g.*, metronidazole or ciprofloxacin); patients with complicated disease and acute inflammation typically require intravenous antibiotics (*e.g.*, ampicillin/sulbactam 1–3 g every 6 hours i.v. or cefotetan, 1–3 g i.v. every 12 hours).

Immunomodulating agents are used in patients requiring frequent or high-dose steroids. Azathioprine (1.5–3.0 mg/kg/ day orally) or 6-mercaptopurine (1.0–2.5 mg/kg/day orally) are used most frequently to induce remission and to reduce steroid requirements. Treatment response may take 2–6 months. Side effects include pancytopenia, severe immunosuppression, and pancreatitis. Methotrexate may be used in patients intolerant of the above drugs. Infliximab (anti-tumor necrosis-α) at a dose of 5 mg/kg i.v. is useful in refractory cases, particularly those with fistulas [4].

Alternative medicine

Recommended use: none.

Common use: quercetin; magnesium; zinc picolinate; vitamin A; vitamin E; fish oil; marshmallow (*Hibiscus mosheutos*); slippery elm bark (*Ulmus rubra*); comfrey root (*Symphtum officinale*).

Caution: magnesium may have cathartic action; comfrey root contains pyrrolidizine alkaloids and may cause liver damage at high dosages.

Treatment aims

To suppress disease activity.
To prevent complications.
To correct nutritional deficiencies.

Other treatments

Whenever possible, medical management is favored over surgery because of the high incidence of recurrent disease after surgery

Surgery is indicated for acute obstruction, peritonitis, or bleeding that is refractory to medical management.

Intra-abdominal abscesses can often be drained under CT guidance without need of surgery.

In select cases, strictures may be balloon dilated by using fiberoptic instruments.

Prognosis

- Improved immunosuppressive regimens, and conservative surgery have greatly decreased the incidence of long-term complications.
- The risk of carcinoma is increased slightly in excluded loops.

Follow-up and management

- Disease activity must be monitored using symptoms, signs, and surveillance of abnormal laboratory studies.
- Signs and symptoms of a disease flare do not typically require restaging of disease unless medical management fails to arrest the disease or surgery is anticipated.

Key references

1. Fiocchi C: Inflammatory bowel disease: etiology and pathogenesis. *Gastroenterology* 1998, **115**:182–205.
2. Hanuer SB: Inflammatory bowel disease. *N Engl J Med* 1996, **334**:841–848.
3. Hanauer SB, Meyers S: Management of Crohn's disease in adults. *Am J Gastroenterol* 1997, **92**:559–564.
4. Present DH, *et al.*: Infliximab for the treatment of fistulas in patients with Crohn's disease. *N Engl J Med* 1999, **340**:1398–1405.

Cushing's syndrome

Diagnosis

Symptoms

Central weight gain: trunk more than arms and legs.

Hirsutism, thin skin, easy bruising, stretch marks, acne on back and chest.

Muscle weakness and aching, back and joint pain.

Menstrual disturbance, impotence, loss of libido.

Depression, anxiety, psychiatric and sleep disturbance.

Signs

Centripetal obesity.

"Moon face," hirsutism, facial plethora.

Supraclavicular filling, "Buffalo hump."

Thin skin relative to age, easy bruising, acne, red or purple wide abdominal striae: not just stretch marks, which are common in obese patients and after pregnancy.

Proximal myopathy: *e.g.*, difficulty rising from squat without assistance.

Hypertension: incidental finding or with symptoms of cardiovascular complications.

Kyphosis, loss of height.

Pedal edema.

Investigations [1–5]

• The diagnosis of Cushing's syndrome is made biochemically, not radiologically. Imaging procedures should be used to confirm and extend the results of biochemical testing.

Screening tests for Cushing's syndrome

24-hour urinary-free cortisol (UFC): usually increased 2–3-fold in Cushing's syndrome. Smaller increases may be due to depression, alcoholism, or obesity (pseudo-Cushing's).

Overnight dexamethasone suppression test: dexamethasone, 1 mg, is given orally at 23.00 hours. Serum cortisol obtained at 08.00 hours the following day will normally be <5 mg/dL. Patients with Cushing's will not suppress. Higher false-positive rate than 24-hour UFC.

Differential diagnosis of Cushing's syndrome

Plasma corticotropin (ACTH) measurement: undetectable concentration confirms an adrenal source (adrenal adenoma or carcinoma). Values >400 ng/L suggest, but do not prove, ectopic ACTH secretion secondary to tumor.

Liddle test (6-day dexamethasone suppression test) [2]: 24-hour UFCs and 17-OH corticosteroids (17-OHS) are measured on 6 consecutive days. Days 1 and 2 are baseline. On days 3 and 4, patients receive dexamethasone, 0.5 mg orally every 6 hours (low dose). On days 5 and 6, they receive 2 mg every 6 hours (high dose). Suppression of UFCs and 17-OHS from the average of the baseline days to day 6 is calculated. Suppression of UFCs by >90% and 17-OHS by >64% is highly suggestive of Cushing's disease (84% sensitivity with 100% specificity).

8-mg overnight dexamethasone suppression test [3] and corticotropin-releasing hormone (CRH) simulation test [4]: newer tests that are emerging as efficient and effective in separating pituitary from nonpituitary causes of Cushing's syndrome.

Petrosal sinus sampling catheterization [5]: confirms pituitary ACTH secretion with high degree of confidence. Simultaneous use of CRH increases accuracy of test. Can also be used to lateralize the pituitary tumor. Requires a well-trained invasive radiologist.

CT or MRI of pituitary gland: if pituitary disease is suspected.

CT or MRI of adrenal glands: if primary adrenal disease is suspected.

CT or MRI of chest and/or abdomen: if ectopic ACTH syndrome is suspected and source of ACTH is unknown.

Complications

Diabetes, infections, osteoporosis, thromboembolism, ischemic heart disease, cerebrovascular disease, peripheral vascular disease.

Differential diagnosis

Simple obesity.

Polycystic ovarian syndrome.

• Few patients with obesity, hirsutism, bruising, stretch marks, hypertension, or diabetes have Cushing's syndrome.

Etiology [1]

ACTH-dependent Cushing's syndrome

• Pituitary Cushing's disease (70% of patients) is usually due to a (basophil) corticotroph microadenoma, but can be due to macroadenoma or very rarely to corticotroph hyperplasia.

• Ectopic ACTH secretion (10%) is usually due to tumors of neuroendocrine origin (carcinoid, metastatic gastrointestinal endocrine tumors).

• Ectopic corticotropin-releasing hormone secretion is rare.

Adrenal Cushing's syndrome

• Causes include adrenal adenoma (10%), adrenal carcinoma (10%), and macro-nodular or micronodular adrenal hyperplasia (rare).

Iatrogenic Cushing's syndrome

• The most common cause of the clinical syndrome, this is due to steroid or ACTH treatment.

Epidemiology

• Endogenous Cushing's syndrome is rare.

• Cushing's syndrome and adrenal adenomas occur more often in women.

Ectopic ACTH syndrome

Occult ectopic ACTH syndrome

• This is usually seen when a neuroendocrine tumor (often carcinoid, of bronchial or thymic origin) secretes large amounts of ACTH and mimics a pituitary adenoma.

• The tumor may be only a few millimeters in diameter and only discovered after intensive imaging over extended periods of time; diagnosis may prove difficult with conventional tests.

Overt ectopic ACTH secretion

• Many malignant tumors secrete ACTH, most often bronchial small-cell carcinoma; usually the tumor is clinically obvious.

• Patients are rarely cushingoid; they may have no endocrine symptoms or may exhibit pigmentation, myopathy, weight loss, and debility, associated with high cortisol and ACTH concentrations and profound hypokalemic alkalosis.

Treatment

Diet and lifestyle

• Patients who maintain regular low-impact exercise and weight control probably have an improved postoperative recovery.

Pharmacological treatment

• Medical treatment for Cushing's syndrome is effective in improving the clinical syndrome but is a short-term measure to prepare the patient for surgery, while awaiting the long-term benefit of other treatment, or in patients with inoperable tumors.

• Drugs include metyrapone, ketoconazole, aminoglutethimide, and mitotane; all have significant problems and should be used only under specialist supervision.

Nonpharmacological treatment

For Cushing's disease

• Selective adenomectomy is the treatment of choice. Transsphenoidal surgery must be performed by a surgeon experienced in locating and removing ACTH-secreting microadenomas. Successful surgery results in temporary adrenal insufficiency due to the suppression of normal hypothalamic–pituitary function.

• Pituitary irradiation is combined with mitotane for patients with inoperable tumors or surgical failures. Bilateral adrenalectomy is reserved for patients who fail transsphenoidal surgery and external radiation therapy.

For ectopic ACTH syndrome

• Surgical excision is the treatment of choice if the hormone-secreting tumor can be localized and is resectable. Chemotherapy should be used when appropriate (*e.g.*, small cell cancers), with radiotherapy reserved for inoperable tumors (rarely effective).

• Long-term medical therapy (2–3 years) can be used with periodic (every 6 months) scanning to localize difficult-to-find tumors. Patients who begin to decompensate during this time due to excessive cortisol secretion should undergo bilateral adrenalectomy. Attempts to identify and resect the tumor should continue even after adrenalectomy.

For adrenal tumors

Excision of adrenal adenomas: usually complete, with cure of clinical syndrome and temporary adrenal insufficiency due to suppression of normal axis.

Excision of adrenal carcinomas: sometimes complete, although these carcinomas are often inoperable and usually recur (in which case, medical treatment is essential).

Micronodular or macronodular adrenal disease: bilateral adrenalectomy cures clinical syndrome and results in permanent adrenal insufficiency requiring hormone replacement (hydrocortisone and, in many cases, Florinef).

Treatment aims

To restore a normally functioning hypothalamo–pituitary axis, without damage to other endocrine axes.

Prognosis

• Young patients with mild Cushing's disease cured by transsphenoidal surgery without recurrence have no long-term sequelae.

• Patients with adrenal carcinoma usually suffer recurrence and death within months–years.

• Before effective treatment was available, 50% of patients with Cushing's syndrome died within 5 years of diagnosis.

• For adrenal adenomas, surgical excision cures most patients.

Follow-up and management

• Follow-up must be life-long because of the risk of recurrence and morbidity.

• Management depends on the individual patient and should be done by specialists.

Key references

1. Tsigos C, Chrousos GP: Differential diagnosis and management of Cushing's syndrome. *Ann Rev Med* 1996, **47**:443–461.
2. Flack MR, Oldfield EH, Cutler GB Jr, *et al.*: Urine free cortisol in the high-dose dexamethasone suppression test for the differential diagnosis of the Cushing syndrome. *Ann Intern Med* 1992, **116**:211–217.
3. Dichek HL, Nieman LK, Oldfield EH, *et al.*: A comparison of the standard high dose dexamethasone suppression test and the overnight 8-mg dexamethasone suppression test for the differential diagnosis of adrenocorticotropin-dependent Cushing's syndrome. *J Clin Endocrinol Metab* 1994, **78**:418–422.
4. Nieman LK, Oldfield EH, Wesley R, *et al.*: A simplified morning ovine corticotropin-releasing hormone stimulation test for the differential diagnosis of adrenocorticotropin-dependent Cushing's syndrome. *J Clin Endocrinol Metab* 1994, **77**:1308–1312.
5. Oldfield EH, Doppman JL, Nieman LK, *et al.*: Petrosal sinus sampling with and without corticotropin-releasing hormone for the differential diagnosis of Cushing's syndrome. *N Engl J Med* 1991, **325**:897–905.

Diagnosis

Symptoms

Cough that produces viscous and purulent sputum, shortness of breath, hemoptysis, wheezing.

Sinusitis, nasal polyposis.

Sterility in males, decreased fertility in females: due to absent or defective vas deferens in males and increased viscosity of vaginal secretions in females.

Signs of congestive heart failure and cor pulmonale in late disease.

Gastrointestinal symptoms: including meconium ileus or distal intestinal obstruction syndrome, malabsorption with weight loss, steatorrhea, failure to thrive in infancy and childhood, rectal prolapse, intussusception, volvulus, recurrent pancreatitis, cirrhosis.

Diabetes mellitus.

Salt depletion, heat stroke.

Signs

Inspiratory and expiratory rhonchi, rales, wheezes; barrel-shaped chest, reduced breath sounds, signs of hyperinflation; cyanosis, presence of *Pseudomonas* spp. in respiratory secretions, clubbing (hypertrophic osteoarthropathy).

Thin, anorexic appearance, weight loss: however, normal size and weight do not rule out a diagnosis of cystic fibrosis.

Right ventricular heave, pedal edema: with cor pulmonale.

Pneumothorax.

Respiratory failure.

Investigations

Sweat chloride testing by quantitative iontophoresis: still the standard for diagnosing cystic fibrosis. A level >60 mEg/L is diagnostic in most patients.

Pulmonary function testing: should be done to document severity of the obstructive respiratory defect. Pulmonary function studies may show airway hyperreactivity. Level of oxygenation by pulse oximetry or arterial blood gases should be done. Po_2 levels may be normal in mild disease, but eventually dip below 55 mm Hg on room air, signaling the need for oxygen supplementation. In end-stage disease, arterial Pco_2 increases.

Pancreatic function studies: may be done to demonstrate steatorrhea, although clinical description suffices in most cases.

Chest radiography: shows hyperinflation increased linear streaking and nodular-cystic pattern, which involve all lung areas, most particularly the right upper lobe.

Complications

Infective exacerbations: common.

Malnutrition with weight loss.

Pulmonary hypertension.

Gastrointestinal obstruction.

Diabetes mellitus.

Atelectasis.

Massive hemoptysis.

Cor pulmonale.

Respiratory failure.

Death.

Differential diagnosis

Asthma.

Chronic bronchitis.

Emphysema.

Bronchiectasis from any other causes.

Chronic pancreatitis.

Hypogammaglobulinemia.

$Alpha_1$-antitrypsin deficiency.

Malabsorption from any other cause.

Cirrhosis from any other cause.

Etiology

• Cystic fibrosis is an inherited disease that follows an autosomal recessive pattern of transmission. It is caused by mutations in the cystic fibrosis transmembrane conductance regulator (CFTR) protein. An abnormality resulting in the loss of phenylalanine residue at position 508 on the long arm of chromosome 7 accounts for ~70% of all cystic fibrosis mutations. More than 600 other abnormalities at this site have been identified with the disease.

Epidemiology

• Cystic fibrosis is the most common life-limiting genetic disease in the United States; its frequency varies with ethnicity.

• The incidence is ~1:3300 white newborns, ~1:15 300 in African-Americans, and 1:32 100 in Asian-Americans.

Treatment

Diet and lifestyle

• Many patients with cystic fibrosis have higher caloric needs both from malabsorption and the increased workload of breathing. Replacement of pancreatic enzymes with normal diets and even increased caloric intake will help to maintain normal or near-normal weight.

• Fat-soluble vitamins (vitamins A, D, E, and K) are recommended as a supplement.

Pharmacological treatment

Antibiotic therapy

• Oral antibiotics are indicated for minor exacerbations of sensitive organisms. Agents selected should reflect the sputum culture and the susceptibilities. Because *P. aeruginosa* is a frequent pathogen, antipseudomonal oral agents are often used.

• Ciprofloxacin, 750 mg twice daily, or ofloxacin, 400 mg twice daily for 2- to 3-weeks, would be common agents used against *Pseudomonas* spp. Patients with staphylococcus infection are often treated with dicloxacillin, 500 mg every 6 hours, or cephalexin, 500 mg every 6 hours.

• Patients with cystic fibrosis will have recurrent exacerbations. For major exacerbation, i.v. antibiotics are indicated; i.v. antibiotics should be chosen reflecting the culture and sensitivity of the sputum. In general, two agents are used, especially to obtain synergy against *Pseudomonas* spp. Popular combinations include ceftazidime/tobramycin or tobramycin/piperacillin. Dosage of aminoglycoside should be determined by monitoring plasma levels.

• Nebulized antipseudomonal antibiotic (tobramycin) can be added as a prophylactic measure to minimize the infective exacerbations. Inhalation tobramycin solution 300 mg twice daily is given every other month.

• Home i.v. antibiotics are becoming increasingly common, and guidelines for this therapy have been established for select candidates.

Bronchodilators

• These include inhaled β-agonists, inhaled anticholinergics (which have been shown to be efficacious in a subset of patients with cystic fibrosis), and theophyllines (occasionally used in patients with cystic fibrosis, especially in the presence of reactive airway disease).

Standard dosage	Inhaled β_2 agonists (*e.g.*, albuterol, metaproterenol, terbutaline), two puffs up to four times daily as needed. Ipratropium bromide inhaler (or another anticholinergic), two puffs four times daily. Theophylline, 300–600 mg daily.
Special points	*Theophylline:* plasma concentrations must be monitored; should be maintained between 10–15 μg/L.
Main drug interactions	*Inhaled β_2 agonists*: none. *Inhaled anticholinergics*: none. *Theophylline:* cimetidine, erythromycin, ciprofloxacin.
Main side effects	*Inhaled β_2 agonists*: tremor. *Inhaled anticholinergics*: dry mouth in rare cases. *Theophylline:* tachycardia and arrhythmias.

Mucolytic therapy

Standard dosage	DNase, aerosolized, 2.5 mg once daily.
Main drug interactions	None.
Special points	An approved nebulizer must be used to ensure adequate delivery.
Main side effects	Dysphagia or hoarseness, seen uncommonly.

Pancreatic enzymes

• Most patients with cystic fibrosis have exocrine pancreatic deficiency. Pancreatic enzymes are useful to minimize malabsorption. Dosing is empiric. Doses >6000 lipase U/kg/meal have been associated with colonic strictures in children. Fat-soluble vitamins (vitamins A, D, E, and K) are recommended.

Treatment aims

To minimize pulmonary exacerbations and forestall lung damage.

To treat the complication of obstruction and infection in the airways, enhance mucous clearance, and improve nutrition.

Other treatments

Chest physiotherapy: percussion and postural drainage are essential to minimize infective exacerbations. Recently, a flutter device has been shown to be effective in promoting pulmonary mucociliary clearance.

Oxygen: long-term oxygen therapy is indicated when the PO_2 drops <55 mm Hg or if there are clinical signs of cor pulmonale.

Transplantation: lung transplantation is a therapeutic option in appropriately selected patients with cystic fibrosis; recurrence of the cystic fibrosis defect does not occur in the transplanted lungs.

Gene therapy: the possibility of gene therapy is undergoing intensive investigation with the hope that it may either cure the disease or alleviate its symptoms.

Prognosis

Comprehensive treatment programs over the past 35 years have increased the overall survival rate of cystic fibrosis patients. The median survival of patients born with cystic fibrosis today is ~30 years. The development of right-sided failure with cor pulmonale is a poor prognostic sign. Elevation of the CO_2 or an FEV_1 of <30% of predicted indicates a mean survival of ~30 months.

Follow-up and management

• Patients should be monitored for pulmonary exacerbation, which will be treated aggressively with i.v. antibiotics.

• Culture and sensitivity of respiratory microbial organisms should guide therapy.

General references

Clinical Practice Guidelines for Cystic Fibrosis. Bethesda: The Cystic Fibrosis Foundation; 1997.

Davis PB, Drumm M, Konstan MW: Cystic fibrosis. *Am J Respir Crit Care Med* 1996, **154**:1229–1256.

Ramsey BW: Management of pulmonary disease in patients with cystic fibrosis. *N Engl J Med* 1996, 335:179–188.

Rosenstein BJ, Cutting GR: The diagnosis of cystic fibrosis: a consensus statement. *J Pediatr* 1998, **132**:589.

Stern RC: The diagnosis of cystic fibrosis. *N Engl J Med* 1997, **336**:487–491.

Cytomegalovirus infection in AIDS

Diagnosis

Symptoms

Loss of vision, floaters, decrease in visual acuity, unexplained fever: indicating retinitis (asymptomatic at early stage).

Fever, anorexia, odynophagia, weight loss, diarrhea, pain, cramps: indicating gastrointestinal tract infection (esophagitis, gastritis, colitis, or biliary involvement).

Fever, lower extremity weakness, headaches, seizures, somnolence: bladder incontinence indicating polyradiculopathy or encephalopathy.

Fever, cough, dyspnea: indicating pneumonitis.

Signs

Fever: in 60%–80% of patients with cytomegalovirus disseminated infection.

Decreased visual acuity: indicating retinitis.

Weight loss, abdominal tenderness, hemorrhages: indicating gastrointestinal tract infections.

Neurological deficit, lethargy, coma: indicating CNS complications.

Bilateral lower extremity weakness: other.

Increase of respiratory rate, minimal findings at auscultation: indicating pneumonitis.

Investigations

• Serological tests do not have diagnostic use.

Fundoscopy: in retinitis, shows hemorrhagic exudates and necrotic areas.

Endoscopy: in gastrointestinal tract infection, shows submucosal hemorrhages, ulceration; each level of tract may be involved, *e.g.*, esophagus, stomach, duodenum, small intestine, or colon.

Ultrasonography: in cholangitis, shows dilatation of biliary tract.

Biopsy: in cholangitis, shows cytomegalovirus inclusions.

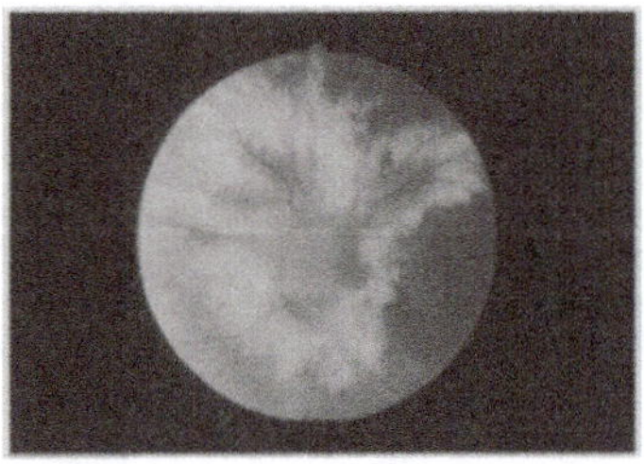

Fundoscopic appearance of cytomegalovirus retinitis. (*See* Color Plate.)

CSF culture: in encephalitis or myelitis, shows increased cells (nonspecific), presence of cytomegalovirus (unusual) in culture or polymerase chain reaction.

CT or MRI: in encephalitis or myelitis, shows ventriculitis or ependymitis, using contrast enhancement.

Transbronchial biopsy: in pneumonitis, shows cytomegalovirus inclusions.

Complications

Loss of vision, retinal detachment, acute retinal necrosis.

Gastrointestinal tract perforation, hemorrhages.

Respiratory failure.

Coma or death.

Differential diagnosis

Retinitis

Cotton-wool spot.

Toxoplasmosis.

Herpes simplex or varicella–zoster virus.

Acute retinal necrosis.

Syphilis.

Pneumocystis carinii choroiditis.

Gastrointestinal tract disorder

Cryptosporidiosis or microsporidiosis.

Giardia, Entamoeba, Shigella, Salmonella, Mycobacterium avium, or *Campylobacter* spp. infection.

Lymphoma.

Kaposi's sarcoma.

Herpes simplex virus.

Aphthous ulcers.

Encephalitis or myelitis

HIV encephalopathy or myelopathy.

Progressive multifocal leukoencephalopathy.

Aseptic meningitis.

Herpes virus encephalitis.

Spinal cord lymphoma.

Pneumonitis

P. carinii infection.

Mycobacteria infection.

Etiology

• Reactivation of latent cytomegalovirus infection due to underlying immune deficiency may be a cause.

Epidemiology

• >90% of homosexual or bisexual men have latent cytomegalovirus infection.

• Cytomegalovirus disease was found in 20%–40% of AIDS patients. The incidence is now lower in patients receiving highly active antiretroviral therapy (HAART).

• End-stage opportunistic infection occurs in 90% of patients with CD4 counts of $<50 \times 10^6$/L (median, 25×10^6/L).

Treatment

Diet and lifestyle

• No special precautions are necessary.

Pharmacological treatment

Choice of treatment

• Systemic treatment is indicated in acute visceral localization. Intravitreal implants may be used to treat retinitis and therefore avoid intravenous treatment; adjunctive oral ganciclovir is indicated to prevent systemic infection. Ganciclovir and foscarnet have similar efficacy: 90% in retinitis, 80%–95% in gastrointestinal tract disorder, 60%–80% in pneumonitis. Cidovofir is effective for treatment of retinitis.

• Maintenance treatment is indicated for retinitis and gastrointestinal tract involvement (nonsystematically). Ganciclovir and foscarnet have similar efficacy: 50% relapse within 4 months.

Ganciclovir

• Intravenous ganciclovir is less toxic than foscarnet.

• Oral ganciclovir may be considered for maintenance therapy.

• It is active against cytomegalovirus and herpesvirus.

• Disadvantages include hemotoxicity and resistance in some strains of cytomegalovirus.

Standard dosage	*Acute:* ganciclovir, 5 mg/kg i.v. twice daily, 20-minute infusion for 2–3 weeks. *Maintenance:* ganciclovir, 5 mg/kg i.v. once daily long term.
Contraindications	Neutropenia, anemia, resistant strains.
Main drug interactions	Zidovudine and other hemotoxic drugs.
Main side effects	Neutropenia, thrombocytopenia (frequent); rash-convulsion (unusual).

• Oral ganciclovir, 3 g daily, reduces progression of cytomegalovirus retinitis after i.v. induction. It may be considered in additon to retinal implants.

Foscarnet

• Foscarnet may be considered in individuals who progress while receiving ganciclovir.

• Advantages include absence of hemotoxicity and anti-HIV effect; disadvantages include the long infusion time.

Standard dosage	*Acute:* foscarnet, 90 mg/kg in 0.75–1.0 L saline isotonic solution i.v. twice daily, 90-minute infusion for 2–3 weeks. *Maintenance:* foscarnet, 90 mg/kg 0.75–1.0 L saline isotonic solution i.v. once daily, 90–120-minute infusion.
Contraindications	Renal impairment, concomitant nephrotoxic drugs.
Main drug interactions	Amphotericin B, i.v. pentamidine.
Main side effects	Nephrotoxicity, hypocalcemia, hypophosphatemia, nausea, genital ulcer.

Cidovofir

• Cidovofir may be considered in individuals who progress while receiving ganciclovir.

Standard dosage	Cidovofir, 5 mg/kg/wk induction × 2–3 weeks; then every other week.
Contraindications	Renal impairment.
Main drug interactions	Amphotericin, pentamidine.
Main side effects	Nephrotoxicity.

Treatment aims

To prevent replication of cytomegalovirus.

To halt progress of disease.

Prognosis

• The incidence of visceral manifestations of cytomegalovirus is approximately 30%; this is reduced with oral ganciclovir

• With maintenance treatment, retinitis relapse rates have been reduced in HAART-treated patients

Follow-up and management

• Patients having acute treatment should be followed up every week.

• Patients having maintenance treatment must be followed up every 2–3 weeks.

General references

d'Arminio Monforte A, Mainini F, Testa L, *et al.*: Predictors of cytomegalovirus disease, natural history, and autopsy findings in a cohort of patients with AIDS. *AIDS* 1997, **11**:517–524.

Jabs D, SOCA group: Mortality in patients with acquired immunodeficiency syndrome treated with either foscarnet or ganciclovir for cytomegalovirus retinitis. *N Engl J Med* 1992, **326**:213–220.

Rodriguez-Barradas MC, Stool E, Musher DM, *et al.*: Diagnosing and treating cytomegalovirus pneumonia in patients with AIDS. *Clin Infect Dis* 1996, **23**:76–81.

Spector SA, McKinley GF, Lalczari JP, *et al.*: Oral ganciclovir for the prevention of cytomegalovirus disease in persons with AIDS. *N Engl J Med* 1996, **334**:1491–1497.

Deep-vein thrombosis

Diagnosis

Symptoms

Asymptomatic

Typical of isolated calf thrombi.

Common in high-risk groups, *e.g.*, patients with acute cerebrovascular accident, spinal cord injuries, or malignancy; those undergoing general surgical or orthopedic surgical procedures; and hospitalized medical patients (*see* Prophylactic treatment).

Lower extremity pain

Dull ache or tightness in the calf or entire leg.

- Pain is generally worse when walking or standing.

Signs

Erythema, tenderness, and edema of the involved calf.

Slight fever and tachycardia.

Distention of superficial venous collateral vessels.

Palpable venous cord.

Homans' sign: limitation of dorsiflexion of the foot secondary to pain (insensitive and unreliable finding).

Phlegmasia cerulia dolens: pale, cool extremity resulting from severe venous obstruction and reflex arterial spasm.

Investigations

Venography: remains the gold standard of diagnosis: can define the location, extent, and degree of attachment of the thrombus; is the only reliable way to detect calf-vein or intra-abdominal thrombosis; limitations include the potential to induce thrombi at the injection site, the risk of contrast reaction, and decreased sensitivity for defining recurrent thrombosis.

Doppler ultrasonography: diagnostic finding is noncompressibility of a venous segment; the addition of Doppler technology to standard two-dimensional ultrasonography allows for detection of sonic differences in flow rates that occur with inspiration. Sensitivity for symptomatic patients is 93% by meta-analysis, and it has been shown to be safe to withhold anticoagulation in patients with serial negative studies (*e.g.*, days 1, 2, and 6) [1]. Specificity is high; positive results are diagnostic and do not require confirmatory studies. Clinical models have been developed to identify low-risk patients with clinically suspected lower extremity deep-vein thrombosis (DVT) [2]. If validated, clinicians will be able to identify persons in whom a single negative Doppler ultrasongraphy result essentially rules out DVT.

Impedance plethysmography: with a proximal venous obstruction there is a delay in the characteristic increase in calf impedance when a thigh cuff is deflated. Sensitivity and specificity are comparable to Doppler ultrasonography in the detection of symptomatic DVT.
Unacceptably low sensitivity for asymptomatic clots.

Complications

Pulmonary embolism.

Postphlebitic syndrome.

Recurrent DVT.

Differential diagnosis

Cellulitis.

Venous stasis or lymphedema.

Popliteal inflammatory cysts (Baker's cysts).

Pathophysiology

Most thrombi originate as a platelet nidus within the valvular sinuses of the calf veins.

Platelets and fibrin aggregate to form a red fibrin clot that either dissolves or becomes organized and adherent to the vessel wall.

At any time during the process the clot may propagate or detach.

Risk factors: Virchow's triad

Trauma: direct lower extremity trauma, surgery (particularly orthopedic surgery), prior DVT, or varicose veins.

Hypercoagulable states: antithrombin III deficiency, protein C deficiency, protein S deficiency, resistance to activated protein C (factor V Leiden), prothrombin 20210 variant, antiphospholipid syndrome, malignancy, hyperhomocysteinemia, estrogen-containing medications, polycythemia.

Stasis: anesthesia, cerebrovascular accident, paraplegia, hospitalized medical patients.

Epidemiology

(Extrapolation to account for clinically unsuspected cases.)

Five million episodes of DVT annually in the United States.

500 000 pulmonary emboli annually.

50 000 attributable deaths annually.

Treatment

Lifestyle management

• Bedrest is recommended with the legs elevated and the knees slightly bent until the local tenderness and swelling have subsided.

• Support stockings should be worn at all times after symptomatic DVT to prevent postphlebitic syndrome and symptomatic recurrences.

Pharmacological treatment

Initial therapy

• Therapy should begin with heparin for an immediate effect (80 U/kg bolus followed by 18 U/kg/h continuous infusion).

• A partial thromboplastin time (PTT) range of 1.5–2.5 times control should be targeted.

• Begin warfarin loading once target PTT is attained on heparin to a target international normalized ratio (INR) of 2.0–3.0.

• Five days of heparin infusion has been shown to be as effective as 10 days in terms of preventing recurrences.

• Thrombolytic agents are more effective at achieving early patency rates but are associated with an unacceptably higher incidence of serious bleeding.

Low molecular weight (LMW) heparin

• Treatment with LMW heparin at home during warfarin loading has been shown to be safe and cost-effective.

• The fixed subcutaneous dosage is higher than dosages used for prophylaxis and varies for different preparations.

• Monitoring of PTT is unnecessary.

Duration of treatment

• Oral anticoagulants should be continued for 3–6 months after an initial episode of DVT.

• Consider indefinite anticoagulation for recurrences and for events in the setting of permanent risk factors if there are no contraindications to anticoagulation.

Prophylactic treatment

Orthopedic surgery

• The rates for DVT are similar for LMW heparin vs. adjusted-dose warfarin to INR 2.0–3.0.

• Both warfarin and LMW heparin have shown limited efficacy in preventing DVT in patients undergoing knee replacement, although recent studies suggest a significant difference favoring LMW heparin (36.9% vs. 51.7% event rate) [3].

• Significantly fewer recurrences occur when prophylaxis with LMW heparin is continued for 1 month postoperatively rather than only during the hospitalization.

General surgery

Early ambulation only for low-risk patients (age <40 years, cases <60 minutes).

Heparin 5000 U twice daily, compression stockings, or intermittent pneumatic compression devices (IPC) for moderate-risk patients (age >40 years, major surgery).

Heparin 5000 U three times daily or LMW heparin for high-risk patients (age >40 years, major surgery, and other risk factors).

LMW heparin or adjusted-dose warfarin with IPC for very high-risk cases (multiple risk factors).

Hospitalized medical patients

• High-risk patients shown to benefit from heparin prophylaxis include intensive care unit patients, those with underlying malignancy, patients with spinal cord injuries or cerebrovascular accident, patients with indwelling catheters, and hospitalized patients aged >65 years.

Treatment aims

To prevent pulmonary embolism.

To prevent recurrent DVT.

To prevent the postphlebitic state.

Other treatment options

Thrombectomy: can achieve high early patency rates; the majority will eventually reocclude; indicated only for phlegmasia cerulea dolens.

Vena caval interruption: Greenfield filter has an extremely low rate of recurrent pulmonary embolism (4%) over 20 years; indicated for recurrent events (DVT or pulmonary embolism while adequately anticoagulated or when there is a contraindication to systemic anticoagulation.

Prognosis

Postphlebitic syndrome: nearly 30% of patients with DVT may develop characteristic changes of pain, swelling, and discoloration after 8 years of follow-up.

Recurrent DVT: rates are estimated to be 20% at 2 years and 30% at 8 years; independent risk factors for increased rates of recurrence include an underlying diagnosis of malignancy, younger age at first presentation, and a history of thrombophilia [4].

Key references

1. Heijboer H, *et al.*: A comparison of real-time compression ultrasonography with impedance plethysmography for the diagnosis of deep-vein thrombosis in symptomatic outpatients. *N Engl J Med* 1993, **329**:1365–1369.
2. Wells PS, Hirsh J, Anderson DR, *et al.*: Accuracy of clinical assessment of deep-vein thrombosis. *Lancet* 1995, **345**:1326–1330.
3. Leclerc JR, Geerts WH, Desjardins L, *et al.*: Prevention of venous thromboembolism after knee arthroplasty: a randomized, double-blind trial comparing enoxaparin with warfarin. *Ann Intern Med* 1996, **124**:619–626.
4. Pradoni P, *et al.*: The long-term clinical course of acute deep venous thrombosis. *Ann Intern Med* 1996, **125**:1–7.

Diagnosis

Definition

• Dementia is the syndrome of impairment in multiple domains of cognition, which must include memory, with intact consciousness.

• Symptoms, signs, and investigations are used to differentiate potentially treatable causes of dementias from the degenerative dementias.

Symptoms

• Patients may be unaware of deficits and deny symptoms (anosognosia); a history from a caregiver is therefore essential.

Memory loss: the most common presenting symptom.

Psychiatric disturbances: including depression, hallucinations, or behavioral changes.

Dysphasia, dyspraxia, visuospatial dysfunction, behavioral change: usually progressive and may occur in any order.

• Additional symptoms depend on the cause, *e.g.*, the following:

Headache: due to space-occupying lesions or temporal arteritis.

Fatigue: due to systemic disease (*e.g.*, HIV, hypothyroidism).

Weight loss: due to neoplasia.

Peripheral neuropathy: due to vitamin B_{12} deficiency, alcohol.

Seizures: may occur in patients with Alzheimer's disease or may have a focal cause.

Gait disturbances: can be seen in normal pressure hydrocephalus.

Focal neurological symptoms: including hemiparesis can be seen in multi-infarct dementia.

Signs

• The primary degenerative dementias (*e.g.*, Alzheimer's disease) have few signs other than those relating to higher cortical function.

Primitive reflexes (grasp, rooting, sucking), spasticity: late in dementia.

More widespread dysfunction: in dementia plus syndromes, *e.g.*, Huntington's disease (dementia plus chorea), multi-infarct dementia (dementia plus focal motor signs).

Papilledema or focal signs: suggesting a potentially treatable intracranial cause.

Investigations [1]

• Few specific tests are available, and none for the most common cause, Alzheimer's disease.

• Investigations are aimed at excluding secondary causes, *e.g.*, cerebral neoplasms, metabolic disturbances.

Psychometry: to assess pattern and severity of cognitive impairment and influence of the affective components.

Complete blood count, ESR measurement, routine biochemistry, serum vitamin B_{12}, thyroid function tests, treponemal serology, and HIV antibody serology: in some patients.

EEG: to exclude Creutzfeldt-Jakob disease or concomitant epilepsy.

CT or MRI: to exclude mass lesions, assess vascular changes, and determine regional atrophy.

PET: if available, to assess regional metabolism.

Lumbar puncture: in selected patients with rapidly progressing symptoms to exclude inflammatory changes.

Cerebral biopsy: rarely used; can provide definitive histological diagnosis.

• Many markers are available (apolipoprotein E, and so on); no clear indication for these.

Complications

Bronchopneumonia: due to aspiration.

Parkinsonism or seizures: can be late complications of several degenerative dementias.

Incontinence.

Differential diagnosis

Acute confusional states or delirium with fluctuating impairment of arousal.

Korsakoff's and Wernicke's syndromes secondary to alcohol abuse.

Focal neuropsychological deficits, *e.g.*, dysphasia.

"Pseudodementia" resulting from impairment of cognitive function by anxiety or depression.

Etiology

• Any disease disrupting the function of corticocortical or subcorticocortical connections can cause dementia, *e.g.*, the following:

Causes of degenerative dementia [2]

Alzheimer's disease, frontal-lobe degeneration, Pick's disease, cortical Lewy body disease, Huntington's disease, prion disease.

• Some hereditary dementias are associated with specific genetic markers, *e.g.*, rare families with Alzheimer's disease and amyloid precursor protein gene mutations, later-onset disease with the apolipoprotein E4 genotype.

• Neuropathologically, dementia of Alzheimer's disease is associated with senile plaques and neurofibrillary tangles in the cerebral cortex.

• ~15% of Alzheimer's disease is familial.

Vascular causes

Multiple cortical or subcortical infarcts, small-vessel disease (Binswanger's disease).

Potentially treatable causes

Neoplasms, normal-pressure hydrocephalus, trauma, subdural and extradural hematomas, drugs or toxins.

Vitamin B_{12} deficiency, hypothyroidism, renal and hepatic dysfunction, inherited metabolic disease.

Multiple sclerosis, temporal arteritis, cerebral vasculitis, sarcoid.

HIV, neurosyphilis, chronic viral encephalitides, chronic meningitides, cerebral Whipple's disease.

Epidemiology

• Dementia is common in elderly patients, occurring in 2%–5% aged >65 years; 20%–40% aged >80 years.

• Alzheimer's disease is the most common cause, accounting for 50% of dementia patients and a further 15%–20% in association with vascular disease.

Treatment

Diet and lifestyle

• Patients must avoid fatigue, alcohol, and centrally active medications unless clearly indicated.

• Patients should use cognitive aids, *e.g.*, clear labeling, diary, calendars.

• Medicalert bracelets should be worn.

• Safety issues including driving, using potentially dangerous equipment, and wandering need to be addressed.

• Supplemental vitamin E, and possibly estrogen replacement, may be helpful.

Pharmacological treatment [3]

• The treatment of dementia is first the treatment of the underlying cause when possible, *e.g.*, removal of meningioma, vitamin B_{12} replacement.

• The degeneration in Alzheimer's disease particularly affects the glutamatergic cortico-cortical association pyramidal neurons and the subcortico-cortical cholinergic projection neurons; cholinergic enhancement can improve memory in cholinergic-deficit states.

• Tacrine may be helpful to slow progression in some early cases [4].

Standard dosage	Tetrahydroaminoacridine (tacrine), 40–160 mg daily in divided doses.
Contraindications	Pregnancy, hepatic disease.
Main drug interactions	None.
Main side effects	Cholinergic effects, hepatotoxicity.

• Donepezil, another cholinesterase inhibitor, may slow progression of mild to moderate (MMSE 10-26) Alzheimer's dementia [5].

Standard dosage	Donepezil, 5 mg at bedtime.
Contraindications	Pregnancy.
Main drug interactions	None.
Main side effects	Nausea, diarrhea, dizziness.

• Other medications are under investigation.

• Many medications can be useful to manage psychiatric and behavioral problems, including antidepressants, anxiolytics, and antipsychotics.

Alternative medicine

Recommended use: none.

Common use: ginkgo (*Ginkgo biloba*); huperzine (*Huperzia serrata*); vitamin C; vitamin E; flaxseed oil; phosphatidylserine; L-acetyl carnitine; thiamin; methylcobalamin.

Caution: ginkgo biloba may cause bleeding.

Treatment aims

To treat the underlying cause, when possible.

To slow progression of disease.

To maintain patient safety and caregiver support.

Prognosis

• Prognosis depends on the causative disease.

Follow-up and management

• Management involves many disciplines: neurologists, psychiatrists, and geriatricians.

• Early involvement of social work and community psychiatric services is important.

Social support

Alzheimer's Association, 919 N. Michigan Ave., Suite 1000, Chicago, IL 60611-1676; phone (312) 335-870 or (800) 272-3900.

Legal issues

• Patients and families need to consider early living wills or medical, legal, and financial designation of power of attorney.

Key references

1. Cummings JL, Benson DF: *Dementia: a Clinical Approach*, edn 2. Oxford: Butterworth–Heinemann; 1992.
2. Geldmacher DS, Whitehouse PJ Jr: Differential diagnosis of Alzheimer's disease. *Neurology* 1997, **48(suppl)**:S2–S9.
3. Rossor MN: Management of neurological disorders: dementia. *J Neurol Neurosurg Psychiatry* 1994, **57**:1451–1456.
4. Knapp MJ, *et al.*: A thirty week randomized controlled trial of high dose tacrine in patients with Alzheimer's disease. *JAMA* 1994, **271**:985–991.
5. Rogers SL, Friedhoff LT: Efficacy and safety of Donepezil in patients with Alzheimer's disease. *Dementia* 1996, **7**:293–303.

Diagnosis

Symptoms and signs

Risk factors for major depressive illness

Prior episodes of depression (especially if age of onset <40 years).
Family history of depressive disorder.
Lack of social support, stressful life events.
Current alcohol or substance abuse.
Stroke.
Disabling chronic diseases.
Prior suicide attempts.
Postpartum period.
Age >75 years.

Unexplained or ill-defined symptoms: *e.g.*, chronic pain, sleep problems, somatic symptoms without organic cause after appropriate investigation.

Major depression [1]

Distinct periods (at least 2 weeks) of depressed mood (sometimes irritability in children or adolescents) or loss or interest of pleasure in usual activities, with at least four of the following:

Change in appetite or weight.
Difficulty in concentrating or making decisions.
Sleep disturbance (insomnia or hypersomnia).
Psychomotor agitation or retardation.
Anergia.
Suicidal thoughts or attempts.
Feelings of hopelessness, worthlessness, or guilt.

Dysthymia

Chronic disturbance with depressed mood, lasting 2 years—symptoms similar to those of a major depressive episode but less severe.

Depression in the elderly

Can manifest as decline in functional or cognitive status, or somatic symptoms, often without depressed mood.

Other forms of depression

- Seasonal (winter) major depressive episodes suggest seasonal affective disorder.
- Symptoms of depression insufficient in number, severity, or duration to meet criteria for major depression or dysthymic disorder are termed "subsyndromal depression."

Investigations

Screening for depression [2]

- Screening instruments (*e.g.*, Centers for Epidemiological Studies-Depression instrument, Beck Depression Inventory) may help identify depression among patients at low to moderate risk.
- Screening instruments are best used to rule out depression (negative result) and to identify patients for further investigation (positive result).

Laboratory investigations

- None are routinely indicated. In middle-aged and elderly patients, especially, investigations to rule out secondary depression (*e.g.*, associated with occult neoplasm or endocrine disturbance) may be warranted if the patient's symptoms suggest physical illness.

Assessment for complicated depression: identify and consider for immediate referral if suicidal thoughts or actions, frank delusions or hallucinations, prominent vegetative symptoms (*e.g.*, profound weight loss), or severe social role dysfunction is present.

Assessment for bipolar illness: symptoms of mania (periods of elevated or irritable mood, accompanied by hyperactivity, pressured speech, flight of ideas, euphoria, reduced sleep, distractability, or recklessness) should prompt consideration of lithium therapy and/or referral.

Screen for comorbid conditions: high prevalence of substance abuse (*e.g.*, alcohol), anxiety disorder, obsessive-compulsive disorder, personality disorder, somatization syndromes.

Complications

High suicide rate: 15%; highest risk groups are adolescents, middle-aged white men, and the elderly.

Distress to others in the patient's social network: *e.g.*, spouse, children.

Impairment in occupational function: *e.g.*, reduced productivity, absenteeism, unemployment.

Death due to dehydration and malnutrion: in elderly patients.

Differential diagnosis

Major depression

Medications: *e.g.*, steroids, antihypertensive agents, sedatives, alcohol, anticonvulsants.

Dementia: in elderly patients.

Schizophrenia, schizoaffective disorder.

Chronic anxiety state.

Uncomplicated bereavement.

Dysthymia

Major depression.

Personality disorder: *e.g.*, dependent, borderline, histrionic.

Normal fluctuation of mood.

Etiology

Biological factors: major depressive and bipolar disorders are familial; activity of biogenic amines (*i.e*, 5-hydroxytryptamine, noradrenaline) is altered in depressive and bipolar conditions.

Psychosocial factors: psychodynamic and cognitive factors and adverse life events have been associated with depressive illness.

Epidemiology

Prevalence of major depressive illness: in community-based populations, 2%–3% among men, 5%–10% among women.

Primary care outpatient settings: 4%–9%.

Patients with one or more general medical conditions: 12%–36%.

Poststroke: 10%–27%.

Subsyndromal depressive disorders: prevalence less well documented; estimated at 8%–10% of primary care patients.

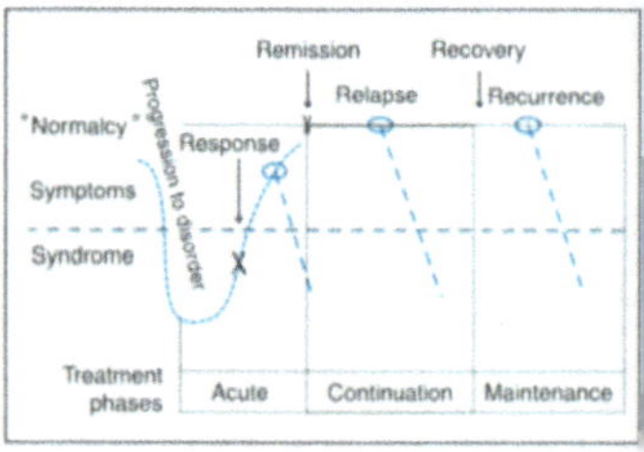

Stages of evaluation for major depression.

Treatment

Diet and lifestyle

• No special precautions are necessary.

Pharmacological treatment [1,3]

• Depression is a recurrent disorder; optimal management is evaluated in terms of the following:

Response to initial therapy: reduction of symptoms with treatment.

Remission: resolution of symptoms for a continuous period in an episode.

Recovery: a stable remission lasting at least 4–6 months.

Relapse: symptoms recur during remission.

Recurrence: a new episode after recovery.

Standard dosage
Selective serotonin reuptake inhibitors (SSRIs), *e.g.*, fluvoxamine, 50–300 mg; paroxetine, 20–50 mg.
Secondary amine tricyclic antidepressants (TCAs): nortriptyline, 25–250 mg; desipramine, 25–300 mg.
Other agents: buproprion, 100–450 mg; nefazodone, 200–600 mg; venlafaxine, 75–375 mg; mirtazapine, 15–45mg.

Contraindications
SSRIs: relate mainly to potential drug interactions (*see* below); pregnancy rating C (fluvoxamine) or B (paroxetine).
TCAs: relatively contraindicated in recent myocardial infarction, ischemic heart disease, heart block; pregnancy rating C (desiprimine) or D (nortryptiline).

Special points
SSRIs: generally have fewer side effects than older agents and may be considered first-line agents, especially for patients on few or no other medications; tricyclics and other new agents should be considered if drug interactions are likely with SSRI, or if no response to adequate doses of SSRIs.

Main drug interactions
All agents: potentially fatal interaction with monoamine oxidase inhibitors (MAOIs).
Tricyclics, SSRIs: potentially fatal interaction with antiarrythmic agents.
Most newer agents (fluvoxamine, nafazodone, paroxetine): hepatic cytochrome P_{450} isoenzyme inhibition, yielding a large number of potential drug interactions [3].
Serotonergic crisis (hypertension, hyperpyrexia, seizures) possible in patients on other serotonergic medications (*e.g.*, MAOIs, lithium, carbamazepine).

Main side effects
SSRIs: gastrointestinal upset, anorexia, vomiting, diarrhea, agitation, insomnia, sexual dysfunction.
TCAs: cardiac dysrhythmias (high levels or underlying cardiac disease), anticholinergic effects (dry mouth, orthostasis, constipation, urinary retention), lower seizure threshold.
Venlafaxine: supine hypertension, sexual dysfunction.
Bupropion: lowers seizure threshold.

Treatment aims

To obtain remission and prevent relapse of major depression.

Other treatments

• Clinical management alone (support, reassurance, education) is most appropriate for patients with mild symptoms.

• Electroconvulsive therapy under the direction of an experienced specialist should be considered for patients with severe or refractory symptoms.

Psychotherapy

• Psychotherapy may be more effective in preventing relapse.

Light therapy

• For patients with seasonal affective disorder, light therapy with ~2500–10 000 lux of full-spectrum light (10–20 times brighter than ordinary indoor light) for 30–60 minutes a day is recommended.

Prognosis

• With one, two, and three major depressive episodes, lifetime risk of recurrence is 50%, 70%, and 90%, respectively.

• Response in ~70% of patients (30% respond to placebo), may take 4–6 weeks.

Follow-up and management

Acute phase

• Provide a limited supply (1 week) of medication to patients with history of suicidal thoughts.

• Follow-up in 1 week after initiating therapy, with phone availability in the interim.

• Provide weekly visits for 6–8 weeks if depression severe, every 10–14 days if less severe.

Continuation phase

• Follow-up every 1–3 months.

• After 4–9 months, consider taper and discontinuation of medication. If symptoms recur, treat as new episode.

Key references

1. Greden J, Schwenk TL; Major mood disorders. In: *Primary Care Psychiatry.* Edited by Knesper DJ, Riba MB, Schwenk TL Philadelphia: W.B. Saunders. 1997
2. Mulrow CD, *et al.*: Case-finding instruments for depression in primary care. *Ann Intern Med* 1995, **122**:913–921.
3. Bhatia SC, Bhatia BK: Major depression: selecting safe and effective treatment. *Am Fam Physician* 1997, **55**:1683–1694.

Diabetes mellitus in children

Diagnosis

Symptoms

• Children may not admit to any symptoms until very late.

Thirst: including unusual forms, *e.g.*, drinking bath water.

Polyuria: bed wetting.

Weight loss.

Decreased appetite.

Vomiting: possibly with abdominal pain.

Confusion: without coma.

Signs

Uncomplicated

Irritability.

Dehydration.

Complicated

Semi-coma.

Deep but rapid respiration: Kussmaul's respiration.

Hypotension.

Infection: in ear, throat, lung, urinary tract.

Investigations (at presentation or with acute illness)

• The urine should be tested for glucose in a sick child with some of the above symptoms or signs, even if atypical.

Blood glucose and plasma sodium, potassium, bicarbonate, and urea measurement: glucose >400 mg/dL; sodium usually within normal range (but is dependent on level of hypoglycemia and dehydration); potassium low, normal, or high (value governs i.v. replacement); bicarbonate low.

Urinalysis: for glucose and ketones.

Blood pH, oxygen, carbon dioxide, acid–base status analysis: if indicated, based on clinical findings and results of blood tests.

Blood, urine, and/or sputum cultures: as clinically indicated.

Chest radiography: to identify consolidation due to pneumonia.

Complications

Hypovolemia, circulatory failure, cardiac arrest.

Cerebral edema: caused by over-rapid correction of hyperglycemia or electrolyte imbalance.

Hypokalemia or hyperkalemia: due to inappropriate i.v. potassium replacement and insulin treatment.

Hypophosphatemia.

Hypoglycemia: due to insulin treatment.

Long-term complications of diabetes (*e.g.*, retinopathy, neuropathy, nephropathy, and macrovascular disease): unusual in childhood.

Differential diagnosis

Newly diagnosed child

Any condition manifest by nausea and vomiting.

Any condition manifest by polyuria.

Any condition manifest by coma.

Previously diagnosed child

Uncontrolled diabetes mellitus due to intercurrent infection.

Coma due to hypoglycemia.

Etiology

Failure of insulin production and secretion due to lymphocytic infiltration and destruction of beta cells of the islets of Langerhans of the pancreas.

Epidemiology

• ~3 in 1000 US children have type 1 diabetes mellitus.

Treatment

Diet and lifestyle

• Parents should work closely with a dietitian to develop a realistic meal plan for their child.

• Meals should be regular, with snacks between main meals and at bedtime.

• Minimal restrictions should be placed on children, but bouts of physical exercise may require additional carbohydrate intake. Hypoglycemia must be avoided during activities in which children are exposed to cold because their thermal regulation fails and hypothermia may occur.

• Glucose in the form of tablets or gel must be carried by a child or an accompanying adult. Parents should be taught to give glucagon, used when a hypoglycemic child cannot take oral glucose.

Pharmacological treatment [1]

• Oral agents have no place in the management of childhood-onset type 1 diabetes mellitus.

• Long- and short-acting insulins are typically injected before meals, at a frequency and combination meant to achieve maximum glycemic control.

• Humalog insulin, with its rapid onset of action, can be administered at the end of a meal. This can be particularly useful for young children with irregular eating habits.

• In small children, insulin therapy may present a problem because of their sleep patterns. The evening injection can be divided so that short-acting insulin is given before the evening meal and intermediate-acting insulin later in the evening; this can be given while the child is asleep.

• Insulin-containing pens are available containing both short- and intermediate-acting insulin.

• Regimens can be altered so that insulin is injected before each meal and intermediate-acting insulin at bedtime, the latter to provide sufficient insulin during sleep.

Standard dosage	Insulin, 0.5–1 U/kg daily, adjusted according to blood glucose concentration.
Contraindications	Very rare hypersensitivity (usually due to preservatives in insulin preparation).
Special points	Home blood glucose monitoring essential for good glucose control.
Main drug interactions	High-dose beta-agonists cause severe insulin resistance.
Main side effects	Hyper- or hypoglycemia due to inappropriate dosing.

• Insulin can also be given by continuous infusions using pumps.

Treatment aims

To return child to health and normal lifestyle.
To achieve glycemic control.

Prognosis

• In the past, life expectancy was reduced by one-third, although this is rapidly improving.

Follow-up and management

• Regular attendance at a combined pediatric and diabetic clinic is vital to monitor growth, provide advice on diet as child gets older, monitor long-term glycemic control, and check for complications [2].

• Management at presentation requires the following:

With hyperglycemia and ketonuria but no vomiting, outpatient management (i.v. fluids not needed).

With vomiting, hospital admission for i.v. rehydration, insulin treatment, and identification of immediate cause of diabetic ketoacidosis.

Frequent visits to specialist diabetic unit or frequent visits of staff of the center to the child's home.

Adjustment of dose of insulin on the basis of blood glucose values.

Two or more s.c. insulin injections daily along with change in diet.

Depending on age, education of child about the diabetic process and basic physiology of glucose homeostasis by a skilled member of the diabetic team, usually a specialist nurse.

Education of parents about their child's disease and its control (treatment of hyperglycemia, hypoglycemia, alteration of diet for physical activities, holidays, and sick days).

Counseling to enable parents to come to terms with their child's illness.

Key references

1. Kostraba JN, *et al.*: Increasing trend of outpatient management of children with newly diagnosed IDDM. *Diabetes Care* 1992, **15**:95–100.
2. Diabetes Control and Complication Trial Group: The effect of intensive treatment of diabetes on the development and progression of longterm complications in insulin dependent diabetes. *N Engl J Med* 1993, **329**:977–986.

Diagnosis

Symptoms

• Symptoms are usually of short duration (days to weeks), often longer in older patients.

Polyuria.

Polydipsia.

Weight loss.

Lethargy.

Diabetic ketoacidosis or coma: if disease undetected or ignored; progression of above symptoms, with vomiting, abdominal pain, increased respiratory rate; may progress to altered mental status, including coma.

Signs

• Initially, few signs may be present.

Mild dehydration, weight loss: early signs.

Shock, severe dehydration, Kussmaul's respiration, ketones on breath (fruity), reduced level of consciousness: later signs.

Investigations

Laboratory blood glucose measurement: essential for diagnosis; in the absence of diabetic ketoacidosis, two fasting glucose levels >126 mg/dL are required for the diagnosis of diabetes [1].

Urinalysis: may show glycosuria; ketonuria may also be present.

Arterial blood gas measurement: shows metabolic acidosis in ketoacidosis.

Electrolyte analysis: wide variation in cases of diabetic ketoacidosis; typical findings include hyponatremia, hyperkalemia, hypophosphatemia, anion gap acidosis, and evidence of dehydration.

Anti-islet cell receptor antibody tests: usually unnecessary; can be used to confirm the diagnosis of type I diabetes.

Complications [2]

• Complications are rare before 5–10 years' duration of type I diabetes. Microvascular complications (retinopathy, nephropathy, and neuropathy) can be prevented or slowed with improved glucose control [3].

Diabetic retinopathy: background changes in >75% by age 30 years, only affects vision if near macula; proliferative affects fewer patients but threatens vision by vitreous hemorrhage/fibrosis; treated by laser; most common cause of new adult blindness in patients <65 years of age.

Diabetic nephropathy: affects up to 40% after age 30 years, but rate probably now falling; proteinuria is hallmark, with progressive renal impairment; can be slowed by early diagnosis (yearly screening for microalbuminuria) and vigorous antihypertensive treatment; angiotensin-converting enzyme inhibitors have been shown to slow the progression of diabetic nephropathy.

Diabetic neuropathy: many forms, most common being symmetrical sensory polyneuropathy leading to loss of temperature, vibration, and pain sense, hence easy progression to foot ulceration; also several painful forms.

Large-vessel disease (coronary, cerebrovascular, peripheral): also much more common, especially when nephropathy is present; possibly more diffuse than nondiabetic large-vessel disease, but otherwise generally similar.

• Other problems include skin disorders, especially necrobiosis, joint disorders, mononeuropathies, and cataracts.

Differential diagnosis

• In patients with altered mental status, the diagnosis of diabetic ketoacidosis is usually straightforward. However, a variety of illnesses can precipitate, exacerbate, or mimic diabetic ketoacidosis. Always consider infection, surgical abdomen, stroke, myocardial infarction, and alcohol and other drugs.

• Deciding whether the patient is insulin-dependent can be difficult if the diagnosis is made early; in case of doubt, short-term insulin treatment should be given.

Etiology

• The process occurs via an autoimmune mechanism with antibodies against pancreatic islet-cells, which show insulitis and are progressively destroyed.

• The triggering environmental agent is not known.

Epidemiology

• Type 1 diabetes mellitus can occur at any age, but onset is frequently in children and young adults (hence the alternative term "juvenile-onset diabetes mellitus").

• It occurs most often in whites, especially in those farthest from the equator (Scandinavia, southern New Zealand); other races differ in genetic susceptibility.

• It affects ~3 in 1000 of the US population and represents ~10% of all patients with diabetes.

Treatment

Diet and lifestyle

• Annual dietary consultation is strongly recommended; the diet should be high in unrefined carbohydrate, low in simple sugars, with high fiber and low fat, spread throughout the day, including three meals and a bedtime snack.

• Normal activity is advised, except for a few career and driving limitations.

Pharmacological treatment [2]

• After insulin dependency has been established, exogenous insulin is required.

Types of insulin

• Mainly human biosynthetic insulins are used; pork and beef insulins are still available in some preparations.

Ultra-short acting: Humalog or H.

Short acting: regular or R.

Intermediate-acting (isophane): NPH or N.

Intermediate-acting (zinc): lente or L.

Long-acting: ultralente or U.

Premixed (NPH/R): 70%/30%, 60%/40%, 50%/50%.

Premixed (N/H): 75%/25%

Types of regimen (a sampling)

Twice-daily: minimum level of therapy, including mixtures of short- and long-acting insulins.

Added bedtime dose: mixture in morning, short-acting before supper, intermediate-acting before bedtime; flexible regimen, especially for patients troubled by overnight hypoglycemia.

Multiple daily injections: long-acting overnight, short-acting boluses before meals.

Insulin pump: continuous s.c. infusion of regular or Humalog insulin with premeal boluses.

Practical issues

Sites of injection: abdomen, leg or buttock, arm (s.c.).

Timing: usually 30 minutes before meal (at mealtime with Humalog).

Exercise: requires either extra food or reduced insulin dose.

Insulin infusion (variable rate): best treatment for ketoacidosis, for unstable diabetes, and during surgery.

Hypoglycemia

• This is the major unwanted effect of insulin treatment and the predominant concern of many patients.

• It is more common with long duration of diabetes and "tight control." Frequent episodes of hypoglycemia can result in subsequent hypoglycemic unawareness.

• Symptoms include sweating, shaking, hunger, palpitation, lack of concentration, confusion, and restlessness. In severe cases, seizure or coma may occur.

• Hypoglycemia should be treated by oral glucose or food (*e.g.*, skim milk or orange juice), i.v. glucose, or i.m. glucagon.

See Hypoglycemia *for details.*

Alternative medicine

Recommended use: none

Common use: chromium; bitter melon (*Momordica charantia*); bilberry (*Vaccinium myrtillus*); garlic (*Allium sativa*); Fenugreek (*Triagonella foenum-gracum*); Goat's rue (*Galega officinalis*); blueberry (*Vaccinium* spp.).

Caution: none.

Treatment aims

To restore normal sense of well-being.

To achieve optimal glycemic control without significant hypoglycemia.

To provide patient education and self-care.

To prevent complications.

Prognosis

• The prognosis is excellent and improving in the short and medium terms. Ketoacidosis and hypoglycemia are now rare causes of death.

• Longer-term prognosis largely depends on long-term glycemic control and compliance with screening and treatment [3].

• Major causes of death are end-stage renal failure and coronary artery disease.

• Major causes of morbidity include proliferative retinopathy leading to blindness, coronary artery disease and peripheral vascular disease, and neuropathy leading to foot ulceration, claudication, or gangrene.

Follow-up and management

• Long-term follow-up is essential for continued education, checks on long-term control (hemoglobin A_{1c}), home capillary blood glucose levels preprandially, and screening for complications (especially eye and foot examination, proteinuria).

• Potentially fertile women should have pre-conception counseling and optimal control before conception.

• Patient and family education by specialist nurses and dietitians is essential.

• Most patients should test their own blood glucose and learn to adjust insulin.

Patient support

American Diabetes Association, 1660 Duke Street, Alexandria, VA 22314; tel 1-800-ADA-DISC.

Key references

1. The Expert Committee on the Diagnosis and Classification of Diabetes Mellitus: Report of the Expert Committee on the Diagnosis and Classification of Diabetes Mellitus. *Diabetes Care* 1997, **20**:1183–1197.
2. American Diabetes Association: *Medical Management of Insulin-Dependent (Type I) Diabetes*, edn 2. Alexandria, VA: American Diabetes Association; 1994.
3. Diabetes Control and Complications Trial Research Group: The effect of intensive treatment of diabetes on the development and progression of long-term complications in insulin dependent diabetes. *N Engl J Med* 1993, **329**:977–986.

Diabetes mellitus type 2 (noninsulin-dependent)

Diagnosis

Symptoms

• ~50% of patients are symptomatic; 50% found on routine or accidental screening.

• Common symptoms, often manifest over many months or years, include the following:

Polyuria, polydipsia.

Candidal vaginitis or balanitis.

Weight loss, fatigue, blurred vision.

Hyperglycemia nonketotic coma, with severe dehydration and hyperosmolality: rare manifestation.

Signs

• Generally, no signs are manifest.

• Patients may present with the following:

Obesity.

Foot ulceration or infection.

Diabetic retinopathy or peripheral neuropathy.

Signs of secondary causes of diabetes: *e.g.*, steroid use, acromegaly, Cushing's syndrome, thyrotoxicosis.

Investigations

Blood glucose measurement: two fasting levels >126 mg/dL is diagnostic; the National Institutes of Health recommends screening fasting glucose levels every 3 years in patients who are ≥45 years of age or at increased risk [1].

Glucose tolerance test: needed when diagnosis in doubt.

Measurement of hemoglobin A_{1c}: elevated concentration is strong evidence for diabetes [2].

Measurement of iron and total iron-binding capacity: to rule out hemochromatosis.

Measurement of thyroxine and thyroid-stimulating hormone: to rule out thyrotoxicosis.

• Glycosuria alone and self-monitoring of blood glucoses should not be considered diagnostic.

Complications

• Complications are often present at the time of diagnosis because patients may have had several years of asymptomatic hyperglycemia.

Diabetic retinopathy: may be present at diagnosis, only affects vision if near macula; macular edema frequent with major reduction of visual acuity; proliferative affects fewer but threatens vision by vitreous hemorrhage/fibrosis; both treated by laser.

Diabetic nephropathy: less common than in insulin-dependent diabetes mellitus, except in nonwhites; can be slowed by vigorous antihypertensive treatment (*e.g.*, angiotensin-converting enzyme inhibitors).

Diabetic neuropathy: many forms, most common being symmetrical sensory polyneuropathy leading to loss of temperature, vibration, and pain sense, hence easy progression to foot ulceration.

Large-vessel disease (coronary, cerebrovascular, peripheral): a very common complication with higher prevalence in patients with diabetic nephropathy; possibly more diffuse than nondiabetic large-vessel disease, but otherwise generally similar; these, especially coronary artery disease, are major causes of premature death.

Insulin

• Insulin is indicated for symptomatic or uncontrolled type 2 diabetes mellitus despite maximal therapy oral agents, in addition to diet.

• Usually needed only once or twice daily; a longer-acting formulation may be used to control basal hyperglycemia.

• *See* Diabetes mellitus type 1 *for details.*

Differential diagnosis

• Diagnosis is not usually problematic, after diabetes mellitus has been considered; possible errors include the following:

Urinary tract infection.

Prostatic hyperplasia.

Primary polydipsia.

Diabetes insipidus.

Etiology [1]

• The cause of type 2 diabetes mellitus is unknown. However, patients have a mixture of progressive insulin deficiency and insulin resistance, with contributions of the two varying widely among individuals.

• A strong familial component is evident.

• A marked link with obesity is seen.

• Very rarely, patients have insulin receptor abnormalities or antireceptor antibodies.

Epidemiology

• The US prevalence of diagnosed diabetes is ~3%, although an additional 3% may go undiagnosed.

• The disease is more common in Asians and blacks.

• It is becoming more common in developing nations.

Treatment

Diet and lifestyle

• Weight loss and exercise are critical components of any treatment plan.

• The diet should be high in unrefined carbohydrate, low in simple sugars, with high fiber and low fat, spread throughout the day.

Pharmacological treatment [3]

• Diet and exercise should be used initially unless the patient is markedly symptomatic or has a significant elevation in hemoglobin A_{1c}.

• Each of the following oral therapies reduces hemoglobin A_{1c} levels by 0.5%–1.5%. Additive effects for some combinations have been reported.

Sulfonylureas

• These medications act as insulin secretagogues.

Standard dosage	Glyburide, 2.5–20 mg orally daily, given once or twice daily. Glipizide, 2.5–20 mg orally daily, given once or twice daily. Glibenclamide, 1–8 mg daily.
Contraindications	Breast-feeding, porphyria, pregnancy; caution in elderly patients and those with renal or hepatic dysfunction.
Main drug interactions	*See manufacturer's current prescribing information.*
Main side effects	Hypoglycemia is common; otherwise occasional rashes, jaundice, headache.

Biguanides

• Metformin reduces hepatic gluconeogenesis and may decrease carbohydrate absorption.

Standard dosage	Metformin, 1–2.5 g daily in divided doses.
Contraindications	Hepatic or renal impairment (creatinine >1.4 mg/dL in men or 1.3 in women), heart failure, pregnancy.
Special points	Does not cause hypoglycemia; may rarely cause lactic acidosis. Should be discontinued prior to and 2 days after any radiological study using i.v. contrast.
Main side effects	Flatulence, anorexia, diarrhea, sometimes transient.

Alpha-glucosidase inhibitors

• Acarbose decreases the rate of glucose absorption, which reduces postprandial rises in glucose.

Standard dosage	Acarbose, 25 mg with meals to start; titrate up to 50 mg with each meal.
Contraindications	*See manufacturer's current prescribing information.*
Special points	Does not cause hypoglycemia; can be used with other oral medications and insulin.
Side effects	Flatulence, diarrhea (usually, but not always, transient).

Insulin sensitizers

• Troglitazone increases insulin sensitivity in multiple tissues, most notably muscle.

Standard dosage	Troglitazone, 200–600 mg daily with food.
Contraindications	*See manufacturer's current prescribing information.*
Special points	Does not cause hypoglycemia; most expensive oral agent.
Drug interactions	Lowers serum levels of administered estrogens by 30%, which may reduce the efficacy of some oral contraceptives.
Side effects	Very well tolerated; however, there is a 2% incidence of elevated liver function tests.

Treatment aims

To restore normal sense of well-being.

To achieve optimal glycemic control without significant hypoglycemia.

To provide patient education.

To prevent complications.

Prognosis

• Mortality is increased primarily as a result of excess cardiovascular disease, myocardial infarction, stroke, and peripheral vascular disease.

• Morbidity is also due to these causes, as well as to retinopathy, renal disease, and foot ulceration.

• Recent studies support that glycemic control does reduce complications in patients with type 2 diabetes, including mortality.

Follow-up and management

• Patients need long-term follow-up for treatment aims and screening for development of complications.

• Hemoglobin A_{1c} is an objective marker of glycemic control.

Patient support

American Diabetes Association, 1660 Duke Street, Alexandria, VA 22314; tel 1-800-ADA-DISC.

Key references

1. The Expert Committee on the Diagnosis and Classification of Diabetes Mellitus: Report of the Expert Committee on the Diagnosis and Classification of Diabetes Mellitus. *Diabetes Care* 1997, **20**:1183–1197.
2. Peters AL, Davidson MB, Schriger DL, Hasselblad V, for the Meta-Analysis Research Group on the Diagnosis of Diabetes Using Glycated Hemoglobin Levels: A clinical approach of the diagnosis of diabetes mellitus. *JAMA* 1996, **276**:1246–1252.
3. American Diabetes Association: *Medical Management of Non-Insulin-Dependent (Type II) Diabetes*, edn 3. Alexandria, VA: American Diabetes Association; 1994.

Diabetic management in pregnancy

Diagnosis

Symptoms and signs

• Diabetes may be a pre-existing condition (pregestational diabetes) or may develop during pregnancy (gestational diabetes). Also, some women with asymptomatic pregestational diabetes are first diagnosed during pregnancy. If this situation is suspected, the patient should be treated as a pregestational diabetic during the pregnancy.

• For women with pregestational diabetes, pre-conception counseling and optimal glucose control are of critical importance. A good rule of thumb is to inquire about contraception and prepregnancy planning at each visit.

• Gestational diabetes is usually asymptomatic; however, some patients may complain of an increase in their baseline polyuria. Because these patients have no history of diabetes, it is not necessary to screen for complications.

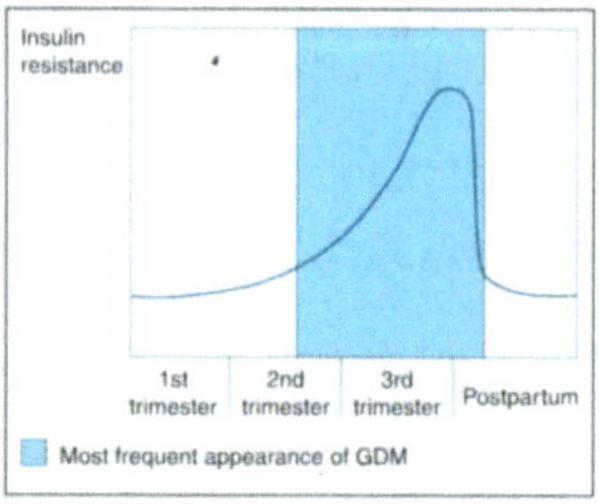

Increase of insulin resistance and the appearance of gestational diabetes mellitus (GDM).

Investigations [1,2]

• All women with risk factors for gestational diabetes mellitus should be screened at 12 weeks.
• All pregnant women should be screened at 24–28 weeks.
• If fasting blood glucose is >90 mg/dL, random blood glucose is >125 mg/dL, or if failed 1-hour screening test, a glucose tolerance test should be considered.

Screening test: give 50 g oral glucose solution and measure plasma glucose at 1 hour. All women with plasma glucose >140 mg/dL at 1 hour should have a 3-hour oral glucose tolerance test (GTT).

3-hour GTT: in pregnancy, 100 g glucose solution with blood glucose measured at fasting and at 1, 2, and 3 hours. Gestational diabetes is diagnosed if two or more values > these parameters: fasting >95 mg/dL; 1 hour >180 mg/dL; 2 hours >155 mg/dL; 3 hours >140 mg/dL.

Evaluation of pregnant women with pregestational diabetes

Hemoglobin A_{1c}: should be checked monthly and kept in the normal range throughout pregnancy; discrepancies between hemoglobin A_{1c} values and self-monitoring of glucoses need to be investigated; usually these can be explained by problems with home monitoring.

Dilated retinal examination (by a qualified examiner): during the first trimester, with follow-up as needed.

Electrolytes, blood urea nitrogen, creatinine, and complete blood count.

24-hour urine for protein and creatinine clearance: if both are normal in the first trimester, there is probably little need to repeat these studies unless specific problems arise.

Ultrasound for fetal abnormalities (including cardiac): performed at ~18 weeks.

Evaluation of all pregnant women with diabetes

Hemoglobin A_{1c}: *see above.*

Self-monitoring of glucoses: at least four times daily; targets vary from center to center, but are generally 65–95 mg/dL before meals, <110 mg/dL before bed, and <120 mg/dL 2 hours after meals.

Third-trimester monitoring of fetal weight and viability: *e.g.*, nonstress tests and biophysical profiles.

Complications

Maternal

Worsening retinopathy, nephropathy.
Worsening macrovascular disease.
Increased pre-eclamptic toxemia.
Hydramnios.
Ketosis, hyperglycemia.
Death.

Fetal

Respiratory distress, jaundice, macrosomia.
Hypoglycemia.
Hypocalcemia.
Polycythemia.
Microcephaly, sacral agenesis.
Congenital malformations.
Congenital heart disease.
Fetal demise.

Differential diagnosis

Not applicable.

Etiology

Causes of gestational diabetes (increased insulin resistance)

Increased concentrations of progesterone, cortisol, prolactin, and human placental lactogen, which also influence postinsulin receptor metabolism.

Poorly understood processes, which increase insulin need 2–3-fold during pregnancy.

Risk factors for gestational diabetes mellitus

Age.
Increasing parity.
Previous gestational diabetes.
First-degree relative with diabetes.
Fasting glycosuria.
Previous unexplained fetal death.
Previous "large for dates" baby.
Previous congenital anomaly.
Maternal obesity.

Epidemiology

• Prevalence of gestational diabetes mellitus is increasing in the United States, and is now about 4% to 5%.
• Prevalence ranges from 2% to 13% depending on the diagnostic criteria and population studied.

Pregnancy counseling [2]

• Diabetic women must be advised of the following:
• The risk of maternal death is slightly higher than in nondiabetic women.
• Pre-existing complications, *e.g.*, retinopathy, nephropathy, and heart disease, may worsen in pregnancy.
• Cesarean section is more likely.
• Numerous antenatal visits and close supervision will be needed.
• Home blood glucose monitoring will be needed several times daily.
• Multiple insulin injections will be needed daily.
• Diet must be adhered to, and smoking and drinking must be stopped.
• The baby may be at increased risk of malformations and serious neonatal complications. However, these risks can be reduced by close supervision and cooperation, and maintenance of euglycemia.

Treatment

Diet and lifestyle

• Known diabetic patients should already have consulted a dietitian; those with gestational diabetes must be referred.

• Patients must ensure that 50% of energy intake is carbohydrate and that their diet contains adequate calcium and vitamins.

• Iron and folate supplements are needed.

• Patients should aim to achieve the normal weight gain in pregnancy by appropriate food intake.

Pharmacological treatment [2]

During pregnancy

• All patients on oral agents [3] should be transferred to insulin, usually given 2–4 times daily; a mixture of short- and intermediate-acting insulin can be used depending on patient needs, or a late dose of intermediate-acting insulin before bed and short-acting insulin before meals.

• Most patients with gestational diabetes mellitus are initially treated by dietary advice; approximately 60% will eventually need insulin, which can be given as a mixture of short- and intermediate-acting insulin twice daily, with possible supplement of short-acting insulin before lunch.

• Insulin needs increase during pregnancy; >100 U daily may be required.

• A sudden decline in insulin requirements in the second or third trimester may be an indication of fetal problems and should be evaluated promptly.

During labor and delivery

• 1–4 U of insulin i.v. are needed hourly; insulin is adjusted based on hourly capillary and/or plasma glucose determination. Insulin requirements fall during and after labor.

• Blood glucose must be maintained at near-normal concentrations.

• In prolonged labor or in high-risk patients, an independent energy source, *e.g.*, 10% dextrose, 100 mL i.v. hourly, is needed.

• Insulin should be delivered by an infusion pump (regular insulin, 50 U in 50 mL normal saline solution).

• Beta-agonists used for premature labor may cause insulin resistance.

• General anesthesia and cesarean section increase insulin needs.

• After delivery, insulin needs fall dramatically.

• Patients with gestational diabetes mellitus usually do not need postpartum therapy, but should have a standard 2-hour glucose tolerance test 6 weeks postpartum.

Other concerns

• Angiotensin-converting enzyme inhibitors are contraindicated in pregnancy and lactation.

• Oral agents are contraindicated in pregnancy and lactation.

• Glucocorticoids may precipitate diabetic ketoacidosis in women with pregestational type I diabetes, particularly when given later in pregnancy to induce fetal lung maturity.

Treatment aims

To maintain preprandial blood glucose at 65–90 mg/dL, 2-hour postprandial blood glucose 120 mg/dL, and hemoglobin A$_{1c}$ in normal range.

To achieve a mature fetus, with no neonatal or maternal complications.

Prognosis

• Retinopathy, nephropathy, and macrovascular disease can worsen during pregnancy, but this can be minimized by good metabolic control and supervision.

• Perinatal mortality is increased in diabetic pregnancies; half of the increase is associated with poor control.

• Maternal mortality is slightly higher than in nondiabetic patients.

Follow-up and management

Initial assessment

• Patients may benefit from a joint clinic with a diabetologist and an obstetrician.

• Patients should be screened for diabetic complications.

• Blood pressure should be monitored at each visit.

Subsequent assessment

• Follow-up should be every 1–2 weeks, depending on the patient's need.

• In gestational diabetes: risk of non–insulin-dependent diabetes mellitus at 5 years is 30%–50%.

Key references

1. The Expert Committee on the Diagnosis and Classification of Diabetes Mellitus: Report of the Expert Committee on the Diagnosis and Classification of Diabetes Mellitus. *Diabetes Care* 1997, **20**:1183–1197.
2. American Diabetes Association: *Medical Management of Pregnancy Complicated by Diabetes*. Alexandria, VA: American Diabetes Association; 1995.
3. Hellmuth E, Damm P, Molsted-Pedersen L: Congenital malformations in offspring of diabetic women treated with oral hypoglycaemic agents during pregnancy. *Diabetic Med* 1994, **11**:471–474.

Diabetic management in surgery

Diagnosis

Symptoms

• Well-controlled diabetic patients having an operation have no symptoms.

Thirst and polyuria: indicating poor control in patients with any type of diabetes.

Nausea and abdominal pain: indicating very poor control in insulin-dependent patients.

Signs

Tachycardia, ketosis, dehydration, hypotension: signs of poor diabetic control in insulin-dependent patients; these will most probably develop following surgery if preoperative control of diabetes was poor.

Investigations [1,2]

For elective surgery

Blood glucose profile: 2 days before patient has a major operation; hemoglobin A_{1c} should ideally be within 10% of normal range.

• Other investigations are the same as for nondiabetic patients.

For emergency surgery

Blood glucose measurement: to assess hyperglycemia.

Electrolytes, blood urea nitrogen analysis: to assess renal function and electrolyte balance.

Blood gas analysis: to assess acid–base balance.

Complications

Cardiovascular problems: particularly myocardial infarction; the major perioperative causes of death in diabetic patients.

Infection and poor wound healing: in poorly controlled diabetic patients [3].

Differential diagnosis

• Acute surgical abdominal disorders can be confused with severely decompensated diabetes in insulin-dependent patients: a medical opinion is essential.

Etiology

• The stress response to surgery and anesthesia is characterized by hyperglycemia, suppression of insulin release, and insulin resistance. This is due to increases in cortisol, catecholamines, and other counterregulatory hormones.

• The stress response is greater with major surgery.

Epidemiology

• 50% of diabetic patients have operations at some point in their lives.

• Patients with macrovascular disease will probably have several operations.

Treatment

Diet and lifestyle

• Major operations are often followed by a period of relative or absolute starvation: adequate energy intake and insulin must be supplied to type I diabetic patients as insulin depletion leads to ketoacidosis.

• Breakfast and oral agents are omitted if the operation is in the morning.

• If the operation is minor, eating and oral agents can soon be restarted.

Pharmacological treatment [1,2]

• Patients with "brittle" diabetes may need a glucose insulin infusion for 24 hours before surgery.

• Regional anesthesia does not produce the same degree of stress response as general anesthesia.

• Infections should be treated aggressively with antibiotics.

For non–insulin-requiring diabetes: preoperative

• Metformin, which may cause lactic acidosis, and chlorpropamide, because its long action may lead to hypoglycemia, should be avoided for at least 48 hours prior to surgery.

• Patients should be given shorter-acting sulfonylureas instead, *e.g.*, glyburide, 2.5–20 mg daily, or glipizide, 2.5–20 mg daily.

• Blood glucose concentration must be monitored.

• The main side effect is hypoglycemia.

For non–insulin-requiring diabetes: perioperative

• Routine use of i.v. solutions containing glucose is not advised unless hypoglycemia is a risk.

• If the operation is major, treatment should be the same as for insulin-requiring diabetes until the stress response of surgery is finished [4].

For insulin-requiring diabetes (type 1 and type 2): preoperative

• Preoperative admission for stabilization may be needed to achieve a blood glucose concentration of 100–180 mg/dL.

• If control is good, the insulin regimen need not be changed until the day of surgery; if control is poor before a meal, short-acting insulin achieves rapid metabolic control.

• Blood glucose concentration must be monitored.

For insulin-requiring diabetes (type 1 and type 2): operative perioperative

Short-acting insulin, 50 U in 50 mL normal saline solution with an infusion pump; continuous insulin infusion is of critical importance to avoid ketoacidosis in type 1 diabetes; if patients are hypoglycemic, dextrose infusion should be increased.

Dextrose solution with 10 mEq/L potassium chloride through a separate infusion pump; start with 5% dextrose at 125 mL/min or 10% dextrose at 60 mL/min.

• Blood glucose concentration should be maintained at 100–180 mg/dL; 1–4 U of insulin may be needed hourly via an infusion pump and can be titrated as needed [4].

• Premixed insulins are unsuitable as insulin need changes rapidly postoperatively.

• Glucoses should be monitored hourly.

• The insulin infusion must be continued until the patient's first meal, when s.c. insulin should be started 1–3 hours prior to cessation of insulin infusion; insulin needs will probably be higher than usual.

Treatment aims

To maintain blood glucose at 100–180 mg/dL during the operation.

Prognosis

• Mortality should be similar to that in nondiabetic patients.

Follow-up and management

• Blood glucose should be monitored 3–4 times daily before the operation.

• During and early after an operation, blood glucose should be monitored at least hourly.

• Creatinine and electrolytes should be followed daily.

Timing of surgery

• Routine surgery should be postponed in newly diagnosed diabetic patients until good control is attained.

• Acute surgical conditions may lead to ketoacidosis; if possible, surgery should be delayed until metabolic control is achieved.

• Surgery should be done in the morning if possible.

Special situations

Cardiac surgery

• Hypothermic bypass surgery with pump priming and inotropic drugs leads to marked insulin resistance and much higher insulin needs.

• The rapidly changing insulin need makes a separate infusion line for insulin essential.

Pregnancy

• Control of diabetes during delivery is critical for mother and fetus. (See Diabetic management in pregnanacy.)

Key references

1. Clark JDA, Currie J, Hartog M: Management of diabetes in surgery: a survey of current practice by anaesthetists. *Diabetic Med* 1992, **9**:271–274.

2. Gill GV: Surgery and diabetes mellitus. In *Textbook of Diabetes* vol 2. Edited by Pickup J, Williams G. Oxford: Blackwell Scientific Publications; 1991:820–825.

3. Sawyer RG, Pruett TL: Wound infections. *Surg Clin North Am* 1994, **74**:523–524.

4. Smith EA, Kilpatrick ES: Intra-operative blood glucose measurements. *Anaesthesia* 1994, **49**:129–132.

Diarrhea & HIV infection

Diagnosis

Symptoms

Watery, large-volume diarrhea: >400 mL daily.

Abdominal pain, severe.

Vomiting.

Signs

Prominent weight loss and dehydration: possibly.

Investigations

Stool culture: for *Salmonella*, *Campylobacter*, and *Shigella* spp.

Stool staining and microscopy: possibly with concentration of stools: Ziehl–Neelsen stain for cryptosporidia, and *Cyclospora* spp.; trichrome or fluorescent stain for microsporidia; microscopy of fresh stool for amoeba and cysts of *Giardia* and *Isopora* spp.

Small-intestinal biopsy: electron microscopy gold standard for diagnosis of microsporidia, cytomegalovirus inclusions and *Mycobacterium avium* cultures.

Biopsy: for cytomegalovirus or *M. avium* complex colitis, or involvement due to lymphoma or Kaposi's sarcoma.

Tests of malabsorption: protozoan infection associated with partial villus atrophy and malabsorption.

Complications

Toxic dilatation: unusual.

Right upper quadrant pain, cholangiographic appearances of "AIDS-related sclerosing cholangitis."

Wasting, inanition, death.

Differential diagnosis

Viral diarrhea: cytomegalovirus infection may be bloody and associated with abdominal pain.

Bacterial diarrhea: *Shigella*, *Salmonella*, and *Campylobacter* spp. cause acute diarrhea with systemic symptoms; opportunistic bacterial infection by *M. avium-intracellulare* causes watery diarrhea in patients with severely reduced CD4 counts ($<100 \times 10^6$/L).

"Pathogen-negative diarrhea": after complete investigation, large-volume diarrhea with no cause is rare; low-volume irritable-bowel diarrhea is more common in patients with CD4 counts $>200 \times 10^6$/L.

Etiology

Infectious

M. avium.

Cryptosporidia.

Microsporidia (at least two species: *Septata intestinalis* and *Enterocytozoon bieneusi*).

Cyclospora spp.

Isospora spp.

Entamoeba spp.

Giardia spp.

Cytomegalovirus.

Noninfectious

Lymphoma.

Kaposi's sarcoma.

Epidemiology

- Cryptosporidiosis is associated with water-borne outbreaks.
- Microsporidiosis occurs only in severely immunosuppressed patients (CD4 lymphocyte count $<100 \times 10^6$/L).
- *Isospora* infection is common in South Americans and Africans; it occasionally occurs in travelers to these continents.
- Infection by *Entamoeba* spp. is common in homosexual men, although these strains are usually not pathogenic.
- *Giardia* infection is common in homosexual men (possible sexual transmission); it is more common in HIV-seropositive men.

Treatment

Diet and lifestyle

- Safe sexual practices reduce sexual transmission.
- Immunosuppressed patients with a CD4 count <200 × 10^6/L should boil drinking water.
- Care must be taken when gardening or handling pets or domestic animals.

Pharmacological treatment

General treatment

- Patients should be rehydrated, usually with oral rehydration fluids.
- Reduction with antimotility agents (*e.g.*, codeine phosphate, 30–80 mg daily) or stronger opiates may cause toxic megacolon.
- Specific vitamin supplementation should be given for malabsorption.
- Transient stool volume can be reduced during treatment by somatostatin analogues (*e.g.*, octreotide, 50–200 μg 2–3 times daily).

For cryptosporidiosis

- No standard treatment is of proven value.

Standard dosage	Paromomycin, 500 mg 4 times daily (not successful). Azithromycin, up to 1.5 g daily, may be used.
Contraindications	None.
Special points	*Paromomycin:* stool volumes reduced by 50%, but cryptosporidia not eradicated.
Main drug interactions	None known.
Main side effects	None known.

For microsporidiosis

- No standard treatment is of proven value.

Standard dosage	Albendazole, 400 mg twice daily, or metronidazole, 400 mg 3 times daily.
Contraindications	None.
Special points	*Albendazole:* eradicates *Septata intestinalis*, less effect on *E. bienusi*. *Metronidazole:* may produce symptomatic benefit.
Main drug interactions	*Metronidazole:* alcohol.
Main side effects	*Metronidazole:* nausea.

For *Entamoeba histolytica* infection

- Metronidazole, 400 mg 3 times daily for 1 week; iodoquinol for 3 weeks.

For giardiasis

- Patients can be given metronidazole, 1.2–2 g daily for 3 days; tinidazole, 2 g initially, repeated if necessary; or mepacrine, 100 mg 3 times daily for 5–7 days, repeated after 2 weeks if necessary.

For isosporiasis and cyclosporiasis

- Trimethoprim-sulfamethoxazole double-strength tablet by mouth twice daily × 2 weeks, then maintenance therapy.

Alternative medicine

Recommended use: none.

Common use: Goldenseal (*Hydrastis canadensis*); *S. boulardie*; Oregon grape (*Mahonia* spp.).

Caution: none.

Treatment aims

To resolve diarrhea.

To eradicate organism.

To promote weight gain or prevent weight loss.

Prognosis

Cryptosporidiosis

- In patients with CD4 counts >200 × 10^6/L, the diarrhea resolves eventually.
- In patients with CD4 counts <200 × 10^6/L, the diarrhea may be chronic.
- Diarrhea usually continues despite treatment.
- In patients with CD4 counts >200 × 10^6/L, the prognosis depends on the CD4 count, rather than on the diarrhea.
- In patients with CD4 counts <200 × 10^6/L, median survival is 1 year.

Microsporidiosis

- Diarrhea usually continues despite treatment.
- Median survival is <1 year.

Other infections

- Diarrhea usually resolves with treatment, but patients may relapse after treatment has stopped.
- The prognosis depends on the underlying CD4 count, rather than on the diarrhea.

Follow-up and management

- Eradication of organism must be checked.
- Continuing diarrhea leads to wasting due to severe anorexia; therefore, the need for supplements, elemental diets, or nasogastric or gastrostomy feeding must be reviewed.

General references

Babameto G, Kotler DP: Malnutrition in HIV infection. *Gastroenterol Clin North Am* 1997, **26**:393–415.

Clayton F, Clayton CH: Gastrointestinal pathology in HIV-infected patients. *Gastroenterol Clin North Am* 1997, **26**:191–240.

Framm SR, Soave R: Agents of diarrhea. *Med Clin North Am* 1997, **81**:427–447.

Diagnosis

Symptoms

Liquid stools: >3 movements and >200 mL per day.

Blood (dysentery): implies active mucosal inflammation.

Abdominal pain: variable and often predefecatory.

Tenesmus: suggests proctitis.

Fever.

Weight loss, malnutrition, dehydration: in prolonged cases.

Oily stools with malabsorbed food: common in giardiasis.

Signs

Pyrexia: suggests active mucosal inflammation.

Clinical evidence of dehydration or malnutrition.

Pallor: patients with chronic anemia or acute blood loss.

Anal rash or excoriation: nonspecific irritation from alkaline stool; however, may also be due to infection by *Enterobius vermicularis* or *Strongyloides stercoralis.*

Arthropathy: occasionally seen with gram-negative infections.

Borborygmi.

Splenomegaly, rose spots: due to *Salmonella typhi* or *paratyphi* infection.

Peritonitis: rare.

Investigations

• Diagnostic investigations are indicated in patients with severe symptoms or signs and in patients with disease processes lasting >1 week [1,2].

Complete blood count: evaluate for anemia, leukocytosis; eosinophilia suggests invasive helminthic infection.

Fecal microscopy for leukocytes: when present, invasive infections/inflammation present; typically negative in viral or self-limited bacterial diarrhea.

Fecal microscopy for ova and parasites: Fresh, warm samples yield highest positivity rates for *Giardia lamblia* and *Entamoeba histolytica*; special stool antigen testing also available for *Giardia*, *Cyclospora*, *Cryptosporidium*, *Microsporidia* spp.

Fecal fat, fecal sodium, potassium, magnesium: in undiagnosed diarrhea lasting longer than 2 weeks; if abnormal, consider noninfectious causes.

***Clostridium difficile* toxin:** In all toxic patients or patients with invasive pattern; with recent use of antibiotics or in immunocompromised

Upper gastrointestinal endoscopy, including duodenal biopsy: for morphology and parasitology in severe cases or when symptoms persist >2 weeks and stool studies are negative.

Small-intestinal radiography: to check for ileocecal tuberculosis in patients at risk for tuberculosis or in those without diagnosis despite extensive evaluation.

Hydrogen breath test: to evaluate for bacterial overgrowth.

HIV serology: in patients with risk factors or otherwise negative evaluation. These patients require evaluation for atypical infections [3].

Complications

Dehydration, electrolyte disturbance.

Anemia: due to hemorrhage in dysentery; malabsorption.

Gram-negative septicemia: rare.

"Hyperinfection syndrome": due to *S. stercoralis* infection.

Ileal perforation, hemorrhage: due to salmonellosis.

Mesenteric adenitis or ileitis, nonsuppurative arthritis, ankylosing spondylitis, erythema nodosum, Reiter's syndrome: due to *Yersinia enterocolitica*, other gram-negative infections.

Perforation, hemorrhage, Reiter's syndrome, hemolytic uremic syndrome: due to shigellosis.

Acute necrotizing colitis, appendicitis, ameboma, hemorrhage, stricture: due to amebic colitis.

Colonic necrosis: due to pseudomembranous colitis.

Differential diagnosis

Inflammatory bowel disease.

Drug-induced diarrhea: laxatives, magnesium compounds, quinidine, prostaglandins.

Lactose intolerance.

Diabetic autonomic neuropathy.

Endocrine-associated diarrhea (*e.g.*, diabetes, hyperthyroidism).

Celiac disease.

Pancreatic insufficiency.

Factitious.

Pheochromocytoma.

Bacterial overgrowth syndrome.

NSAID enteropathy.

Etiology

Bacteria: *Aeromonas* spp., *Campylobacter* spp., *Clostridium difficile, Escherichia coli* (including O157:H7), *Mycobacterium tuberculosis, Plesiomonas shigelloides, Salmonella* spp., *Shigella* spp., *Vibrio* spp., *Y. enterocolitica, T. whippeli.*

Viruses: adenovirus, astrovirus, Norwalk virus, rotavirus, HIV.

Protozoa: *E. histolytica, G. lamblia, Isospora belli, Cryptosporidium* spp., *Mycobacterium avium-intracellulare, cyclospora spp., microsporidia spp.*

Helminths: *Capillaria philippinensis, E. vermicularis, Fasciolopsis buski, Schistosoma mansoni, Schistosoma japonicum, Strongyloides stercoralis, Taenia* spp., *Trichuris trichiuria, Ascaris* spp.

Travelers' diarrhea: clinical syndrome with many causes, including viruses, bacteria, and protozoa.

Food poisoning.

Immunosuppression (AIDS enteropathy).

Epidemiology

• Intestinal infection occurs worldwide.

• Fecal–oral transmission.

• Travelers' diarrhea occurs more often in people who have travelled to an area where socioeconomic standards and hygiene are compromised (including most tropical and subtropical countries).

Treatment

Diet and lifestyle

• Food hygiene must be strictly observed: most intestinal infections result from a contaminated environment, commonly food or drink (especially drinking water).

• Avoidance of milk and dairy products is advised during diarrhea because of secondary hypolactasia complicating an intestinal infection of any cause.

• Aggressive intake of fluids while avoiding alcohol and caffeine is advised.

• Good handwashing must be stressed to avoid passage of the infection to others.

Pharmacological treatment

• Most infectious diarrheas are self-limiting and require no pharmacological management.

Enteric fever, sepsis should always be treated with antibiotics; dysentery (except with enterohemorrhagic *E. coli*) should usually be treated with antibiotics

• Travelers' diarrhea: prophylaxis with bismuth subsalicylate; hydration only for loose stools; ciprofloxacin for toxic patients (fever, dehydration) or dysentery, which may require treatment with metronidazole if entamoeba a consideration.

Infections usually requiring antibiotics

C. difficile infection: vancomycin, 125 mg every 6 hours for 10 days, or metronidazole, 500 mg 3 times daily for 10 days.

E. histolytica infection: metronidazole, 500 mg 3 times daily for 10 days.

G. lamblia infection: metronidazole, 250–500 mg 3 times daily for 7 days.

I. belli infection: trimethoprim-sulfamethoxazole, 160 mg/800 mg 3 times daily for 10 days, then twice daily for 3 weeks.

S. typhi or *paratyphi* infection: ciprofloxacin, chloramphenicol, trimethoprim-sulfamethoxazole, or amoxicillin.

S. mansoni, japonicum, mekongi, intercalatum, or *matthei* infection: praziquantel.

S. stercoralis infection: albendazole or thiabendazole.

Cholera, watery (enterotoxigenic) diarrheas: oral rehydration (i.v. in extreme cases, *e.g.*, infection by *Vibrio cholerae*).

Selected regimens

Amoxicillin, 500 mg 3 times daily for 14 days (in *S. typhi* infection, reduced after defervescence).

Ampicillin, 1 g 4 times daily for 14 days.

Chloramphenicol, 50 mg/kg daily in 4 divided doses for 14 days.

Ciprofloxacin, 500–750 mg twice daily for 3 days for severe travelers' diarrhea; for 14 days for *Salmonella* spp.

Albendazole, 400 mg twice daily for 1–3 days; with *S. stercoralis* infection, 3-day course repeated after 3 weeks.

Mebendazole, 100 mg initially (for ascariasis second dose may be needed).

Thiabendazole, 25mg/kg twice daily for 3 days (longer in "hyperinfection syndrome").

Praziquantel, 40–50 mg/kg initially; for *S. japonicum* infection, 60 mg/kg in three divided doses on a single day.

See manufacturer's current prescribing information *for further details.*

Treatment aims

To relieve diarrhea, abdominal colic, and other intestinal symptoms.

To rehydrate patient as rapidly as possible, preferably orally.

To ensure bacteriological or parasitic cure.

To return patient's nutritional status to normal, especially when clinically overt malabsorption has accompanied infection.

To prevent recurrences, especially of *Salmonella typhi* or *paratyphi* infections.

To relieve symptoms in untreatable immunosuppressed patients.

Prognosis

• In some severe infections (*e.g.*, shigellosis, *E. histolytica* colitis), specific chemotherapy results in complete recovery in almost all patients.

• If surgery is necessary for complications, the prognosis is less favorable.

Follow-up and management

• Most intestinal infections are acute; follow-up is unnecessary.

• *S. typhi* or *paratyphi* infections should be followed up in order to establish that the carrier state has not ensued.

• Patients with overt malabsorption as a secondary manifestation of an intestinal infection should be followed up for maintenance therapy and ascertainment of ultimate cure.

Key references

1. Aranda-Michel JA, Gianella RA: Acute diarrhea: a practical review. *Am J Med* 1999, **106**:670–676.
2. Miner PB: Evaluation of the patient with diarrhea. *Curr Pract Med* 1998, **1**:712–722.
3. Goodgame RW: Gastrointestinal disease in patients with AIDS. *Curr PractMed* 1998, **1**:904–909.
4. Banerjee S, LaMont JT: Treatment of gastrointestinal infections. *Gastroenterology* 2000, **118**:S48–S67.

Diagnosis

Symptoms

• Disseminated intravascular coagulation occurs in a spectrum of guises: from a chronic syndrome, diagnosed on laboratory tests, with no symptoms or signs (compensated), to an acute florid clinical bleeding state (uncompensated).

• It is always associated with an underlying disorder.

• The major symptoms are those of the underlying disorder.

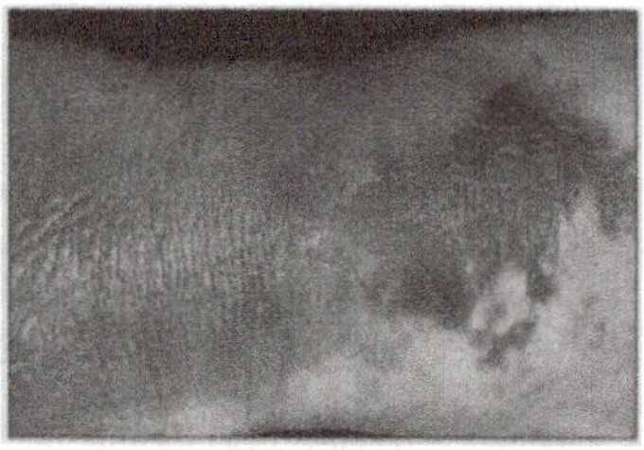

Purpura fulminans, with surrounding extensive subcutaneous hemorrhage. (*See* Color Plate.)

Generalized bruising: especially over dependent areas.

Bleeding at surgical sites and incisions, around venipuncture sites, indwelling lines, and drainage tubes.

Hematemesis, melena, hemoptysis, hematuria, and vaginal bleeding.

Gangrene of fingers and toes, purpura fulminans, hemorrhagic bullae: microthrombotic lesions in 5%–10% of patients.

Signs

Evidence of bleeding: as detailed under symptoms, when present.

Investigations [1,2]

• Simple screening tests show reduced levels of clotting factors and platelets.

• Disseminated intravascular coagulation cannot be ruled out by a single set of normal results; serial values may be needed to show consumption.

Measurement of prothrombin time, activated partial thromboplastin time, thrombin time: all times prolonged; prolongation of thrombin time best guide to clinical significance of raised fibrinogen degradation products and low fibrinogen; thrombin time twice normal control value indicates impending overt clinical bleeding.

Fibrinogen measurement: concentration low.

Fibrinogen degradation products and D-dimers measurement: concentrations raised; fibrinogen degradation products sensitive but not specific for disseminated intravascular coagulation; D-dimer specific but not as sensitive.

Platelet count: low.

Blood film: many patients have associated microangiographic hemolytic anemia; erythrocytes fragmented by passing through deposited fibrin strands.

Complications

Uncontrollable hemorrhage.

Microvascular blockage and tissue necrosis of heart, liver, kidney, and brain.

Acute respiratory distress syndrome.

Differential diagnosis

• Simple screening tests and the clinical picture are usually diagnostic.

Vitamin K deficiency: normal platelet count.

Liver disease: raised factor VIII concentrations.

Lupus anticoagulant and thrombocytopenia: normal fibrinogen, inhibitor present.

Thrombotic thrombocytopenic purpura: clotting tests usually normal, florid microangiopathic changes on blood film.

Massive transfusion: clinical history.

Etiology [1,2]

Causes and associated disorders

Infections: meningococcal septicemia, gram-negative septicemia, malaria, virus (purpura fulminans).

Malignancy: disseminated metastatic carcinomas, myeloid leukemia, promyelocitic leukemia.

Obstetric complications: septic abortion, amniotic fluid embolism, placental abruption, eclampsia, retained dead fetus and placenta.

Tissue injury: severe burns or trauma, extensive surgery, hypo- or hyperthermia, shock.

Immunological phenomena: anaphylaxis, incompatible transfusion, allograft rejection.

Miscellaneous: liver disease and ascitic fluid shunts, extracorporeal circuits, certain snake and insect bites, vascular malformations.

Pathogenesis

• Disseminated intravascular coagulopathy is triggered by inappropriate and continued activation of clotting pathways.

• This leads to excessive thrombin generation, coagulation factor consumption, and platelet aggregation.

• Thrombin also activates protein C and fibrinolytic systems via secondary generation of plasmin.

• Natural inhibitors of the clotting cascade are overwhelmed.

• Coagulation factor consumption, consumptive thrombocytopenia, and hyperfibrinolysis lead to bleeding.

• Uncontrolled fibrin deposition leads to microthrombosis.

Epidemiology

• 60% of clinical cases of disseminated intravascular coagulation are associated with septicemic infection, usually due to gram-negative bacteria.

• Most acute cases are encountered in severely ill patients in intensive care.

Treatment

Diet and lifestyle

• No special precautions are necessary.

Pharmacological treatment [1,2]

Anticoagulants

• Although controversial, anticoagulants may have a role in acute promyelocytic leukemia (M3), acute intravascular hemolysis (incompatible blood transfusion), and purpura fulminans.

Standard dosage	Heparin, 300–500 U/h continuous i.v. infusion.
Contraindications	Florid bleeding.
Special points	Requires antithrombin III for its action, which is often low in patients with disseminated intravascular coagulation; fresh frozen plasma may also be needed to supply antithrombin III to maintain effective heparinization. May increase bleeding tendency; close monitoring and specialist advice needed.
Main drug interactions	Other anticoagulants.
Main side effects	Bleeding (with overdose).

Fibrinolytic inhibitors

• Because of increased deposition, fibrinolysis is protective against microvascular organ damage in disseminated intravascular coagulation; inhibitors of fibrinolysis are therefore generally contraindicated. In special circumstances of predominant fibrinolysis, however, they may be useful.

• Specialist advice must be sought before use.

Nonpharmacological treatment [1,2]

See Transfusion medicine *for further details.*

Fresh frozen plasma

• Fresh frozen plasma supplies all clotting factors and naturally occurring inhibitors of coagulation.

• Initially, 10–15 mL/kg should be given.

• It may cause fluid overload.

Cryoprecipitate

• Cryoprecipitate supplies fibrinogen and factor VIII.

• It is used, at a rate of 1 U/5 kg, when substantial fibrinogen replacement is needed.

Platelet concentrates

• Platelet concentrates are needed when consumptive thrombocytopenia is present.

• They are given, at a rate of 4 U/m^2 body surface area, if the platelet count falls below 50 x 10^9/L and overt bleeding occurs.

Packed red blood cells

• Packed red blood cells are needed to treat associated hemolysis or anemia at a rate sufficient to maintain hematocrit >0.3.

• Virus transmission is a risk with any blood product.

• Fluid overload may also be a problem.

Treatment aims

To treat the underlying disorder.

To reverse the coagulopathy (by replacement of clotting factors and platelets or use of pharmacological inhibitors of coagulation).

To provide general supportive care for acutely ill patients.

Prognosis

• The mortality in severe disseminated intravascular coagulation is high and may exceed 80%.

• Death is usually due to progression of the underlying disease; elimination or amelioration of the cause is of utmost importance.

Follow-up and management

• Coagulation screening tests should be repeated to assess the effect of replacement therapy; the aim is a prothrombin time within 3 seconds of control, partial thromboplastin time within 10 seconds of control, and fibrinogen >1.0 g/L.

• The need for further replacement should be judged by the results of screening tests and degree of clinical bleeding.

• Laboratory abnormalities correct with successful treatment of the underlying disorder.

Key references

1. Levi M, ten Cate H: Disseminated intravascular coagulation. *N Engl J Med* 1999, **341**:586–592.

2. Carey MJ, Rodgers GM: Disseminated intravascular coagulation: clinical and laboratory aspects. *Am J Hematol* 1998, **59**:65–73.

Diverticular disease of the colon

Diagnosis

Symptoms

• Diverticulosis (*i.e.*, the presence of diverticular disease within the colon) is found in the majority of older adults but causes symptoms or signs of disease in only a minority [1].

Symptomatic diverticular disease

• Symptomatic diverticular disease may present with the following:

Fever, left lower quadrant abdominal pain (acute diverticulitis).

Constipation, obstruction (stricture from chronic diverticulitis).

Maroon stools or frank rectal bleeding (bleeding diverticula).

Signs

Symptomatic diverticular disease

Fever with abdominal tenderness, most often in the left lower quadrant: suggestive of diverticulitis.

Shock, peritoneal signs, or a palpable inflammatory mass: suggests severe disease (*e.g.*, abscess or perforation) [2].

Hypotension, tachycardia, red blood per rectum: suggestive of significant diverticular bleeding (*i.e.*, more than 1-2 units of packed red blood cells), which is typically painless (or associated with cramping as the colon expels the blood). Occult gastrointestinal bleeding or transient hematochezia with an otherwise normal bowel movement suggests an alternative diagnosis.

Investigations

• Symptomatic diverticular disease is a clinical diagnosis that relies more on presenting symptoms and signs as opposed to investigative studies of the colon. An imaging study of the colon is indicated in the evaluation of all patients with symptomatic diverticular disease to exclude other conditions, such as inflammatory bowel disease or malignancy. Intraluminal colonic pressure from fiberoptic scopes or barium enemas may further complicate acute diverticulitis and should be postponed until inflammation is controlled.

Complete blood count: to identify anemia due to bleeding or elevated leukocyte count from inflammation. Microcytic anemia suggests an alternative diagnosis.

Liver chemistry tests: to exclude biliary disease, which can occasionally mimic symptomatic diverticular disease.

Urinalysis: to exclude active renal inflammation from continguous diverticulitis.

Plain abdominal radiography: may show features of ileus or perforation.

Barium enema: may show obstruction or stricture; sensitive for demonstrating the presence of diverticula.

Colonoscopy: indicated in all patients with suspected diverticular bleeding; done to attempt endoscopic measures to achieve hemostasis and exclude other causes for bleeding [3].

Tagged red blood nuclear scan: to investigate patients with ongoing bleeding despite supportive management alone. Once a region is identified on a nuclear scan, angiography can be pursued to further localize the bleeding vessel.

Sigmoidoscopy: to exclude colitis or malignancy.

CT of abdomen and pelvis: useful to diagnose diverticular abscess or perforation.

Complications

Life-threatening gastrointestinal bleeding.

Abscess formation or perforation: leading to subphrenic or pericolic collections.

Intestinal obstruction.

Stricture formation.

Fistula: connection to bladder or vagina.

Differential diagnosis

General

Carcinoma of colon.

Inflammatory bowel disease.

Pseudomembranous colitis.

Ischemic colitis.

Abscess or perforation

Pelvic inflammatory disease.

Pyelonephritis.

Perforated peptic ulcer.

Ischemic colitis.

Appendicitis.

Crohn's disease.

Hemorrhage

Angiodysplasia.

Upper gastrointestinal tract bleeding.

Stricture

Radiation damage.

Ischemic colitis.

Endometriosis.

Etiology

Diverticula result from altered colonic wall tension, probably as a result of low dietary fiber intake.

Diverticular bleeding occurs from rupture of an injured artery adjacent to the lumen of an individual diverticulum.

Diverticulitis results from abrasion and microperforation of the diverticulum from inspissated stool.

Bleeding more commonly results from diverticula in the right colon, whereas diverticulitis more commonly originates in the left colon.

Epidemiology

• Colonic diverticula occur in 33% of people >40 years and 50% of people >70 years.

• Diverticulosis appears to be more common in developed countries.

• It is rare for diverticulitis and diverticular bleeding to coexist.

Treatment

Diet and lifestyle

• Increased dietary fiber intake may help some patients, especially those with marked constipation.

• Excessive dietary fiber is contraindicated in patients with excessive narrowing or stricture formation from previous inflammation.

• Regular exercise improves bowel function.

Pharmacological treatment

Diverticulitis

Antibiotics are administered to patients with acute inflammation for at least 2 weeks. Many regimens may be used depending on the patient.

Patients with significant fever, peritoneal signs, or evidence of systemic toxicity should initially begin receiving intravenous antibiotics with broad-spectrum coverage for aerobic and anaerobic bacteria (*e.g.*, ampicillin/sulbactam 1–3 g every 6 hours i.v. or cefotetan, 1–3 g every 12 hours i.v.).

For milder disease or after improvement with intravenous medications, therapy with oral antibiotics can be initiated; however, two agents are typically required to achieve the broad coverage that is necessary (*e.g.*, ciprofloxacin, 500 mg orally every 12 hours plus metronidazole, 500 mg orally every 6 hours). Metronidazole should be completely avoided in pregnant women or in patients who cannot completely abstain from alcohol during the treatment course.

Diverticular bleeding

• Therapy is supportive, with volume expansion and blood products as necessary.

• Antibiotics have no role in the management of patients with diverticular bleeding.

Nonpharmacological treatment

• For perforated diverticular disease of the colon: emergency decompression of the colon by colostomy, followed by elective resection of the diseased segment [4]. Abscess formation, sepsis, or failure to respond to medical therapy should prompt surgical consultation.

• For life-threatening hemorrhage from diverticular disease. Therapeutic colonoscopy should first be attempted [3]. If bleeding persists, surgical control or embolization therapy at the time of selective mesenteric arteriography.

• Surgical resection of structures; consideration of endoscopic dilation in select cases.

Alternative medicine

Recommended use: none.

Common use: colocynthis, homeopathic; bryonia, homeopathic; belladonna, homeopathic; wild yam (*Dioscorea villosa*); German chamomile (*Matricaria chamomile*); marshmallow root (*Hibiscus mosheutos*); calamus root (*Acorus calamus*).

Caution: none.

Treatment aims

To relieve acute symptoms.

To improve bowel function.

To reduce incidence of further symptom attacks.

Prognosis

• 70%–80% of patients with diverticular bleeding have spontaneous cessation, with recurrence in <50%.

• Most patients with diverticulitis respond to antibiotic management alone; a small subset will require drainage of an abscess or surgical management of strictures.

Follow-up and management

• Recurrent symptoms are common, but new or different symptoms need further investigations.

• If symptoms are relieved by fiber supplementation, long-term treatment must be continued.

Key references

1. Cheskin LJ, Bohlman M, Schusler MM: Diverticular disease in the elderly. *Gastroenterol Clin North Am* 1990, **19**:391–403.
2. Jones DJ: Diverticular disease. *BMJ* 1992, **304**:1435–1437.
3. Jensen DM, Machicado GA, et al.: Urgent colonoscopy for the diagnosis and treatment of severe diverticular hemorrhage. *N Engl J Med* 2000, 342:78–82.
4. Acute appendicitis and diverticular disease of the colon. *Curr Pract Med* 1998, 1(4):835.

Duodenal ulcer

Diagnosis

Symptoms

Epigastric pain: often described as dull or burning; occurring on an empty stomach and relieved with eating or antacids; pain may awaken patient from sleep during the early morning hours; pain may radiate to the back.

Hematemesis or melena: patients may present with gastrointestinal bleeding as their first symptom of peptic ulcer disease.

Anorexia and occasional vomiting in patients with outflow obstruction.

Weight loss.

Signs

• Most patients with duodenal ulcer disease have a normal examination. Epigastric tenderness is not a reliable measure for the presence or absence of duodenal ulcer disease.

• Abnormalities, when present, may include the following:

Melena.

Hemetemesis.

Pallor and clinical evidence of anemia.

Peritonitis: patients who present with perforation (<5% of patients).

"Succussion splash" of gastric outflow obstruction: <5% of patients.

Investigations [1]

"Test and treat" strategies in young, uncomplicated patients with dyspepsia involve testing for *Helicobacter pylori* (using serology or breath test) and treating positive patients with an eradication program; this is a cost-effective approach to the empiric treatment of patients with suspected peptic ulcer disease (*see* Nonulcer dyspepsia).

• An imaging study of the gastroduodenal lumen is required to render a specific diagnosis of duodenal ulcer disease.

Contrast radiography: a barium upper gastrointestinal series is relatively inexpensive and safe; however, small lesions may be missed and tissue biopsies are not feasible.

Fiberoptic endoscopy: esophagogastroduodenoscopy typically is performed under i.v. sedation and allows direct visualization of ulcers with biopsy and local treatment for bleeding when present. *H. pylori*, the greatest risk factor for duodenal ulcer disease, may be identified from tissue samples immediately at the time of endoscopy (*e.g.*, CLO test) or histologically on formalin-fixed biopsy specimens.

Testing for *H. pylori* in patients who have ulcer but no tissue studies for *H. pylori*: urea breath test, serology for *H. pylori*. (Note: patients may remain seropositive 1 mg after eradication.) Urea breath testing performed 1 month after completion of an eradication program, is the best test to confirm adequate treatment of an *H. pylori* infection. However, patients must be off of proton-pump inhibitors for at least 2 weeks before breath testing to prevent false-negative results.)

Complete blood count: to evaluate for anemia or systemic evidence of inflammation.

Serum gastrin levels: in patients with unexplained recurrent disease or severe disease without evidence of nonsteroidal drug ingestion or *H. pylori*.

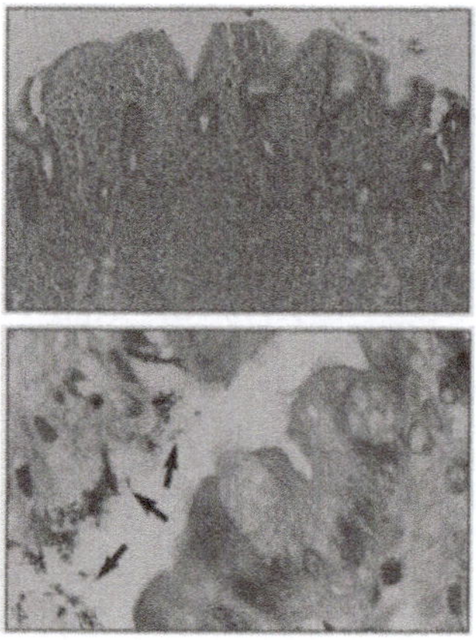

Histologic specimen of gastric mucosa with Helicobacter pylori infection. (*Top*) Gastritis is shown because the mucosa is heavily infiltrated with acute and chronic inflammatory cells. (*Bottom*) High power showing bacteria stained with silver (*arrows*). (*Courtesy of* R. Genta, Houston, TX.)

Complications

Acute hemorrhage: in 10% of patients.

Perforation: in 1% (often asymptomatic in elderly or immunosuppressed patients).

Penetration: pancreatitis.

Outlet obstruction from scarring of the duodenum.

Differential diagnosis

Nonulcer dyspepsia.
Gastric ulcer.
Gastroesophageal reflux disease.
Irritable bowel syndrome.
Pancreatitis.
Gallstone disease.
Carcinoma of stomach.
Pancreatic carcinoma.
Hepatobiliary carcinoma.
Crohn's disease.
Peritonitis.
Ischemia.
Lymphoma.
Acute myocardial infarction.
Aortic dissection.

Etiology

• Causes include the following:

H. pylori infection: 90% of patients.
NSAIDs (a common cause).
Increased basal acid secretion: in 30% of patients; consider gastrinoma.
Increased nocturnal acid secretion.
Smoking.

Epidemiology

• 10% of the population has a duodenal ulcer at some point in their lives.

• Duodenal ulcers occur almost as often in women as in men.

Treatment

Diet and lifestyle

• Patients should restrict alcohol consumption, eat balanced meals daily with no bedtime snacks, avoid aspirin and other NSAIDs, and stop cigarette smoking.

• Bland or milk diets have not been shown to decrease acidity, promote healing, or relieve symptoms.

Pharmacological treatment

H. pylori–positive patients [2]

Numerous regimens are available for eradication of *H. pylori*. They all rely on three or four drug regimens that are optimally taken for 14 days. Compliance with these regimens must be carefully stressed and continuously evaluated.

Factors involved in selecting a regimen include local costs of component medications, patient hypersensitivities, and local patterns of *H. pylori* resistance (most important for metronidazole and clarithromycin)

Common regimens (all for 14 days):

Triple drug regimens:

A twice-daily dose of a proton-pump inhibitor (see below) or ranitidine bismuth citrate plus two of the following: amoxicillin, 1 g twice daily; metronidazole, 500 mg twice daily; clarithromycin, 500 mg twice daily.

Quadruple drug regimens:

A proton-pump inhibitor (twice daily) plus tetracycline, 500 mg four times daily; bismuth, 2 tablets four times daily; metronidazole, 500 mg three times daily.

H. pylori–negative patients (*e.g.*, those with NSAID-related ulcers) [3]

Ideally, stop NSAID use during treatment period. Replace with acetaminophen (safest alternative) or with one of the new cyclo-oxygenase-2 inhibitors (rofecoxib, celecoxib), which are significantly less ulcerogenic.

Healing can be achieved with a 4–6 week course of an H_2-receptor antagonist or proton-pump inhibitor.

Sulcrafate (2 g twice daily taken on empty stomach) for 6–8 weeks is also effective (80% healing at 4 weeks); antacids are much less convenient because of the aggressive dosing schedule (30–60 mL, 1 and 3 hours after eating and at bedtime) required to achieve healing.

In patients who must continue to receive NSAIDs, healing can be promoted and recurrent ulcers minimized with concurrent use of omeprazole (20–40 mg daily) or high-dose famotidine (40 mg twice daily). Misoprostol (200 µg 4 times daily) is also of benefit in minimizing the development of ulcers in patients who require NSAIDs.

H_2-receptor antagonists [4]

• These relieve symptoms in days and cause ulcer healing in 80% of patients at 4 weeks and 95% at 8 weeks; they are also used as maintenance treatment to prevent recurrence at half the usual dose.

Standard dosage	Ranitidine, 300 mg; cimetidine, 800 mg; famotidine, 40 mg; nizatidine, 300 mg given once in the evening.
Contraindications	Rare hypersensitivity; avoid in pregnancy and lactation.
Main drug interactions	*Cimetidine:* oral anticoagulants, theophylline, phenytoin, warfarin.
Main side effects	Altered bowel habits, headache (both rare). *Cimetidine:* gynecomastia, confusion in elderly.

Proton-pump inhibitors [4]

• Proton-pump inhibitors are associated with faster healing (*e.g.*, 93% healing after 4 weeks of treatment). They should be ingested just before breakfast and should not be crushed or chewed. Twice-daily dosing or addition of an evening H_2-receptor antagonist can also be pursued for refractory cases.

Standard dosage	Omeprazole, 20 mg daily; lansoprazole, 30 mg daily; pantoprazole, 40 mg daily; rabeprazole, 20 mg daily.
Contraindications	Pregnancy and lactation.
Main drug interactions	Consider agent choice carefully in patients receiving digoxin, itraconazole, ketoconazole, benzodiazepines, phenytoin, or warfarin.
Main side effects	Diarrhea, headache, rash (all rare); increased risk of enteric infection.

Treatment aims

To relieve pain.

To heal ulcer.

To prevent recurrence and complications.

To eradicate *H. pylori* infection.

Other treatments

Surgery: for uncontrollable bleeding, second major bleeding, perforation or penetration, outlet obstruction.

• Elective surgery is very rarely necessary.

Prognosis

• Excellent when underlying cause (*e.g.*, *H. pylori* infection, NSAID use) has been addressed.

• Untreated, most patients with duodenal ulcers relapse within 1–2 years of initial healing, particularly the elderly, NSAID users, and smokers.

Follow-up and management

• If symptoms continue after 8 weeks of full-dose H_2 blockade, patients should be checked with endoscopy, and the ulcer and antrum should be biopsied.

• Eradication of *H. pylori* should be verified with urea breath testing in patients with recurrent disease.

• Maintenance with half-dose H_2 antagonist should be considered to prevent recurrence for patients with a history of aggressive ulcer (*e.g.*, previous bleeding), the elderly, or those with other illnesses.

Key references

1. Graham DY: Peptic ulcer disease. *Curr Pract Med* 1998, **1**:765–773.
2. Wolfe MM, Lichtenstein DR, Sing G: Gastrointestinal toxicity of nonsteroidal antiinflammatory drugs. *N Engl J Med* 1999, **340**:1888–1899.
3. Graham DY: Therapy of *Helicobacter pylori*: current status and issues. *Gastroenterology* 2000, **118**:S2–S8.
4. Wolfe MM, Sachs G. Acid suppression: Optimizing therapy for gastroduodenal ulcer healing, gastroesophageal reflux disease, and stress related erosive syndrome. *Gastroenterology* 2000, **118**:S9–S31.

Dyslipoproteinemia

Diagnosis

Symptoms

Myocardial infarction, angina, claudication, transient ischemic attacks, cerebrovascular accident: indicating accelerated atheroma.

Pancreatitis, confusional states: rare, caused by chylomicronemia.

• Adverse lipid profiles without symptoms are often revealed by well-person screening or through other risk association, *e.g.*, bad family history.

Signs

• Ectopic lipid deposits should be sought because they suggest the duration of lipidemia (and thus the degree of risk) and alert to asymptomatic lipidemia

Corneal arcus: traces in 50% of adults by age 50 years; heavy or early presence can reveal hypercholesterolemia; differential arcus can reveal carotid stenosis.

Tendon xanthomas: heels, knees, knuckles; indicating long-standing severe hypercholesterolemia, almost always familial.

Xanthomas of soft tissues: elbows, eyelids, palmar creases, rarely elsewhere; typical of mixed lipidemia and triglyceride excess.

Lipidemia retinalis and eruptive xanthomas: indicating chylomicronemia.

Corneal clouding: rare major disorder of high-density lipoprotein.

Carotid bruit, poor or absent peripheral pulses: vascular abnormalities.

Investigations

• The aim of investigations is to clarify the pattern of lipid abnormality and its cause.

• Lipid profiles can be disturbed and difficult to interpret for up to 3 months after myocardial infarction.

Lipid profile: for concentrations of cholesterol, triglycerides (TG), and high-density lipoprotein cholesterol (HDL-C) after overnight fasting: random sample adequate for cholesterol. Since laboratory and biological variability is considerable (up to 10% for low-density lipoprotein cholesterol (LDL-C), 20%–25% for TG and 3%–5% for NDL-C, at least two sets of lipids should be obtained before initiating therapy. LDL-C cannot be estimated when TG level remains above 400 mg/dL. Options include measurement after treating elevated TG level or direct LDL-C measurement.

Second-level tests: apolipoprotein E typing for moderate mixed excess or palmar xanthomas, fibrinogen levels, platelet function, and lipoprotein (a) concentration also of interest.

Special procedures: for major hypertriglyceridemia, measurement of apolipoprotein CII and lipoprotein lipase; for major HDL deficiency, measurement of lecithin cholesterol acyltransferase activity, and apolipoprotein AI and DNA studies.

Family screening: to review suspected genetic problem, notably polygenic or familial hypercholesterolemia.

Other problems: notably blood pressure, cardiac status, cigarette smoking, and fibrinogen concentration, should be considered in the overall assessment of clinical risk and options for benefit.

Complications

Progressive atheromatous disease.

Graft or angioplasty restenosis.

Attacks of abdominal pain and pancreatitis.

Differential diagnosis

Other causes of premature vascular disease, pancreatitis, corneal clouding.

Etiology

Genetic causes

Monogenic dominant forms of heterozygous familial hypercholesterolemia (rare homozygotes) and familial combined hypercholesterolemia.

Recessive: most causes of familial dysbetalipoproteinemia (type III).

Polygenic

Secondary causes

Hypothyroidism in older hypercholesterolemic women.

Alcoholism.

Diabetes or impaired glucose tolerance in older men or women with mixed lipidemia.

Chronic renal or liver disease.

Etretinate sensitivity.

Unknown causes

Includes diet-dependent effects and possible genetic basis ("common hypercholesterolemia").

Epidemiology

• US cholesterol levels are high by world standards; roughly 20% of the US adult population has a total cholesterol level >240 mg/dL and another 30% has borderline triglyceridemia (200–240 mg/dL).

• HDL-C levels are higher and LDL-C levels are lower in women than in men.

• HDL-C levels are not affected by age after puberty; LDL-C levels continue to increase in women and young men.

• Heterozygous familial hypercholesterolemia is present in 0.2% of live births and 6% of patients aged < 50 years admitted to coronary care units.

• Major apolipoprotein E variants are present in 1.7% of live births (type III lipemia), but only 1% of these patients have major pulmonary vascular or cardiovascular disease as adults; a secondary problem (*e.g.*, alcohol) is usually needed to provoke clinical expression.

Treatment

Diet and lifestyle

Reduction in total dietary fat; weight loss; smoking cessation; regular physical exercise; reduction in excess alcohol intake.

Pharmacological treatment

• Drug therapy should be reserved for patients with: known coronary heart disease/ atherosclerotic coronary vascular disease after cardiac transplantation; increased risk for coronary heart disease after not reaching LDL-C targets with lifestyle modifications.

• Some groups have recommended restricting drug therapy to patients with a 10% or more 5-year risk for coronary heart disease. This can be easily calculated:

Patient risk profile	LDL-C for dietary therapy	LDL-C for drug therapy	Treatment aims
F1 CHD risk*	≥ 160	≥ 190†	< 160
≥CHD risks	≥ 130	≥ 160	< 130
CHD or arteriosclerotic CVD or type 2 diabetes	≥ 100	≥ 130	< 100

*Risks include men ≥ 45 years of age; women ≥ 55 years of age or women with premature estrogen without estrogen placement, family history of premature coronary heart disease (CHD), current smoker, hypertension, LDL-C level < 35 mg/dL, and diabetes mellitus.

† Men < 35 years of age and premenopausal women with ≤ 2 risk factors are at extremely low short-term risk; medication should be deferred until LDL-C level is > 200 mg/dL.

Hydroxymethylglutaryl coenzyme A (HMG-CoA) reductase inhibitors (statins)

• These drugs are the best studied and show most benefit in reducing LDL-C levels and improving patient outcome. Statins have been considered to have a class effect.

• Atorvastatin is the most potent agent. Pravastatin is not metabolized by the liver and has fewer drug interactions. Cerivastatin uses two enzyme pathways and also carries low risk for drug interaction. Lovastatin is the oldest and will be generic soon.

• Adverse effects include gastrointestinal disturbances, muscle aches, rash, headache, rhabdomyolysis.

• Patients not achieving target LDL-C levels with full-dose statins would benefit from niacin or resin. Niacin and fibrates with statins increase the risk for hepatitis and rhabdomyolysis.

Contraindications: Statins are contraindicated in pregnancy.

Bile acid resins

• Cholestyramine and colestipol have been shown to reduce LDL-C levels in 10%–20% of patients, depending on dose. They act by binding cholesterol in the gut and interfering with absorption; are available in powder and pill form; raise TG levels and should be avoided in patients with hypertriglyceridemia.

Adverse effects: include bloating, nausea, constipation, and abdominal pain. Side effects can be reduced by slowly uptitrating the dosage. Resins interfere with absorption of fat-soluble vitamins and drugs; should be taken 1 hour before or 4 hours after other medications.

Fibrates

• Include gemfibrozil and fenofibrate.

• Used to lower TG levels and raise HDL-C levels. Gibrozil has no significant effect on LDL-C. Fenofibrate has been shown to lower LDL-C, but the impact on cardiac outcome and mortality is unknown. Both agents have been shown to have benefits on angiography.

Adverse events: generally gastrointestinal, including nausea, dyspepsia, and change in bowel habits. The risk of cholestasis and cholecystectomy is increased. When fibrates are used with statins, the risk of rhabdomyolysis and hepatitis is increased.

Contraindications: severe renal or liver disease, preexisting gall bladder disease, pregnancy.

Niacin

Niacin improves all aspects of lipid profile, including lipoprotein (a); shown to reduce cardiac events and mortality after 9 years of therapy.

Adverse effects: include flushing, pruritus, gastrointestinal disturbances, fatigue, glucose intolerance, gout, and peptic ulcer. Hepatic toxicity has been reported.

• Available in generic immediate-release (IR) and sustained-release (SR) formulations. Niaspan has been shown to have fewer side effects than IR niacin.. SR niacin is considered twice as potent.

Treatment aims

To improve overall lipid profile in patients with or at risk of coronary heart disease.

To reduce coronary progression and improve outcomes, including survival.

Prognosis

• Increase in HDL-C levels is associated with plaque regression.

Follow-up and management

• Dietary support must be reinforced and be enthusiastic and family based.

• For patients in whom lipid response fails, compliance and the prospect of a second lipid-related disorder (*e.g.*, hypothyroidism, alcoholism) must be checked.

Diet or medication changes must be given time to act (*e.g.*, review after 4 months).

Alternative medicine

Recommended use: flaxseed oil; niacin; pantethine.

Common use: garlic (Allium sativum or A. cepa); guggul (Commiphora mukul).

Caution: with niacin, use inositol hexaniacinate to avoid flushing; with guggul, crude preparation may cause skin rashes or diarrhea.

Key reference

1. *Circulation* 1998,**97**:1837–1847.

General references

Rubenfire M, *et al.*: Treatment strategies for management of serum lipids: lessons learned from lipid metabolism, recent clinical trials, and experience with HMG CoA reductase inhibitors. *Prog Cardiovasc Dis* 1998, **41**:95–116.

Rubins HB, *et al.*: Gemfibrozil for the secondary prevention of coronary heart disease in men with low levels of HDL-C. *N Engl J Med* 1999, **341**:410–418.

Scandinavian Simvastatin Survival Study Group: randomised trial of cholesterol lowering in 4444 patients with coronary heart disease (4S). *Lancet* 1994, **344**: 383–389.

Shepard J, *et al.*: Prevention of coronary heart disease with pravastatin in men with hypercholesterolemia. *N Engl M Med* 1995, **333**:1301–1307.

Diagnosis

Symptoms

Itching (often worse at night).

Signs

There are two clinical forms: infantile and adult.

Infantile:

- Most common on face, scalp, extensor surfaces, groin; perioral and diaper area usually spared; may be generalized.

Adult:

- Most common on flexural creases, neck, dorsa of hands and feet; may be generalized.

Lesions may be further classified into acute, subacute, and chronic eczema:

- Acute flares may present as poorly defined edematous and erythematous patches, vesicles, papules, or plaques. Lesions may be weepy, and excoriations are not uncommon.
- Subacute lesions are crusted and scaling, but still red and pruritic.
- Chronic eczema is characterized by well-demarcated, dry, scaly, lichenified plaques with fissures and erosions; hyperpigmentation or hypopigmentation may be present.

Other associated features: xerosis, keratosis pilaris, Dennie–Morgan lines (infraorbital fold of skin), "allergic shiners" (infraorbital darkening secondary to venous congestion), follicular prominence, pityriasis alba, accentuation of palmar creases.

Investigations

- Atopic eczema is a clinical diagnosis, although family history is helpful.
- Patients often have all or part of the atopic triad (*i.e.*, asthma, allergic rhinitis, atopic eczema).

Skin scrapings: to rule out scabies or dermatophyte infections.

Cultures: to rule out staphylococcal superinfections.

Skin biopsy: rarely performed by experienced clinicians.

Complications

Secondary infection: may occur because of the impaired skin barrier function.

- Bacterial: usually with *Staphylococcus aureus* (golden crusting or oozing may be present).
- Viral: Kaposi's varicelliform eruption is herpes simplex disseminated over the involved cutaneous surface (unlike with classic herpes simplex, the findings may be subtle; look for multiple pinpoint erosions within the areas of atopic dermatitis or the sudden onset of pain in lesions; may be very severe in children); molluscum contagiosum is also not uncommon (multiple pearly umbilicated papules).

Erythroderma (exfoliative erythroderma): possible in severe cases; requires hospital admission with close monitoring to fluid and electrolyte status as well as treatment of any secondary infection that could have triggered the flare.

Differential diagnosis

Scabies.

Tinea.

Psoriasis.

Ichthyosis.

Dermatitis herpetiformis.

Acrodermatitis enteropathica.

Neurodermatitis.

Contact dermatitis.

HIV infection (especially in children).

Seborrheic dermatitis in infants.

Etiology

- Although a host of immunological abnormalities have been identified, there is no real consensus as to the cause of atopic dermatitis; it is probable that many factors play a role.

Immunological abnormalities have included the following:

Elevated serum IgE levels.

Reduced cell-mediated immunity.

Slowed chemotaxis of neutrophils and monocytes.

Epidemiology

- Prevalence of atopic dermatitis (atopic eczema) is 7–24 per 1000.
- The highest prevalence is in children.
- Onset of disease is in the first year of life in ~50% of patients and before the age of 5 years in 85% of patients.

Treatment

Diet and lifestyle

• Rare patients have a definite cutaneous response to certain foods, which obviously should be avoided.

• Children as well as adults should be educated regarding the disease and taught how to apply emollients when they "itch" instead of scratching.

• Encourage brief lukewarm baths or showers with limited use of mild soaps, followed by liberal use of emollient creams or ointments (more moisturizing than lotions).

• Avoid irritants (*e.g.*, dry ambient environment, contact with wool, fragrances [in detergents and fabric softener], scratching).

• Trimming the fingernails may help.

• Stress can exacerbate atopic dermatitis.

• Symptoms may fluctuate seasonally; most symptoms worsen in winter with a dry, harsh environment; some worsen in summer with heat and sweating.

Pharmacological treatment

Topical

• Emollients are the mainstay to prevent dryness.

• In patients refractory to treatment, consider the possibility of allergic contact dermatitis, which may even result from topical emollients or medications.

• Steroids may be used at mild, intermediate, or most potent strength; ointments are the vehicle of choice:

Mild potency: topical steroids, over-the-counter or prescription, 1%–2.5% hydrocortisone; class VI and VII steroids.

Intermediate potency: triamcinolone, flurandrenolide, fluocinolone; class III–V steroids.

Most potent: desoximetasone, clobetasol, betamethasone; class I and II steroids.

Standard dosage	All topical steroids should be applied once or twice a day; intermediate and potent topical steroids should not be used for more than a few days on the face, axillary region, or groin.
Contraindications	None.
Special points	Potent topical steroids should be tapered off as soon as possible to avoid side effects.
Main side effects	Atrophy of the skin, steroid folliculitis, systemic absorption (especially in children).

Systemic therapy

• Systemic treatment is used only in the following situations:

Acyclovir: for secondary infection with herpes.

Antibiotics: for secondary bacterial infection.

Systemic steroids: used only in exceptional cases.

Antihistamines: to relieve prurius.

• Immunosuppressive therapy (cyclosporine, tacrolimus, azathioprine) has shown some success in refractory atopic dermatitis.

• Ultraviolet radiation: may be a useful adjunct in the treatment of chronic recalcitrant dermatitis. Artificial UVB or PUVA (oral or topical psoralens followed by UVA) requires 2–3 treatments per week under professional supervision.

Treatment aims

To decrease pruritus.

To prevent secondary infection.

To educate patients so that they can control the disease.

• The main objective is to control, not cure, the disease, as it is a chronic skin disease.

Prognosis

Resolves in approximately 40% of patients by adulthood.

• The remainder of patients have a chronic course characterized by intermittent flares and remissions.

Follow-up and management

• Most patients are treated with topical agents and are followed up until their disease clears.

• Some physicians continue to follow-up at 3- to 6-month intervals to educate their patients appropriately.

General references

Bork K, Brauninger W: Increasing incidence of eczema herpeticum: analysis of seventy-five cases. *J Am Acad Dermatol* 1988, **19**:1024–1029.

Correale CE, *et al.*: Atopic dermatitis: a review of diagnosis and treatment. *Am Fam Physician* 1999, **60**:1191–1198.

Friedmann PS: Allergy and the skin. II—Contact and atopic eczema. *BMJ* 1998, **316**:1226–1229.

Van der Heijden FL, *et al.*: High frequency of IL-4-producing CD4 positive allergen-specific T-lymphocytes in atopic dermatitis lesional skin. *Invest Dermatol* 1991, **97**:389–394.

Diagnosis

Definition

Eisenmenger's complex
• Originally described by Eisenmenger; pulmonary hypertension at systemic levels due to raised pulmonary vascular resistance, with reversed shunting through a large ventricular septal defect and in the absence of pulmonary stenosis.

Eisenmenger's syndrome
• Term first used by Paul Wood includes all defects associated with pulmonary hypertension at systemic levels and pulmonary vascular disease.

Symptoms
• Symptoms may not appear until the early part of late childhood or early adulthood.

• In many patients, pulmonary congestion in early infancy resolves in early infancy or early childhood as pulmonary vascular resistance increases and magnitude of shunting decreases.

• Occasionally, patients have no history of pulmonary congestion or a murmur in childhood.

• Cyanosis appears as right-to-left shunting develops.

Dyspnea: on exercise; impaired exercise tolerance.

Palpitations: common and usually due to atrial fibrillation or flutter.

Angina of effort.

Hemoptysis: may result from pulmonary infarction or rupture of dilated pulmonary arteries or aorticopulmonary vessels.

Syncope: due to inadequate cardiac output or, less commonly, arrhythmia.

Symptoms of hyperviscosity: visual disturbances, fatigue, headache, dizziness, and paraesthesia.

Symptoms of heart failure: uncommon until the disease is in advanced stages

Signs
Digital clubbing, central cyanosis, arterial pulses (small volume).

Jugular venous pressure: may be normal or elevated, and prominent V waves are seen if tricuspid regurgitation is present.

Heart
Right parasternal heave due to right ventricular hypertrophy.

Loud pulmonary component of S2, often palpable.

Right-sided S4.

Second sound: in ventricular septal defect, a single sound; in atrial septal defect, a fixed wide split S2; and in patent ductus arteriosus, either normally split or reverse splitting.

• Murmur caused by a ventricular septal defect, patent ductus arteriosus, or atrial septal defect disappears; many patients have a decrescendo diastolic murmur caused by pulmonary regurgitation or a holosystolic murmur caused by tricuspid regurgitation.

Investigations
ECG: right ventricular hypertrophy; atrial arrhythmias, particularly in atrial septal defect.

Chest radiography: conspicuous dilatation of the pulmonary artery with narrowed "pruned" peripheral vessels; slight to moderate enlargement of the heart may be seen in atrial septal defect, whereas the size of the heart is normal in ventricular septal defect or patent ductus arteriosus.

Transthoracic echocardiography: evidence of right ventricular overload and pulmonary hypertension; underlying cardiac defect can be visualized; contrast echocardiography permits localization of shunt.

Cardiac catheterization: to assess severity of pulmonary vascular disease and to quantify magnitude of intracardiac shunting; reversibility of shunting assessed with pulmonary vasodilators.

Complications
Right ventricular failure.

Cerebrovascular accidents.

Sudden death.

Brain abscess.

Bleeding and thrombosis.

Paradoxical embolization.

Infective endocarditis.

Hyperuricemia.

Recurrent hemoptysis.

Differential diagnosis
Tetralogy of Fallot.

Transposition with pulmonary stenosis.

Primary pulmonary hypertension.

Secondary pulmonary hypertension: *e.g.*, pulmonary vasculitis or pulmonary thromboembolic disease.

• Any of these may coexist with a patent foramen ovale and may confuse the significance of the defect.

Etiology
• Associated defects include the following:

Ventricular septal defect.

Atrial septal defect.

Patent ductus arteriosus.

Aortopulmonary defect.

Double outlet right ventricle.

Truncus arteriosus.

Transposition of great vessels.

Epidemiology
• The incidence of congenital heart disease is ~10 in 1000 live births; only a few of these progress to Eisenmenger's syndrome.

Treatment

Diet and lifestyle

- Pregnancy carries significant mortality and should be avoided.
- Travel to high altitude is extremely poorly tolerated.
- Strenuous exertion and competitive sports must be avoided.
- Oxygen should be given during flights and dehydration avoided.

Pharmacological treatment

Diuretics

- Standard diuretic treatment is appropriate for right ventricular failure, but care must be taken to avoid dehydration.

Digoxin

- Digoxin remains the mainstay for rate control of atrial fibrillation. Role of primary antiarrhythmic agents such as amiodarone has been little studied.

Standard dosage	Digoxin, 0.0625–0.25 mg daily.
Contraindications	Renal failure.
Special points	Hypokalemia must be avoided.
Main drug interactions	None.
Main side effects	Anorexia, nausea, vomiting, arrhythmias.

Antibiotics

- Antibiotics are indicated for invasive procedures and to treat infective endocarditis (*see* Endocarditis *for specific details)*.

Anticoagulants

- Anticoagulants are indicated when thromboembolism is clinically evident (*e.g.*, transient ischemic attacks) and for patients with atrial fibrillation and are frequently prescribed for severe pulmonary hypertension to prevent in situ thrombosis.

Standard dosage	Warfarin guided by INR.
Contraindications	Pregnancy, peptic ulcer, severe hypertension.
Main drug interactions	*See manufacturer's current prescribing information.*
Main side effects	Hemorrhage.

Other options

- Nonpharmacological methods of contraception are preferred, but the progesterone-only pill may be used.
- No effective pulmonary vasodilators can be recommended routinely; controlled trials on an individual patient basis may be appropriate. Early experience with continuous infusion of prostacyclin is encouraging.
- Hemoptysis should be treated as a medical emergency; specialist treatment at a cardiac center is recommended.

Treatment aims

To improve symptoms and prolong survival.

Other treatments

- Hyperviscosity: phlebotomy with isovolumic replacement. Prophylactic phlebotomy should be considered in preparation for noncardiac surgery (usually 1–2 units of blood with isovolumic replacement) is recommended for patients with hematocrit >65%.
- Heart-lung transplantation: limited success; patients should be carefully selected.

Prognosis

- Survival is 80% 10 years after diagnosis, 77% at 15 years, and 42% at 25 years.
- Death is usually sudden; other causes include heart failure, hemoptysis, brain abscess, and stroke.
- Poor prognostic factors include syncope, clinically evident right ventricular systolic dysfunction, low cardiac output, and severe hypoxemia.

Follow-up and management

- Patients need careful follow-up.
- Attention must be paid to hematocrit and phlebotomy in polycythemic patients.
- Cardiological input to all aspects of the patient's medical care is essential (*e.g.*, contraception and pregnancy, noncardiac surgery, infections).

General references

Brickner ME, Hillis LD, Lange RA: Congenital heart disease in adults. *N Engl J Med* 2000, **342**:334–343.

McLaughlin VV, Genthner DE, Panella MM, *et al.*: Compassionate use of continuous prostacyclin in the management of secondary pulmonary hypertension: a case series. *Ann Intern Med* 1999, **130**:740–743.

Rosenzweig EB, Kerstein D, Barst RJ: Long-term prostacyclin for pulmonary hypertension with associated congenital heart defects. *Circulation* 1999, **99**: 1858–1865.

Wood P: The Eisenmenger syndrome or pulmonary hypertension with reversed central shunt. *BMJ* 1958, **2**:755–762.

Diagnosis

Symptoms

Headache, behavioral abnormality, fever, photophobia, drowsiness; may progress to confusion, coma, convulsions.

Speech disturbance, limb weakness, incoordination, involuntary movements: indicating focal cerebral involvement.

Seizures.

Signs

Drowsiness, confusion, irritability, coma.

Neck stiffness: due to associated meningeal inflammation (may be absent).

Associated focal cerebral hemisphere signs: *e.g.*, hemiparesis and dysphasia (consider herpes simplex encephalitis).

Ataxia, nystagmus, myoclonus, involuntary movements, extensor plantar responses.

Investigations

CT and MRI of brain: help to exclude other causes and may show brain edema; focal inferior temporal and orbital frontal damage with herpes simplex can take several days to become apparent on plain CT but may be seen earlier on contrast-enhanced CT.

Lumbar puncture and CSF analysis: CSF may be under increased pressure and usually shows lymphocytic pleocytosis, modestly elevated protein, and normal glucose concentration. Enzyme-linked immunoassays for viral antigens and gene amplification with polymerase chain reaction are increasingly available to aid early specific diagnosis [1,2], especially in cases of cytomegalovirus or herpes simplex virus.

EEG: shows widespread slow activity with diffuse brain disorder and may show periodic complexes or focal slowing over temporal region in herpes simplex encephalitis.

Complications

Seizures and status epilepticus: often occur and need vigorous treatment.

Cerebral edema: may cause herniation and calls for measures to reduce intracranial pressure.

Differential diagnosis

Meningitis: bacterial, tuberculous, fungal, or viral.

Acute disseminated encephalomyelitis.

Toxic encephalopathy with systemic infection.

Metabolic encephalopathy: usually no fever, headache, or CSF abnormality.

Cerebral abscess, empyema, subdural hematoma, and other mass lesions.

Meningeal carcinomatosis.

Etiology

- Viral invasion of brain parenchyma causes an inflammatory reaction of varying intensity, associated with perivascular cuffing with lymphocytes and other mononuclear cells and with destruction of nerve cells and glia; hemorrhagic necrosis may occur.

Epidemiology [3,4]

- Herpes simplex virus is the most common cause of sporadic encephalitis.
- Other herpes viruses, especially herpes zoster, cytomegalovirus, and Epstein-Barr virus, are common causes, particularly when immunity is impaired, as in transplant or AIDS patients.
- Arboviral encephalitis occurs in epidemics in which mosquitoes bite humans.
- Mumps encephalitis and subacute sclerosing encephalitis have declined in incidence with vaccination; the latter is a progressive late complication of measles infection.
- Progressive multifocal leukoencephalopathy, common in AIDS patients, is due to a human polyoma virus (JC) complicating immunodeficiency.
- HIV may cause meningoencephalitis at seroconversion and, later, a slowly progressive dementia.

Treatment

Diet and lifestyle

Not relevant.

Pharmacological treatment

• No effective treatment is available against many of the viruses causing encephalitis; often, the specific causative virus is not identified.

• Seizures need prompt anticonvulsant administration to reduce the deleterious effects of further seizures.

• Full supportive measures are necessary during what is often a self-limiting illness with good recovery.

• Ventilation, mannitol, and dexamethasone can be used acutely to manage edema.

• Intravenous acyclovir started early reduces the morbidity and mortality of herpes simplex encephalitis; treatment should not await the outcome of brain biopsy, which is seldom appropriate [2].

Standard dosage	Acyclovir, 10 mg/kg i.v. infusion every 8 hours for 14 days (adults), 500 mg/m^2 every 8 hours (children aged 3 months–12 years).
Contraindications	Hypersensitivity.
Special points	Renal impairment necessitates dose reduction.
Main drug interactions	Possible interaction with zidovudine.

• Ganciclovir may be of benefit when cytomegalovirus is the probable cause.

• Improvement of HIV encephalopathy has been reported with zidovudine.

Treatment aims

To treat herpes simplex or cytomegalovirus encephalitis.

To prevent recurrent seizures.

To control raised intracranial pressure.

To provide optimal rehabilitation when necessary.

Prognosis

• The outcome varies with different causative viruses, the age of the patient, and associated underlying disease.

• Death and serious residual disability are frequent with herpes simplex when the diagnosis and treatment are delayed.

Follow-up and management

• Specialized neurological rehabilitation may be important for patients with residual disability in the wake of the illness.

Key references

1. Aurelius E, *et al.*: Rapid diagnosis of herpes simplex encephalitis by nested polymerase chain reaction assay of cerebrospinal fluid. *Lancet* 1991, **337**:189–192.
2. Whitley RJ: Viral encephalitis. *N Engl J Med* 1990, **323**:242–250.
3. Skoldenberg B: Herpes simplex encephalitis. *Scand J Infect Dis* 1996, **100**:8–13.
4. Armbas JR, Storch GA, Clifford DB, Tselis AC: Cytomegalovirus encephalitis. *Ann Intern Med* 1996, **125**:577–587.

Endocarditis

Diagnosis

Definition

• Endocarditis is an infection of the lining of the heart; the hallmark is endocardial vegetation consisting of platelet or fibrin thrombi with bacteria and mononuclear cells.

Subacute endocarditis: low-virulence organisms on previously abnormal valves.

Acute endocarditis: high-virulence organisms on previously normal valves.

Culture-negative endocarditis: negative blood cultures may be due to previous partial treatment, infection by an unusual organism, or noninfective endocarditis.

Noninfective endocarditis: Libman-Sacks endocarditis in SLE; noninfected vegetations occur with valvular stenosis or regurgitation.

Marasmic endocarditis in terminal illnesses: sterile vegetations, rarely embolizing, postmortem findings often seen by chance.

Symptoms

Fever, malaise, anorexia, weight loss, rigors: nonspecific symptoms of inflammation.

Progressive heart failure: due to valve destruction (can be dramatic).

Stroke, pulseless limb, renal infarction, pulmonary infarction: due to embolization of vegetations.

Arthralgia, loin pain: due to immune-complex deposition.

Signs

Fever: unless patient is moribund or immunosuppressed.

Murmurs: except in right-sided endocarditis.

Pallor, purpura, petechiae, vasculitis, splinter hemorrhage, erythematous nodules in finger pulps (Osler's nodes), flat red spots on palms and soles (Janeway lesions), hemorrhagic retinal infarctions, exudative lesions on the retina (Roth spots).

Rashes.

Heart failure.

Clubbing, café-au-lait pigmentation, splenomegaly: if disease is chronic.

Investigations

• Diagnosis depends on a high index of suspicion; no single test is "diagnostic."

Blood culture: at least three sets of cultures 1 hour apart from separate venipuncture sites.

Complete blood count: shows anemia, raised leukocyte count, hemolysis.

Urinalysis: shows microscopic hematuria, proteinuria.

Urea and creatinine: concentrations raised with glomerulonephritis.

CRP, ESR, plasma viscosity analysis: raised as markers of inflammation.

ECG: may reveal conduction disturbances indicative of septal abscess formation.

Two-dimensional echocardiography: may reveal vegetations to support diagnosis; can be used to assess valvular regurgitation or heart chamber size; may detect early complications.

Transesophageal echocardiography: more sensitive than two-dimensional; indicated if diagnosis is in doubt and in patients with prosthetic valves.

Serologic tests.

Complications

Valve destruction.

Congestive heart failure.

Embolism.

Local extension of infection.

Septic emboli to vasa vasorum.

Distal infection (metastatic).

Candidal endocarditis.

Glomerulonephritis.

Differential diagnosis

Pyrexia of unknown origin, tuberculosis, staphylococcal septicemia, paraneoplastic phenomenon (lymphoma, carcinoma).

Systemic vasculitis.

Chordal rupture, aortic dissection, left atrial myxoma.

Etiology

• Damaged valves carry small, short-lived, sterile platelet or fibrin thrombi on their surfaces; these thrombi become infected during transient ischemia.

• Bacteremia can result from dental manipulations (*Streptococcus viridans*), genitourinary instrumentation or surgery (*Escherichia coli*, *Streptococcus faecalis*), mucosal damage due to carcinoma of the colon (*Streptococcus bovis*) or insertion of intravenous lines or injections (*Staphylococcus aureus* or *epidermidis*).

• Alpha hemolytic (*S. viridans* group) accounts for 50% of patients.

• Other bacteria include *Streptococcus pyogenes*, *Haemophilus parainfluenzae*, and *Neisseria*, *Pseudomonas*, and *Brucella* spp.

• Nonbacterial organisms include fungi (*e.g.*, *Candida* spp., *Aspergillus* spp.), chlamydiae (*e.g.*, *Chlamydia psittaci*), and rickettsiae (*e.g.*, *Coxiella burnetii*).

• Groups at risk include the following: patients with previously damaged endocardium (75% of cases: 25% with rheumatic heart disease, 25% with prosthetic heart valves, 15% with bicuspid aortic valve, mitral valve prolapse; 10% with congenital heart disease), intravenous drug abusers, patients with long-standing i.v. lines (*e.g.*, for feeding chemotherapy or hemodynamic monitoring), recurrent bacteremia, immunosuppression, and valve trauma caused by the line itself.

Epidemiology

• An average community hospital admits one patient with endocarditis each month.

• An average primary care physician sees one patient with endocarditis every 10 years.

• The yearly incidence is ~15 000 to 20 000 new cases.

Treatment

Diet and lifestyle

• No special precautions are necessary.

Pharmacological Treatment

• The key is accurate, early diagnosis and close cooperation among cardiologist, infectious disease specialist, and cardiac surgeon.

•Patients presenting with fever and suspected endocarditis do not need emergency antibiotic treatment (unless they are acutely unwell); a delay of 48–72 hours allow efforts to make an accurate diagnosis.

• Positive blood cultures allow the initiation of i.v. antibiotic treatment based on probable sensitivities while awaiting laboratory confirmation.

• If the blood culture is negative, appropriate serology for culture-negative organisms should be obtained while the "best bet" i.v. antibiotics are given. Empirical antibiotics should be active against staphylococci, streptococci, and enterococci. Nafcillin or oxacillin, 1.5 g every 4 hours, plus penicillin, 2–3 MU every 4 hours (or ampicillin, 1.5 g every 4 hours), plus gentamicin, 1 mg/kg every 8 hours, is effective. Vancomycin, 15 mg/kg every 12 hours, may be used instead of penicillin in patients allergic to penicillin.

• Successful treatment should result in a reduction in fever within 10 days and a decrease in CRP level within 2 weeks.

Nonpharmacological treatment

• If the portal of entry was bad teeth, these should be removed.

• After the need for surgery has been identified, treatment should not be delayed.

• Surgery is indicated in the following situations:

Failure of medical treatment to control infective process (possible abscess formation), indicated by continuing fever > 10 days, rising CRP concentration, worsening nephritis.

Indications of abscess formation, *e.g.*, conduction abnormalities, cavity on echocardiography, or prosthetic valve dehiscence.

Hemodynamic deterioration, *e.g.*, pulmonary edema or increasing cardiomegaly.

Infection by organisms that are difficult to eradicate, *e.g.*, *Staphylococcus aureus, Candida spp., Aspergillus spp.*

Infection on a prosthetic valve.

Recurrent embolization or enlarging, large vegetations while patient is receiving effective antimicrobial therapy.

Treatment aims

To eradicate infection and prevent valve damage

Prognosis

• Despite advances in diagnosis and treatment, mortality remains high at >20%; avoiding delay before diagnosis, isolating an organism, using high-dose antibiotics, and appropriately using cardiac surgery should reduce this figure.

• Some patients have recurrent infection (<10%), and all are at risk of reinfection.

Follow-up and management

• Blood culture, blood count, CRP concentrations, and echocardiogram should be checked 3–4 weeks after apparently successful antibiotic treatment has been stopped.

• Removal of the predisposing factor (e.g., ventricular septal defect, patent ductus arteriosus) should be considered. This will, however, probably prevent only 10% of cases.

Prevention

• High-risk categories include prosthetic cardiac valves, previous bacterial endocarditis, complex cyanotic congenital heart disease, surgically constructed systemic pulmonary shunts or conduits. Endocarditis prophylaxis is recommended in these patients.

• Patients at risk should maintain good dental hygiene and receive antibiotic prophylaxis for potentially bacteremic maneuvers, e.g., tooth extraction, rigid bronchoscopy, sclerotherapy, endoscopic retrograde cholangiopancreatography with biliary obstruction, biliary tract surgery, genitourinary surgery, instrumentation. This will, however, probably prevent only 10% of the cases.

General references

Bayer AS, Bolger AF, Taubert KA, *et al.*: Diagnosis and management of infective endocarditis. *Circulation* 1998, **98**:2936–2948.

Dajani AS, Taubert KA, Wilson W, *et al.*: Prevention of bacterial endocarditis: recommendations of the American Heart Association. *Circulation* 1997, **96**:358–366.

Epilepsy

Diagnosis

Symptoms

Seizures: usually abrupt onset, transient, stereotyped, and recurrent.

Somatic, visual, auditory, olfactory, gustatory, or visceral sensations.

***Déjà vu, jamais vu*, macropsia, micropsia.**

Abnormal posture, tone, movements.

Loss of or altered awareness.

Incontinence or oral trauma with ictus.

Signs

- Usually no signs are manifest.
- Patients should be checked for the following:

Mental status and cognitive function.

Focal neurological deficit, head circumference, hemiatrophy.

Evidence of raised intracranial pressure.

Evidence of adverse effects from antiepileptic drugs.

Cutaneous lesions suggestive of tuberous sclerosis, neurofibromatosis.

Investigations [1]

EEG: routine, with hyperventilation and photic stimulation; if normal and diagnosis in doubt, sleep-deprived and sleep EEG, 24-hour ambulatory tape, video-EEG monitoring can be considered (if episodes frequent); yield increased with repeat EEG up to 4.

Neuroimaging: MRI superior to CT, necessary for intractable partial seizures or focal deficit, if CT normal or unclear, or if surgical treatment of epilepsy contemplated.

Antiepileptic drug concentration measurement: if prescribed treatment, to check compliance and to assess role of medication levels in symptoms and seizure control.

Blood chemistry: fasting glucose, liver, renal, and complete blood count profiles.

Lumbar puncture: for acute assessment where indicated.

Neuropsychology: if cognition or memory causes concern.

Chest radiography, ECG, HIV, and syphilis serology: can also be considered.

Complications

Trauma.

Status epilepticus.

Sudden unexpected death, atrial arrhythmias.

Psychosocial handicap.

Differential diagnosis

Altered or lost awareness

Syncope, vagal overactivity, breath holding (children), arrhythmia, cardiac outflow obstruction, drug abuse, hypoglycemia, toxic confusional state, narcolepsy or cataplexy, sleep attacks, transient global amnesia, psychologically mediated disorders.

Abnormal movements

Paroxysmal movement disorder, oculogyric crisis, tetany from hyperventilation, psychologically mediated disorders.

Neurological deficit

Transient ischemic attack, stroke, migraine, psychologically mediated disorders.

Nocturnal spells

Parasomnias, paroxysmal nocturnal dystonia.

Etiology

- Causes include the following:

Cryptogenic.
Idiopathic (often familial).
Hippocampal sclerosis.
Cortical dysplasia.
Tumor.
Trauma.
Infection: encephalitis, bacterial meningitis.
Vascular: infarct, hemorrhage.
Hypoxia.
Granuloma: tuberculosis, cystercercosis or other infections
Autoimmune cerebral vasculitis.

Epidemiology

- 1 person in 40 has a nonfebrile seizure at some time in his or her life.
- The prevalence of active epilepsy (seizure within past 2 years) is 1 in 200 of the general population and 1 in 150 people aged <15 years.

Classification

- Classification of epilepsy is important for investigation, treatment, and prognosis.

Partial epilepsy

Seizures arising from one or more discrete foci with mixture of simple partial, complex partial, and secondarily generalized seizures.

Generalized epilepsy

Primary: normal cerebral function with normal background EEG, high incidence of familial and young onset, absence, myoclonic tonic–clonic seizures.

Secondary: abnormal cerebral function, slowed EEG, mixed tonic, atypical absence, myoclonic, or tonic–clonic seizures.

Treatment

Diet and lifestyle

- Patients must avoid sleep deprivation.
- Alcohol lowers seizure threshold and may affect antiepileptic levels.
- Patients are not allowed to drive, swim, go to heights alone, or operate dangerous tools.
- Strobe lights may activate epilepsy.

Pharmacological treatment [2]

- Drug interactions are complex.
- The following doses are for adults.

First line

Phenytoin: for all seizure types; may give 20 mg/kg loading dose; i.v. phosphenytoin now available with less toxicity (maintenance 300–500 mg/day).

Carbamazepine: for simple, complex, or secondarily generalized partial seizures and for tonic or clonic generalized seizures; 100 mg initially, average maintenance dose 600–2400 mg daily in 3–4 doses. Available in long-acting equivalent twice-daily dose.

Clonazepam: for myoclonic seizures (second-line treatment for absences, atonic seizures); 0.5 mg initially, average maintenance dose 0.5–3.0 mg daily in 1–2 doses.

Ethosuximide: for absences only; 250 mg initially, average maintenance dose 500–1500 mg daily in 1–2 doses.

Valproate: primarily for generalized or myoclonic seizures; also useful for some partial epilepsies; 750 mg initially, average maintenance dose 1500–3000 mg daily in 3 divided doses.

Second line

Gabapentin: for partial seizures; 300 mg initially, average maintenance dose 1800–3600 mg daily in 3 doses.

Lamotrigine: for partial seizures, tonic, clonic, tonic-clonic, or atonic seizures, and absence or atypical absence; 25 mg initially, average maintenance dose 300–500 mg daily in 2 doses; if combined with valproate, initial dosage should be 25 mg increasing on alternate weeks.

Phenobarbitol: for partial seizures, tonic, clonic, tonic-clonic, atonic, and atypical absences; 60 mg initially, average maintenance dose 60–180 mg daily as single dose.

Topirimate: for partial seizures, 50 mg increasing gradually up to 400 mg daily.

General adverse effects

Acute, dose-related: sedation, dizziness, nausea, headaches, sometimes tremor.

Idiosyncratic: skin rash, severe bone-marrow suppression, diplopia, liver failure, behavioral disorder, weight gain, tremor, gingival hyperplasia, soft-tissue changes, peripheral neuropathy.

Treatment aims

To control seizures without drug side effects.

Other treatments

- In patients with refractory mesial temporal lobe epilepsy, anterior temporal lobectomy produces an 80% chance of remission, in well-chosen patients.
- Lesional and extratemporal partial epilepsy remission rate is 30%–50% after surgery.

Prognosis

- Remission occurs in 70%–80% of patients in 2–5 years; patients have a 30% chance of remission if epilepsy is active for 5 years.
- After the patient is in remission, the overall risk of relapse is 20% in 2 years if the patient remains on medication, and 40% if medication is tapered.
- Risk factors for relapse include early onset, frequent generalized seizures, generalized spike-wave on EEG, structural brain damage, and difficulty obtaining seizure control.

Follow-up and management

Staged treatment strategy

- This can be followed as far as necessary.

1. Minimizing of epileptogenic stimuli: fever (in children), alcohol, excessive fatigue, epileptogenic drugs, photosensitivity.
2. Initial small dose of first-line drug.
3. Dosage increase if needed, up to maximum tolerated dose.
4. Review of diagnosis, cause, and compliance if no response after treatment.
5. Trial of other drugs alone or combined (80% of patients best treated by monotherapy, 10%–15% by two drugs).
6. Gradual withdrawal of unhelpful drugs or drugs causing adverse effects.
7. Referral for investigational drugs.
8. Referral for possible neurosurgical treatment of partial epilepsies.
9. Gradual drug withdrawal considered in patients free of seizures for 2–3 years.

Essential counseling

- Patients should be advised of the need to take medication regularly, driving regulations, contraception and pregnancy, safe bathing, and safe cooking with a microwave.

Key references

1. Wylie E: *The Treatment of Epilepsy*. Philadelphia: Lea and Febiger; 1993.
2. MacDonald RL, Greenfield LJ Jr: Mechanisms of action of new antiepileptic drugs. *Curr Opin Neurol* 1997, **10**:121–128.

Erectile dysfunction

Diagnosis

Symptoms

Erectile dysfunction: sexual dysfunction of any degree related to achieving adequate erection with associated satisfactory performance; includes flaccidity, loss of erection, semirigid erection, loss of nocturnal erection, anorgasmia, unsatisfied sexual partner, loss of libido, marital/relationship discord, anxiety, depression.

Impotence: the inability to obtain and sustain an erection to orgasm during ≥75% of attempts.

• Patients are frequently reluctant to express symptoms without direct questioning.

Signs

• Direct signs of impotence/erectile dysfunction are infrequently elicited in the office, even in specialized clinics.

• Indirect signs of possible contributing factors include evidence of peripheral vascular disease (audible bruits, palpable thrills), signs of peripheral neuropathy, or central nervous system disease/injury including absence of a normal bulbocavernosus reflex.

Investigations

All patients

Serum testosterone, serum prolactin, glycohemoglobin level: screen for hypogonadism, hyperprolactinemia, diabetes as contributors.

Selected patients

Nocturnal penile tumescence, postage stamp test, Rigi-scan: to determine presence or absence of any erectile function.

Cavernosography, cavernosometry, ultrasonography: specialized examination to rule out venous leak as cause.

Pelvic electromyography: advised when neurogenic cause is possible but not clearly demonstrable on examination.

Complications

• These relate mainly to the deterioration of quality of life, with possible reactive psychiatric sequlae and loss of self-esteem.

Differential diagnosis

• Erectile dysfunction may be a presenting symptom for a variety of chronic and/or subacute medical and psychiatric conditions or as a result of their treatment.

Psychogenic: anxiety, depression, psychosis, alcoholism.

Hormonal: hypopituitarism, hyperprolactinemia, hypogonadism, diabetes.

Neurological: spinal cord injury, multiple sclerosis, stroke, peripheral neuropathy.

Vascular: atherosclerosis, hypertension.

Etiology

• 75% of cases have primary organic/ physiologic cause; 25% have primary psychological cause.

• Most cases should not be considered psychological in cause/nature.

Medications: particularly antihypertensive drugs and those with anticholinergic activity or side effects; many others may also contribute.

Alcohol use/abuse: with or without associated hormonal disturbance.

Vascular atherosclerosis: commonly associated with chronic diabetes and hypertension.

Venous leak: commonly affects younger men.

Neurological: >50% of patients with spinal cord injury affected; peripheral neuropathies of many types may contribute.

Psychiatric: reactive and endogenous syndromes (particularly depression and anxiety) and/or their treatment.

Postoperative: as a complication of urologic surgery.

Epidemiology

Common in elderly population: one-third of men aged >65 years are affected by impotence.

• ~30 million Americans are affected by impotence.

• 52% of men aged 40-70 years will suffer erectile dysfunction.

Treatment

Diet and lifestyle

• The centerpiece of managing this condition is involvement of the patient and his sexual partner.

• Alcohol intake should be restricted.

• Adequate, quality sleep time, and absence of excessive fatigue improve management.

Pharmacological treatment

Standard dose	Sildenafil (Viagra), 50–100 mg orally as needed 1 hour before anticipated encounter. Safety, effectiveness, and ease of administration have made it the drug of choice in initial treatment of erectile dysfunction.
	Alprostadil (prostaglandin E_1), used in an injectable form and as an intraurethral suppository. Effective and reasonably safe, but its use is limited because of discomfort caused by the methods of administration. A lack of response to alprostadil treatment suggests that venous leak may be cause of erectile dysfunction.
Contraindications	*Sildenafil:* contraindicated in patients with known coronary artery disease who are using nitrate therapy. Studies are underway to determine safety in patients with coronary artery disease not using nitrates.
	Itracavernosal and intraurethral alprostadil: contraindicated in conditions predisposing to priapism (*e.g.*, sickle cell disease), anatomic deformation of the penis (*e.g.*, Peyronie's disease).
Main drug interactions	Nitrate therapy *(sildenafil).*
Main side effects	*Sildanafil:* visual disturbance (blue halo seen around objects).
	Prostaglandin: penile pain, prolonged erections.
	Urethral burning: intraurethral prostaglandin.

Other treatment options

• Referral is recommended if suspected cause is venous leak or psychological, or if implantable prosthesis is the preferred treatment option.

Sex therapy

• Sex therapy is a strongly recommended adjunct to any successful intervention.

• The drawback is limited availability of qualified experts.

Vacuum erection device

• This is indicated regardless of cause.

Implantable penile prosthesis

• This is indicated regardless of cause and is very effective.

• The drawback is expense, and surgical revision is required in 10%–50% of cases.

Alternative medicine

Recommended use: none.

Common use: Ginkgo biloba; yohimbe (Pausinystalia yohimbe); ginseng (Panax ginseng); Saw palmetto (Serenoa ripens).

Caution: yohimbe may cause anxiety, tachycardia, hypertension, flushing, headache, or hallucination; do not combine with sildenafil.

Treatment aims

To ensure patient and sexual partner satisfaction with sexual performance.

To improve quality of life.

To limit effects from treatment.

Prognosis

• Response rates are high for one or more of available treatment options. Patients' and their partners' satisfaction rates are 70% with vacuum erection device, 80% with injection therapy, and 90% with inflatable prosthesis.

• Success rates with sildenafil range from 60% to 70%.

Follow-up and management

• Priapism resulting from PGE1 therapy is a medical emergency and deserves immediate referral to a well-qualified urologic surgeon.

• Reassurance and indicating concern are reason enough for frequent follow-up with the patient and sexual partner after treatment has been prescribed.

General references

Dewire DM: Evaluation and treatment of erectile dysfunction. *Am Fam Physician* 1996, **53**:2101-2106.

Impotence. NIH Consensus Statement (http://odp.od.nih.gov/consensus/) 1992, **10**:1-31.

Nehra A, *et al.*: Pharmacotherapeutic advances in the treatment of erectile dysfunction. *Mayo Clin Proc* 1999, **74**:709–721.

Perring M, Moran J: Holistic approach to the management of erectile disorders in a male sexual health clinic. *Br J Clin Pract* 1995, **3**:140-144.

Erythema multiforme & Stevens–Johnson syndrome

Diagnosis

Symptoms

• Erythema multiforme (EM) and Stevens–Johnson syndrome (SJS) were previously thought to form a spectrum of diseases ranging from mild to life-threatening. Current opinion suggests that these conditions are distinct cutaneous reactions to underlying conditions. Both exhibit mucosal erosions and targetoid lesions, but they do so with different patterns of involvement.

Erythema multiforme
Asymptomatic: often.
Pain or pruritus: due to skin lesions; pain caused by oral mucosal erosions.
Pain or paresthesias: from preceding herpes simplex virus infection.
Stevens–Johnson syndrome
Nonspecific upper respiratory symptoms: prodrome may be present.
Pain: from mucosal erosions or skin bullae.
Fever, malaise, myalgias: from systemic reaction.

Signs

Erythema multiforme

Mild, self-limited; recurrences are not uncommon.

Classic "target" lesions: develop abruptly and symmetrically; heaviest peripherally; often involve palms and soles.
Oral mucosal lesions: may be present; usually manifest as erosions.
Vesicles and bullae: may develop in existing lesions as a result of intense inflammation at the dermal-epidermal junction.

• Diagnosis can be made clinically if classic target lesions are present.

Biopsy: helpful in cases with atypical target lesions; histological findings vary with evolution of skin lesions.
Serology: for herpes simplex virus, *Mycoplasma pneumoniae*.
Viral culture: may be useful to detect herpes simplex virus.

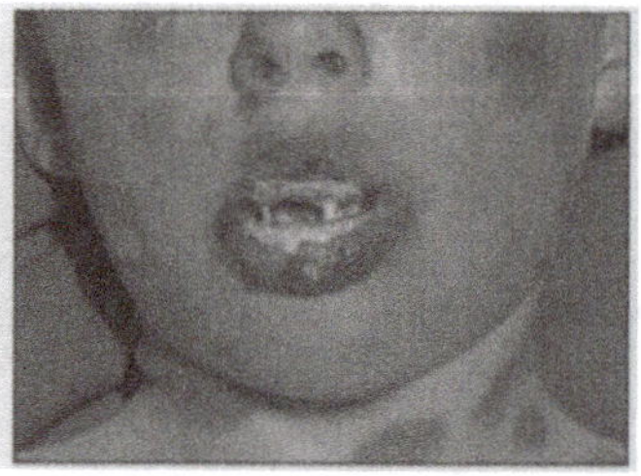

Buccal mucous membrane involvement. (*See* Color Plate.)

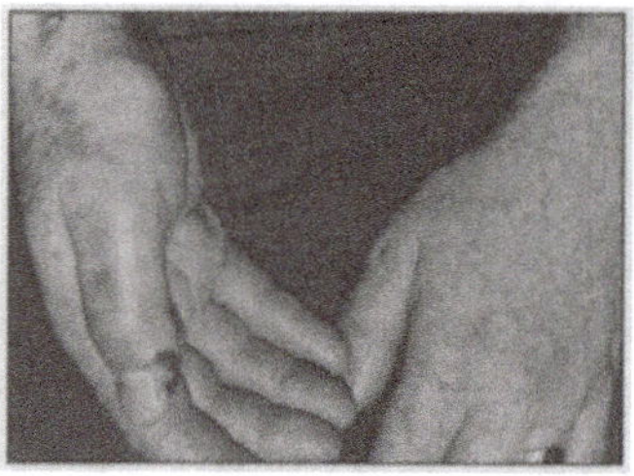

Typical "target" lesions on hands. (*See* Color Plate.)

Stevens–Johnson syndrome

Severe and potentially life-threatening.

Atypical target lesions or purpuric macules: may be present with vesicles and bullae; cutaneous involvement is usually widespread or truncal.
Painful mucosal lesions: arise abruptly 1–14 days after other symptoms; typically involving two or more mucosal surfaces (*e.g.*, oral, conjunctival, urethral, vulvo-vaginal); may result in painful or impaired alimentation, respiration or micturition; conjunctival involvement can be severe.
Pulmonary disease, renal failure, diarrhea, and polyarthritis: all may occur.

History of drug ingestion: very important.
Biopsy: may help diagnosis.
Serum electrolyte and albumin measurement: to monitor fluid and electrolyte status in extensive disease.

Complications

Secondary infection/sepsis.
Dehydration/electrolyte imbalances: in severe SJS.
Ocular complications: in SJS.
Acute respiratory distress syndrome: from diffuse interstitial pneumonitis in SJS.
Postinflammatory hyperpigmentation.

Differential diagnosis

Drug eruption.
Erythema chronicum migrans (Lyme disease).
Erythema annulare centrifugum.
Bullous pemphigoid.
Pemphigus vulgaris.
Chronic urticaria.
Toxic epidermal necrolysis.
Staphylococcal scalded skin syndrome.

Etiology

• Both conditions are produced by a hypersensitivity reaction to some inciting factor.

Erythema multiforme

• Most cases are associated with herpes simplex virus infection (which may be subclinical). This is true particularly in cases of recurrent EM.

• Other potential causes: malignancy, hormonal factors, other infections (*M. pneumoniae*)

• In some cases, no inciting agent is found.

Stevens–Johnson syndrome

• Most cases are related to drug ingestion. The most common culprits are antibiotics (penicillins, sulfonamides), anticonvulsant agents (phenytoin, carbamazepine, phenobarbital, lamotrigine), NSAIDs, and allopurinol.

Epidemiology

• Erythema multiforme and SJS account for up to 1% of dermatology outpatient consultations.

• In EM, children <3 years and adults >50 years are rarely affected.

• Seasonal epidemics may occur, related to the provoking agents (*e.g.*, *Mycoplasma* spp.).

Treatment

Diet and lifestyle

•A special diet may be needed in the case of mucosal erosions.

Pharmacological treatment

Erythema multiforme: prophylaxis

• Anti-herpes virus therapy is useful to suppress recurrent EM.

Standard dosage	Acyclovir, 400 mg twice daily. Valacyclovir, 1000 mg daily.
Contraindications	*Acyclovir:* renal impairment, severe dehydration. *Valacyclovir:* patients with advanced HIV disease or transplant recipients may develop thrombotic thrombocytopenic purpura or hemolytic uremic syndrome.
Main side effects	Generally well tolerated.

Erythema multiforme: treatment of acute episode

Standard dosage	Acyclovir, 200 mg five times daily for 5 days. Valacyclovir, 500 mg twice daily for 5 days.
Contraindications	*Acyclovir:* renal impairment, severe dehydration. *Valacyclovir:* patients with advanced HIV disease or transplant recipients may develop thrombotic thrombocytopenic purpura or hemolytic uremic syndrome.
Main side effects	Generally well tolerated.

• In cases precipitated by *M. pneumoniae* infection, consider antibiotic therapy with a macrolide or tetracycline.

•Topical steroids or antihistamines may be helpful for relieving symptoms.

Stevens–Johnson syndrome

• Withdrawal of any drug precipitant and treatment of infective causes are vital.

• The use of oral prednisone is controversial because no well-controlled trials are available.

• Fluid and electrolyte status must be carefully monitored.

• Any sign of secondary infection must be aggressively treated.

Other treatments

• For ocular lesions, refer the patient to an ophthalmologist.

• Careful skin nursing is essential to prevent secondary infection.

Treatment aims

To remove or treat underlying "triggers."

To provide adequate pain relief for mucosal involvement.

To provide symptomatic relief for generalized skin involvement.

To maintain nutrition and fluid replacement.

Prognosis

Erythema multiforme

Disease is normally mild and self-limited, with complete recovery in 2–3 weeks.

EM associated with herpes simplex virus may recur with reactivation of the virus.

Stevens–Johnson syndrome

Untreated SJS has a 5%–15% mortality rate; sepsis is the most common cause of death.

Serious sequelae may occur depending on the extent of involvement.

Follow-up and management

• Prophylaxis against herpes simplex virus is important if the virus precipitates erythema multiforme.

• Follow-up should be based on the severity of disease.

General references

Assier H, *et al.*: Erythema multiforme with mucous membrane involvement and Stevens-Johnson syndrome are clinically different disorders with distinct causes. *Arch Dermatol* 1995, **131**:539–543.

Imafuku S, *et al.*: Expression of herpes simplex virus DNA fragments located in epidermal keratinocytes and germinative cells is associated with the development of erythema multiforme lesions. *J Invest Dermatol* 1997, **109**:550–556.

Kerob D, *et al.*: Recurrent erythema multiforme unresponsive to acyclovir prophylaxis and responsive to valacyclovir continuous therapy. *Arch Dermatol* 1998, **134**:876–877.

Renfro L, *et al.*: Controversy: are systemic steroids indicated in the treatment of erythema multiforme? *Pediatr Dermatol* 1989, **6**:43–50.

Tatnall FM: A double-blind placebo controlled trial of continuous acyclovir therapy of recurrent erythema multiforme. *Br J Dermatol* 1995, **132**:267–270.

Wong KC, *et al.*: Clinical manifestations and outcomes in 17 cases of Stevens-Johnson syndrome and toxic epidermal necrolysis. *Australas J Dermatol* 1999, **40**:131–134.

Erythema nodosum

Diagnosis

Symptoms

Tender subcutaneous nodules: pain worse on weight-bearing.

"Crops" of lesions: occurring at different times, so that lesions may manifest at different stages of evolution.

Fever, arthralgias, and malaise: variable but may precede lesions by 1–7 days,

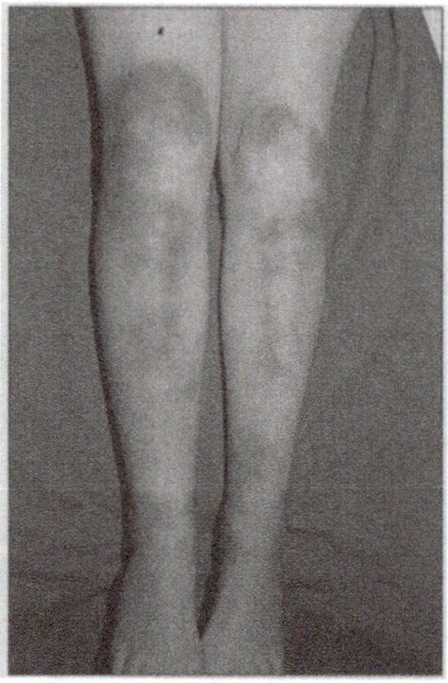

Classic lesions over pretibial region. (*See* Color Plate.)

Signs

Tender subcutaneous erythematous nodules: usually asymmetric and bilateral over pretibial areas; no ulceration or blistering; spontaneous involution over 3–6 weeks; may involve any body area with subcutaneous fat.

Arthropathy: seen in 70% of patients; may persist longer than cutaneous eruption.

Investigations

• Diagnosis can usually be made clinically; deep skin biopsy, including subcutaneous tissue, may be needed.

• Determination of the underlying cause is crucial.

• Discovering the cause is important because treatment of this prevents recurrences.

Extensive history: for drugs, infection, inflammatory disease.

ESR, acute-phase reactants: raised.

CBC: leukocytosis.

Purified protein derivative test: positive in tuberculosis.

Bacteriology: sputum or early morning urine for acid/alcohol-fast bacilli; throat swab or antistreptolysin O titer for evidence of streptococcal infection; stool culture.

Chest radiography: to detect features of sarcoidosis, tuberculosis, disseminated fungal infection.

Complications

• Complications relate to the underlying condition; if this is not controlled, the skin lesions may recur.

Differential diagnosis

Cellulitis.

Thrombophlebitis.

Other panniculitides (lupus panniculitis, nodular vasculitis).

Erythema nodosum leprosum.

Etiology

• Erythema nodosum is a septal panniculitis and represents a hypersensitivity reaction to an underlying stimulus.

• Causes include the following:

Drugs: *e.g.*, sulfonamides, oral contraceptive pill.

Infections: *e.g.*, tuberculosis, streptococci, *Yersinia, Salmonella, Campylobacter* spp., deep fungal infection, including Histoplasmosis, coccidiodomycosis, leprosy.

Inflammatory conditions: *e.g.*, sarcoidosis, inflammatory bowel disease, Behçet's syndrome.

Epidemiology

• The most common cause in children is streptococcal pharyngitis.

• The peak age is 20–30 years, but it can occur at any age.

• The female:male ratio is 3:1.

• Fever and systemic reactions occur more often and persist longer in older patients.

Treatment

Diet and lifestyle

- During the acute phase of the inflammation, prolonged weight-bearing should be avoided.

Pharmacological treatment

- Treatment of skin lesions is primarily symptomatic because spontaneous resolution usually occurs.
- Treatment should be aimed at the underlying cause.
- If lesions are severe or recur, other therapy may be indicated.

NSAIDs: may relieve symptoms.

Standard dosage	Naproxen, 250–500 mg twice daily.
	Indomethacin, 25–50 mg one to three times daily.
Contraindications	Peptic ulcer disease, previous hypersensitivity reaction, renal insufficiency.
Main drug interactions	Warfarin may exacerbate peptic ulcer disease.
Side effects	Gastrointestinal.

Treatment aims

To relieve symptoms.

To remove or treat underlying cause.

Other treatments

Systemic steroids are rarely used and may be dangerous if underlying infection is present.

Potassium iodide.

Prognosis

- Spontaneous resolution usually occurs in 3–6 weeks.

Follow-up and management

- The most important aspect of erythema nodosum management is diagnosis of any underlying precipitant.

General references

Cribier B, *et al.*: Erythema nodosum and associated diseases: a study of 129 cases. *Int J Dermatol* 1998, **37**:667–672.

White WL, Hitchcock MG: Diagnosis: erythema nodosum or not? *Semin Cutan Med Surg* 1999, **18**:47–55.

Esophageal carcinoma

Diagnosis

Symptoms

Dysphagia: solids > liquids is the classic presentation.

Weight loss, fatigue.

Unexplained cessation of reflux symptoms: in patients with untreated pyrosis.

• Gastrointestinal bleeding occasionally is the chief presenting symptom.

Signs

• Most typically, patients have a normal physical examination on presentation. When present, abnormalities may include the following items:

Clinical evidence of weight loss (*e.g.,* muscle wasting).

Pallor when anemia is present.

Supraclavicular or cervical lymphadenopathy.

Hepatomegaly secondary to metastasis.

Respiratory findings (*i.e.,* rales or rhonchi) from aspiration.

Investigations

• Primary investigation should be directed at imaging the of the esophageal lumen.

Barium swallow (esophagram): least expensive imaging modality but does not allow tissue identification of the lesion or therapeutic dilation if necessary; malignant findings must be confirmed with biopsy.

Upper endoscopy: offers direct examination of the lesion and allows sampling of abnormalities for histological confirmation.

Endoscopic ultrasonography: allows staging of the tumor in patients who are potential candidates for surgical resection.

Thoracic-abdominal CT scanning: best initial study to determine the extensiveness of disease once malignancy has been identified.

Complete blood count: may reveal iron-deficiency anemia.

Liver chemistry tests: may reveal metastatic disease to the liver with elevated alkaline phosphatase or amino transfecase levels.

Complications

Esophageal obstruction.

Malnutrition.

Bleeding.

Fistula to bronchial tree: cough with swallowing.

Invasion of mediastinum.

Aspiration: recurrent pneumonia.

Differential diagnosis

Benign esophageal stricture.

Motility disorders, particularly achalasia.

Extrinsic compression of esophagus: *e.g.,* carcinoma of bronchus.

Schatzki's ring.

Risk factors

Squamous carcinoma: most common in African-American males; associated with alcohol and tobacco use; previous caustic ingestion.

Adenocarcinoma: most common in whites with a slight predominance in males; reflux predisposes to Barrett's esophagus (premalignant tissue of specialized columnar epithelium in the distal esophagus that may progress to adenocarcinoma of the esophagus) [1,2].

• Achalasia and previous caustic ingestion injuries predispose to later development of esophageal malignancies.

Epidemiology [1]

• Esophageal carcinoma is one of the most common cancers in the world, but wide geographical variations are found.

• Environmental factors are poorly characterized (*e.g.,* high-risk regions in Iran, China, and Russia identified).

• It is relatively less frequent in western Europe and North America (incidence, 5 in 100 000).

Histological types

• Worldwide, squamous carcinoma predominates, accounting for 90% of esophageal malignancies.

• Adenocarcinoma of the stomach cardia and distal esophagus is increasing in frequency, probably because of the association with gastroesophageal reflux and Barrett's esophagus.

Treatment

Diet and lifestyle

• Adequate nutrition should be ensured, preferably orally (soft foods and high-calorie nutritional supplements should be emphasized).

• The need for a fine-bore enteral feeding tube or percutaneous endoscopic gastrostomy tube should be anticipated, and the tube should be placed prior to high-grade obstruction of the esophagus.

Pharmacological treatment [4,5]

• Simple analgesics are used for pain control in the early stages, but opiates are needed later.

• Avoid prokinetic agents such as metoclopramide or cisapride, which may potentiate dysphagia.

Standard dosage	Morphine, 5–10 mg every 4 hours, titrate as needed.
Contraindications	Raised intracranial pressure.
Special points	Concerns about side effects should not deter use.
Main drug interactions	Synergistic effect with other CNS depressants.
Main drug effects	Constipation, nausea, drowsiness.

• Chemotherapy is reserved for patients who are not surgical candidates and involves 5-fluorouracil- and cisplatin-based protocols that are ideally used concomitantly with radiation therapy [4].

Nonpharmacological treatment

• Curative surgery is attempted whenever possible, but most patients have evidence of extensive disease on presentation and are suitable for only palliative treatment.

Surgical resection: suitable in only about one-third of patients; esophagectomy with primary esophagogastrostomy most frequently chosen. Investigational protocols involving perioperative radiation and/or chemotherapy show some promise but are often quite cumbersome for the patient [5].

Endoscopic palliation: simple dilatation (by bougie or balloon), endoscopic intubations (prosthetic stents available), laser therapy, thermal devices (*e.g.*, bipolar coagulation) may be used to facilitate patency of the esophageal lumen allowing maintenance of hydration and nutrition [3].

Palliative radiation therapy: intracavitary irradiation with cobalt or iridium or external-beam irradiation; can be beneficial for pain from mediastinal extension.

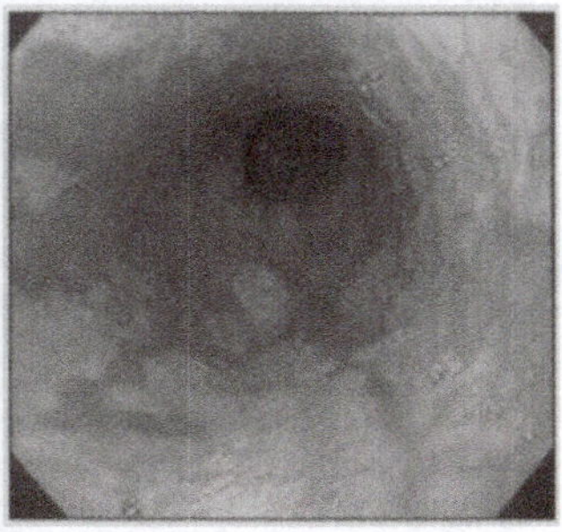

Esophageal stricture with ulcer at the squamocolumnar junction.

Treatment aims

To delay physical deterioration by improving and maintaining swallowing and nutrition.

To diminish pain.

To avoid respiratory complications.

Prognosis

• The 5-year survival for patients with esophageal cancer is <10% and most patients die within 4–12 months of diagnosis. Radiation and/or chemotherapy can offer only modest improvements in this prognosis.

• Patients who are candidates for surgical resection have a 5-year survival of ~20%. This may be further enhanced with perioperative chemotherapy/radiation investigational protocols. Perioperative mortality in general is <15% and attributed to cardiopulmonary complications, sepsis, and anastamotic leaks with malnutrition as an additional potentiating influence.

Follow-up and management

• Patients who have had curative treatment should be monitored for features of relapse with CT scans and imaging studies of the esophageal lumen.

• A fistula communicating with the bronchial tree should be considered in patients with progressive disease who develop a cough; stent placement may be beneficial in these patients.

Key references

1. Blot WJ: Esophageal cancer trends and risk factors. *Semin Oncol* 1994, **21**:403–410.
2. Griffin SM, Robertson CS: Nonsurgical treatment of cancer of the oesophagus. *Br J Surg* 1993, **80**:412–413.
3. Sontag St. Gastroesophageal reflux disease. Current Practice of Med 1998, **1**:733–740.

Diagnosis

Symptoms

• Symptoms do not predict the severity of mucosal inflammation.

Heartburn: retrosternal or epigastric burning is the most common symptom; dull ache may resemble angina.

Regurgitation of food, acid, or bitter juice: may be confused with "vomiting" (but usually without nausea).

Respiratory symptoms: *e.g.*, nocturnal cough or asthma often a dominant symptom.

Hoarseness.

Dysphagia: stricture or motility disorder.

Odynophagia (painful swallowing): suggests alternative diagnosis (*e.g.*, pill-induced esophageal ulcer, esophageal infection).

Signs

• Signs are frequently absent.

Pulmonary consolidation or bronchospasm: rarely, if aspiration has occurred as a result of regurgitation.

Melena or hematochezia.

Investigations

• Uncomplicated reflux esophagitis often requires no diagnostic testing before initiation of therapy; for patients with dysphagia, weight loss, bleeding, or refractory symptoms, diagnostic imaging must be performed.

Endoscopy: preferred to radiography because it offers visualization of mucosa and option of obtaining cytology and histology; allows determination of severity of esophagitis.

Barium radiography: not reliable for showing esophagitis (particularly mild forms) or reflux; may be of some use in assessing esophageal motility.

24-hour pH monitoring: not required in most cases; useful to diagnose reflux in the absence of esophagitis on endoscopy, for evaluating therapy in complicated patients, or for evaluation before surgical management for reflux disease.

Manometry: useful to exclude associated motility disorders before antireflux surgery.

Cardiac tests: to exclude cardiac disease as a source of symptoms.

Complete blood count: in complicated cases to evaluate for anemia or systemic manifestations of inflammation.

Complications

Ulcerations.

Stricture [1].

Barrett's esophagus, Barrett's adenocarcinoma.

Aspiration, leading to night cough, bronchospasm, pneumonia, asthma.

Bleeding: may be life-threatening.

Differential diagnosis

Peptic ulcer disease.

Esophageal malignancy.

Esophageal motility disorder.

Gallstone disease.

Ischemic heart disease.

Etiology

• Reflux esophagitis is caused by prolonged exposure of esophageal mucosa to gastric contents, the most important of which is acid.

Adenocarcinoma: more common in white population and in males.

Barrett's esophagus is a preneoplastic lession associated with the transformation of lower-esophageal mucosa to specialized gastric mucosa, usually as a result of acid reflux (see figure).

• Reflux symptoms are often erroneously attributed to hiatal hernia, a common condition that is most often asymptomatic.

Epidemiology

• Two-thirds of the population may suffer from reflux at some time, but only a small proportion seek medical advice.

• Mechanical and hormonal factors make reflux common during pregnancy.

• Infectious esophagitis is a common component of HIV infections.

• Pill-induced ulcers of the esophagus are most common in bedridden patients with medications such as NSAIDs, tetracyclines, quinidine.

Savary-Miller endoscopic classification

Grade I: nonconfluent mucosal lesions.

Grade II: confluent mucosal lesions.

Grade III: circumferential mucosal lesions.

Grade IV: deep ulcer, stricture, or Barrett's esophagus.

Treatment

Diet and lifestyle

• Reducing weight, stopping smoking, eating small meals, avoiding certain foods (*e.g.*, chocolate, coffee, mints, alcohol), and sleeping with the head of the bed raised (4–6 inches) are crucial measures that decrease reflux [1,2].

• Patients should be advised to remain upright for 2–4 hours after a meal.

• NSAIDs, slow-release potassium chloride, theophylline, nitrates, and calcium-channel blockers (*e.g.*, nifedipine) may also aggravate symptoms.

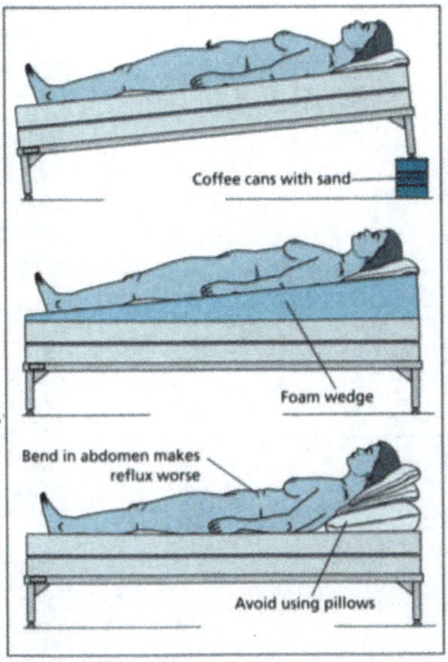

Appropriate method for elevation of the head of the bed.

Pharmacological treatment [3]

Acid reduction: general principles

Antacids may provide reasonable but short-lasting relief for mild disease; frequent dosing required.

Proton-pump inhibitors provide better healing rates than H_2-receptor antagonists and are the first agents of choice in moderate or severe disease.

Short-term treatment typically lasts 6–8 weeks.

Empiric response to proton-pump inhibitors used diagnostically to confirm diagnosis [4].

Combination therapy consisting of proton-pump inhibitor in morning and H_2-receptor antagonist in evening is useful in refractory disease.

H_2-receptor antagonists and proton-pump inhibitors are generally safe medications with occasional side effects of diarrhea, skin reactions, blood dyscrasias (rare).

Long-term therapy often required; no definitive serious long-term sequelae of prolonged use has been demonstrated with these medications.

Motility enhancing (prokinetic) agents

Not often used because of side effects (metoclopramide: central nervous system/extrapyramidal effects, particularly in the elderly; cisapride: is associated with multiple drug–drug interactions that place patients at risk for cardiac arrhythmias and sudden death and is contraindicated in patients with heart disease or prolonged QT intervals [the latter should be monitored shortly after initiation of drug therapy]).

Alternative medicine

Recommended use: none.

Common use: licorice (*Glycyrrhiza glabra*); comfrey (*Symphytum officinale*); althea (*Althaea officinalis*); calendula (*Calendula officinalis*); *Matricaria recutita*.

Caution: licorice at high doses can cause hypertension and hypokalemia.

Treatment aims

To control symptoms.

To prevent complications, especially for stricture formation [5].

Other treatments

Antireflux surgery

• Nissen fundoplication and its modifications using a laparoscopic approach are the most popular techniques.

• Surgery is indicated for the following: refractory, debilitating symptoms that are complicated by bleeding, asthma, or severe strictures or that are refractory to aggressive medical management.

• Prevention is most important in patients with Barrett's esophagus who should undergo surveillance endoscopy with biopsies every 2–3 years. Consider case finding for Barrett's esophagus with screening endoscopy in patients with reflux symptoms for more than 5 years.

Prognosis

• This is a chronic and relapsing condition, but up to 40% of patients remain in remission.

Follow-up and management

• Permanent reflux-reducing measures (particularly weight reduction) must be implemented in order to avoid relapse. Some form of treatment may be necessary to maintain remission.

• Long-term treatment is indicated in patients who have had frequent relapse.

• Identification of Barrett's esophagus is an indication for more careful monitoring for esophageal malignancy. Esophago-gastroduodenoscopy with biopsies are routinely performed every 1–3 years.

Key references

1. Marks AD, Richter JE: Peptic strictures of the esophagus. *Am J Gastroenterol* 1993, **88**:1160–1173.
2. Cameron AJ: Management of Barrett's esophagus. *Mayo Clin Proc* 1998, **73**:457–461.
3. Richter JE: Esophageal chest pain: current controversies in pathogenesis, diagnosis, and therapy. *Ann Intern Med* 1989, **110**:66–78.
4. Cooper JS, *et al.*: Chemoradiotherapy of locally advanced esophageal cancer. *JAMA* 1999, **281**:1623–1627.
5. Kelsen DP, *et al.*: Chemotherapy followed by surgery compared with surgery alone for localized esophageal cancer. *N Engl J Med* 1998, **339**:1979–1984.

Fibromyalgia

Diagnosis

Symptoms [1,2]

Total body aches.

Total body exhaustion.

Fatigue.

Intractable chronic pain.

Myalgias, arthralgias.

Low-grade fever.

Exercise limitation.

Sleep disturbance.

Signs

Absence of objective inflammation.

Trigger points.

Normal range of motion.

Investigations

Normal complete blood count.

Normal serologies: Westegren erythrocyte sedimentation rate, rheumatoid factor, antinuclear antibodies.

Electromyography.

Radiography.

Complications

Impaired quality of life.

Deconditioning.

Work limitation.

Analgesic dependency.

Depression.

• Chronic deformity and/or crippling does not occur with fibromyalgia.

Differential diagnosis

Chronic fatigue syndrome.

Depression.

Osteoarthritis.

Rheumatoid arthritis.

Systemic lupus erythematosus.

Terminology issues

The term "fibrositis" should be avoided because inflammation is not present in this condition; "myofascial pain syndrome" is an acceptable alternative.

Etiology [1,2]

Unknown.

• Hypotheses include the following:

A disorder of central pain perception.

Abnormal muscle metabolism.

Abnormality of nonrestorative deep sleep.

Epidemiology

Prevalence: 5% of patients in general medicine practice, 2%–4% of the general population.

More common in women.

Age of onset 20–45 years of age.

Overrepresented in highly educated, high-achieving, perfectionistic individuals.

Treatment

Diet and lifestyle

• A gentle, continuous exercise program may be the most helpful intervention overall. Rigorous exercise programs are uniformly poorly tolerated (and abandoned early).

Pharmacological treatment [2,3]

• Low-dose antidepressants, *e.g.*, amitriptyline, 10–25 mg daily, may be helpful in 20%–30% of patients. It may work via effects on central pain, biochemical pathways, and sleep disturbance. Main side effects include dry mouth, fatigue, and somnolence. The low dosages help to minimize these side effects.

Nonpharmacological treatment

Reassurance: nondestructive, not deforming.

Chronic pain management: referral may be very helpful, including techniques such as visual imagery, relaxation, meditation, etc.

Physical therapy: gentle, long-term exercise program with special emphasis on evidence of injury and exhaustion.

Treatment aims

To control pain.

To improve sense of well being.

To improve exercise tolerance.

To improve work tolerance.

Prognosis

• The prognosis is highly variable.

• It is controversial whether life expectancy is normal or slightly diminished.

Follow-up and management

• The primary care provider can follow the patient at mutually agreeable intervals.

• Narcotic analgesia should be avoided (and frequently does not significantly reduce pain).

Key references

1. Krsnich-Shriwise S: Fibromyalgia syndrome: an overview. *Phys Ther* 1997, **77**:68–75.
2. Simms RW: Fibromyalgia syndrome: current concepts in pathophysiology, clinical features, and management. *Arthritis Care Res* 1996, **9**:315–328.
3. Goldenberg D, Mayskiy M, Mossey C, *et al.*: A randomized double-blind crossover trial of fluoxetine and amitriptyline in the treatment of fibromyalgia. *Arthritis Rheum* 1996, **39**:1852–1859.
4. Tavoni A, Vitalic, Bombardier: S, Pasero G: Evaluation of S-adenosylmethionine in primary fibromyalgia: a double-blind crossover study. *Am J Med* 1987, **83(5A)**:107–110.

Fungal infections, invasive

Diagnosis

Symptoms and signs

Candida infections

White plaques in mouth or tongue, angular cheilitis.
Vulvovaginal discharge, pruritus.
Cutaneous candidiasis, intertrigo, folliculitis, balanitis, perianal or interdigital infection, diaper rash.
Paronychia or onychomycosis.
Cystitis, urethritis.
Disseminated candidiasis involving several organs; endophthalmitis, endocarditis, cerebral or hepatosplenic microabscesses.
Pneumonia, allergic wheeze, breathlessness.
Peritonitis, esophagitis.

Aspergillus infections

Wheeze, breathlessness: indicating allergic bronchopulmonary aspergillosis.
Fever, cough, hypoxia, chest discomfort or pleuritic pain, hemoptysis, pneumonia: indicating invasive aspergillosis.
Blocked nose, facial pain, nasal discharge, chronic headache: indicating allergic or saprophytic sinus infection.
Chronic otitis media or externa, meningitis or cerebral microabscesses, endocarditis, endophthalmitis, osteoarticular disorders.

Focal neurologic signs: CNS diseases.

Cryptococcal infections

• Onset is insidious.

Fever, headache, nausea, vomiting, neck stiffness, photophobia: indicating meningitis.
Dyspnea, cough: indicating pneumonia.

Histoplasmosis, coccidiodomycosis, blastomycosis

Breathlessness, lung infiltrates: indicating pulmonary histoplasmosis.
Pancytopenia, pneumonia, lymphadenopathy, hepatosplenomegaly oral or gastrointestinal ulcers, adrenal masses: indicating disseminated histoplasmosis.
Enlarged lymph glands: indicating lymphadenopathy.

Agents of mucormycosis (zygomycosis)

Headache, facial pain, orbital cellulitis, lower cranial nerve palsies: indicating rhinocerebral infection.
Pneumonia, disseminated disease.

Investigations

Biopsy of tissue and bone marrow with culture and histology (histoplasmosis only), lysis-centrifugation culture of blood (histoplasmosis), culture of sputum, fluid (including CSF), and sinuses.
Antigen tests: for cryptococcal infections.
CT for *Aspergillus* infections: of thorax for aspergilloma and invasive infections; of sinuses for allergy, saprophytic, acute invasion; of brain for brain abscess.
Endoscopy, colonoscopy, barium meal, swallow, follow-through: for esophagitis, gastritis, small and large bowel plaques, and ulceration.
Radiography of chest, thorax, and sinuses.
Bronchoscopy: lavage, biopsy, for pulmonary disease and diagnosis.
Serology: fungal immunodiffusion testing and serum cryptococcal antigen.
Antigen test: for histoplasmosis.

Complications

Candida infections

Esophageal candidiasis, azole-resistant thrush, endometritis, ascending renal infection in intensive care or surgical patients, prostatitis, multiple organ involvement, hepatosplenic candidiasis in leukemic patients.

Other infections

Pulmonary fibrosis: after 5–10 years; complication of allergic bronchopulmonary aspergillosis.
Hemoptysis: in *Aspergillus* infections and zygomycosis.
Hydrocephalus, impaired mental function, blindness: complications of cryptococcal infections; hydrocephalus usually communicating.

Differential diagnosis

Other infections.
Lymphoma.
Tuberculosis.

Etiology

• Predisposing causes include the following:

Superficial *Candida* infections
Antibiotics, steroids, diabetes mellitus, AIDS, pregnancy, oral contraceptives, macerated skin, occupation, abnormal T-cell response to *Candida* antigens.

Systemic *Candida* infections
Urinary catheterization, immunosuppression, surgery, burns, premature birth, endocarditis, valvular heart disease, prosthetic valves, peritoneal dialysis, abdominal surgery, bowel perforation, hematological malignancies, CSF shunts, antibiotic use.

***Aspergillus* infections**
Asthma, cystic fibrosis, neutropenia, organ transplantation, AIDS, steroids, chronic granulomatous disease, previous pulmonary tuberculosis, sarcoidosis, bronchiectasis, chronic lung disease, diabetes mellitus, alcoholism, previous ear disease, i.v. drug abuse, valve replacement, antibiotic use.

Cryptococcal infections
AIDS, lymphoma, steroids, sarcoidosis.

Histoplasmosis, coccidiodomycosis, blastomycosis
History of exposure, e.g., endemic area, bat caves (acute), emphysema (chronic), AIDS.

Mucormycosis
Acidosis, diabetes mellitus, neutropenia, bone-marrow transplantation, i.v. drug abuse, deferoxamine treatment.

Epidemiology

Environmental saprophytes.
• Vaginal candidiasis affects 70% of all women, and 5% have frequent recurrences.
• Oral thrush affects 90% of AIDS patients and 15%–30% of leukemia patients.
• Invasive aspergillosis affects 5%–40% of immunocompromised patients.
• Cryptococcal meningitis affects 4%–35% of AIDS patients, depending on country.

Treatment

Diet and lifestyle

• No special precautions are necessary.

Pharmacological treatment

Amphotericin B

• Amphotericin B is indicated for the following:

Candida infections (oropharyngeal, urogenital tract, candidemia, endocarditis, pneumonia, visceral, CNS).
Aspergillus infections (invasive or chronic necrotizing aspergillosis, acute invasive sinus, or paranasal granuloma).
Cryptococcal infections (meningitis).
Histoplasmosis (chronic pulmonary, disseminated).
Agents of mucormycosis (rhinocerebral).

Standard dosage	Amphotericin B, 0.5–1.5 mg/kg i.v.
Contraindications	Hypersensitivity.
Special points	Resistant strains include *Candida krusei*, *Fusarium* spp., *Pseudallescheria boydii*, *Trichosporon beigelii*, Mucorales (limited activity).
Main drug interactions	Increased nephrotoxicity with aminoglycosides or cyclosporine.
Main side effects	Infusion-related fever or rigors, nausea, phlebitis, renal toxicity, anemia, electrolyte disturbances.

Azoles

• Fluconazole is indicated for *Candida* infections (oropharyngeal, vulvovaginal, nail infections, chronic mucocutaneous candidiasis, urogenital tract, visceral candidiasis) and for cryptococcal infections (meningitis in AIDS).

• Itraconazole is indicated for *Aspergillus* infections (pulmonary, acute invasive sinus, paranasal granuloma) and for histoplasmosis (severe acute, chronic pulmonary, less seriously ill, disseminated; maintenance in AIDS and coccidiodomycosis).

Standard dosage	Fluconazole, 50–400 mg orally or i.v. daily. Itraconazole, 100–200 mg orally daily; 200 mg loading doses 3 times daily initially in severe or life-threatening disease. Ketoconazole, 200–400 mg orally daily.
Contraindications	Azole hypersensitivity.
Special points	*Fluconazole:* resistant strains include *Histoplasma capsulatum*, Mucorales, *Candida krusei* and *glabrata*, *Aspergillus* and *Fusarium* spp. *Itraconazole:* resistant strains include *C. glabrata*, *Fusarium* spp., Mucorales. *Ketoconazole:* resistant strains include *C. glabrata*, *Cryptococcus neoformans*, *Aspergillus* and *Fusarium* spp.
Main drug interactions	Altered azole or drug concentrations with phenytoin, cyclosporine, rifampin, phenobarbital, carbamazepine, warfarin, astemizole, digoxin.
Main side effects	*Fluconazole:* nausea, rash, liver dysfunction (rare). *Itraconazole:* gynecomastia, peripheral edema, hypokalemia, liver dysfunction (rare). *Ketoconazole:* liver dysfunction, nausea, reduced libido, menstrual irregularities, gynecomastia.

Other drugs

Flucytosine, 100 mg/kg orally daily in 4 divided doses only in combination with amphotericin B: for cryptococcal infections (candidemia, endocarditis, CNS infections), *Aspergillus* infections (invasive aspergillosis), and cryptococcal infections (meningitis).

Topical nystatin: for mucosal *Candida* infection.

Topical antifungals: for cutaneous *Candida* and dermatophyte infections.

Inhaled steroids, bronchodilators: for allergic pneumonitis.

Oral steroids: for exacerbations of allergic bronchopulmonary aspergillosis.

Treatment aims

To eradicate infection.
To prevent recurrence of infection.
To remove underlying cause.

Other treatments

Removal or replacement of catheter or shunt.
Surgery: for invasive aspergillosis, aspergilloma, allergic sinus infection, fungus ball, paranasal granuloma, rhinocerebral infection (radical clearance).
Removal of CSF in cryptococcal meningitis.

Prognosis

• In patients with candidemia, overall mortality is 55%; in surgical patients with candidal peritonitis, mortality is 37%.
• In patients with invasive aspergillosis, mortality is 30%–90%, depending on the host group: poor prognosis in patients with late-diagnosis and persistent neutropenia, 85%–90% in bone-marrow transplant recipients, 95% in patients with disseminated disease or cerebral aspergillosis.
• In patients with hemoptysis resulting from aspergilloma, mortality is 10%; spontaneous resolution is 10%.
• 50% of leukemia patients with acute invasive *Aspergillus* sinus infection relapse.
• In patients with meningitis, acute mortality is 15%–20%, lower if intracranial hypertension is treated aggressively.
• More than one-third of patients who have had meningitis relapse without prophylaxis.

Follow-up and management

• Patients with life-threatening invasive fungal infections should have specialist treatment and prolonged follow-up.

General references

British Society for Antimicrobial Chemotherapy Working Party: Antifungal chemotherapy in patients with acquired immunodeficiency syndrome. *Lancet* 1992, **340**:648–651.

Denning DW, Stevens DA: Antifungal and surgical treatment of invasive aspergillosis: review of 2121 published cases. *Rev Infect Dis* 1990, **12**:1147–1201.

Minamoto GY, Rosenberg AS: Fungal infections in patients with aquired immunodeficiency syndrome. *Med Clin North Am* 1997, **81**:381–409.

Fungal nail infection

Diagnosis

Symptoms

Social embarrassment.

Mechanical problems: onychodystrophic nails get snagged on clothing; pressure and irritation from footwear; pain.

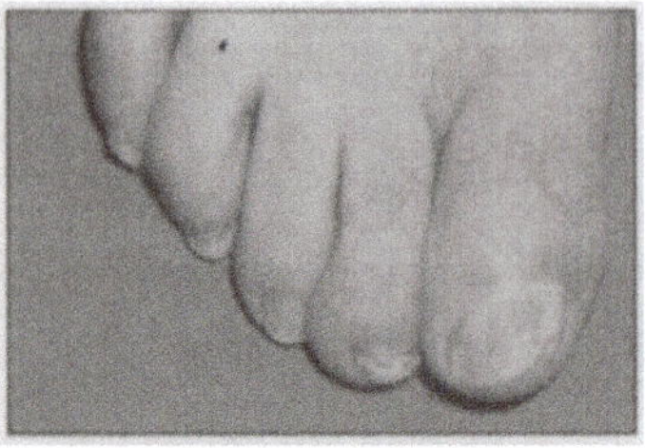

Distal and lateral subungual onychomycosis secondary to dermatophyte infection. (*See* Color Plate.)

Signs

• Signs can be divided into three varieties of clinical manifestations based on the type of nail infection: distal, proximal, or superficial infection.

Distal infection

Onychodystrophy: dystrophic changes in fingernails or toenails.

Onycholysis: distal or distal-lateral nail separation from the nail bed.

Subungual hyperkeratosis: hyperkeratotic subungual debris, crumbling friable nails.

Proximal infection

Discoloration: white to yellow, affecting the proximal ventral nail plate; extends distally and toward the dorsal surface of the nail plate but rarely involves the whole nail (least common type); may be seen in immunosuppressed patients.

Superficial infection

Discoloration: patchy chalk-white, mainly of toenails, known as "superficial white onychomycosis."

Investigations

Microscopic examination: potassium hydroxide preparation of subungual debris (as proximal as possible) will be positive only in 50% of cases.

Culture: positive in only 50% of cases in which microscopy is positive.

Complications

Spread of infection: to other nails or adjacent skin (causing tinea pedis).

Secondary pseudomonas infection (green nail syndrome).

Complete onycholysis: disruption and separation of the entire nail plate from the nail bed.

Differential diagnosis

Psoriasis.

Lichen planus.

Trauma.

Drug-induced photoonycholysis.

Etiology

• With the rare exception of immunosuppressed patients, patients with mucocutaneous candidiasis, and patients with chronic paronychia, most cases are caused by dermatophyte infection.

• *Trichophyton rubrum, Trichophyton mentagrophytes*, and *Epidermophyton floccosum* are the most common organisms; *T. mentagrophytes* is usually the cause in superficial white onychomycosis.

• *Candida* infection is rare and usually occurs when there is candidal chronic paronychia.

Epidemiology

• Infection most likely spreads from skin to nails.

• It is a very common problem, especially in the elderly (extremely rare in children). Onychomycosis accounts for 50% of all nail disorders and affects 2%–18% of the world's population.

• Toenail infection is more prevalent than fingernail infection.

• It appears to be more common in men than in women.

Treatment

Diet and lifestyle

• Prophylaxis using antifungal foot powder and prevention of overhydration of feet in occlusive, nonbreathing footwear undoubtedly has merit.

Pharmacological treatment

Topical treatment

• Topical treatment is used only to control or prevent tinea pedis.

• Superficial white onychomycosis can be treated by simply scraping off the superficial fungi from the nail.

Systemic treatment

• Allylamines (terbinafine) and triazoles (itraconazole and fluconazole) are much more effective over a much shorter treatment period than is griseofulvin.

Standard dosage Terbinafine, 250 mg daily for 6 weeks in fingernail disease and for 12 weeks in toenail disease.

Itraconazole (pulse therapy), 400 mg daily once a week each month for 2 months in fingernail disease and for 3 months in toenail disease.

Itraconazole (continuous therapy), 200 mg daily for 8 weeks in fingernail disease and for 12 weeks in toenail disease.

Fluconazole, 150–300 mg once weekly for up to 12 months.

Contraindications Pregnancy, hepatic disease.

Main drug interactions *Terbinafine:* potential for drug interactions is much lower than with the azoles because terbinafine does not significantly alter the P-450 enzyme system.

Itraconazole: inhibitor of P-450 enzyme system; specifically contraindicated with the use of cisapride terfenadine, astemizole, simvastatin, lovastatin, midazolam, and triazolam. Should be closely monitored when used with digoxin, cyclosporine, and warfarin.

Fluconazole: same profile as itraconazole; less inhibition of P-450.

Main side effects *Terbinafine*: gastrointestinal upset, neutropenia and thrombocytopenia (rare), taste disturbance.
Itraconazole: nausea, gastrointestinal upset, elevated liver function tests (0.3%–5% of patients).
Fluconazole: gastrointestinal upset.

Alternative medicine

Recommended use: tea tree oil (*Melaleuca alternifera*); **Common use:** myrrh (*Commiphora* spp.); garlic (*Allium sativa*); citrus seed oil extract.

Caution: tea tree oil may cause skin irritation.

Treatment aims

To eradicate the infection.

To prevent recurrence.

Other treatments

• Amorolfine 5% nail lacquer may be an alternative to systemic therapy, especially when the nail matrix is not involved.

Nail avulsion combined with systemic therapy.

Prognosis

Better for fingernail involvement.

High relapse rate.

Follow-up and management

• It is important to monitor liver function tests because of the possibility of hepatotoxicity.

General references

Gupta A, Sauder D, Shear N: Antifungal agents: an overview. Part II. J Am Acad Demerol 1994, **30**:911-933.

Jaffe R: Onychomycosis: recognition, diagnosis, and management. *Arch Fam Med* 1998, **7**:587–592.

Raza A: Ecology and epidemiology of dermatophyte infections. J Am Acad Dermatol 1994, **31**:521-525.

Roberts DT: Oral therapeutic agents in fungal nail disease. J Am Acad Dermatol 1994, **31**:578-581

Scher RK: Onychomycosis: therapeutic update. *J Am Acad Dermatol* 1999, **40(6 Pt 2)**:S21–S26.

Gallstones, cholesterol

Diagnosis

Symptoms

• Up to 70% of patients are asymptomatic or have nonspecific dyspeptic symptoms.

Uncomplicated

Biliary colic: sudden-onset severe epigastric or upper right quadrant abdominal pain, lasting for several hours, usually radiating to back, sometimes associated with nausea and vomiting.

Complicated

Fever, persistent abdominal pain, nausea and vomiting: indicating acute cholecystitis.

Fever, pain, jaundice: indicating acute cholangitis.

Abdominal pain radiating to the back, vomiting: suggests acute pancreatitis.

Signs

Uncomplicated

• Few signs are manifest.

Tenderness in right upper quadrant: usually during or after episodes of biliary colic.

Complicated

Jaundice: indicating stone impaction in common bile duct.

Murphy's sign (a halt in deep inspiration when deep palpation in the right upper quadrant results in pain): indicating acute cholecystitis.

Hypotension: suggests acute pancreatitis or sepsis from cholangitis.

Investigations

Ultrasonography: first choice test to identify stones; may also detect small stones and biliary sludge; detects dilated bile ducts and can occasionally identify disease in the liver, pancreas, or kidneys.

• Gallstones are frequently found incidentally by ultrasonography or abdominal radiography (if calcified).

• Endoscopic retrograde cholangiopancreatography: an appropriate next step in patients suspected of having gallstones within their biliary ducts (*e.g.*, dilated ducts on ultrasonography) if sphincterotomy can be performed for stone removal.

Laboratory tests are not diagnostic but are useful for identifying complications and excluding other abnormalities.

Serum alkaline phosphatase and bilirubin measurement: elevation suggests biliary tract disease.

Leukocyte count: frequently elevated with inflammation of the biliary tract.

Serum amylase measurement: elevation suggests acute pancreatitis.

Antimitochondrial antibody tests: in atypical cases (*e.g.*, pruritus, painless jaundice) to exclude primary biliary cirrhosis.

Plain abdominal radiography: identifies stones that are calcified (~20%).

Oral cholecystography: identifies radiolucent stones, good for determining gallbladder contraction and cystic duct patency and for identifying anatomical abnormalities in gallbladder; not sensitive for detecting small stones and invalid in case of nonopacifying gallbladder.

CT: less sensitive than ultrasonography for detecting gallbladder stones or bile duct dilatation.

Cholescintigraphy: using ^{99m}Tc-HIDA (hepatic iminodiacetic acid) helpful in suspected acute cholecystitis (*i.e.*, gallbladder does not fill); parenchymal liver disease or significant cholestasis may lead to false-positive results.

Complications

Acute cholecystitis.
Acute cholangitis.
Acute pancreatitis.
Hydrops, empyema of gallbladder.
Malignancy of gallbladder.
Perforation.
Internal and external biliary fistulas.
Gallstone ileus.
Hemobilia.
Choledocholithiasis.

Differential diagnosis

Obstructive jaundice

Pancreatic neoplasm.

Bile-duct stricture.

Cholestatic hepatitis

Biliary colic

Pancreatitis.

Esophagitis.

Peptic ulcer.

Irritable bowel syndrome.

Etiology [1]

• No unifying cause has been found, but the following may have a role:

Pathogenesis

Cholesterol supersaturation of bile.

Impaired gallbladder emptying.

Rapid cholesterol nucleation.

Predisposing factors

Obesity.

High-fat diet.

Disease: cirrhosis of liver, ileal dysfunction.

Drugs: *e.g.*, octreotide, oral contraceptives.

Epidemiology

• 10%–15% of the adult population has cholesterol gallstones.

• The incidence is 0.6% of the population.

• Gallstones occur more often in women, and their occurrence increases with age.

Treatment

Diet and lifestyle

• No evidence suggests that diet high in fiber and low in cholesterol dissolves stones or prevents their recurrence.

• Patients at risk of gallstones should avoid obesity.

• Rapid weight reduction should be avoided.

• Diets high in polyunsaturated fat should be avoided.

Pharmacological treatment

• Dissolution therapy with oral agents is indicated for patients with other major medical problems that are contraindications for nonpharmacological treatment; radiolucent stones and functioning gallbladder must be verified.

• Bile-acid treatment is used for patients with small stones (<15 mm diameter); bile acids dissolve cholesterol gallstones by micellar solubilization or liquid crystal formation; they also reduce cholesterol absorption by intestine or secretion by liver [2].

Standard dosage	Ursodeoxycholic acid (UDCA), 10 mg/kg daily. Chenodeoxycholic acid (CDCA), 15 mg/kg daily. UDCA and CDCA, 5 mg/kg each daily. All as single bedtime dose for up to 2 years.
Contraindications	Pregnancy and lactation. *CDCA:* chronic liver disease or diarrhea. *UDCA:* active peptic ulcers.
Special points	Dissolution of stones requires 12 months or more of treatment, and recurrence is common when the medication is discontinued; UDCA or combination better than CDCA alone.
Main drug interactions	Sex hormones, oral contraceptives, blood cholesterol-lowering agents.
Main side effects	*CDCA:* diarrhea, hypertransaminasemia (reversible and dose-dependent). *UDCA:* gallstone calcification resulting in treatment failure.

Nonpharmacological treatment

Surgery

• Surgery (laparoscopic cholecystectomy) is the preferred management for almost all patients with symptomatic gallstones.

Endoscopic retrograde cholangiography with sphincterotomy and stone extraction

• This treatment is for patients with choledocholithiasis.

• It is often performed in conjunction with laparoscopic cholecystectomy [3].

Extracorporeal shock-wave lithotripsy

• Lithotripsy is possible for 1–3 stones <30 mm in diameter; however, surgical management or dissolution therapy is the preferred approach.

• Expensive equipment is needed.

• The incidence of biliary colic and hematuria hematobilia is higher than with other approaches.

• It is contraindicated in hemolytic disorders.

Alternative medicine

Recommended use: none.

Common use: lecithin; fish oils; dandelion (*Taraxacum officinale*); boldo (*Peumus boldo*); milk thistle (*Silybum marianum*); artichoke (*Cynara scolymus*); turmeric (*Curcuma longa*).

Caution: "liver flush" (olive oil plus lemon juice) may precipitate cholecystitis or increase gall stones.

Treatment aims

To dissolve stones, with consequent relief of symptoms and prevention of complications [4,5].

Prognosis

• Gallstones recur after dissolution therapy in 50% of patients within 5 years.

• If recurrent stones are detected early and treated, >80% of patients remain gallstone-free in the long term.

Follow-up and management

• Regular ultrasonography is needed every 6–12 months after dissolution to detect early recurrence.

• Bile acid treatment (full dose) is needed for recurrent stones.

Causes of pharmacological treatment failure

Patients' noncompliance with treatment.

Presence of radiolucent pigment stones or subradiographic calcification of stones.

Development of nonfunctioning gallbladder.

Inadequate dose (especially in obese patients).

Key references

1. Jonston DE, Kaplan MM: Pathogenesis and treatment of gallstones. *N Engl J Med* 1993, **328**:412–421.
2. Jazrawi RP, ***et al.***: Optimum bile acid therapy for rapid gallstone dissolution. *Gut* 1992, **33**:381–386.
3. Cuschieri A, ***et al.***: The European experience with laparoscopic cholecystectomy. *Am J Surg* 1991, **161**:385–387.
4. Sauerbruch T, Paumgartner G: Gallbladder stones: management. *Lancet* 1991, **338**:1121–1124.
5. Ransohoft DF, ***et al.***: Treatment of gallstones. *Ann Intern Med* 1993, **119**:606–619.
6. Brugge WR, Van Dam J: Pancreatic and biliary endoscope. *N Engl J Med* 1999, **341**:1808–1816.

Diagnosis

Symptoms [1]

Epigastric pain: often aggravated by eating.

Weight loss.

Early satiety, fullness.

Dysphagia: with adeocarcinoma of the cardia or distal esopohagus.

Vomiting.

Hematemesis or melena.

Signs

• Typically, no signs are manifest.

Pallor: due to anemia.

Abdominal epigastric mass: palpable gastric tumor (uncommon).

Nodular, enlarged liver: with metastatic disease.

Succussion splash: suggests gastric outlet obstruction.

Hard fixed supraclavicular node: sentinel node of Virchow; in left supraclavicular fossa.

Rectal mass: rectal shelf of Blumer; on digital examination (uncommon).

Infiltration of the umbilicus: "Sister Joseph's" nodule (uncommon).

Investigations

• Laboratory tests are not diagnostic but may suggest bleeding or liver metastases.

Complete blood count: to identify anemia.

Liver chemistry tests: raised alkaline phosphatase level common with metastatic disease.

Fiberoptic endoscopy: allows direct visualization of cancer and assessment of obstruction to cardia or pylorus; allows biopsy (a minimum of eight tissue samples should be obtained, especially from the edge) and cytology; infiltrating cancer (linitis plastica) and lymphoma may need deep or large biopsies at repeated endoscopy to establish the diagnosis; superficial cancers may be difficult to recognize.

Double-contrast barium meal: blunting, fusion, clubbing, or tapering of mucosal folds suggests cancer; less accurate than endoscopy.

CT: to assess extent of disease, metastases.

Ultrasonography: conventional abdominal ultrasonography helpful when assessing for liver metastases; endoscopic ultrasonography is very useful for determining resectability if other imaging studies are negative for metastatic disease.

Complications

Obstruction.

Hemorrhage.

Tumor spread: lymphatic, hematogenous (liver, lungs, bone, adrenals), local dissemination into esophagus, invasion of adjacent organs (pancreas, mesocolon, liver).

Differential diagnosis

Ulcer or nonulcer dyspepsia.

Reflux esophagitis.

Ischemic gastropathy.

Hepatic or pancreatic cancer.

Anemia of other causes.

Depression.

NSAID gastropathy.

Gastro paresis.

Etiology

• Risk factors include the following:

Helicobacter pylori infection [2].

Smoked foods, salt fish, pickled foods. Inverse association with refrigeration, vitamin C, fresh fruit and vegetable intake.

Genetic factors: including blood group A, family history, and Lynch syndrome II.

Epidemiology

• In the United States, the annual incidence is 10 cases per 100 000 population; more common in patients from Japan and other regions of east Asia.

• The male:female ratio is 2:1.

• The incidence of gastric cancer has declined considerably over the past 30 years.

• Patients with early gastric cancer are, on average, 8 years younger than those with advanced disease [3].

Pathology

Malignant neoplasm of stomach

90% adenocarcinoma; 5% lymphoma; 5% others (carcinoid, leiomyosarcoma, squamous, liposarcoma).

• Advanced cancer may be polypoidal or fungating, ulcerating with a raised border, or diffusely infiltrating (linitis plastica).

Early gastric cancer

Confined to gastric mucosa or submucosa, irrespective of lymph-node invasion.

Three types: protruded (type I), superficial (type II, most common), excavated (type III).

Premalignant conditions

Chronic atrophic gastritis/achlorhydria.

Pernicious anemia.

Dysplasia.

Adenomatous polyps.

Previous gastrectomy (*i.e.*, 20 years after Billroth II).

Hypertrophic gastropathy (Menetrier's disease).

Treatment

Diet and lifestyle

- Patients with dysphagia should have a semi-liquid diet, with enteral feeding supplements.
- After gastrectomy, patients are at risk for dumping syndrome. Liquids should be taken before a meal but not during or immediately after ingestion of solid food. Patients should be advised to ingest frequent, small meals. Lying down immediately after a meal may be helpful.

Pharmacological treatment

- Chemotherapy has not been shown in trials to increase survival; it can produce effective reduction in tumor size and has been used for palliation. A combination of fluorouracil, doxorubicin, and mitomycin yields some tumor response in patients with advanced disease.
- Symptoms may respond to treatment, as follows:

Ulcer-type pain: H_2 blockers (*e.g.*, ranitidine, cimetidine, nizatidine, or famotidine) or proton-pump inhibitors (*e.g.*, omeprazole, lansoprazole, pantoprazole, or rabeprazole).

Thrush or odynophagia pain: nystatin or fluconazole if candidal infection is present.

Infiltrative pain: narcotic analgesics.

Constipation: laxatives.

Vomiting (infiltrative: incompetence of gastroesophageal sphincter): metoclopramide or cisapride (condition rarely responds to these drugs; drugs may aggravate obstructive symptoms).

Nonpharmacological treatment [3]

- Curative resection: for the 30%–50% of patients without evidence of distant metastases. [4,5]

Total gastrectomy: if tumor is extensive or close to cardioesophageal junction; higher mortality and morbidity than partial gastrectomy; side effects include small reservoir or bilious vomiting, diarrhea, and malabsorption.

Partial gastrectomy: for early gastric cancer or infiltrative advanced cancer with 5 cm distance clear of cancer from the cardia; side effects include weight loss and altered eating ability.

Dissection of lymph glands draining stomach: important even in early gastric cancer.

Palliation of symptoms, as follows:
Gastric bypass surgery: for obstructive pain or obstructive vomiting due to pyloric stenosis.
For dysphagia: laser treatment or repeat dilation.
For bleeding: surgery, endoscopic laser or electrocautery treatment.
For depression, anxiety, or anger: careful discussion, enlistment of family, and palliative care team support with appropriate use of antidepressants, anxiolytics, and analgesics.

- Palliative surgery for locally advanced disease involving adjacent organs may benefit patients with bleeding or pyloric obstruction even with metastatic spread.
- Complications after surgery include anastomotic leakage and small gastric reserve.

Treatment aims

To provide curative resection when still possible.

To provide effective symptomatic palliation when cure not possible [6].

Prognosis

- In patients with unresectable disease, mean survival is 4–12 months, with almost no 5-year survivors.
- In patients having apparent curative resection, mean survival is 28 months, and the 5-year survival rate is 40%.
- The prognosis of early gastric cancer is much better, with a 5-year survival rate of 80%, compared with 20% for advanced gastric cancer after resection (types I and II better prognosis than type III) [7,8].

Follow-up and management

- Gastrectomy patients may need iron and vitamin B_{12} or vitamin D supplements.
- Some total gastrectomy patients need careful nutritional support.
- Endoscopy, ultrasonography, or CT may be needed during follow-up to diagnose local or distant recurrence.

Key references

1. Takemoto T, *et al.*: Impact of staging on treatment of gastric carcinoma. *Endoscopy* 1993, **25**:46–50.
2. Scheiman JM, Cutler AF: *Helicobacter pylori* and gastric cancer. *Am J Med* 1999, **106**:222–226.
3. Lechago J, Correa P: Prolonged achlorhydria and gastric neoplasia: is there a causal relationship? *Gastroenterology* 1993, **104**:1554-1557.
4. Cushieri A: Gastrectomy for gastric cancer: definitions and objectives. *Br J Surg* 1986, **73**:513-514.
5. Gouzi JL, *et al.*: Total versus subtotal gastrectomy for adenocarcinoma of the gastric antrum. *Ann Surg* 1989, **2**:162-166.
6. Valen B, *et al.*: Treatment of stomach cancer: a national experience. *Br J Surg* 1988, **75**:708-710.
7. Thompson GB, van Heerden JA, Sarr MG: Adenocarcinoma of the stomach: are we making progress? *Lancet* 1993, **342**:713-718.
8. Green PHR, *et al.*: Increasing incidence and excellent survival of patients with early gastric cancer. *Am J Med* 1988, **85**:658-661.

Gastric ulcer

Diagnosis

Symptoms

Often clinically indistinguishable from duodenal ulcer (*See* Duodenal Ulcer *and* Nonulcer Dyspepsia [1]).

Epigastric pain: described as dull, burning discomfort; variably affected by food; relieved by antacids; nocturnal pain common.

Nausea, early satiety, or vomiting: with gastric outflow obstruction.

Hematemesis or melena.

Weight loss: suggesting malignant gastric ulceration.

Signs

• Most commonly, the physical examination is normal; epigastric tenderness on physical examination is an unreliable measure of disease activity.

Signs of hemodynamic compromise: tachycardia, orthostatic hypotension in acute hemorrhage.

Local or generalized peritonitis: if ulcer has perforated.

Upper abdominal distension, succussion splash: with gastric outflow obstruction.

Hematemesis or melena with gastrointestinal bleeding.

Investigations

• Gastric ulcer can be diagnosed only after imaging the gastric lumen.

Fiberoptic endoscopy: esophagogastroduodenoscopy (EGD) is the investigation of choice (biopsy and cytology essential to exclude malignancy); allows direct visualization of ulcer; may help to diagnose small lesions or mucosal abnormalities; allows histological confirmation of diagnosis; allows assessment of *Helicobacter pylori* status.

Contrast radiography: barium upper gastrointestinal studies compare favorably with EGD at a lower cost, although small lesions may be missed and biopsies are not possible.

Complete blood count: to detect anemia or systemic evidence of inflammation.

Serum gastrin measurement: to evaluate for Zollinger-Ellison syndrome in recurrent or multiple ulceration not due to NSAID gastropathy or *H. pylori* [1].

• Patients with gastric ulcers should be tested for *H. pylori* (*see* Duodenal ulcer).

Complications

Perforation.

Hemorrhage.

Gastric outflow obstruction.

Differential diagnosis

Duodenal ulceration.

Nonulcer dyspepsia.

Pancreatic carcinoma.

Gastroesophageal reflux disease.

Erosive NSAID gastrophy.

Irritable bowel syndrome.

Biliary disease.

Pancreatitis.

Gastric carcinoma.

Ischemic gastropathy.

Lymphoma.

Etiology

Basal and peak acid secretion usually within normal range; mucosal defenses impaired, with subsequent back-diffusion of acid into mucosa.

• Causes include the following:

NSAIDs inhibiting protective prostaglandin synthesis.

H. pylori infection in 70% of patients.

Epidemiology

• The incidence of gastric ulceration increases with age.

• The male :female ratio is equal.

• Gastric ulceration is more prevalent in low socioeconomic groups.

• The ratio of duodenal to gastric ulcers is 9:1.

Treatment

Diet and lifestyle

- Bland diets, spicy foods, acid-containing fruits do not affect the healing process.
- Caffeine, ethanol, and smoking should be avoided.
- Patients must be explicitly asked about NSAID use and instructed to refrain from all such medications except acetaminophen.

Pharmacological treatment

- If *H. pylori* is present in patients with gastric ulcers, the organism should be eraticated (*see* Duodenal ulcer *for further details*).

H. pylori–negative patients (*e.g.*, NSAID-related ulcers)

Ideally, stop NSAID use during treatment period. Replace with acetaminophen (safest alternative) or with one of the new cyclo-oxygenase-2 inhibitors (rofecoxib, celecoxib), which are significantly less ulcerogenic [2].

An 8-week treatment course of an H_2-receptor antagonist or proton-pump inhibitor is advised [3].

In patients who must continue to receive NSAIDs, healing can be promoted and recurrent ulcers minimized with concurrent use of omeprazole (20–40 mg daily) or high-dose famotidine (40 mg twice daily). Misoprostol (200 μg four times daily) is also of benefit in minimizing the development of ulcers in patients who require NSAIDs.

In patients with a single or atypical-appearing gastric ulcer, particularly in the absence of NSAID use, malignancy must be excluded. Eight biopsy samples should be obtained from the ulcer edge and base. Healing must be confirmed with a follow-up study.

H_2-receptor antagonists

- The mainstay of treatment, these relieve symptoms within days and have ulcer healing rates of 80% at 4 weeks and 90% at 8 weeks [4].

Standard dosage Ranitidine, 300 mg; cimetidine, 800 mg; famotidine, 40 mg; all given as single dose at night.

Contraindications Known hypersensitivity (rare), pregnancy and lactation.

Main drug interactions *Cimetidine:* oral anticoagulants, theophylline, phenytoin.

Main side effects *Cimetidine:* headache, constipation or diarrhea, gynecomastia (all unusual).

Proton-pump inhibitors

- Proton-pump inhibitors are associated with faster healing (*e.g.*, 93% healing after 4 weeks of treatment), but they are not approved for long-term treatment.

Standard dosage Omeprazole, 20 mg daily, lansoprazole, 30 mg daily.

Contraindications Pregnancy and lactation.

Main drug interactions Diazepam, phenytoin, warfarin.

Main side effects Diarrhea, headache, rash (all rare); increased risk of enteric infection.

Prostaglandins

- Prostaglandins are probably most useful as prophylatic agents in patients with peptic ulcer disease who require ongoing NSAID treatment. Healing rates are inferior to those of H_2 antagonists or proton-pump inhibitor.

Standard dosage Misoprostol, 400 μg daily in 4 divided doses.

Contraindications Pregnancy or planned pregnancy.

Special points Small doses of synthetic prostaglandins have been shown to exhibit a cytoprotective effect and to inhibit gastric acid secretion.

Main drug interactions None known.

Main side effects Diarrhea, abdominal pain, flushing, menorrhagia.

Treatment aims

To relieve symptoms.

To heal ulcer.

To exclude malignancy.

Other treatments

- Surgery is indicated for uncontrolled ulcer-related hemorrhage (early operation important in elderly patients), perforation, malignant ulceration, delayed healing, or gastric outlet obstruction due to structure.

Prognosis

- After completion of a healing course of H_2 antagonists, the chance of recurrence in 1 year is 50% unless predisposing factors (NSAIDs, *H. pylori*) are removed.

Follow-up and management

- Endoscopic confirmation of mucosal healing at 8–12 weeks is essential, with repeated biopsy and further endoscopy if ulcer healing has not occurred.
- After ulcer healing, treatment is usually discontinued unless an obvious and continuing predisposing factor is present.
- Recurrence of symptoms must be reassessed with further endoscopy.
- Significant gastrointestinal bleeding is managed by maintenance treatment with half-dose H_2 blockade and the therapeutic treatment regimen is completed.

Key references

1. Graham DY: Peptic ulcer disease. *Curr Pract Med* 1998, **1**:765–773.
2. Wolfe MM, Lichtenstein DR, Sing G: Gastrointestinal toxicity of nonsteroidal antiinflammatory drugs. *N Engl J Med* 1999, **340**:1888–1899.
3. Wolfe MM, Sachs G: Acid suppression: optimizing therapy for gastroduodenal ulcer healing, gastroesophageal reflux disease, and stress related erosive syndrome. *Gastroenterology* 2000, **118**:59–S31.
4. Maton RP: Omeprazole. *N Engl J Med* 1991, **324**:965–975.

Glomerulonephritis

Diagnosis

Definition

• Glomerulonephritis is an immunologically mediated glomerular injury, often with associated tubulointerstitial lesions that may be chronic or acute.

Nonproliferative

Minimal-change disease: normal on light microscopy; no immune complexes.

Focal segmental glomerulosclerosis: mesangial and capillary loop scarring.

Membranous glomerulonephritis: thick-basement membranes, subepithelial immune complexes.

Proliferative: endocapillary

Proliferative glomerulonephritis: inflammatory cells in immune complexes in subendothelial and mesangial compartments; can also be subepithelial.

IgA nephropathy: large IgA immune complexes in mesangium.

Membranoproliferative glomerulonephritis: thick capillary loops with expanded overcellular mesangium.

Focal necrotizing glomerulonephritis: segment of necrosis in peripheral capillary loop, often associated with vasculitis.

Proliferative: extracapillary

Crescentic glomerulonephritis: layers of macrophages and other cells in Bowman's proliferative glomerulonephritis; usually with rapidly progressive glomerulonephritis.

Symptoms and signs

Proteinuria: nephrotic range >73.5 g/24 hours.

Hematuria: microscopic (detected by dipstick test); macroscopic (smoky urine).

Hypertension.

Acute renal failure.

Chronic renal failure.

Peripheral edema.

Associated symptoms can include: fever, hemoptysis, arthralgias, skin rash.

Investigations

Urine microscopy: dysmorphic erythrocytes and erythrocyte casts imply glomerular inflammation.

24-hour urinalysis: for creatinine clearance and urine protein.

Blood urea nitrogen and creatinine measurement.

Renal biopsy (light, electron, and immunofluorescent microscopy needed): necessary to diagnose and manage almost all types of glomerulonephritis.

Albumin and lipid measurement.

Tests for lupus and vasculitis: *e.g.*, antinuclear antibody, anti-double-stranded DNA antibody, antineutrophil cytoplasmic antibody (ANCA).

Antiglomerular basement membrane antibody measurement.

Investigation for appropriate associated infections (*see* Etiology).

Complement studies: CH50, C3, C4.

Ultrasonography to assess kidney size, scarring.

Hepatitis C and B serologic testing.

Cryoglobulin levels.

Complications

Hypertension: can be severe.

Acute or chronic renal failure.

Nephrotic syndrome: venous and arterial thromboses, pleural effusions, ascites, intravascular volume depletion, infection, accelerated atherosclerosis, hypercholesterolemia, volume overload.

Differential diagnosis

Nephritic syndrome

Severe hypertension.

Scleroderma renal crisis.

Thrombotic microangiopathies (*e.g.*, hemolytic uremic syndrome).

Acute interstitial nephritis.

Nephrotic syndrome

Pre-eclampsia.

Amyloidosis.

Diabetes mellitus.

Congestive heart failure.

Cirrhosis with edema and ascites.

NSAID use.

Other

Orthostatic proteinuria.

Other causes of hypertension or acute or chronic renal failure.

Etiology

Immunopathogenesis

Immune complex: in situ formation (built up within glomerulus) or, less commonly, deposition of preformed immune complexes from circulation.

Direct antibody-mediated injury: antiglomerular basement membrane antibody (Goodpasture's syndrome); rare.

Unknown; probably cell-mediated; no immune complexes; probably important in many forms of glomerulonephritis.

Associated diseases

Primary: no known association (idiopathic).

Secondary: associated with infections, *e.g.*, viruses, (hepatitis B and C, HIV), bacterial (poststreptococcal), syphilis, protozoal (malarial); drug-induced, *e.g.*, gold or penicillamine; vasculitis; neoplasia; systemic lupus erythematosus; cryoglobulinemia.

Epidemiology

• Glomerulonephritis is a common cause of chronic renal failure.

• Minimal-change glomerulonephritis is the most common cause of nephrotic syndrome in children.

• IgA nephropathy is the most common cause of glomerulonephritis.

• Membranous glomerulonephritis is the most common idiopathic glomerulopathy in older adults.

Treatment

Diet and lifestyle

- Patients must not have added salt if they have edema or hypertension.
- Nephrotic patients should have a normal protein intake.
- Oral intake of fluids should be restricted if the patient is edematous.
- Pregnant patients are at increased risk of pre-eclampsia (high risk if creatinine raised).
- Pregnant patients often experience deterioration of renal function.

Pharmacological treatment

Immunosuppression

- Patients are chosen on the basis of clinical syndrome and histology. Consultation with a nephrologist is essential.
- Aggressive treatment is indicated for heavy proteinuria or falling glomerular filtration rate.
- Histology is most helpful for choosing treatment.

For minimal-change glomerulonephritis:
remission induction: high-dose steroids, cyclosporine;
maintenance: low-dose steroids or cyclosporine;
prevention of relapse: cyclophosphamide.

For membranous glomerulonephritis: cyclophosphamide or chlorambucil with corticosteroids in selected patients.

For focal segmental glomerulosclerosis: high-dose steroids or cyclosporine, or both in selected patients.

For mesangial IgA disease: fish oil (eicosapentaenoic acid).

For glomerulonephritis associated with infections: treat infection.

For membranoproliferative glomerulonephritis: no treatment effective; trial of immunosuppression in selected patients.

For focal necrotizing or crescentic glomerulonephritis: steroids with cyclophosphamide (pulse i.v. methylprednisolone for 3 days may help); additional plasma exchange in selected patients (immediate plasma exchange mandatory in Goodpasture's syndrome).

Supportive

Control of fluid balance: diuretics (combinations may be needed).

Control of proteinuria: angiotensin-converting enzyme inhibitors or angiotensin receptor blockers; even in normotensive patients, if tolerated.

Aggressive treatment of intercurrent infections (cellulitis, pneumonia, spontaneous bacterial peritonitis).

Anticoagulation: should be considered for nephrotic patients, especially if they are immobile.

Control of hypertension: angiotensin-converting enzyme inhibitors as first choice; others as needed.

Treatment aims

To suppress glomerular inflammation.

To prevent progressive glomerular scarring and progression to chronic renal failure.

To minimize proteinuria.

To control hypertension and fluid balance.

To avoid overimmunosuppression.

Prognosis

- A poor prognosis is associated with severe hypertension, heavy persistent proteinuria, and raised creatinine.
- Prognosis is closely related to histology, *e.g.:*

Minimal-change glomerulonephritis: excellent, resolves despite relapses.
Membranous glomerulonephritis: 30% resolve, 30% remain static, 30% progress to CRF.
IgA nephropathy: 25% progress to CRF.
Postinfectious diffuse proliferative glomerulonephritis: >90% resolve.
Membranoproliferative glomerulonephritis: >75% progress to CRF.

Follow-up and management

- Strict control of blood pressure is needed, use angiotensin-converting enzyme inhibitors whenever possible
- Immunosuppressive drugs must be titrated to disease activity.
- Lipids must be controlled.
- All patients should be managed in consultation with a nephrologist.

General references

Couser WG: Glomerulonephritis. *Lancet* 1999, **353**:1509–1515.

Gaskin G: Management of rapidly progressive glomerulonephritis. *J R Coll Physicians Lond* 1997, **31**:15–18.

Kluth DC, Rees AS: Antiglomerular basement membran disease. *J Am Soc Nephrol* 1999, **11**:2446–2453.

Maschio G, Albert D: Effect of the angiotensin-converting enzyme inhibitor benazepril on the progression of chronic renal insufficiency. *N Engl J Med* 1996, **334**:939–945.

Reisman L, *et al.*: Renal biospy: why and when. *Mt Sinai J Med* 1996, **63**:178–190.

Wasserstein AG: Membranous glomerulonephritis. *J Am Soc Nephrol* 1997, **4**:664–674.

Gout

Diagnosis

Symptoms

Acute pain in a single joint: usually base of great toe; often starting at night; self-limiting but tendency to recur.

Mild systemic disturbance, with irritability and low-grade fever.

Polyarticular attacks: in 5%–10% of patients (50% of elderly patients).

Chronic asymmetrical polyarthritis: after repeated acute attacks.

Signs

Exquisite tenderness.

Swollen, shiny, red, tender joints.

Desquamation: as attack subsides.

Tophi in helix of ear, elbow, and over small joints of hands and feet: in severe cases.

Olecranon bursitis: "imbiber's elbow"; common.

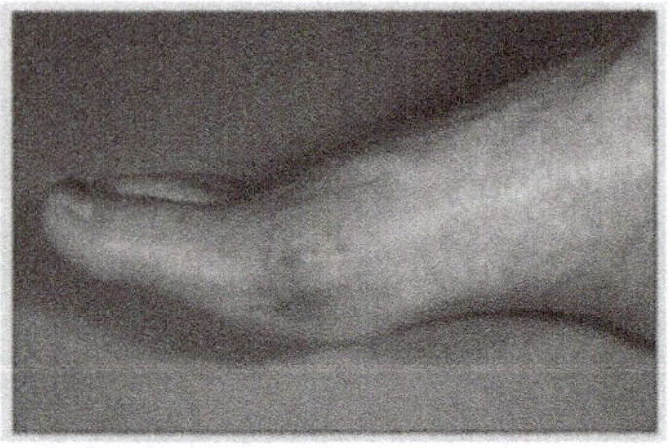

Acute gout in big toe. (*See* Color Plate.)

Investigations

Polarized light microscopy: needle-shaped, negatively birefringent crystals in synovial fluid from the affected joint are diagnostic.

Serum uric acid measurement: concentration usually raised but may fall to normal during acute attack.

Complete blood count: to exclude secondary cause, *e.g.*, lymphoproliferative disorder.

ESR measurement: may be raised during acute attack.

Creatinine measurement: renal failure may result from or be caused by hyperuricemia.

Fasting lipids measurement: hyperlipidemia common.

Urinary urate excretion measurement: differentiates overproducers from underexcretors (while on low-purine diet).

Radiography: may show characteristic juxta-articular punched-out erosions without accompanying osteoporosis around joints ("overhanging edges") in patients with chronic arthritic gout.

Complications

Prolongation of acute attack: by incorrect use of allopurinol.

Gastrointestinal bleeding: due to high-dose NSAIDs.

Renal impairment: due to drug interference with renal cortical blood flow.

Differential diagnosis

Acute gout

Septic arthritis.

Cellulitis.

Pyrophosphate arthritis ("pseudogout").

Chronic tophaceous gout

Rheumatoid arthritis.

Septic arthritis.

Hyperlipidemia with xanthomata.

Nongout

Painful bunion with asymptomatic hyperuricemia.

Etiology

- Gout is often precipitated by alcohol overindulgence, surgery, or intercurrent illness.
- Primary gout may be caused by a genetic predisposition to overproduction or underexcretion of urate or failure to inhibit crystallization in tissues.
- Secondary gout may be caused by diuretics (particularly in older women), renal impairment, diet (high purine intake coupled with obesity), high cell turnover (malignant disease), alcohol excess, or heavy-metal poisoning, especially lead (saturnine gout).

Epidemiology

- Gout is particularly prevalent in middle-aged men, postmenopausal women, and patients with renal insufficiency (controversial).

Treatment

Diet and lifestyle

• Patients with associated obesity may benefit from caloric restriction.

• Alcohol intake should be moderated because alcohol inhibits urate excretion by the kidney and is often associated with acute attacks [1].

• Consumption of high-purine foods (*e.g.*, shellfish) should be restricted because they may provoke acute attacks; a purine-free diet is impractical.

Pharmacological treatment

For acute attack

Standard dosage	Rapidly acting NSAID, *e.g.*, indomethacin, 25–50 mg initially, followed by 25–50 mg 3 times daily until attack starts to subside, then reduced dose [1,2]. Colchicine, 0.5 mg hourly to a maximum of 6 mg in first 24 hours; do not repeat dose for 7 days.
Contraindications	*Indomethacin:* peptic ulcer, anticoagulants, renal impairment. *Colchicine:* hypersensitivity.
Special points	*Colchicine:* can be used to prevent recurrence at 0.5 g once or twice daily. Alternatives for resistant or difficult cases include intra-articular or oral steroids.
Main drug interactions	*Indomethacin:* warfarin.
Main side effects	*Indomethacin, diclofenac:* indigestion, gastric bleeding, headache, nausea, dizziness (worse with indomethacin). *Colchicine:* nausea, diarrhea.

For hyperuricemia

• Treatment can be considered between attacks if the serum urate concentration remains raised [1,2].

• Allopurinol is indicated for recurrent attacks of gout, chronic tophaceous gout, renal impairment due to hyperuricemia, induction of chemotherapy, and asymptomatic hyperuricemia (>12 mg/dL) or for any gouty patient with a history of renal stones.

Standard dosage	Allopurinol, 300 mg initially; reduce dosage for renal insufficiency.
Contraindications	Acute gout, hypersensitivity.
Special points	Lower dose in renal failure to prevent build up of metabolites; additional prophylactic NSAID or colchicine for first 3 months to prevent multiple attacks of gout.
Main drug interactions	Azathioprine, cyclosporin.
Main side effects	Rash.

• Uricosuric agents (sulfinpyrazone, probenecid).

Special points	Can be used safely only if 24-hour urine collection shows <30 mg uric acid excretion (or increasing risk of kidney stone formation).

Treatment aims

To control inflammation during acute attack.

To prevent recurrent acute attacks and chronic gouty arthritis by lowering serum urate concentrations.

Prognosis

• The prognosis is excellent; with modern hypouricemic treatment, most patients are effectively cured.

Follow-up and management

• Patients are usually followed up by the primary care physician, who should monitor serum urate concentrations to adjust the dose of hypouricemic treatment and to ensure compliance.

• Referral to a specialist is indicated if the diagnosis is in doubt, response to treatment is poor, or drug sensitivity develops.

Key references

1. Star VL, Hockberg MC: Prevention and management of gout. ***Drugs*** 1993, **45**:212–222.
2. Tan N, Lertratanakul W, Barr WG: Acute gouty arthritis: modern approaches to an ancient disease. ***Postgrad Med*** 1993, **94**:73–75; 78; 83–84.

Gram-negative septicemia

Diagnosis

Symptoms

Sweats, chills, or rigors.

Cough, possibly with sputum, pleuritic chest pain, breathlessness.

Dysuria, urinary frequency.

Abdominal pain, nausea, vomiting, diarrhea.

Headache, neck stiffness, confusion.

Signs

• Focal clinical signs, if present, may help to localize the site of infection.

Tachycardia: >90 beats/min.

Tachypnea: >20 breaths/min.

Temperature >38°C or <35.6°C: hypothermia associated with worse prognosis.

Hypotension: systolic blood pressure <90 mm Hg or fall of 40 mm Hg from baseline.

Oliguria: <20 mL/h.

Petechial or purpuric skin rash: suggesting meningococcal septicemia; ecthyma gangrenosum associated with *Pseudomonas* infection in neutropenic patients.

Investigations

• Investigations are directed toward ascertaining the microbiology, site of infection, severity, and complications of gram-negative sepsis.

• Ideally, culture specimens should be taken before antimicrobial treatment, but treatment should not be unduly delayed in seriously ill patients.

Blood cultures: at least two, preferably three.

Urine microscopy and culture.

Gram stain and culture of available pus or body fluids: may provide rapid diagnosis.

Chest radiography, further radiography directed by clinical picture.

Hemoglobin level: to detect severe anemia (may need to be corrected).

Leukocyte count: to detect neutrophil leukocytosis or toxic granulation; leukopenia associated with poor prognosis.

Platelet count and coagulation studies: for evidence of disseminated intravascular coagulation.

Arterial blood gas analysis: shows respiratory alkalosis early and metabolic acidosis later; possibly hypoxia.

Liver function tests: abnormal results in 40%–60% of patients; abdominal ultrasonography or CT scan if indicated.

Complications

Renal failure: acute tubular necrosis, usually reversible.

Disseminated intravascular coagulation.

Acute respiratory distress syndrome: in 15%–40% of patients.

Hepatic failure.

Differential diagnosis

• More than one factor may contribute to shock in an individual patient.

Other causes of shock: cardiogenic, hypovolemic, redistribution of fluid (*e.g.*, burns, pancreatitis, anaphylaxis), toxins.

Other infections: *e.g.*, gram-positive bacteria, fungi, malaria, or viral infections, staphylococcal or streptococcal toxic shock syndrome.

Etiology

• Gram-negative septicemia is usually associated with *Escherichia coli, Klebsiella, Enterobacter, Serratia, Proteus, Pseudomonas* spp., and *Neisseria meningitidis;* enteric gram-negative bacteria account for most cases.

• The most common sources are intra-abdominal or urinary tract infections and pneumonia.

• Host risk factors include the following:

Surgery (especially gastrointestinal, genitourinary, hepatobiliary).

Abnormalities of genitourinary tract.

Intravenous lines.

Hospitalization.

Cancer.

Neutropenia.

Immunosuppression.

Epidemiology

• Gram-negative septicemia and shock have been increasing over the past 30 years.

• Bacteremia is found in ~7 in 1000 hospital admissions.

• Septic shock complicates 20% of bacteremias.

Pathogenesis of gram-negative shock

• Bacterial endotoxin (lipopolysaccharide) and other bacterial products initiate the release of inflammatory mediators from monocyte/macrophages, endothelial cells, and polymorphonuclear leukocytes.

• The interaction of these mediators leads to an "inflammatory cascade" of reactions, leading to widespread endothelial damage, hypotension, refractory shock, multiorgan failure, and death.

Treatment

Diet and lifestyle

• No special precautions are necessary.

Pharmacological treatment

Indications

• Antibiotic treatment depends on the site of the infection and host and environmental factors.

Urinary tract (community-acquired): quinolone.

Urinary tract or pneumonia (hospital-acquired): ceftazidime, or piperacillin with gentamicin.

Intra-abdominal: cefotaxime with metronidazole, or piperacillin with gentamicin.

Biliary tract: piperacillin with gentamicin.

Cefotaxime or ceftazidime

Standard dosage	Ceftriaxone, 1–2 g daily, or ceftazidime, 1–2 g every 8 hours.
Contraindications	Previous cephalosporin hypersensitivity.
Special points	Dose adjusted in moderate to severe renal failure.
Main drug interactions	None.
Main side effects	Rashes, diarrhea, hemolysis, or raised transaminases (rare).

Gentamicin

Standard dosage	Gentamicin, 4 mg/kg daily (normal renal function).
Contraindications	Myasthenia gravis, pre-existing renal failure.
Special points	Concentrations must be monitored before and after dose.
Main drug interactions	Loop diuretics, curare-type anesthetic agents.
Main side effects	Nephrotoxicity, ototoxicity.

Quinolones

Standard dosage	Ciprofloxacin, 500 mg twice daily.
Contraindications	Pregnancy, childhood.
Special points	Dose adjusted in severe renal failure.
Main drug interactions	None.
Main side effects	Diarrhea, renal failure.

Piperacillin

Standard dosage	Piperacillin, 2 g every 6 hours.
Contraindications	Penicillin hypersensitivity.
Special points	Dose adjusted in moderate to severe renal failure.
Main drug interactions	Inactivates aminoglycosides if mixed in solution.
Main side effects	Hypersensitivity, hepatotoxicity in 3% of patients, platelet dysfunction.

Treatment aims

To control infection.
To maintain organ perfusion and tissue oxygen delivery.
To minimize complications

Other treatments

Drainage of infected collections of pus.
Surgical debridement of dead or infected material.

Prognosis

• Mortality is 10%–20% in patients with bacteremia, 40%–60% in those with shock, and >90% in those with multiorgan failure.

Follow-up and management

• Patients need careful management in the convalescent stage, which may be prolonged after acute septic shock; they may relapse if the predisposing condition remains.

Management of gram-negative bacterial shock

• Monitoring of the following is needed:
Systolic blood pressure (must be kept >90 mm Hg or high enough to maintain renal perfusion).
Central venous pressure or postcapillary wedge pressure (to exclude hypovolemia).
Cardiac output.
Systemic vascular resistance (normal, >1000; in septic shock, generally <1000).
Catheterization (for urine measurement).
Oxygen saturation (arterial pressure falls, venous pressure rises because of failure in tissue oxygenation).
• Treatment includes the following:
Colloid to restore intravascular volume (blood for severe anemia).
Pressor or inotropic agents, if necessary.
Renal dopamine 2–4 μg/min to maintain renal perfusion.
Inspired oxygen at minimum to maintain arterial oxygenation.
Nutritional support.

General references

Edwards JD: Management of septic shock. *BMJ* 1993, **306**:1661–1664.

Parillo JE: Pathogenetic mechanisms of septic shock. *N Engl J Med* 1993, **328**:1471–1477.

Pollack M, Ohl CA: Endotoxin-based molecular strategies for the prevention and treatment of gram-negative sepsis and septic shock. *Curr Top Microbiol Immunol* 1996, **216**:275–297.

Diagnosis

Symptoms

Height less than the third height centile or short for family.

Delayed puberty: in some patients.

Signs

- Signs are not always manifest.
- Features of hypothyroidism with or without goiter may be seen.

Disproportionate growth: *e.g.*, short legs.

Dysmorphic features: *e.g.*, in Turner's syndrome, intrauterine growth retardation.

Investigations [1,2]

Anthropometry: height of child should be recorded on at least two occasions separated by at least 3 months to calculate growth velocity; assessments of nutrition (weight, skinfold thickness) helpful; Tanner stages of puberty must be elicited; heights of parents should be measured.

Radiography: bone age; skeletal survey (for disproportionate short stature); pituitary MRI (if hypothalamic or pituitary dysfunction is suspected).

Hematology: to identify anemia (vitamin B_{12}, folate, ferritin malabsorption).

ESR measurement: to exclude inflammatory disease.

Chemistries: standard chemistry panel including electrolytes, blood urea nitrogen, creatinine, calcium, and liver function tests; growth hormone and/or somatomedin C (insulin-like growth factor-1); thyroid function tests (thyrotropin, free thyroxine); luteinizing hormone, follicle-stimulating hormone, gonadal steroids, prolactin (if delayed puberty is suspected).

Karyotyping: XO in Turner's syndrome.

Complications

Premature fusion of epiphyses: through injudicious treatment with gonadal steroids.

Differential diagnosis

- The vast majority of short children have no abnormalities and will go on to achieve their normal adult heights. These children, and particularly their parents, should be reassured following an appropriate medical evaluation.

Etiology [1,2]

- All disease in childhood causes a decrease in growth velocity that ultimately becomes manifest as short stature.
- The following may play a role:

Nutritional disorders: in infants.

Diminished growth hormone secretion: in the absence of physical signs in children (hypoglycemia may sometimes be present).

Delayed or absent puberty.

Some hypothalamic–pituitary disorders associated with obesity and short stature (*e.g.*, Prader Willi).

Epidemiology

- Boys with delayed puberty (and its consequent short stature) outnumber girls by 20:1.

Treatment

Diet and lifestyle

• In infants, adequate nutrition must be promoted, including correction of malabsorption.

Pharmacological treatment [1,2]

• In childhood, growth hormone is appropriately prescribed to correct insufficiency; sex steroids are otherwise appropriate first-line treatment (*see* below).

• Long-term alleviation of short stature is achievable only when an abnormal growth velocity can be corrected; the height of a normal child cannot be increased.

Thyroxine: 100 μg/m² orally as single daily dose for children with hypothyroidism.

• The following should be prescribed by the appropriate specialist:

Growth hormone: 0.04 mg/kg daily.

Ethinyl estradiol: initially 2 μg daily, increased to 5, 10, 15, 20, and 30 μg daily at 6-monthly intervals; progestogen added when dose of 15 μg achieved or if breakthrough bleeding occurs earlier; use caution if family history of thrombotic disorder is present.

Testosterone: initially 50 mg testosterone esters at 4-weekly intervals, increased to 100 mg every 4 weeks after 6 months; increased to 3-weekly intervals over a further 6 months and then to 2-weekly intervals; causes accelerated fusion of epiphyses.

Treatment aims

To redress abnormal growth.

To reassure patients and parents.

Prognosis

• Medical therapy does not turn normal short children into tall children.

• Adult height is fixed once epiphyses have fused.

• Early diagnosis and treatment maximizes the chances of achieving maximal potential adult height.

• Best case scenario with treatment is achieving expected height based on parents' height.

Follow-up and management

• Anthropometry is needed every 6 months to record effects on growth and to readjust doses for increase in size.

Key references

1. Brook CGD: ***A Guide to the Practice of Paediatric Endocrinology.*** Cambridge: Cambridge University Press; 1993.

2. Brook CGD (ed.): ***Clinical Paediatric Endocrinology,*** edn 3. Oxford: Blackwell Scientific Publications; 1995.

Growth abnormalities, tall stature

Diagnosis

Symptoms

- Symptoms are usually minimal (other than being tall for one's age).

Signs

- Tall children usually look normal.

Signs of precocious puberty or thyrotoxicosis.

Signs of virilization (in girls): pubic hair, acne, cliteromegaly; adrenal androgen excess should be ruled out.

Joint hypermobility, arachnodactyly, iridonodesis, high arch palate: signs of Marfan syndrome.

Investigations [1]

- Height and weight should be monitored on standard growth charts. Patients whose height and weight percentiles remain constant over time are less likely to have a pathological cause of tall stature.
- Tall stature associated with true precocious puberty must be fully investigated.

Anthropometry: height of child and both parents should be measured; Tanner stages of puberty should be recorded; arm measurement of sitting height to determine leg length more helpful than measurement of span.

Radiography: assessment of skeletal maturity (including bone age) enables height prediction.

Special tests: measurement of thyroxine and thyroid-stimulating hormone may reveal thyrotoxicosis; gigantism is associated with elevated somatomedin-C levels and may also be accompanied by hypogonadism (resulting in nonclosure of epiphyses).

Complications

- There are no complications in normal tall individuals.
- Complications are related to underlying disease in patients with pathological tall stature.
- Patients with tall stature due to congenital adrenal hyperplasia or precocious puberty may complete puberty early, resulting in a short final adult height.

Differential diagnosis

Not applicable.

Etiology [1]

Normal growth rate and appearance

Tall parents.

Obesity of infantile onset.

Marfan, Klinefelter's, or Sotos' syndrome.

Excessive growth rate

Early puberty or premature adrenarche.

Androgen secretion (congenital adrenal hyperplasia, adrenal neoplasm).

Thyrotoxicosis.

Growth hormone excess.

Epidemiology

- 1% of the population is tall.

Treatment

Diet and lifestyle

• No special precautions are necessary.

Pharmacological treatment [1]

• Precocious puberty and adrenal, thyroid, and pituitary conditions should be referred for appropriate treatment, including surgery.

• Patients with Klinefelter's syndrome and inadequate puberty need androgens to prevent gynecomastia and osteoporosis.

• Sex steroids can be used to accelerate epiphyseal closure in tall children with hypogonadism or delayed puberty.

• The following should be prescribed by the appropriate subspecialist:

Ethinyl estradiol: initially 2 µg daily, increased to 5, 10, 15, 20, and 30 µg daily at 6-monthly intervals; progestogen added when dose of 15 µg achieved or if breakthrough bleeding occurs earlier; contraindicated if family history of thrombotic disorder.

Testosterone: initially 50 mg testosterone esters at 4-weekly intervals, increased to 100 mg every 4 weeks after 6 months; increased to 3-weekly intervals over a further 6 months and then to 2-weekly intervals; causes accelerated fusion of epiphyses.

Treatment aims

To reduce adult stature.

Prognosis

• The prognosis depends on the diagnosis.

Follow-up and management

• Children with Marfan syndrome need ophthalmological and cardiac evaluation.

Key reference

1. Brook CGD (ed.): ***Clinical Paediatric Endocrinology***, edn. 3. Oxford: Blackwell Scientific Publications; 1995.

Guillain–Barré syndrome

Diagnosis

Symptoms [1]

Ascending, symmetrical weakness in all limbs: legs usually affected first, with patient initially noticing difficulty climbing stairs, rising from sitting, and, eventually, walking and standing.

Paresthesias of extremities, with distal sensory loss: in 95% of patients.

Neck, shoulder, back, and sciatic pain: may be severe.

Diplopia, drooling, nasal regurgitation of food or drink, slurred speech, weak cough: indicating cranial nerve involvement.

Dyspnea: late symptom, reflecting intercostal and diaphragmatic weakness.

Fatigue: possibly profound and often persisting after return of muscle strength.

Hesitancy and urinary retention: usually when weakness more advanced (vs acute myelopathy, in which sphincter symptoms appear early).

Signs

Weakness in limbs: flaccid, usually symmetrical, arms usually less severely affected.

Cranial nerve palsies: facial nerve most often affected, followed by bulbar muscles.

Hyporeflexia, areflexia: early.

Sensory deficit: may be absent or minor despite prominent symptoms.

Profound sensory loss: in some patients.

Ataxia, ophthalmoplegia, areflexia, with little or no weakness: Miller–Fisher syndrome; rare.

Investigations

Initial

Lumbar puncture: classically, raised protein concentration associated with normal cell count (albuminocytological dissociation); protein possibly normal within first week.

Serum potassium measurement: to exclude hypo- or hyperkalemic paralysis.

Antinuclear antibodies analysis: positive in rare cases associated with SLE.

Liver function tests: often abnormal.

Heavy metal screening: only if clinically indicated.

Porphyrin screening: positive in acute intermittent porphyria, which may manifest like Guillain–Barré syndrome.

Lyme titers.

Stool *Campylobacter* antibodies analysis: associated with axonal involvement.

Specialist

Nerve conduction studies: to identify multifocal conduction block and slowed conduction, confirming demyelinating neuropathy; studies early in disease may be only mildly abnormal, *e.g.*, delayed or absent F waves; axonal degeneration may also occur [2].

Electromyography: in patients without sensory involvement, to help to rule out neuromuscular conduction block or muscle disease and to document axonal degeneration.

Antiganglioside antibody analysis: anti-GM_1 antibodies present in 20%–30% of patients; anti-GQ1b antibodies associated with Miller–Fisher syndrome.

Complications

Death: if airway not adequately protected.

Atelectasis, pneumonia, deep venous thrombosis, pulmonary embolism, joint contractures, pressure sores, anxiety and depression, pain.

Cardiac arrhythmias, including bradycardic and asystolic episodes, labile blood pressure: due to autonomic instability.

Differential diagnosis

Brain stem encephalitis or infarct.

Acute myelopathy.

Poliomyelitis.

Other neuropathies: porphyria, vasculitis, critical-illness neuropathy, drug-induced neuropathy, toxins (*e.g.*, heavy metals, organophosphates), Lyme disease, or HIV.

Neuromuscular conduction block: myasthenia gravis, botulism.

Muscle disease: hypokalemia (with or without periodic paralysis), polymyositis, acute rhabdomyolysis.

Functional disease: hysteria, malingering.

Etiology

- The cause of Guillain–Barré syndrome is unknown, but, in 60%–70% of patients, it is associated with antecedent infection.
- Inflammatory demyelination with variable axonal degeneration in the peripheral nervous system due to autoimmune mechanisms is triggered by many different agents, including the following:

Viruses: cytomegalovirus, Epstein–Barr virus, HIV (usually around seroconversion).

Bacteria: *Mycoplasma pneumoniae, Campylobacter jejuni.*

Vaccines against rabies or swine influenza.

Surgery.

Epidemiology

- Guillain–Barré syndrome has become the most frequent cause of acute generalized neuromuscular paralysis in developed countries since the virtual eradication of poliomyelitis.
- The incidence is 1–2 in 100 000 population.
- More men than women are affected.
- The disease occurs more often in young women and elderly patients.
- It is not contagious.
- No seasonal variation is evident.

Treatment

Diet and lifestyle

- No special precautions are necessary.

Pharmacological treatment

General measures

Frequent measurement of vital capacity and continuous ECG monitoring during progressive phase.

Admission to intensive care unit if vital capacity falling rapidly or patient unable to swallow saliva.

Regular turning, mouth and eye care, aspiration of secretions.

Heparin, 5000 units s.c. twice daily.

Nasogastric feeding if patient has bulbar palsy or is too weak to eat.

Plasma exchange

- Plasma, 50 mL/kg, exchanged five times over 5–10 days is indicated for any patient unable to walk unaided.
- Treatment should be initiated as soon as the diagnosis is made because it is more effective in early disease.

Immunoglobulin [3]

Standard dosage	Immunoglobulin, 0.4 g/kg i.v. daily for 5 days or 1 g/kg daily for 2 days.
Contraindications	IgA deficiency due to circulating anti-IgA antibodies, congestive heart failure.
Special points	May cause aseptic meningitis and acute or chronic renal failure and exacerbate underlying ischemic disease.
Main side effects	Fever, hypersensitivity reactions, fluid overload.

Treatment aims

To prevent respiratory failure.

To relieve pain.

To prevent complications of immobility.

To optimize functional recovery.

Other treatments

Early tracheostomy: to assist tracheal toilet and increase patient comfort.

Ventilatory assistance: if vital capacity 20 mL/kg or falling rapidly (oxygen saturation best monitored by pulse oximetry) or patient unable to protect airway.

Endocardial pacemaker: for episodes of bradycardia or sinus arrest.

Prognosis

- ~5% of patients relapse; 80% make a good recovery (median time to full independence, 9 months); 20% have permanent disability; 5% die.
- Poor prognostic indicators include age >40 years, rapid onset of weakness, ventilation, high titers of IgG anti-ganglioside GM_1 antibodies, and previous diarrheal illness.

Follow-up and management

- A high level of vigilance must be maintained until recovery has started and the tracheostomy has been closed.
- The patient should be reassured that recovery is probable and is nearly complete in most cases.
- Rehabilitation, *e.g.*, physical therapy, must be continued after discharge.
- Immunization injections must be avoided, especially tetanus toxoid, which has been associated with relapse.

Key references

1. Fulgram JR, Wijdicks EF: Guillain-Barré syndrome. *Crit Care Clin* 1997, **13**:1–15.
2. Albers JW: Acquired inflammatory demyelinating polyneuropathies: clinical and electrodiagnostic features. *Muscle Nerve* 1989, **12**:435–451.
3. van der Meché FGA, Schmitz PIM, the Dutch Guillain–Barré Study Group: A randomized trial comparing intravenous immune globulin and plasma exchange in Guillain–Barré syndrome. *N Engl J Med* 1992, **326**:1123–1129.

Heart block

Diagnosis

Definition

- Heart block is a disturbance of conduction of electrical impulse from atrium to ventricle.
- Failure of the sinus impulse to penetrate the atrium (sinoatrial block) and bundle-branch block are not considered here.

First-degree atrioventricular (AV) block: delayed conduction of impulses from the sinus node to ventricle: prolonged PR interval but all impulses are conducted.

Second-degree AV block: intermittent complete failure of conduction of atrial impulse to ventricle, with dropped (nonconducted) P waves on ECG.

Mobitz type I (Wenckebach): Stable PP interval and a progressive increase in the PR interval until a P wave fails to conduct. The PR increment usually decreases with each beat in the cycle, so that the RR interval shortens. After the blocked P wave, the next PR interval returns to initial value.

Mobitz type II: There is a stable PP interval with no measurable prolongation of the PR interval before an abrupt conduction failure.

In AV block with a 2:1 conduction ratio or higher (*e.g.*, 3:1 or 4:1), it is impossible to observe prolongation of the PR interval before the block, so a designation of type I or type II is inappropriate. In 2:1 block, a narrow QRS complex and associated periods of Wenckebach block, or simultaneous sinus slowing suggest that atrioventricular block is present; a wide QRS complex suggests the presence of infranodal block.

Third-degree AV block: often referred to as "complete" heart block. In such cases, atrial activity and ventricular activity are independent of each other. The location of the block is deduced from the escape rhythm. A wide QRS escape rhythm suggests that the block is located in the His-Purkinje system. A narrow QRS complex, implies the presence of AV nodal block.

Symptoms

First-degree and Mobitz type I: Patients are usually asymptomatic but may progress to higher-grade atrioventricular block. Some patients with marked first-degree atrioventricular block have symptoms owing to a loss of atrioventricular synchrony that resolve with pacing.

Mobitz type II and complete heart block: *Syncope (Stokes-Adams attack):* loss of consciousness is abrupt, without warning, and the patient appears pale; rare in Mobitz type II. Presyncope and dizzy spells, fatigue, dyspnea, sudden death.

Signs

First-degree: no signs are manifest. **Mobitz type I:** irregular pulse with dropped beats. **Mobitz type II:** occasional dropped beats; irregular pulse. **2:1/3:1 block, etc.:** bradycardia, edema, raised venous pressure. **Complete heart block:** bradycardia, large-volume pulse, raised venous pressure with occasional cannon waves, variable intensity of S1, peripheral edema.

Investigations

Resting ECG.

First-degree AV block: PR interval >0.20 second; every P wave followed by a QRS complex.

Second-degree AV block: *Mobitz Type I (Wenckebach block):* progressive lengthening of PR interval and shortening of RR interval until a P wave is blocked: PR interval after blocked beat is shorter than preceding PR interval; *Mobitz type II:* intermittently blocked P waves, PR interval on conducted beats is constant; *Second-degree, high-grade AV block:* conduction ratio of 3:1 or more, PR interval of conducted beats constant; *Third-degree AV block:* dissociation of atrial and ventricular activity, atrial rate is faster than ventricular rate, which is of junctional or ventricular origin.

24-hour Holter monitoring: if heart block is intermittent; continuous "event recorder" if symptoms are infrequent.

Complications

Injury: from syncope.

"Heart failure": underlying ventricular function may be normal, but low cardiac output due to bradycardia and loss of atrioventricular synchrony may mimic ventricular disease.

Ventricular tachycardia and fibrillation: leading to sudden death, may complicate complete heart block.

Differential diagnosis

- ECG diagnosis is usually definitive; the only difference should be the cause.

Etiology

Idiopathic fibrosis: increasing frequency with age.

Ischemic heart disease: particularly after myocardial infarction.

Calcific aortic stenosis: involvement of ring close to atrioventricular node.

Drug toxicity: many antiarrhythmic, agents, including digoxin and calcium-channel blockers.

Postoperative: especially aortic valve replacement.

Complex complete heart block.

Complex congenital heart disease.

Infection: aortic valve endocarditis with root abscess, diphtheria, Lyme disease, rheumatic fever.

Multisystem disease: sarcoidosis, amyloidosis, ankylosing spondylitis, Reiter's syndrome, rheumatoid arthritis, scleroderma, SLE.

Muscular dystrophy, myotonic dystrophy, Refsum's disease.

Epidemiology

- >200 000 permanent pacemakers are implanted worldwide each year; most of these are for heart block.

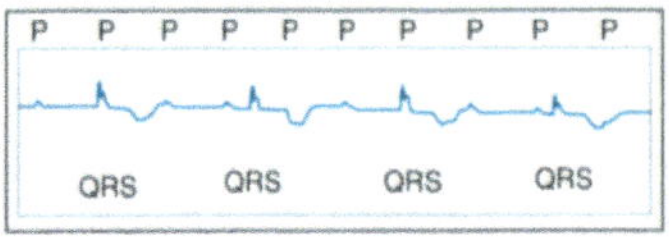

Rhythm strip of ECG for complete heart block demonstrating complete dissociation between P waves and QRS complexes and slow ventricular escape rhythm of 32 beats/min.

Treatment

Diet and lifestyle

• Patients should lead a normal life after heart block has been treated.

• Permanent pacemaker implantation places certain restrictions on patients, *e.g.*, avoidance of contact sports that might damage the device or lead.

Pharmacological treatment

• Atropine (0.5–1 mg i.v. bolus) and isoproterenol (200 μg i.v. bolus or 0.5–10 μg/min infusion) may be used as temporary measures before temporary or permanent pacemaker implantation or when heart block requires treatment during resuscitation; external temporary pacing should also be considered in such circumstances.

Nonpharmacological treatment

• The management of heart block is determined by the severity of symptoms, the degree of correlation between symptoms and confirmed bradycardia, and the presence of potentially reversible causes.

• In asymptomatic patients, the American College of Cardiology/American Heart Association guidelines for implantation of pacemakers in asymptomatic patients include: third-degree atrioventricular block with documented asystole lasting ≥3 seconds (in sinus rhythm) or escape rates F 40 beats/min in patients while awake.

Treatment aims

To return patient to a full and active life.

Prognosis

• Implantation of a permanent pacemaker dramatically improves the prognosis of patients with complete heart block.

Follow-up and management

• Patients with first-degree or second-degree Mobitz type I heart block should be observed carefully to check for development of higher-grade atrioventricular block.

• Patients with permanent pacemaker need regular follow-up in a pacemaker clinic to ensure continued normal function of the device.

• Permanent pacemakers must be changed every 7–10 years.

General reference

Mangrum JM, DiMarco JP: The evaluation and management of bradycardia. *N Engl J Med* 2000, **342**:703–709.

Diagnosis

Definition

• Hemolytic uremic syndrome (HUS) is a syndrome, not a disease; it is defined by the following:

Acute renal insufficiency.

Microangiopathic hemolytic anemia.

Thrombocytopenia.

• Thrombotic thrombocytopenic purpura (TTP) is closely related and often indistinguishable from HUS; the term should be reserved for the following:

A relapsing form of HUS.

Associated fever and fluctuating CNS signs.

• Both HUS and TTP are associated with normal clotting times. Thrombocytopenia and a microangiopathic hemolytic anemia with prolonged clotting times indicate septicemia and disseminated intravascular coagulation.

Symptoms

Malaise, nausea, tiredness: nonspecific symptoms of renal insufficiency.

Oliguria, discolored urine, difficulty concentrating, other subtle CNS changes.

Abdominal cramps; watery diarrhea, then bloody diarrhea; fever <38°C: indicating infection by *Escherichia coli*.

Signs

Pallor: from anemia.

Yellow tinge: occasionally, from the hemolysis.

Purpura, petechia, or prolonged bleeding: if thrombocytopenia is severe.

Investigations

Complete blood count: thrombocytopenia; schistocytes seen on film.

Clotting times: prothrombin time and partial thromboplastin time typically normal.

Biochemistry: raised urea, creatinine, and urate concentrations, hyponatremia, hypoalbuminemia in severely ill patients.

Renal biopsy: usually not needed in children; contraindicated during severe thrombocytopenia; may show glomerular and arteriolar thrombosis, acute tubular necrosis, intimal proliferation of preglomerular arterioles and small arteries, varying degrees of glomerular endothelial injury.

Stool culture for *E. coli* O157:H7 and isolation of verotoxin: can confirm diagnosis in patients with associated diarrhea.

Serology: for neutralizing antibodies to *E. coli* O157:H7.

Hemolysis studies: increased lactate dehydrogenase, increased free hemoglobin, decreased serum haptoglobin.

Complications

Bloody diarrhea, gut infarction, rectal prolapse: in patients with associated diarrhea.

Severe malignant hypertension, cardiomyopathy: in patients without diarrhea.

Irritability, restlessness, twitching, generalized or focal seizures, transient visual disturbance, drowsiness, cerebellar ataxia, reduced level of consciousness, decerebrate spasms, coma.

Differential diagnosis

Septicemia associated with disseminated intravascular coagulation

Gram-negative bacilli.

Infection by *Staphylococcus aureus*, *Pneumococcus* spp., or *Meningococcus* spp.

Psittacosis.

Mycoplasma.

Viral and other diseases: thrombocytopenia without hemolysis

Hantavirus infection.

Dengue hemorrhagic fever.

Malaria.

Leptospirosis.

Snake bite.

Associated with pregnancy (associated with disseminated intravascular coagulation)

Septic abortion.

Amniotic fluid embolus.

Prolonged intrauterine fetal death.

Antepartum hemorrhage.

Other medical conditions

Organ and bone-marrow transplantation.

Scleroderma crisis.

Delayed postpartum or contraceptive pill–associated HUS.

Mytomycin-C cancer chemotherapy.

Etiology

Infectious causes

E. coli associated with diarrhea (in most patients): infection acquired from contaminated beef or dairy products.

Shigella spp.

HIV.

Sporadic, noninfectious causes

Idiopathic or familial disorders, drugs (mitomycin, cyclosporine), tumors, pregnancy, SLE, transplantation, scleroderma, malignant or accelerated hypertension.

Epidemiology

• Patients with diarrhea-associated HUS are usually aged <5 or >65 years.

Treatment

Diet and lifestyle

• No special precautions are necessary.

Pharmacological treatment

Intravenous saline solution and furosemide: to correct circulating volume and reverse prerenal failure and to establish diuresis.

Antiplatelet drugs (*e.g.*, aspirin, dipyridamole): have a logic but no proven benefit.

Prostacyclin infusions: of theoretical value and useful to control hypertension.

Nonpharmacological treatment

Red blood cell transfusion: for anemia.

Hemodialysis: when indicated, *i.e.*, for volume overload, hyperkalemia, "uremia," acidosis.

The utility of fresh frozen plasma and/or plasmapheresis is not predictably clear.

Infusions of fresh frozen plasma: may induce remission; amount necessary not known but probably 1–2 L daily; mechanism of benefit not known but may include neutralizing toxins, restoring antioxidant activity, and inducing prostacyclin synthesis; infusions should be continued until erythrocyte fragmentation ceases and platelet count rises ~100×10^9/L.

Plasma exchange: typically used to create intravascular space for repeated infusions of fresh frozen plasma, and may be of benefit by removing humoral factors. Treatment course is typically 6–12 exchanges, the total number depending on response to therapy, *i.e.*, increasing platelet count, decreasing LDH.

Treatment aims

To establish diuresis if possible.

To provide dialysis if necessary.

To control blood pressure.

To try to induce hematological remission.

To prevent seizures.

Prognosis

• The natural history of HUS, when preceded by a diarrheal illness and associated with glomerular thrombi, is one of spontaneous recovery, although patients may have some residual injury; most children are in this category.

• Idiopathic patients, particularly adults, often have major preglomerular vascular disease and irreversible renal failure.

• 3%–25% of patients die during the acute illness (usually from CNS involvement); 10%–20% remain dependent on dialysis; 10% have long-term neurological sequelae; 70% recover with no residual evidence of renal disease.

Follow-up and management

Recovery of renal function and disappearance of proteinuria.

Long-term follow-up if persistent renal insufficiency.

• Blood pressure should be controlled by ACE inhibitors.

General references

Conlon PJ, Howell DN, Macik G, *et al.*: The renal manifestations and outcome of thrombotic thrombocytopenic purpura/hemolytic uremic syndrome in adults. *Nephrol Dial Transplant* 1995, **10**:1189–1193.

Gordjani N, Sutor AH: Coagulation changes associated with the hemolytic uremic syndrome. *Semin Thrombos Hemost* 1998, **24**:577–582.

Kaplan BS, Meyers KE, Schulman SL: The pathogenesis and treatment of hemolytic uremic syndrome. *J Am Soc Nephrol* 1998, 1126–1133.5

Ruggenenti P, Lutz J, Remuzzi G: Pathogenesis and treatment of thrombotic microangiopathy. *Kidney Int Suppl* 1997, **58**:S97–S101.

Siegler RL: The hemolytic uremic syndrome. *Pediatr Clin North Am* 1995, **42**:1505–1529.

Siegler RL, Pavia AT, Cook JB: Hemolytic-uremic syndrome in adolescents. *Arch Pediatr Adolesc Med* 1997, **151**:165–169.

Hemophilia & von Willebrand's disease

Diagnosis

Symptoms

Hemophilia

Episodic spontaneous hemorrhage: into joints and muscles.

Deep-tissue hematoma: particularly after trauma or surgery.

Von Willebrand's disease

Bruising.

Epistaxis and melena.

Excessive bleeding after dental extraction or surgery.

Postpartum bleeding, rarely hemarthroses and muscle hematomas.

Signs

Hemophilia

Acute: hot, swollen, painful joint; unexpected bleeding after surgery.

Chronic: crippling joint deformity.

Investigations

Hemophilia

Activated partial thromboplastin time measurement: prolonged.

Hemophilia A, factor VIII; hemophilia B, factor IX; and hemophilia C, factor XI assays: all three show low values.

Coagulation factor activity measurement: correlated with disease severity in hemophilia A and B (normal range, 50–150 U/dL):
<2 U/dL indicates severe disease, manifest as frequent spontaneous bleeding episodes, joint deformity, and crippling;
2–5 U/dL indicates moderate disease, manifest as posttraumatic bleeding, occasional spontaneous episodes;
5–20 U/dL indicates mild disease, manifest as posttraumatic bleeding.

Von Willebrand's disease [1]

Bleeding time measurement: prolonged.

Factor VIII clotting activity, von Willebrand factor antigen and activity measurement: low values.

Platelet function tests: reduced aggregation of platelets with ristocetin.

• Von Willebrand's disease is classified on the basis of the type of protein abnormality; this is important for deciding treatment.

Complications

Transfusion-transmitted disease

Hepatitis A: has been a problem with a solvent detergent sterilized product; all patients with bleeding disorders should be vaccinated.

Hepatitis B: although all blood donors are tested for this, sterilization processes for clotting factor concentrate cannot be regarded as 100% safe; vaccination mandatory in patients with bleeding disorders [2].

Hepatitis C: all patients treated by unsterilized clotting factor concentrates have been infected (sterilization introduced in 1985); some patients progress to chronic liver disease; treatment by interferon may normalize transaminases; HIV co-infection results in faster progression of hepatitis C liver disease [2].

HIV infection: occurred in patients receiving concentrates between 1979 and 1985 [3,4].

Inhibitors

Neutralizing antibodies: occurring after infusion of concentrates.

Chronic arthropathy

Chronic disabling arthritis: caused by recurrent hemarthroses.

Differential diagnosis

Other clotting factor deficiencies or platelet function disorders.

Etiology

Causes of hemophilia

Quantitative deficiency of clotting factors.

Factor VIII: hemophilia A (most common).

Factor IX: hemophilia B.

Factor XI: hemophilia C.

Causes of von Willebrand's disease

Quantitative or qualitative deficiency of von Willebrand factor, important in primary platelet hemostasis, acting as an adhesive protein and a carrier protein for factor VIII.

Genetics

Hemophilia A and B: X-linked (men affected, but some women carriers may need concentrate for surgery or trauma).

Von Willebrand's disease: autosomal-dominant.

Hemophilia C (severe disease): autosomal-recessive or compound heterozygote.

Epidemiology

• 1 in 5000 men is affected by hemophilia A or B; 1 in 6 patients with hemophilia has hemophilia B.

• Hemophilia C is common in Ashkenazi Jews; it may occur in any ethnic group.

• Von Willebrand's disease is the most common inherited bleeding disorder if all grades of severity are considered; clinically significant disease occurs in ~125 in 1 million population.

Carrier detection and antenatal diagnosis [5]

• Carrier status and presence of the disorders in fetuses can be detected by the following:

Restriction fragment length polymorphisms.

Variable-number repeat sequences.

Direct mutational analysis.

Chorionic villus sampling before 10 weeks (for carriers with a molecular marker).

Fetal sexing and choriocentesis (for carriers without a molecular marker).

Treatment

Diet and lifestyle

• Patients should avoid contact sports, but regular exercise, *e.g.*, swimming, should be encouraged.

Pharmacological treatment

• Intramuscular injections must be avoided in patients with bleeding disorders.

• Aspirin or NSAIDs that impair platelet function must also be avoided.

Indications

For hemophilia A: factor VIII concentrate or DDAVP (desmopressin).

For hemophilia B: factor IX concentrate.

For hemophilia C: factor XI concentrate or fresh frozen plasma [6].

For von Willebrand's disease: factor VIII concentrate rich in von Willebrand's factor or DDAVP, depending on the type of von Willebrand's disease.

Clotting factor preparations [7]

Recombinant: Recombinate (VIII), Kogenate (VIII), Benefix (IX).

Extracted by immunoaffinity chromatography: Hemofil M (VIII), Antihemophilic factor (American Red Cross) Monoclate P (VIII), Mononine (IX), Humate P (von Willebrand's factor).

Extracted by conventional separation: *very high purity (>100 U/mg):* Alphanine (IX) SD; *intermediate purity (<50 U/mg):* Humate P (von Willebrand's factor) (VIII).

• The units of clotting factor needed, x, can be calculated by the following equation:
$x = [\text{rise in clotting factor required } (\%) \times \text{weight (kg)}] \div K$
where K = 1.5 for factor VIII, 1 for factor IX, and 2 for factor XI.

• Approximate levels for hemostasis are as follows:

15–20 U clotting factor/dL plasma for minor spontaneous hemarthroses and hematomas.

20–40 U clotting factor/dL plasma for severe hemarthroses and muscle hematomas, minor surgery.

80–100 U clotting factor/dL plasma for major surgery or intracranial/intra-abdominal hemorrhage.

DDAVP

• DDAVP releases von Willebrand's factor from endothelial cells.

• It is used to raise endogenous factor VIII von Willebrand's levels during minor procedures in patients with mild hemophilia and von Willebrand's disease.

• It is not indicated for severe hemophilia or type III form of von Willebrand's disease.

Standard dosage	DDAVP, 0.3 µg/kg in 100 mL normal saline solution i.v. infusion over 20 minutes.
Contraindications	Vascular disease, type II B von Willebrand's disease [8].
Special points	Response should be monitored using factor assays.
Main drug interactions	None.
Main side effects	Hyponatremia and seizures (in children aged <2 years), coronary occlusion (in patients aged >60 years).

Tranexamic acid and aminocaproic acid

• Tranexamic acid and aminocaproic acid, an inhibitor of fibrinolysis, reduces blood loss, particularly in mucosal bleeding, *e.g.*, oral surgery, epistaxis, and tonsillectomy.

Standard dosage	Tranexamic acid, 1 g orally or i.v. 3–4 times daily; in children, 25 mg/kg 3 times daily. Aminocaproic acid, 5–30 g in divided doses every 3–6 hours for 5–7 days.
Contraindications	*Tranexamic acid and aminocaproic acid:* hematuria, risk of "clot colic."
Special points	*Tranexamic acid and aminocaproic acid:* dose should be reduced in patients with renal impairment.
Main drug interactions	None.
Main side effects	*Tranexamic acid and aminocaproic acid:* nausea, dizziness.

Treatment aims

To prevent spontaneous bleeds and to make surgery safe.

Prognosis

• With the advent of virally safe blood products and home-treatment programs, many severely hemophilic patients can lead a relatively normal life.

• Mild disease, whether hemophilia or von Willebrand's disease, may impinge little unless an injury occurs or surgery is planned.

Follow-up and management

• All patients with bleeding disorders should be registered and regularly reviewed at a designated hemophilia center; regular review and access to treatment are of paramount importance for the successful long-term management of these patients.

Key references

1. Nichols WC, Ginsburg D: von Willebrand disease. *Medicine* 1997, **76**:1–20.
2. Lee CA, Dusheiko G: Hepatitis and hemophilia. In *Viral Hepatitis*. Edited by Zuckerman AJ, Thomas HC, New York: Churchill Livingstone; 1993.
3. Goerdert JJ, *et al.*: A prospective study of human immunodeficiency virus type I infection and the development of AIDS in subjects with hemophilia. *N Engl J Med* 1989, **321**:1141–1148.
4. Lee CA, *et al.*: Progression of HIV disease in a hemophilic cohort followed for 11 years and the effect of treatment. *BMJ* 1991, **303**:1093–1094.
5. Peake I: Molecular genetics and counselling in haemophilia. *Thromb Haemost* 1995, **74**:40–44.
6. Bolton-Maggs PHB, *et al.*: Production and therapeutic use of a factor XI concentrate from plasma. *Thromb Haemost* 1992, **67**:314–319.
7. DiMichele D, Neufeld EJ: Hemophilia: a new approach to an old disease. *Hematol Oncol Clin North Am* 1998, **12**:1315–1344.
8. Holmberg L, Nilsson IM, Borge L, *et al.*: Platelet aggregation induced by 1-desamino-8-D-arginine vasopressin (DDAVP) in type IIB von Willebrand's disease. *N Eng J Med* 1983, **309**:816–821.

Diagnosis

Symptoms

Painless bleeding: blood typically on surface of stool or toilet paper from an otherwise normal bowel movement; occult blood loss should never be attributed to hemorrhoids without excluding more serious diseases (*see* Differential diagnosis).

Protruding tissue following defecation.

Perianal irritation, pruritis.

Acute, severe perianal pain: suggests acute thrombosis or strangulation.

Signs

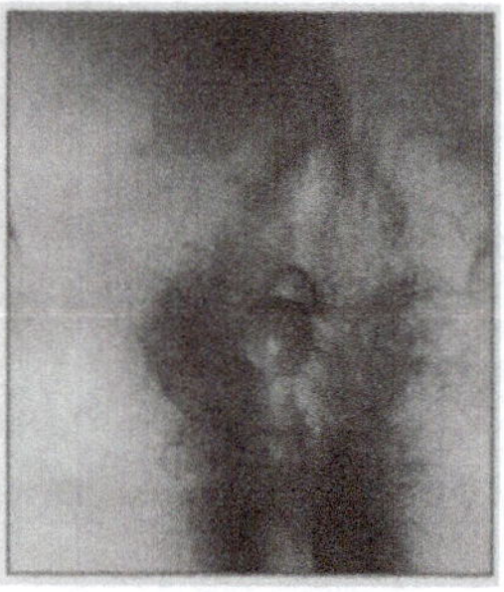

An acutely thrombosed external hemorrhoid. (*See* Color Plate.)

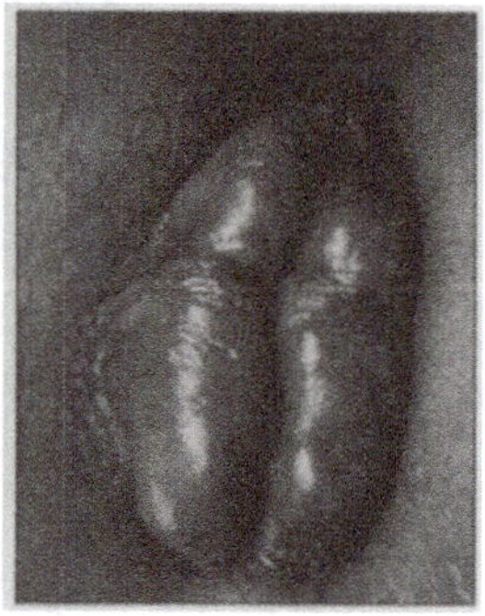

Acutely prolapsed large, bilateral external and internal (mixed) hemorrhoids. (*See* Color Plate.)

Internal hemorrhoids: visible and occasionally palpable hemorrhoidal plexus above the dentate line (seen best with an anoscope).

External hemorrhoids: palpable venous engorgement below the dentate line, covered by squamous epithelium; exquisitely tender when thrombosed, which eventually results in small, benign-appearing external skin tags.

Perianal inflammation: attributed to compromised hygiene because of redundant tissue.

Investigations

Anoscopy: should be performed to assess the nature and severity of hemorrhoids, although patients with acute thrombosis or strangulation will not be able to tolerate this procedure because of extreme tenderness.

Sigmoidoscopy: required to exclude other competing diagnoses, *e.g.*, malignancy; visualization of the entire colon by colonoscopy or air-contrast barium enema should also be performed in patients >45 years of age, patients with a family history of colonic malignancy, and patients who do not respond to conservative therapy.

Complications

Thrombosis resulting in severe pain.

Strangulation of internal hemorrhoids with possible gangrene and life-threatening infection: rare.

Differential diagnosis

Proctocolonic neoplasia (polyp or cancer).
Perianal abscess or fistula.
Anal fissure.
Pilonidal disease.
Proctocolitis.
Condyloma acuminata.
Rectal varices.
Rectal prolapse.
Pruritis ani.

Etiology

Enlargement of vascularized anal cushions with redundant perianal tissue in patients with altered pelvic venous pressures that may occur with the excessive straining that accompanies constipation or pregnancy.

Epidemiology

- Prevalence in the United States has been estimated as high as 50%.

Treatment

Diet and lifestyle

- Patients should be placed on a high-fiber diet.
- Patients should avoid excessive straining during defecation.
- Sitz baths will reduce pain of acute thrombosis.

Pharmacological treatment [1]

- Stool softening agents (*e.g.*, synthetic mucilloids or psyllium preparations) should be titrated at a dose that will minimize straining and achieve 1–2 soft bowel movements each day. A typical starting dose consists of one heaping tablespoon in 8 oz of water once or twice each day. The patient should be instructed to drink the preparation immediately after mixing. A few days of increased flatus or bloating is commonly experienced at the start of therapy.
- Topical emollients with local anesthetics (*e.g.*, benzocaine, witch hazel) may be used to relieve symptoms but do not contribute to a reduction in the hemorrhoids or control of bleeding. Preparations containing a topical steroid (*e.g.*, 1% hydrocortisone) are efficacious in reducing the symptoms of perianal inflammation. Patients should be instructed to apply these preparations locally twice daily as needed for symptom control.

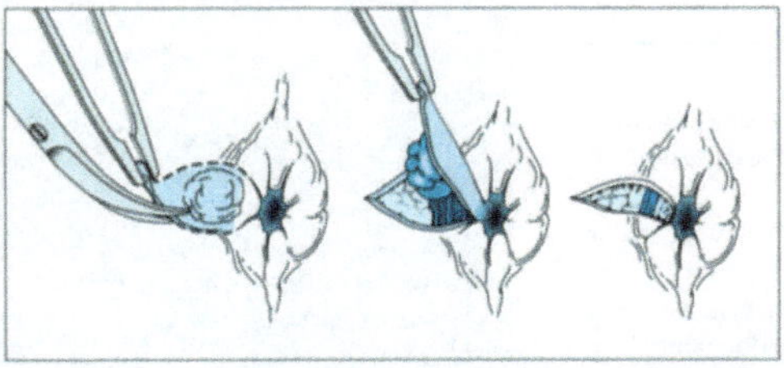

An elliptic incision is used to repair a thrombosed external hemorrhoid.

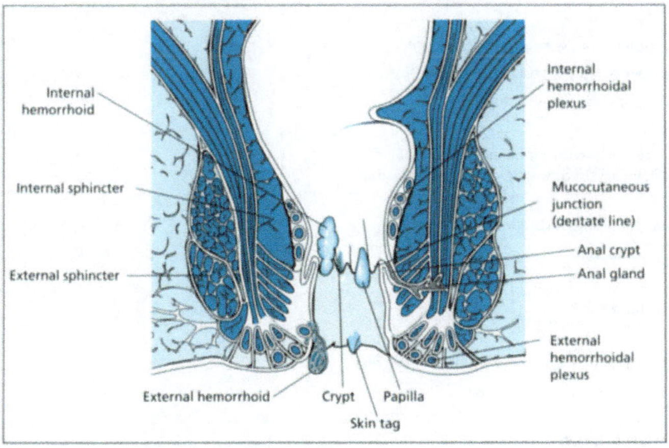

Anal anatomy with external and internal hemorrhoids.

Treatment aims

To reduce pain, bleeding, and perianal inflammation.

Other treatment options [2]

- Rubber band ligation is perhaps the most popular treatment for symptomatic internal hemorrhoids, although injection sclerotherapy, cryosurgery, electro-coagulation, or laser obliteration are alternatives; the innervation of the covering squamous epithelium prevents the use of these modalities in the management of external hemorrhoids.
- The acute pain of a thrombosed external hemorrhoid may be managed with injection of local anesthesia and a limited decompression if performed within the first 48 hours of symptoms. It is often difficult to evacuate the hematoma and achieve optimal control of bleeding after this time period. Surgical therapy of internal hemorrhoids is usually reserved for persistent symptoms despite the use of the conservative approaches noted previously or strangulation.

Prognosis

- Hemorrhoidal disease can be a nuisance but rarely has a significant effect on an individual's health.
- The presence of palpable or visual hemorrhoids alone is not an indication for treatment and is not predictive of future symptoms.

Follow-up and management

- Routine follow-up of hemorrhoidal disease is not typically required; the nature of the patient's symptoms rather than the presence of hemorrhoids should direct the management plan of the physician.

Key references

1. Johnson JF, Rimm A: Optimal nonsurgical treatment of hemorrhoids. *Am J Gastroenterol* 1992, **87**:1601–1605.
2. Barnett JL: Anorectal disease. In *Textbook of Gastroenterology*, edn 2. Edited by Yamada T. Philadelphia: Lippincott Williams & Wilkins; 1999; 2083–2106.

Henoch–Schönlein purpura

Diagnosis

Symptoms

• In most patients, symptoms occur 24–48 hours after infection (usually upper respiratory tract infection) or drug ingestion (antibiotics).

• ~50% of adults develop only the characteristic rash and malaise.

Florid palpable purpuric skin rash: predominantly on lower legs but also on buttocks and arms (cardinal symptom).

Cramping abdominal pains: in 60%–70% of patients.

Joint pains: in 60%–70%.

Blood in urine or stool: in 20%–30%.

Symptoms of intestinal obstruction: due to intussusception, in young children.

Fever and toxicity: if severe.

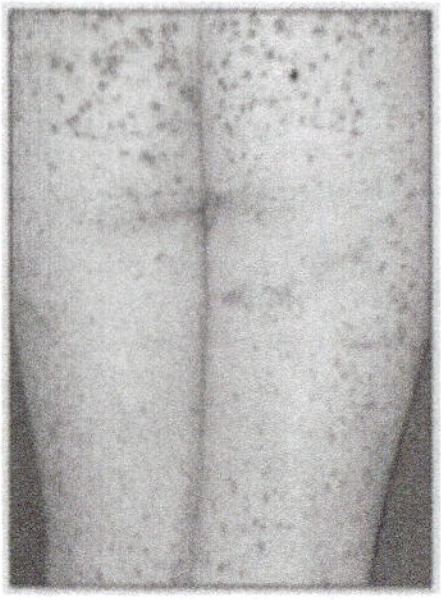

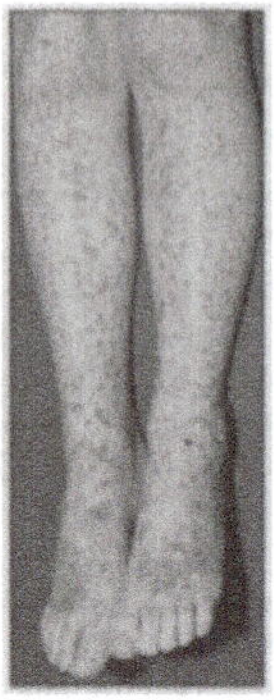

Typical purpuric lesions on buttocks (*left*) and pretibial areas and lower legs (*right*). (*See* Color Plates.)

Signs

Rash: "papular purpura" lesions that do not blanch on pressure, some forming a necrotic center that may vesiculate, usually on buttocks, gluteal cleft, and extremities; usually painless; in adults, may persist or recur for up to 2 months.

Joint involvement: mild to moderate symmetrical arthropathy in 60%–70%; some periarticular swelling; a few patients also have angioedema of hands and feet.

Gut involvement: cramping abdominal pain, and some rebound tenderness in 25%; frank blood in stool in 10%–20%; obstructive symptoms (intussusception) or perforation.

Renal involvement: ~30% of patients develop nephritis.

Investigations

Skin biopsy: may show cutaneous necrotizing venulitis but does not indicate cause.

History: may be positive for recent infective episodes or drug ingestion (antibiotic).

Complete blood count: may show mild polymorphonuclear leukocytosis.

Serology: for recent viral or streptococcal infection.

Stool and urine analysis: regularly during and after rash, with formal microscopy if positive; 30% of patients show evidence of erythrocytes, raised protein concentration, and casts on urinalysis.

Formal renal investigations, including biopsy: if findings indicate renal disease.

Complications

• In children, this condition is often thought of as "harmless."

Secondary infection of vasculitic lesions.

Glomerulonephritis, IgA nephropathy: in ~30% of patients; 15%–20% of these progress to renal failure in 6 months (adults).

Renal failure: in 5%–10% of all patients.

Gastrointestinal or surgical problems: *e.g.*, intussusception or perforation in young children; of the 60%–70% of patients with gastrointestinal complications, a few develop intramural hematomata, associated with intussusception, infarction, or gut perforation; protein-losing enteropathy.

Renal problems: *e.g.*, immunoglobulin nephropathy in older children and adults.

Differential diagnosis

Other forms of vasculitic or purpuric rash (*e.g.*, meningococcal septicemia).

Embolic phenomena from acute or subacute bacterial endocarditis.

Systemic gram-negative sepsis.

Collagen vascular disease, especially polyarteritis nodosa.

Etiology

• Henoch–Schönlein purpura is essentially idiopathic.

• Triggers include the following:

Nonspecific upper respiratory tract infection (in ~33% of patients).

Sulfonamide or penicillin treatment.

Streptococcal infection.

Streptokinase treatment for myocardial infarction.

Epidemiology

• Henoch–Schönlein purpura can occur at any age, but it predominantly affects children.

• It has a seasonal variation, occurring most often in winter months in temperate climates.

Treatment

Diet and lifestyle

• Other than bed rest during the acute phase, no special precautions are necessary.

Pharmacological treatment

• Treatment is symptomatic and does not alter the course or outcome of the condition or its complications.

• Local treatment of the rash, if needed, should be designed to prevent secondary infection, *e.g.*, potassium permanganate soaks.

• Steroids have no effect on renal abnormalities and are associated with a significant incidence of gastrointestinal side effects.

For pain relief

Standard dosage	NSAIDs, *e.g.*, naproxen, 250 mg every 6–8 hours (adults).
Contraindications	Active peptic ulceration.
Special points	Asthma may be exacerbated.
Main drug interactions	Oral anticoagulants.
Main side effects	Gastrointestinal disturbances, discomfort, nausea, or ulceration.

For joint abnormalities

Standard dosage	Corticosteroids, *e.g.*, prednisolone, 40–60 mg daily.
Contraindications	Active peptic ulceration.
Special points	Possible adrenal suppression on sudden withdrawal.
Main drug interactions	NSAIDs, oral anticoagulants.
Main side effects	Cushing's syndrome, growth retardation in children, osteoporosis.

Treatment aims

To prevent secondary infection in vasculitic skin lesions.

To relieve symptoms of joint or abdominal pain.

Other treatments

• Renal replacement therapy may be needed in the 5%–10% of patients who develop renal failure or nephrotic syndrome.

Prognosis

• The prognosis of the rash alone is good.

• Crops of lesions may recur within 4–8 weeks, especially in adults.

• Spontaneous remission is the norm.

• Relapses of the rash alone often occur in adults.

• 15%–20% of adults with IgA nephropathy progress to renal failure in 6 months.

• Generally, 5%–10% of patients develop renal failure; this is most probable in adults or adolescents.

Follow-up and management

• Renal function or urinary sediment must be monitored for evidence of renal involvement.

• If renal involvement is detected, full renal investigation, including biopsy is needed.

General references

Fogazzi GB, *et al.*: Long term outcome of Schönlein Henoch nephritis in the adult. *Clin Nephrol* 1989, **31**:60–66.

Ford EG, Jennings LM, Andrassay RJ: Management of Henoch–Schönlein purpura and polyarteritis nodosum. *Tex Med* 1987, **83**:54–58.

Schreiner DT: Purpura. *Dermatol Clin* 1989, **7**:481–490.

Szer IS: Henoch-Schönlein purpura: when and how to treat. *J Rheumatol* 1996, **23**:1661–1665.

Hepatic encephalopathy

Diagnosis

Definition

• Hepatic encephalopathy is a reversible neuropsychiatric syndrome that is a complication of fulminant or chronic liver disease [1].

• Hepatic encephalopathy may also be present in the rare cases of urea-cycle enzyme defects and portosystemic shunting in the absence of liver disease.

• Latent encephalopathy is a subclinical form occurring in chronic liver disease, only detected by psychometric testing.

Symptoms

• Wide differences are seen in presentation and evolution (*see* Classification).

Inversion of normal sleep pattern.

Deterioration of intellectual function: forgetfulness, disorientation, coma.

Slurred speech.

Tremor: absent at rest.

Personality changes: features of frontal-lobe syndrome, agitation, irritability.

Symptoms of precipitating causes: *e.g.*, infection or gastrointestinal bleeding.

Signs

• Patients with impaired consciousness have intact pupillary reflexes.

Asterixis.

Fetor hepaticus.

Constructional apraxia.

Brisk tendon reflexes: except in coma.

Increased muscle tone and rigidity.

Hyperventilation in deep coma.

Signs of precipitating causes: *e.g.*, spontaneous bacterial peritonitis.

Investigations

• No single measure confirms the diagnosis.

• The underlying liver disease or its complications must be identified.

• A precipitant cause (*e.g.*, metabolic abnormalities, bleeding, dehydration) must always be sought.

• A careful evaluation for infection is warranted, including paracentesis, if ascites is present.

Psychometric testing: essential to detect subclinical encephalopathy; number connection test (Reitan trail) [3] and drawing a clock face easiest to perform; patient is timed for task completion. This measurement serves as a benchmark for disease progression or treatment response.

EEG: slowing of normal frequency to severe slowing; characteristic triphasic waves; (5 cycles/sec) changes appearing first in frontal regions, delta activity with coma.

CT of head: to exclude subdural hematomas and other intracranial diseases; some atrophy of brain usually manifest, particularly in chronic encephalopathy.

Blood ammonia measurement: concentration usually raised, but false-positive and false-negative results may occur. As such, blood ammonia is of little clinical utility in the evaluation of management of these patients.

Complications

Increase in intracranial pressure: in patients with fulminant liver failure; due to cerebral edema, which can lead to brain death.

Complications of coma: *e.g.*, aspiration in patients with encephalopathy.

Structural neuronal damage: with demyelination and a spastic paraplegia, in patients with chronic encephalopathy (rare); chronic cerebellar or basal ganglia signs may also be present with Parkinsonian features.

Focal seizures: rare, other causes must be sought.

Differential diagnosis

Alcohol withdrawal syndrome.

Wernicke's encephalopathy.

Chronic subdural hematoma or other space-occupying lesion.

Other causes of metabolic coma.

Postictal state.

Meningitis, encephalitis.

Etiology

• Precipitant causes include the following:

1. Infection.
2. Dehydration; hypoxia.
3. Diarrhea and vomiting.
4. Gastrointestinal bleeding.
5. Azotenia; electrolyte abnormalities.
6. Dietary indiscretion (protein excess).
7. Acute worsening of chronic liver disease.
8. Sedative and opiate drugs.
9. Uncontrolled diabetes or hypoglycemia.
10. Surgery; portosystemic shunts.

Epidemiology

• Chronic liver disease is usually progressive, so that most patients develop hepatic encephalopathy at some time, particularly secondary to a precipitant cause.

• Intermittent encephalopathy is the most common pattern.

Classification

Mental status

Grade 1	Mild confusion Slowness in mentation Slurred speech Euphoria
Grade II	Increased confusion Disoriented to time Lethargy
Grade III	Somnolent but arousable Marked confusion Incoherent speech
Grade IV	Coma

Signs

None	Ataxia
Mild apraxia	Asterixis
Impaired handwriting	Babinski's sign
	Clonus
Brisk reflexes	Absent reflexes
Increased tone	Decerebrate
Asterixis	

Treatment

Diet and lifestyle

• Careful attention must be paid to adequate nutrition with a daily protien intake of 0.8–1.0 g/kg.

• Protein restriction (*e.g.*, <30 g/day) is required in only a subset of patients with encephalopathy that is difficult to control pharmacologically.

• The early warning signs of encephalopathy must be explained to patients and their families so that early medical attention can be obtained.

Pharmacological treatment

• Encephalopathy typically resolves when the precipitating cause is corrected [2].

For acute encephalopathy in chronic liver disease

Lactose or sorbitol administered by nasogastric tube or enema.

Correction of electrolyte abnormalities.

Intravenous thiamine in alcoholics (*e.g.*, 100 mg daily for 3 days).

Long-term treatment

Standard dosage	Lactulose or sorbitol, 30 mL 4 times daily initially and titrated to produce two to four soft bowel movements daily.
Contraindications	Known hypersensitivity.
Special points	Electrolyte abnormalities and dehydration must be avoided.
Main drug interactions	None known.
Main side effects	Abdominal bloating, flatulence.

• Oral nonabsorbable antibiotics (*e.g.*, neomycin) may be considered for patients refractory to treatment with lactulose or sorbitol.

Encephalopathy of fulminant liver failure

Correction of hypoglycemia: 20% dextrose i.v.

Correction of electrolyte abnormalities.

Bowel decontamination: oral antibacterial agents (*e.g.*, neomycin, 1 g orally every 4 to 6 hours; watch renal function carefully).

Early treatment of infection.

Treatment aims

To correct or remove precipitating cause.

To prevent recurrence.

Other treatments

Refashioning, embolization, or ligation of surgical shunt (if present).

Liver transplantation: for recurrent acute or chronic encephalopathy, and fulminant liver failure with adverse prognostic factors.

Prognosis

• Prognosis is determined by the underlying liver disease and avoidance of precipitating factors.

Follow-up and management

• Follow-up depends on the severity of the underlying liver disease, but clinic visits every 1–3 months are common; patients usually should keep a 3-monthly diary and stool chart.

• Family members must be educated as to the early signs and symptoms so that prompt medical attention may be obtained.

Key references

1. Riordan SM, Williams R: Treatment of hepatic encephalopathy . *N Engl J Med* 1997, **337**:473–479.
2. Butterworth RF: Pathogenesis and treatment of portal-systemic encephalopathy. *Dig Dis Sci* 1992, **37**:321–327.
3. Conn HO: The trailmaking and number connection tests in the assessment of mental state in portal systemic encephalopathy. *Am J Dig Dis* 1977, **22**:541–550.

Hepatitis, acute viral

Diagnosis

Symptoms

• Acute hepatitis is often asymptomatic (hepatitis C is typically asymptomatic).

• Symptoms, when present, may include malaise, headaches, myalgias, arthralgias, anorexia, nausea, right upper quadrant discomfort, fever, jaundice, pruritis, dark urine, acholic stools.

• Children <2 years of age rarely develop symptoms with hepatitis A virus (HAV) or hepatitis B virus (HBV) infection, but most adults who become infected develop symptoms [1].

Signs

• Signs are usually absent but may include the following:

Jaundice, right upper quadrant tenderness, hepatomegaly.

Hepatic encephalopathy, asterixis, fetor hepaticus: rare, associated with acute hepatic failure.

Skin rash secondary to leukocytoclastic vasculitis: less common symptoms.

Investigations [2]

Biochemical assays: should confirm hepatitis, with elevated serum transaminases, mild increase in alkaline phosphatase, variable increase in bilirubin; as disease progresses, cholestatic picture may evolve before recovery.

Complete blood count or blood film: not usually helpful; features consistent with hypersplenism, however, suggest underlying chronic liver disease.

Prothrombin time: If elevated, fulminant hepatic failure should be watched for; underlying chronic liver disease should be considered.

Virology tests: should be ordered on the basis of probable cause.
Hepatitis A: check for IgM antibody (indicates acute infection; IgG antibody present for life and suggests previous infection) [3].
Hepatitis B: check for IgM anticore antibody (develops early in illness) and surface antigen (present in most symptomatic patients but may be eliminated quickly) [4]. Anti-hepatitis b surface antigen suggests previous infection or vaccination.
Hepatitis C: antibody may take several months to convert, although most patients become positive within 2 months (hepatitis C virus RNA using polymerase chain reaction is positive early in the infection) [5].
Hepatitis D: presence of anti-hepatitis D virus antibody indicates infection: as coinfection with acute hepatitis B infection or as a superinfection in a chronic carrier of HBV.
Hepatitis E: can be sought by enzyme-linked immunosorbent assay (very rare) [6].
Cytomegalovirus and Epstein-Barr virus: should be sought when viral cause suspected and the results of other serological tests are negative.
Hepatitis G: probably does not cause clinical disease and should not be tested for at this time.

Liver biopsy: may be indicated in rare circumstances when diagnostic confusion exists or when underlying liver damage is suspected.

Complications

Fulminant liver failure: in 1%–5% of cases.

Progression to chronic hepatitis: may occur with hepatitis B (~10%), hepatitis C (50%–70%); chronic infection never occurs in hepatitis A.

Anemia.

Aplastic anemia, vasculitis, cryoglobulinemia: rarely, in cases of hepatitis B or C.

Arthritis.

Renal disease.

Differential diagnosis

Gall stone disease.

Budd-Chiari syndrome.

Alcoholic liver disease.

Nonalcoholic steatohepatitis.

Hepatic cancer.

Acute manifestations of chronic liver disease.

• Autoimmune hepatitis, Wilson's disease, hemochromatosis, a1-antitrypsin deficiency.

Etiology and epidemiology

HAV: transmitted by fecal-oral route; infection associated with foreign travel, consumption of shellfish, and some sexual practices; often, no source identified.

HBV: often transmitted sexually; vertical transmission (maternal-perinatal) also important; i.v. drug users at risk; no identifiable risk factors in 50%.

Hepatitis C virus: associated with i.v. drug use and transfusion; less effectively transmitted vertically or sexually compared to hepatitis B; no identifiable risk factor in 50%.

Hepatitis D virus: hepatitis D transmitted predominantly by i.v. drug use, occurs only in patients with concomitant hepatitis B infection.

Hepatitis E virus: transmitted by fecal-oral route in developing countries (in epidemics, pregnant women most vulnerable).

Epstein-Barr virus, cytomegalovirus (particularly in immunosuppressed patients).

Treatment

Diet and lifestyle

• Abstinence from alcohol until recovery should be recommended.

• Excessive amounts of acetaminophen (>4 g/day) should be avoided.

• Rest is recommended; many patients are unable to return to work for weeks or months and, even after return, may need time before normal function fully returns.

• Patients must understand the routes by which the hepatitis infection has been acquired and may therefore be transmitted; this may place certain restrictions on professional or sexual activities in the short term.

• Avoid hospitalization (unless patient is progressing to hepatic failure with increasingly prolonged prothrombin time, has altered mental status, requires intravenous hydration, or develops a superimposed bacterial infection).

Pharmacological treatment

• The onset of jaundice is often associated with loss or significant reduction of infectivity in patients with hepatitis A and B; no specific treatment is available for acute viral hepatitis.

• Symptoms may be alleviated in patients with prolonged cholestasis by use of ursodeoxycholic acid, 600 mg at night.

• For HAV, an effective vaccine is available for protective immunization; immunoglobulin has a well-defined role in short-term prophylaxis and for household contacts of patients with acute hepatitis. (*See* Appendix C.)

• For HBV, an effective vaccine is available; vaccination soon after exposure may still be effective; hepatitis B immunoglobulin is given with vaccination to infants born of mothers who are hepatitis B surface antigen–positive and for postexposure prophylaxis. (*See* Appendix C.)

• Acute hepatitis C infection is rarely diagnosed. Given the high rate of chronic hepatitis C infection and its uncertain prognosis, interferon, 3 MU 3 times a week, should be considered in acute infection.

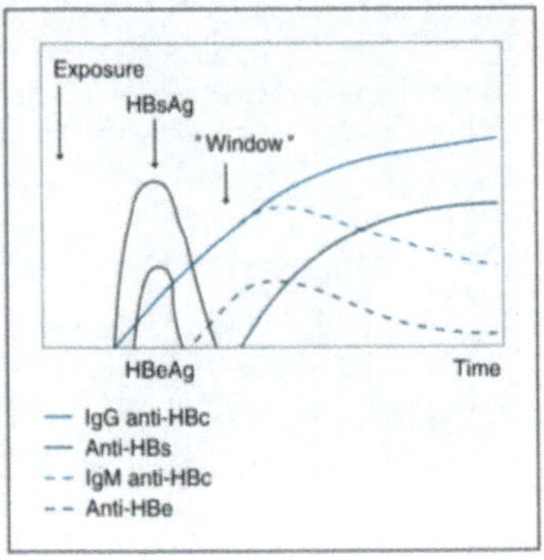

Serological diagnosis of acute hepatitis B (HB) infection. HBeAg, HBe antigen; HBsAg, HB surface antigen.

Treatment aims

To palliate symptoms.

To observe for progression to fulminant hepatic failure.

Prognosis

• Acute hepatitis is often a debilitating illness, but recovery is usual, although patients may experience fatigue for several months before full recovery.

• Over 40% of patients infected by hepatitis C virus and ~10% infected by hepatitis B become carriers; for the latter, chronic infection is less common after a severe, acute illness.

• The immediate prognosis for patients with hepatitis C who become carriers is excellent; chronic liver disease often develops, however.

Follow-up and management

• Patients with acute hepatitis A, B, or E should be followed until the liver function tests have returned to normal.

• Patients with hepatitis B should also be followed until hepatitis B surface antigen is eliminated; persistence of hepatitis Be antigen beyond 6 weeks suggests that a carrier state may be evolving.

• For hepatitis D, the prognosis depends ultimately on the outcome of the hepatitis B infection; a patient who remains hepatitis B surface antigen–positive may develop chronic liver disease.

• In the present state of uncertainty about the prognosis of patients with hepatitis C, they should be followed every 6–12 months unless evidence for persistent hepatitis C is lacking, *i.e.*, disappearance of hepatitis C virus antibody or RNA.

Key references

1. Lieberman JM: Hepatitis A and B vaccines in children. *J Pediatr Infect Dis* 1996, **11**:333–363.
2. Sjogren MH: Serologic diagnosis of viral hepatitis. *Med Clin North Am* 1996, **80**:856–929.
3. Ross BL, *et al.*: Hepatitis A virus and hepatitis A infection. *Ad Virus Res* 1991, **39**:209–257.
4. Brown JL, *et al.*: The hepatitis B virus. *Baillières Clin Gastroenterol* 1990, **4**:721–747.
5. Sharara AI: Hepatitis C. *Ann Intern Med* 1996, **125**:658–668.
6. Krawczynski K: Hepatitis E. *Hepatology* 1993, **17**:932–941.

Hepatitis, chronic

Diagnosis

Symptoms

• Most patients with chronic hepatitis are asymptomatic.

Fatigue, malaise: most common symptoms.

Gastrointestinal bleeding, altered mental status, abdominal pain or distention: in patients with long-standing chronic hepatitis who progress to end-stage liver disease.

Signs

• If signs are present, they usually indicate advanced liver disease.

Muscle wasting, ascites, palmar erythema, Dupuytren's contracture.

Spider telangiectasis, splenomegaly, testicular atrophy, gynecomastia, encephalopathy, caput medusae.

Investigations

Liver chemistry tests: ALT and AST typically elevated to a greater degree than alkaline phosphatase; elevation in bilirubin variable.

An AST level greater than ALT level with AST elevations less than 250 U/L is the classic pattern for alcoholic liver inflammation.

Coagulation screening: impaired hepatic synthetic function causes prolonged prothrombin time in addition to low albumin.

Complete blood count: hypersplenism may result in leukopenia and thrombocytopenia.

Liver ultrasonography or CT: often normal but may show small liver with splenomegaly.

Additional diagnostic investigations: directed at identifying either infectious causes or treatable causes (*e.g.*, hemochromatosis, autoimmune liver disease, Wilson's disease, alcoholic liver disease, or drug-induced hepatotoxicity). These include:

• Hepatitis C serology: interpreted as follows:
Positive, active disease: ELISA+, RIBA+ (2–4 bands), ALT increased, RNA+.
False-positive: ELISA+, RIBA- or indeterminate (1 band), ALT normal, RNA-.

• Hepatitis B serology: interpreted as follows:
Immune, postvaccination: sAb+, sAg–, cAb–, eAg–, eAb–, DNA–.
Immune, past exposure to hepatitis B virus: sAb+, sAg–, cAb+, eAg–, eAb+, DNA–.
Infected, carrier: sAb–, sAg+, cAb+, eAg–, eAb+, DNA–.
Infected, high risk of transmission: sAb–, sAg+, cAb+, eAg+, eAb–, DNA+.

• Hepatitis D (delta) serology: hepatitis D can present as coinfection with hepatitis B virus (HBV) or as superinfection of a HBV carrier; anti-hepatitis D antibody positive indicates superinfection.

• Serum ferritin: elevated in hemochromatosis. Iron saturation (*i.e.*, iron/transferrin) >60% should be evaluated with liver biopsy for quantitative iron.

• Autoantibody analysis: antinuclear antibody, double-stranded DNA, and smooth-muscle antibody often positive in autoimmune disease.

• Serum protein electrophoresis: loss of alpha spike in α-1 antitrypsin deficiency; immunoglobulins elevated in chronic liver disease but particularly prominent in autoimmune hepatitis (especially IgG).

• Ceruloplasmin: decreased and 24-hour urine copper increased in Wilson's disease.

• Liver biopsy for histology: shows the following:
Hepatitis B/D virus: inflammatory cells spreading into parenchyma from enlarged portal tracts; hepatitis B sAg on immunohistochemistry; hepatitis D infection increases severity and can be detected by immunohistochemistry.
Hepatitis C virus: usually mild chronic hepatitis with lobular component, prominent lymphoid follicles in portal tracts, acidophile body formation, focal hepatocellular necrosis; no immunohistochemical staining currently available.
Autoimmune disease: periportal inflammatory infiltrate and piecemeal necrosis; negative to hepatitis B/D staining on immunohistochemistry.

Complications

Cirrhosis: in 20%–50% of patients.
Variceal bleeding, encephalopathy, ascites: due to portal hypertension.
Hepatocellular carcinoma: increased incidence in patients with cirrhosis.

Definition

Hepatic dysfunction (*i.e.*, abnormal liver enzyme levels, often with progression to abnormal synthetic function) of at least 6 months' duration secondary to inflammation of the hepatic parenchyma [1].

Differential diagnosis

Alcoholic cirrhosis.
Hepatic neoplasm.
Primary biliary cirrhosis.
Primary sclerosing cholangitis.
Granulomatous hepatitis: multiple granulomata (on liver biopsy), sarcoid, tuberculosis, histoplasmosis, Q fever, brucella, lymphoma.

Etiology

Hepatitis C virus, 34%.
Alcohol, 38%.
Unknown, 17%.
Nonalcoholic steato-hepatitis, 5%–10%.
HBV, 9%.
Autoimmune, 1%.
• Remaining causes include drugs, Wilson's disease, hemochromatosis, and α_1-antitrypsin deficiency.

Abbreviations

ALT	alanine aminotransferase (SGPT)
AST	aspartate aminotransferase (SGOT)
cAb	Hepatitis B core antibody
eAb	Hepatitis B e antibody
eAg	Hepatitis B e antigen
ELISA	enzyme-linked immunosorbent assay
RIBA	recombinant immunoblot assay
sAb	Hepatitis B surface antibody
sAg	Hepatitis B surface antigen

Treatment

Diet and lifestyle

• Alcohol must be avoided.

• Patients infected by HBV should be advised on barrier methods of contraception unless the partner is vaccinated; sexual transmission of hepatitis C occurs, but at a much lower frequency.

• Avoid excessive amounts of acetaminophen (>4 g/day).

• Patients with nonalcoholic steatohepatitis typically have improvement in ALT and AST in response to weight loss; this is a useful diagnostic and therapeutic approach when other competing diagnoses have been excluded.

Pharmacological treatment

• Treatment should be given under specialist supervision.

For HBV infection

• Treatment is indicated for patients who have histological evidence of chronic hepatitis and are positive for hepatitis B e antigen or virus DNA [2].

• Meaningful remission can be achieved in 40%–50% of patients with HBV.

Standard dosage	Interferon-α, 10 MU s.c. 3 times a week for 4–6 months [2] or lamivudine 100 mg orally each day for one year [5].
Contraindications	Hypersensitivity, evidence of liver failure (*e.g.*, ascites, varicies, thrombocytopenia is a relative risk factor; autoimmune hepatitis).
Main side effects more common with interferon	*Induction:* low-grade fever, malaise, arthralgia, myalgia, headache, anorexia, nausea, vomiting, diarrhea. *Maintenance:* fatigue, anorexia, weight loss, alopecia, depression, neutropenia, thrombocytopenia, exacerbation of autoimmune disease, induction of thyroid disease, myalgia.

For hepatitis C virus infection

• Treatment is indicated for patients with histological evidence of hepatitis who are positive for recombinant immunoblot assay (2–4 bands) or virus RNA by the polymerase chain reaction.

• Sustained response rates of 30%–60% can be achieved with combination therapy of interferon plus ribavirin.

• Hepatitis C genotype 1 has a lower response rate than genotypes 2 or 3.

Standard dosage Interferon-α (3 million U s.c. three times weekly) and ribavirin (600 mg orally twice daily if patient weighs >75 kg; if patient weighs <75 kg, 400 mg orally in morning and 600 mg orally in evening); all regimens given for 6 months.

Contraindications Hypersensitivity; autoimmune hepatitis; decompensated liver disease.

Special points This treatment arena is rapidly changing, and new recommendations are anticipated.

Main interactions Captopril, enalapril, live vaccines, rotavirus vaccine, theophylline, zidovudine.

Main side effects Anemia, insomnia, irritability, depression, headache, nausea.

For autoimmune disease

• Treatment is indicated for patients with raised ALT, AST, and IgG, histological evidence of chronic hepatitis, and serologic test results consistent with autoimmune hepatitis (*e.g.*, ANA, SMA, LKM antibodies) [4].

Standard dosage	Prednisone, 20–40 mg initially, reduced gradually (depending on clinical response); 5–10 mg daily maintenance dose may be needed. Azathioprine, 50–70 mg orally daily as adjunct.
Contraindications	Systemic infection; previous serious reaction to corticosteroids (*e.g.*, psychosis).
Main drug interactions	None.
Main side effects	*Steroids:* osteoporosis, proximal myopathy, skin thinning, cataracts, diabetes mellitus, weight gain, amenorrhea, depression, hypertension. *Azathioprine:* pancreatitis, bone-marrow suppression.

Alternative medicine

Recommended use: none.

Common use: licorice (*Glycyrrhiza glabra*); milk thistle (*Silybum marianum*).

Caution: licorice at high doses can cause hypertension and hypokalemia. Silymarin may cause loose stools; if this occurs, combine with bile-sequestering fiber compound.

Treatment aims

To induce remission and thus prevent progression to cirrhosis.

To eliminate active replication of viruses.

Surgical treatment

Orthotopic liver transplantation: liver transplantation is a treatment option for all patients with end-stage liver disease from chronic hepatitis; the 5-year survival rate is 50%–70% depending on the cause.

For HBV patients, recurrence of HBV accompanied by aggressive progression of liver disease is common [6].

Follow-up and management

• During interferon-α treatment, patients must be monitored closely for leukopenia and thrombocytopenia.

• Thyroid function must be checked because autoimmune disease can be exacerbated.

• Patients on long-term corticosteroid treatment should be monitored for steroid side effects and should have annual bone densitometry to check for osteoporosis.

• Patients who have progressed to cirrhosis are at risk of hepatocellular carcinoma; some investigators advocate surveillance with alpha fetoprotein and ultrasound evaluations every 6 months.

• Relatives of patients with hemochromatosis, Wilson's disease, and α-1-antitrypsin disease should be carefully evaluated.

Key references

1. Scheuer PJ: Classification of chronic viral hepatitis: a need for reassessment. *J Hepatol* 1991, **13**:372–374.
2. Perillo RP: Interferon in the management of chronic hepatitis B. *Dig Dis Sci* 1993, **38**:577–593.
3. Poynard P: Meta-analysis of interferon randomized trials in the treatment of viral hepatitis C: effects of dose and duration. *Hepatology* 1996, **24**:778–789.
4. Johnson RL, *et al.*: The natural course and heterogeneity of autoimmune chronic active hepatitis. *Semin Liver Dis* 1991, **11**:187–196.
5. Lai CL, *et al.*: A one-year trial of lamivudine for chronic hepatitis B. *N Engl J Med* 1998, **339**:61–68.
6. Schalm SW, *et al.*: Interferon-ribavirin for chronic hepatitis C with and without cirrhosis: analysis of individual patient data of six controlled trials. *Gastroenterology* 1999, **117**:408–413.

Hepatocellular carcinoma

Diagnosis

Symptoms

• Small hepatocellular carcinomas (<3 cm diameter) are usually asymptomatic; symptoms have insidious onset and usually consist of the following:

Upper abdominal pain: right hypochondrial or epigastric.

Weight loss, weakness, anorexia.

Abdominal swelling: may be due to ascites or enlarged liver.

Low-grade pyrexia.

Features of cirrhosis.

Metastatic symptoms: *e.g.*, bone pain.

Signs

• The liver is often enlarged and tender but may be normal when the tumor is relatively small.

Stigmata of chronic liver disease.

Arterial bruit: heard in 20% of patients.

Ascites.

Splenomegaly: in 20% to 30%.

Wasting: with more advanced disease.

Jaundice: in later stages of illness.

Investigations

Biochemistry: elevation of alkaline phosphatase without elevation in bilirubin common; aspartate aminotransferase and alanine aminotransferase elevations often mild.

Hematology: may show evidence of pancytopenia (hypersplenism) or erythrocytosis.

Alpha-fetoprotein: elevated in > 80% of cases; alpha fetoprotein possibly normal in small hepatocellular carcinoma; can be falsely elevated in patients with chronic hepatitis; used by some to annually screen patients with chronic liver disease for hepatoma.

Chest radiography: may show raised right hemidiaphragm or metastases.

CT: useful to stage tumor; MRI can be used to complement CT and is of particular use in differentiating hemangiomas from other tumors.

Ultrasonography: may be useful for screening patients with cirrhosis for small hepatocellular carcinoma; 1-cm lesions can be detected, often as hypoechoic lesions.

Celiac axis angiography: tumors usually hypervascular; useful for staging disease that does not appear confined or in distinguishing benign nodules from malignant lesions.

Lipiodol CT: sensitive method for detecting small hepatocellular carcinoma; lipiodol, an oil contrast medium, cleared by hepatocytes but not by hepatocellular carcinoma; CT done 2 weeks after intra-arterial injection.

Liver biopsy: directed biopsy usually indicated; aspiration biopsy can be performed but is less diagnostic.

Complications

Acute intraperitoneal hemorrhage: often the terminal event.

Intravascular and intraductal growth.

Portal vein, inferior vena cava, and right atrial involvement.

Metastases: lung, bone, skin, brain, adrenal, and lymphogenous.

Hypoglycemia, hypercalcemia, polycythemia, hyperlipidemia.

Hepatic failure.

Variceal bleeding.

Differential diagnosis

Cystic lesions, hepatic metastatic carcinoma from other sites, abscess, adenoma, focal nodular hyperplasia.

Benign hemangioma.

Etiology

• Most cases of hepatocellular carcinoma develop in the setting of cirrhosis, including disease caused by the following [1]:

Chronic hepatitis B or C virus infection.

Alcoholic liver disease.

Autoimmune hepatitis or primary biliary cirrhosis.

Hemochromatosis.

Other inherited disorders of metabolism.

Tyrosinosis, α_1-antitrypsin deficiency.

Environmental carcinogens: aflatoxin is a potent chemical carcinogen, produced by *Aspergillus flavus*, which contaminates food in high-incidence areas; genetic changes have been documented.

Membranous inferior vena cava obstruction.

Androgenic anabolic steroids.

Contraceptives (controversial).

Epidemiology

• Areas of high, intermediate, and low incidence correspond crudely to prevalence of hepatitis B and C infection; low-incidence areas include northern Europe and North America.

• Hepatocellular carcinoma is more frequent in immigrants from high- and intermediate-prevalence countries (sub-Saharan Africa, China, southern and eastern Europe, Middle East).

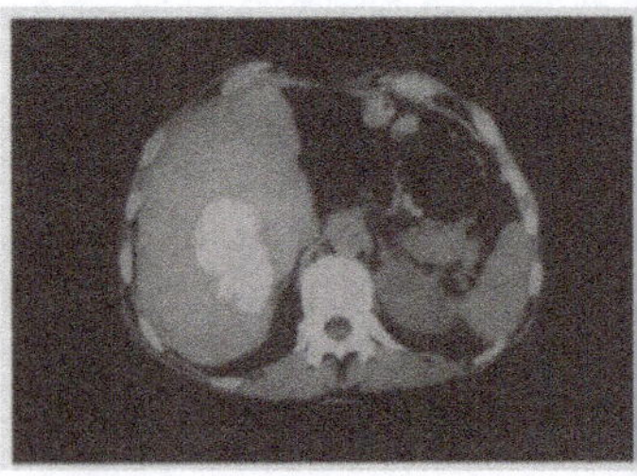

Retention of lipiodol within a hepatocellular carcinoma.

Treatment

Diet and lifestyle

• No special precautions are necessary.

Surgical treatment [2–5]

• Surgical resection is the treatment of choice for hepatocellular carcinoma when possible. Resection is recommended for solitary lesions without vascular evasion or extrahepatic metasasis: extensive resection is not recommended for patients with cirrhosis.

Orthotopic liver transplantation: for patients with underlying cirrhosis, orthotopic liver transplantation can be performed with solitary lesions <5 cm or with three tumor nodules each <3 cm.

Pharmacological treatment

Chemotherapy for palliation

• The response rate and survival in patients undergoing chemotherapy have been disappointing. Treatment should be given under special supervision.

Standard dosage	Doxorubicin, epirubicin, cisplatin, mitoxantrone every 3–4 weeks.
Contraindications	*All:* hypersensitivity. *Doxorubicin:* bone-marrow suppression, buccal ulcerations (after first dose). *Cisplatin:* pre-existing renal impairment, hearing disorders, bone-marrow suppression.
Special points	Other adjunctive agents, *e.g.*, tamoxifen, interferon, and interleukin-2, may be used. *Doxorubicin:* ECG, ejection fraction, and echocardiogram must be monitored. *Cisplatin:* hydration must be maintained; blood count, serum creatinine, and blood urea nitrogen must be monitored; audiometry needed.
Main drug interactions	*Cisplatin:* use with aminoglycoside or cephalosporins may cause increased ototoxicity or nephrotoxicity.
Main side effects	*Doxorubicin:* mucositis, bone-marrow suppression, alopecia, nausea, vomiting, diarrhea, cardiotoxicity. *Cisplatin:* nephrotoxicity, myelosuppression, neurotoxicity, ototoxicity, immunosuppression, nausea, vomiting. *Mitoxantrone:* leukopenia, thrombocytopenia, anemia, nausea, vomiting, alopecia, diarrhea, mucositis, cardiovascular effects (rare), blue-green discoloration of urine.

Percutaneous ethanol injection [6]

• Percutaneous ethanol injection is most effective in solitary tumors <3 cm (injection of tumor using alcohol or lipiodol, *e.g.*, alcohol, 10–20 mL intratumoral injection 3 times weekly for 12 treatments). This form of palliative treatment has become widely used in the past several years. Injection therapy is recommended for those patients with cirrhosis who are not good surgical candidates.

Treatment aims

To cure disease or prolong survival without recurrence.

To alleviate symptoms.

Other treatments

Transcatheter arterial embolization: for unresectable carcinoma, not for portal-vein thrombosis or Child's C cirrhosis; side effects include abdominal pain and fever; can be used with lipiodol-targeted chemotherapy.

Prognosis

• <25% of patients have partial responses to current chemotherapeutic regimens.

• 60% 5-year survival rates have been reported after intratumoral injection of alcohol for small tumors, but injection is without benefit in other series.

• 1-year survival rates as high as 78% after transcatheter arterial embolization have been reported.

• The 5-year survival rate after surgery is 25%; patients with encapsulated tumors, negative resection margins, no intracapsular or intravascular invasion of tumor cells, and Child's class A have better prognosis for surgical management [4].

Follow-up and management

• Serial imaging of the liver, lung, and bones is suggested to detect recurrence.

• Serial alpha-fetoprotein concentrations should be measured if initially high.

Key references

1. Schafer DF, Sorell MF: Hepatocellular carcinoma. Lancet 1999, **353**:1253–1257.
2. Dusheiko GM, *et al.*: Treatment of small hepatocellular carcinomas. *Lancet* 1992, **340**:285–288.
3. Di Bisceglie AM, *et al.*: Hepatocellular carcinoma. *Ann Intern Med* 1988, **108**:390–401.
4. Okuda K: Hepatocellular carcinoma: recent progress. *Hepatology* 1992, **15**:948–963.
5. Mazzafermo V: Liver transplantation for treatment of small hepatocellular carcinomas in patients with cirrhosis. *N Engl J Med* 1996, **334**:693–699.
6. Bruix J: Treatment of hepatocellular carcinoma. *Hepatology* 1997, **25**:259–262.

Herpes simplex infection

Diagnosis

Symptoms

Pain, burning, itching, tingling lasting 6–12 hours, vesicles (generally ulcerating or crusting within 48 hours): recurrent orolabial herpes (cold sores).
Fever, malaise, headache, altered personality, confusion, convulsions, paresis, paralysis, or coma: herpes encephalitis.
Fever, malaise, headache, nausea, vomiting, photophobia, neck stiffness: herpes meningitis.
Pain, photophobia, edema of the eyelid, lacrimation, blurring of vision: ocular herpes (spectrum ranges from superficial infections to stromal keratitis and iridocyclitis affecting inner eye).
Fever, sore mouth, swelling of gums, vesicles, ulceration in anterior half of mouth, tender anterior cervical lymph nodes: primary gingivostomatitis (frequently asymptomatic).
Pain, burning, itching, tingling, vesicles followed by ulcers and crusts in perineum, vaginal discharge, dysparunia: genital herpes; symptoms vary in severity, extent, and duration, depending on whether the infection is primary (usually most severe) or recurrent; may be asymptomatic.
Vesicles, ulcers, crusts, malaise, fever, lymphadenopathy: eczema herpeticum.
Pruritus, severe localized pain, vesicles, ulcers, crusts, fever, lymphadenopathy: other cutaneous herpes infections (herpes whitlow or gladiatorum, herpetic nipple).

Signs

Erythema progressing to vesicles, ulcers, and crusts: cutaneous lesions.
Altered personality, fluctuating levels of consciousness, focal or generalized convulsions, focal neurological findings, drowsiness, stupor, coma: herpes encephalitis.
Neck stiffness, positive Kernig's test: herpes meningitis.
Small blister or predendritic ulcers on cornea: ocular herpes; dendritic ulcers have serpentine branching appearance on fluoroscopy after fluorescein instillation.

Investigations

Cutaneous lesions

- Laboratory tests are usually not needed because symptoms and signs are diagnostic.

Tzanck test: may show multinucleated giant cells.
Immunofluorescence: can show viral antigens in cell smears.
Virus culture: from vesicle fluid or ulcers.

Herpes encephalitis

CT, MRI, EEG: show temporal lobe localization; EEG shows temporal spike and slow wave activity in 80% of patients.
CSF analysis: shows pleocytosis, usually 50–500 cells/mm^3, with lymphocyte predominance; erythrocytes often present, specimen may be xanthochromic; protein or erythrocyte count may be raised, sugar usually normal; CSF can be examined for virus DNA (polymerase chain reaction) or viral antigens (immunology), but treatment should not await results.

Herpes meningitis

Lumbar puncture: to show CSF abnormalities of aseptic meningitis; herpes meningitis assumed when findings accompany mucocutaneous herpes, usually primary genital.
EEG: localized abnormalities in temporal lobe.

Ocular herpes

Ophthalmic examination and fluorescein: show presence of dendritic ulceration.
Abrasion of corneal cells: shows viral antigens; can be used for virus isolation.

Complications

Erythema multiforme, aseptic meningitis, urethritis, urinary retention, myelitis: due to mucocutaneous herpes.
Death, severe neurological sequelae: due to herpes encephalitis.
Visual loss, rupture of the globe (rare): due to recurrent ocular herpes.

Differential diagnosis

Mucocutaneous lesions
Causes of gingivitis and stomatitis.
Aphthous ulceration.
Coxsackievirus infection (hand, foot, and mouth).
Behçet's syndrome.
Inflammatory bowel disease.
Varicella–zoster virus.
Sexually transmitted disease.

Herpes encephalitis
Other encephalitides.
Space-occupying lesions (*e.g.*, abscess, tumor, tuberculoma).

Herpes meningitis
Other causes of meningitis (*e.g.*, viruses, bacteria, fungi).

Ocular herpes
Ocular infections.

Etiology

Herpes simplex virus types 1 and 2: enveloped DNA viruses.
Exposure to strong sunlight, ultraviolet light, pneumonia, meningitis, and malaria: cause reactivation (cold sores).
Fever, stressful events, depression, menstruation, sexual activity: causes of recurrences of genital herpes.
Immunosuppression: cause of mucocutaneous herpes.
Inoculation of virus into a finger or direct contact: cause of herpetic whitlow and herpes gladiatorum.
Bites and other traumatic forms of viral inoculation (*e.g.*, from needles, razors, contaminated finger nails): causes of herpetic nipple.

Epidemiology

- Seroepidemiological studies show that 30%–50% of patients in higher socioeconomic groups and 100% of those in lower groups are infected with herpes simplex virus 1 by puberty.
- The prevalence of antibodies to herpes simplex virus 2 varies from 3% in nuns to ~70% in prostitutes.
- The prevalence of herpes encephalitis is 0.1–0.4 in 100 000 people.

Treatment

Diet and lifestyle

• Parents or grandparents with cold sores should not kiss young children.

• Laboratory tests have shown latex condoms to be effective mechanical barriers to herpes simplex virus.

Pharmacological treatment

• Acyclovir is of proven clinical value in some infections.

• It is not recommended for orolabial herpes.

• Famcyclovir or valciclovir is now available and has equivalent effect for cutaneous herpes infections.

Standard dosage	*For initial genital herpes:* acyclovir, 200 mg 5 times daily for 10 days. *For recurrent genital herpes (prophylaxis):* acyclovir, 400–800 mg daily in 2–4 divided doses (continuous suppressive therapy). *For mucocutaneous herpes in immunocompromised patients:* acyclovir, i.v. or oral. *For herpes encephalitis:* acyclovir, 10 mg/kg i.v. 3 times daily for 10 days. *For ocular herpes simplex:* acyclovir, 400 mg 5 times daily, more effective than 3% ointment.
Contraindications	Hypersensitivity.
Special points	Limited experience in pregnancy and lactation so should be used only when potential benefits outweigh risks. Bioavailability of drug possibly reduced in patients being treated for malignancy so i.v. route advised.
Main drug interactions	Probenecid increases acyclovir half-life. No detrimental interactions recognized.
Main side effects	Raised urea and creatinine concentrations due to deposition of acyclovir crystals in tubules after rapid bolus doses, occasional nausea and vomiting, inflammation and ulceration at site of infusion if extravasation of drug occurs.

Alternative medicine

Recommended use: None.

Common use: lLysine; calendula (*Calendula officinalis*); aloe vera; echinacea (*Echinacea angustifolia*); licorice root (*Glycyrrhiza*).

Caution: licorice at high doses can cause hypertension, hypokalemia.

Treatment aims

To accelerate healing.

To reduce virus replication and dissemination.

To prevent recurrence, death and neurological complications, and blindness.

Prognosis

• Treatment of mucocutaneous herpes results in accelerated healing and reduced viral shedding.

• Treatment of herpes encephalitis results in reduced mortality and morbidity, especially in young patients with high Glasgow Coma Scale scores who are treated early.

• Treatment of ocular herpes has varying outcomes, depending on previous inflammation and scarring.

• Prophylactic treatment reduces the incidence and severity of recurrences in patients with recurrent genital herpes and viral shedding in immunocompromised patients.

Follow-up and management

• Pregnant women should inform their obstetrician of a history of genital herpes.

General references

Conant MA, Berger TG, Coates TJ, *et al.*: Genital herpes: an integrated approach to management. *J Am Acad Dermatol* 1996, **35**:601–605.

Prober CG, *et al.*: The management of pregnancies complicated by genital infections with herpes simplex virus. *Clin Infect Dis* 1992, **15**:1031–1038.

Woo SB, Sonis ST: Recurrent aphthous ulcers: a review of diagnosis and treatment. *J Am Dent Assoc* 1996, **127**:1202–1213.

Herpes zoster & varicella

Diagnosis

Symptoms

Chickenpox (varicella)

Fever and malaise: in prodromal phase, variable.

Headache, myalgia.

Vesicular rash: frequently itchy.

Shingles (herpes zoster)

Pain in affected dermatome: may precede rash by a few days.

Mental confusion, depression: common in elderly patients.

• Symptoms often continue for weeks or months.

Signs

Chickenpox

Vesicular rash: maximal on face and trunk; rapidly evolving from macules and papules to vesicles and crusts; crops of new vesicles continuing to appear for 3–4 days; drying up in 7–10 days; possibly involving conjunctivae, oropharynx, vulva, vagina; larger lesions and slow evolution suggest underlying immune deficiency.

Shingles

Unilateral, segmental skin rash: lesions similar to chickenpox but often confluent; possibly ulcerating; often a few scattered lesions elsewhere: severe multiple dermatome or recurrent disease suggests underlying immune deficiency, including HIV infection.

Investigations

• Virological investigations are needed only when the clinical diagnosis is uncertain.

Tzanck smear: of material from vesicular skin lesions for rapid confirmation of herpes virus infection.

Tissue culture: to distinguish varicella-zoster virus from herpes simplex virus.

Complications

Chickenpox

Secondary bacterial infection of skin: usually *Staphylococcus aureus* or *Streptococcus pyogenes*.

Chickenpox pneumonia: particularly in adults and pregnant women.

Systemic spread: to liver, brain, lung of immunocompromised patients.

Hemorrhagic rash: in immunocompromised patients.

Encephalitis, polyneuritis, transverse myelitis: rare.

Reye's syndrome: in children, rare.

Hemolytic anemia, coagulopathy with hemorrhagic rash: rare.

Shingles

Uveitis, keratitis: in patients with ophthalmic herpes zoster.

Lower motor neuron paralysis.

Ramsey Hunt syndrome: herpes zoster of geniculate ganglion, with facial palsy, loss of taste, ipsilateal oral ulcers and skin lesions in pinna of ear.

Bowel and bladder dysfunction: in patients with sacral herpes zoster infection.

Encephalitis: rare.

Cerebral vasculopathy: trigeminal herpes zoster virus infection, with delayed cerebral infarction and hemiplegia; rare.

Differential diagnosis

Herpes simplex virus.

Other vesicular rashes, especially erythema multiforme.

Etiology

• Chickenpox is caused by direct contact or airborne transmission of varicella-zoster virus from either chickenpox or shingles.

• After primary infection, the virus probably incorporates its DNA into the satellite cells of dorsal-root or cranial-nerve ganglion cells.

• Later reactivation causes shingles.

Epidemiology

• 2% of cases of chickenpox but 25% of deaths due to the disease occur in people aged >20 years.

• The prevalence of shingles rises steadily with age, 1 in 100 people >80 years being affected.

• Shingles in infants and young children probably is caused by a reactivation of intrauterine infection.

• Both chickenpox and shingles are cross-infection hazards in hospitals.

Infection in pregnancy

• Chickenpox in pregnant women may be severe and complicated by varicella pneumonia; patients should be monitored closely.

• Intrauterine infection may damage the fetus and cause limb scarring and hypoplasia, microcephaly or hydrocephalus, and eye abnormalities.

• This fetal varicella syndrome has an incidence of 1%–3% in the first trimester (much lower risk in subsequent trimesters).

• Termination of pregnancy on the grounds of maternal chickenpox is not indicated, because the risk to the fetus is small and unpredictable.

• Maternal herpes zoster infection is not a risk to the fetus.

Infectivity

Incubation period (chickenpox): 17 days.

Infectivity: from 2 days before onset of rash until lesions have dried.

Increased infectivity and susceptibility with immunodeficiency or immunosuppression.

Treatment

Diet and lifestyle

• Patients should avoid contact with susceptible individuals (*e.g.*, immunocompromised) until their skin lesions have dried.

Pharmacological treatment

Acyclovir

• Acyclovir is a highly selective antiviral agent that inhibits viral DNA polymerase and causes premature DNA chain termination.

Standard dosage *For chickenpox and shingles in immunocompromised patients, chickenpox pneumonia:* acyclovir, 10 mg/kg i.v. 8-hourly.
For cutaneous shingles: acyclovir, 800 mg orally 5 times daily for 7 days (started within 72 hours of rash onset).
For ophthalmic shingles: acyclovir orally as above for 10 days.
For severe maternal or neonatal chickenpox: acyclovir i.v.

Contraindications Hypersensitivity.

Special points High cost; no effect on latency or recurrence; not licensed for uncomplicated chickenpox.

Main drug interactions Extreme lethargy has been reported on administration of zidovudine with i.v. acyclovir.

Main side effects Rashes and gastrointestinal disturbances (occasionally), alterations in biochemical and hematological indices (more rarely), headaches and neurological reactions, particularly with i.v. administration, some risk of crystalluria and renal impairment at high dose (maximum oral dose in renal failure, 800 mg 3 times daily).

Varicella-zoster immune globulin

• This is distributed by the Public Health Laboratory Service (in short supply).

• It is used for highly susceptible contacts of chickenpox or shingles, including the following:

Bone-marrow transplant recipients (despite history of previous chickenpox).
Patients with debilitating disease (despite history of previous chickenpox).
HIV-positive patients with symptoms but no known varicella-zoster virus antibody.
Pregnant women without antibody (patients without a definite history of previous chickenpox must be screened for antibody).
Immunosuppressed patients who have been treated by high-dose steroids within the 3 months before contact (screened first).
Neonates up to 4 weeks of age whose mothers develop chickenpox between 1 week before and 1 month after delivery or those in contact with chickenpox or shingles whose mothers have no history of previous varicella-zoster infection or no antibody.
Premature babies <30 weeks gestation or weighing <1 kg at birth in contact with chickenpox.

Standard dosage Varicella-zoster immune globulin, depending on age:
0–5 years, 250 mg; *6–10 years,* 500 mg; *11–14 years,* 750 mg; *≥15 years,* 1000 mg.

Contraindications Hypersensitivity to human immunoglobulin.

Special points Must be given as soon as possible and not more than 10 days after exposure.

Main drug interactions None.

Main side effects Hypersensitivity reactions (rare).

• Live attenuated varicella vaccine is available, on a named-patient basis, for immunocompromised patients, especially children with leukemia.

Treatment aims

Chickenpox

To relieve symptoms in previously healthy patients.

To contain infection and reduce morbidity and mortality in immunocompromised patients or those with chickenpox pneumonia or maternal or neonatal infection.

Shingles

To accelerate healing and curtail pain.

To prevent complications in patients with ophthalmic herpes zoster.

To prevent progressive disease in immunocompromised patients.

Prognosis

• Mortality from chickenpox is increased in patients aged >20 years.

• Morbidity and mortality are reduced by acyclovir treatment in immunocompromised patients.

Follow-up and management

• Patients must be monitored for the development of complications.

• Pain continuing at the site of herpes zoster infection 30 days or more after an acute attack indicates postherpetic neuralgia, which should be treated by amitriptyline or sodium valproate. See Neuralgia, postherpetic *for details.*

General references

Anonymous: Acyclovir in general practice. *Drug Ther Bull* 1992, **30**:101–104.

Arvin AM: Varicella-zoster virus: overview and clinical manifestations. *Semin Dermatol* 1996, **15(suppl)**:4–7.

Bowsher D: Neurogenic pain syndromes and their management. *Br Med Bull* 1991, **47**:644–666.

Flamholc L: Neurological complications in herpes zoster. *Scand J Infect Dis* 1996, **100(suppl)**: 35–40.

Gilbert GL: Chickenpox during pregnancy. *BMJ* 1993, **306**:1079–1080.

Wallace MR, *et al.*: Treatment of adult varicella with oral acyclovir. A randomized, placebo-controlled trial. *Ann Intern Med* 1992, **117**:358–363.

Hip disorders

Diagnosis

Symptoms

Localized

Pain: important to distinguish exact location among and between:

- Groin, anterior thigh, medial knee (hip).
- Buttock (LS spine).
- SI joint.
- Lateral hip (trochonteric bursitis).
- Deep pelvic pain (pelvic fracture, Paget's, ilio-inguinal bursitis).
- Falls/ "buckling"

Limp (antalgic gait).
Sleep disturbance.

Generalized

"Lameness."
Weakness.
Difficulty tying shoe laces.
Inability to sit cross-legged.
Inability to crouch.
Sexual dysfunction.

Signs

Groin tenderness.
Range of motion (flexion, extension, internal rotation, external rotation, log-rolling, abduction).
Trochanteric tenderness.
Antalgic gait.
Normal back examination.
Normal knee examination.
Normal pelvic compression test.
Normal SI joint.
Provocative maneuvers: Fabere's, Patrick's test, SCR.
Normal straight leg raising.

Investigations

Radiographs: to rule out osteoarthritis, fracture, Paget's disease.

Bone scan.

Magnetic resonance imaging: for earliest evidence of avascular necrosis.

Computer tomography: for early osteomyelitis.

Ultrasound: for cartilaginous assessment.

Joint aspiration (fluoroscopic guidance): to rule out sepsis.

Intraosseous pressure measurement: by orthopedics, to confirm and possibly alleviate early avascular necrosis.

Arthrography: to prove bursitis.

Arthroscopy: for loose bodies.

Complications

Fracture.
Falls.
Chronic pain.
Sleep disturbance.
Work impairment.
Limb length discrepancy.
Referred pain.
Secondary problems with low back and knee pain.
Exercise limitation.

Differential diagnosis

Osteoarthritis
Rheumatoid arthritis.
Avascular necrosis.
Fracture.
Paget's disease.
Osteoporosis.
Bursitis.
Low back pain.
Neoplasm.
Septic arthritis.
Childhood hip synovitis.
Endometriosis.
Reflex sympathetic dystrophy.
Spinal stenosis.
Piriformis syndrome.
Meralgia paresthetica.
Lateral femoral cutaneous nerve entrapment.
Tensor fascia lata syndrome.
Hemachromatosis.
Gaucher's disease.
Congenital hip dislocation (unrecognized).

Etiology

Moderate obesity is a primary risk factor and predictor for osteoarthritis of hip, especially in adolescents and young adults.
Weight-bearing degenerative changes.
Seated occupations.
Immobility.
Inflammation.
Infections.
After fracture.

Epidemiology

Osteoarthritis of the hips is extremely common.
Hip replacement is one of the most common elective surgeries of adulthood.
Hip fracture surgery is a major source of morbidity and mortality in the elderly.
Avascular necrosis is commonly diagnosed as steroid dosage increases; magnetic resonance imaging availability leads to earlier diagnosis.

Treatment

Diet and lifestyle

Weight reduction: modest decrease in weight (10 to 20 pounds) may be associated with significant improvement.

Exercise: walking, swimming, low-impact aerobics.

Joint-protection techniques.

Fall prevention.

Adaptive equipment: cane, walker, wheelchair.

Pharmacological treatment

COX-2 inhibitors.

Nonsteroidal antiinflammatory drugs.

Acetaminophen.

Topical agents: of little benefit.

Glucosamine/chondroitin sulfate supplementation: controversial.

Nonpharmacological treatment

Exercise.

Physical therapy: modalities, gait training.

Surgery: hip arthoplasty.

Treatment aims

To reduce pain.

To restore and maintain function.

To improve sleep.

To improve quality of life.

To prevent falls and fractures.

Prognosis

Varies widely with causation, severity, comorbidities, age of onset, activity level maintained, patient expectations, and longevity.

General references

Benson, ER, Schutzer SF: Posttraumatic piriformis syndrome: diagnosis and results of operative treatment. *J Bone Joint Surg Am* 1999, **81**:941-949.

Gennari C, Nuti R, Anusdei D, Camporeale A, Martini G: Management of osteoporosis and Paget's disease: an appraisal of the risks and benefits of drug treatment. *Drug Saf* 1994, **11**(3):179-195.

Ledwith CA, Fleisher GR: Slipped capital femoral epiphysis without hip pain leads to missed diagnosis. *Pediatrics* 1992, **89** (4 pt 1):660-662.

Minor MA: Exercise in management of osteoarthritis of the knee and hip. *Arthritis Care Res* 1994, **7**(4):198-204.

Ritter MA, Helphinstine J, Keating EM, Faris PM, Meding JB: Total hip arthroplasty in patients with osteonecrosis: the effect of cement techniques. *Clin Orthop* 1997, May:94-99.

Van Schaardenburg D, Van den Brande KJ, Ligthart GJ, Breedveld FC, Hazes JM: Musculoskeletal disorders and disability in persons aged 85 and over: a community survery. *Ann Rheum Dis* 1994, **53**(12): 807-811.

Wolfe F, Kong SX: Rasch analysis of the Western Ontario MacMaster questionnaire (WOMAC) in 2205 patients with osteoarthritis, rheumatoid arthritis, and fibromyalgia. *Ann Rheum Dis* 1999, **58**:563-568.

Diagnosis

Symptoms

- The usual presentation is a lymph-node mass noticed by the patient.
- Fluctuation in size is not unusual.
- ~25% of patients have other symptoms.

"B" symptoms: unexplained temperature >38°C, loss of >10% body weight in 6 months, night sweats.

Pruritus: may lead to extensive excoriation from scratching.

Alcohol-induced nodal pain: rare and nonspecific.

Anorexia, lethargy.

Signs

Palpable lymphadenopathy: usually; careful examination of all node-bearing areas essential.

Extranodal involvement: *e.g.*, bone-marrow, liver, CNS; in 10%–20% of patients.

Investigations

- Initially, a good biopsy specimen must be carefully examined to make the diagnosis. Reed–Sternberg cells are the hallmark of Hodgkin's disease and the putative malignant cell.
- Investigation is then systematic to "stage" the disease.

Full blood count: possible neutrophilia, eosinophilia, lymphopenia, leukoerythroblastic picture if bone marrow is involved.

ESR measurement: rate sometimes raised; can be useful disease marker and prognostic feature.

Liver function tests: abnormalities raise possibility of liver involvement.

Lactate dehydrogenase measurement: useful disease marker and prognostic feature.

Chest radiography: to look for nodal and pulmonary disease.

CT of chest and abdomen: to detect nodes; poor at detecting hepatic and splenic disease.

Lymphangiography: in centers with expertise, better than CT for assessing retroperitoneal nodes.

Bone-marrow examination: with trephine; rarely reveals unsuspected bone-marrow involvement.

Staging laparotomy: controversial now; in theory, might detect unsuspected splenic disease and change treatment plan.

Complications

Infection related to underlying defect in cell-mediated immunity: herpes zoster seen in 20%, and tuberculosis not unusual.

Differential diagnosis

Non-Hodgkin's lymphoma.

Infections, *e.g.*, Epstein-Barr virus, toxoplasma, cytomegalovirus.

Angioimmunoblastic lymphadenopathy.

Etiology [1]

- The origin of the Reed-Sternberg cell, the putative malignant cell, is still debated; cell surface marker CD15 is usually expressed; T- or B-lymphocyte markers are also sometimes expressed.
- Recent evidence implicates Epstein–Barr virus (EBV) in the cause of some cases of Hodgkin's disease; the EBV genome has been found incorporated into DNA in Reed–Sternberg cells, and serological evidence links EBV with Hodgkin's disease.

Epidemiology [1]

- Hodgkin's disease has a bimodal distribution, with a first peak at 15–40 years, then increasing incidence with increasing age.
- Male patients are more frequently affected than female patients.
- The incidence is higher in whites.

Classification

Based on the Rye system:

1. Nodular sclerosing (>80% of patients): dense bands of collagen with nodules of tumor.
2. Lymphocyte predominant: infiltrate of small lymphocytes.
3. Mixed cellularity: pleomorphic infiltrate.
4. Lymphocyte depleted: few Reed–Sternberg cells seen.

Staging

- Hodgkin's disease appears to start unifocally and to spread to adjacent lymph nodes in an orderly fashion. Staging (based on the Ann Arbor Scheme) is important for rational planning of treatment.

Stage I: involvement of single lymph-node region.

Stage II: two or more lymph-node regions on same side of diaphragm.

Stage III: lymph-node involvement on both sides of diaphragm, including spleen.

Stage IV: diffuse involvement of extranodal sites.

Suffix A: no systemic symptoms.

Suffix B: "B" symptoms as described earlier.

Treatment

Diet and lifestyle

• Some patients continue a normal lifestyle during chemotherapy; others feel quite unwell.

Pharmacological treatment

• Hodgkin's disease is a chemo- and radiosensitive disease.

• Treatment decision depends on accurate staging and should also take into account current clinical trials.

Radiotherapy [2]

• Patients with stage I and IIA disease and no other adverse prognostic features can be cured by radiation therapy alone.

• This is usually given to an extended field beyond the area of overt nodal disease over 1 month.

• Initial treatment with combined chemotherapy and radiation therapy provides no survival advantage in early-stage disease and may lead to increased toxicity.

• Radiation therapy is typically administered after completion of chemotherapy for bulky disease to decrease the risk of local recurrence.

Chemotherapy [3,4]

•As an alternative therapy for early stage disease and for more advanced disease, several standard four-drug combinations are used, *e.g.*, MOPP (mechlorethamine, vincristine, procarbazine, prednisone), ABVD (doxorubicin, bleomycin, vinblastine, dacarbazine), or combinations of MOPP and ABVD.

• Precise details of treatment should always be decided by an experienced hematologist or oncologist.

• Good i.v. access is needed because some drugs, particularly vinca alkaloids and anthracyclines, are vesicant.

• Admission to the hospital is not usually required for treatment, although treatment should commence as soon as practical after initial diagnosis and staging.

Treatment after relapse

• Relapse after initial treatment may still be compatible with long-term survival.

• Patients who relapse after radiation therapy can be "salvaged" with chemotherapy with overall survival similar to that in patients who were initially treated with both modalities; the converse is rarely true.

• The longer the duration of first remission, the greater is the chance of obtaining a second remission on standard treatment.

• Increasing dose intensity of treatment is of benefit in Hodgkin's disease; ~50% of patients resistant to standard treatment can still achieve long-term survival with high-dose chemotherapy regimens such as BEAM (BCNU [carmustine], etoposide, cytarabine, melphalan) and autologous hematopoietic stem cell support [5,6].

Complications of treatment

Skin reactions and pneumonitis after radiation therapy.

Myelosuppression, emesis, hair loss, and neurotoxicity after chemotherapy.

Second malignancy: lung cancer, breast cancer, soft tissue sarcomas, coronary artery disease, acute myeloid leukemia (~1%), peak incidence 4–11 years after initial treatment.

Impaired fertility after chemotherapy: consideration of sperm banking should be discussed with male patients before initiation of therapy.

Pulmonary fibrosis.

Treatment aims

To cure the disease with minimal toxicity from the treatment.

Prognosis

• The overall survival at 10 years is ~60%

• Poor prognostic features include:

Older age.

Presence of B symptoms.

Mixed cellularity/lymphocyte-depleted histology.

Stage III or IV disease at presentation.

ESR >40 mm/h.

Lactic dehydrogenase >normal.

Mass >10 cm.

Failure to obtain complete remission after adequate first-line treatment.

Follow-up and management

• Regular review during treatment is essential to detect complications and assess response.

• Full blood count is mandatory before administration of each cycle of treatment.

• After treatment is finished, full restaging is needed.

• Follow-up interval may gradually lengthen but should be continued indefinitely to detect late complications of treatment or relapse.

Key references

1. Collins RH Jr: The pathogenesis of Hodgkin's disease. *Blood Rev* 1990, **4**:61–68.
2. Mendenhall NP: The role of radiation in the management of Hodgkin's disease: an update. *Cancer Invest* 1999, **17**:47–55.
3. DeVita VT Jr, Hubbard SM: Drug treatment: Hodgkin's disease. *N Engl J Med* 1993, **328**:560–565.
4. Linch DC, *et al.*: Dose intensification with autologous bone marrow transplantation in relapsed and resistant Hodgkin's disease: results of a BNLI randomised trial. *Lancet* 1993, **341**:1051–1054.
5. Diehl V, Engert A (eds.): Proceedings of the Third International Symposium on Hodgkin's Lymphoma. *Ann Oncol* 1996, **7(suppl 4)**:1–143.
6. Horning SJ, Chao NJ, Negrin RS, *et al.*: High-dose therapy and autologous hematopoietic progenitor cell transplantation for recurrent or refractory Hodgkin's disease: analysis of the Stanford University results and prognostic indices. *Blood* 1997, **89**:801–813.

Hypercalcemia

Diagnosis

Symptoms

• Hypercalcemia causes no symptoms or nonspecific symptoms, such as:

Tiredness and lethargy.

Nausea and vomiting.

Constipation.

Polydipsia and polyuria.

Muscle weakness.

Impaired mental function and occasional loss of consciousness: in severe cases.

Signs

• Specific signs of hypercalcemia are rare.

Signs of dehydration: caused by moderate to severe hypercalcemia.

Nephrolithiasis: may be seen in hyperparathyroidism.

Corneal and soft-tissue calcification.

Investigations

Serum calcium measurement: total serum calcium influenced by serum protein concentration, especially albumin. Measurements of ionized serum calcium are unaffected by levels of serum proteins.

Parathyroid hormone measurement: high concentration indicates probable hyperparathyroidism; measurement of intact parathyroid hormone molecule is preferred.

Tests for anemia, liver function tests, alkaline phosphatase and serum protein electrophoresis: malignancy more probable if concentrations are abnormal or raised.

Chest and skeletal radiography: indicated if malignancy probable.

• Specific investigations of other causes of hypercalcemia are indicated when the more common causes have been excluded.

Complications [1]

Dehydration: common and, unless corrected, causes worsening of hypercalcemia.

Bone pain: common in malignancy, rare in hyperparathyroidism.

Pancreatitis: rare complication of chronic hypercalcemia.

Differential diagnosis

Not applicable.

Etiology

• 97% of cases of hypercalcemia in general medical practice are due either to primary hyperparathyroidism or to malignancy, which is usually disseminated.

• Other causes include the following:

Severe thyrotoxicosis.

Vitamin D excess.

Vitamin A excess.

Calcium treatment to bind phosphate in chronic renal failure.

Sarcoidosis.

Familial benign or hypocalciuric hypercalcemia.

Diuretic phase of acute renal failure.

Milk-alkali syndrome.

Addison's disease.

Epidemiology

• Primary hyperparathyroidism increases markedly after middle age and is three times more common in women than in men.

• Hyperparathyroidism is typically present in multiple endocrine neoplasia type I (90%–95%), but is less common in type II (20%–30%).

• Many malignancies can be complicated by hypercalcemia.

Treatment

Diet and lifestyle

• A low-calcium diet is of little value in treating hypercalcemia, although high calcium intake exacerbates the disorder.

• Patients with hyperparathyroidism treated conservatively should be advised to maintain an adequate fluid intake, especially when they are unwell.

Pharmacological treatment [2]

For hyperparathyroidism [3]

• The only definitive treatment of hypercalcemia due to primary hyperparathyroidism is surgical.

• Estrogen therapy helps to maintain bone mass in women with hyperparathyroidism.

For malignancy [3]

• Intravenous rehydration *followed* by diuresis is of primary importance.

• The bisphosphonate drugs are frequently first-line pharmacological therapy for significant hypercalcemia.

Standard dosage	Pamidronate, 60–90 mg i.v. by continuous infusion.
	Etidronate, 5–10 mg orally daily, can also be used.
Contraindications	Caution in renal failure.
Special points	Serum calcium falls to or toward normal within 3–5 days. IV bisphosphonates are typically more effective than oral preparations.
Main drug interactions	Oral bisphosphonates must be taken on an empty stomach.
Main side effects	Gastrointestinal upset.

For sarcoidosis

• Hypercalcemia responds rapidly to steroids.

Standard dosage	Prednisone, 20 mg daily, reduced to lowest dose that controls hypercalcemia.
Contraindications	Systemic infections; caution in peptic ulceration or diabetes.
Main drug interactions	None.
Main side effects	Cushingoid appearance (with maintained high doses), dyspepsia.

Adjunctive therapy

• Calcitonin may be used early as an adjunct for rapid treatment of hypercalcemia.

Standard dosage	Calcitonin, 4 IU/kg s.c. or i.m. every 12 hours; dose may be increased to 8 IU/kg every 12 or every 6 hours if necessary.
Contraindications	Allergy to synthetic salmon calcitonin.
Main drug interactions	Effective within 12 hours but effectiveness greatly diminished by 72–96 hours.
Main side effects	Hypocalcemia.

Nonpharmacological treatment

For hyperparathyroidism

• Surgery should be seriously considered for all younger patients and those with complications of the disease (*e.g.*, renal stones).

• Elderly asymptomatic patients can be followed conservatively [4].

• Surgery *must* be done by an experienced parathyroid surgeon.

• After successful surgery, serum calcium is usually normal or low within 24 hours.

• Transient hypocalcemia may occur; rarely, permanent hypoparathyroidism may follow.

For malignancy

• Surgical cure is rare because of early metastases.

Treatment aims

Hyperparathyroidism

To cure disease by surgery.

To monitor asymptomatic patients.

Malignancy

To alleviate symptoms.

Prognosis

Hyperparathyroidism

• Effective surgical treatment of hyperparathyroidism is associated with a normal life expectancy.

• After a patient has been cured, a recurrence of hypercalcemia is unusual, except when hyperplastic glands are present, as in multiple endocrine neoplasia syndromes.

Malignancy

• In hypercalcemia of malignancy, unless effective chemotherapy can be offered, the prognosis is poor, with recurrent hypercalcemia and most patients dying within 6 months.

Follow-up and management

• Follow-up of the malignant disease is essential, to check for recurrence of hypercalcemia if the malignancy has not been cured.

Key references

1. Larsson K, *et al.*: The risk of hip fractures in patients with primary hyperparathyroidism: a population based cohort study with a follow-up of 19 years. *J Int Med* 1993, **234**:585–593.
2. Bilezikian JP: Management of hypercalcaemia. *J Clin Endocrinol Metab* 1993, **77**:1445–1449.
3. Heath DA: The treatment of hypercalcaemia of malignancy. *Clin Endocrinol* 1991, **34**:155–157.
4. Proceedings of the NIH Consensus Development Conference on diagnosis and management of asymptomatic primary hyperparathyroidism. Bethesda, Maryland, October 29–31, 1990. *J Bone Miner Res* 1991, **6(suppl 2)**:81–166.

Hyperglycemic emergencies

Diagnosis

Symptoms

Hyperglycemia

Polyuria, thirst, polydipsia.

Weight loss.

Lassitude, general malaise.

Decreasing level of consciousness.

Ketoacidosis

Nausea, vomiting, abdominal pain.

Dyspnea.

Precipitating cause

Symptoms of infection, myocardial infarction, or other illness.

Signs

General

Dehydration: particularly marked in hyperosmolar coma.

Hypotension.

Variable level of consciousness.

Signs of precipitating cause, especially fever: however, infection may be present in absence of fever in patients with ketoacidosis.

Ketoacidosis

Kussmaul's respiration, ketones on breath.

Peripheral vasodilatation, warm skin, tachycardia, generalized abdominal tenderness.

Investigations [1,2]

To rapidly establish diagnosis

Capillary blood glucose analysis.

Urinalysis: for glucose, ketones.

To confirm diagnosis

Laboratory blood glucose analysis.

Serum sodium, potassium, bicarbonate, phosphate, blood urea nitrogen, and creatinine measurement.

Arterial blood gas: if indicated.

To identify precipitating cause

Complete blood count: to look for anemia or leukocytosis.

Blood, urine, and throat cultures.

ECG: may show acute myocardial infarction or signs of electrolyte disturbance.

Chest radiography: may show infection or pulmonary edema.

Abdominal ultrasonography or paracentesis: to exclude acute abdominal disease if abdominal signs do not resolve quickly.

Complications

Cardiac arrest.

Thromboembolism: particularly if patient is hyperosmolar.

Aspiration pneumonia.

Renal failure.

Rhabdomyolysis: rare; may result from hypophosphatemia.

Differential diagnosis

Ketosis

Hyperventilation, chest infection, lactic acidosis, sepsis.

Acute abdominal disease.

Nonketotic

Hypercalcemia.

Cerebrovascular disease.

Thyrotoxicosis.

Etiology [2]

- Causes include the following (in both type I and II diabetes):

Initial presentation of diabetes.

Physical stressors, precipitating rise in counter-regulatory hormones and relative deficiency of insulin (*e.g.*, infection, myocardial infarction, stroke).

Omission of insulin.

Epidemiology

- Incidence not declining, despite advances in diabetes education.
- 3–8 episodes occur in 1000 diabetic patients each year.

Treatment

Diet and lifestyle

• Patients should be told not to stop insulin treatment if they become acutely ill. Instead, they should call their physician for "sick-day" management.

Pharmacological treatment [3]

• Rehydration and correction of electrolyte imbalance must begin immediately.

• A central venous pressure measurement may be a useful guide to fluid replacement in elderly patients or those with cardiac or renal disease.

• If the patient is comatose, a nasogastric tube should be passed.

• Urinary catheterization may be needed to allow accurate monitoring of urinary output.

Rehydration

0.9% saline solution, 1 L in first hour to restore circulating volume, raise blood pressure, and open renal circulation; then infusion rates should be adjusted as clinically indicated.

• 0.45% saline solution should be used if serum sodium is >155 mEq/L.

• Colloid solution can be given if the patient remains hypotensive.

Insulin

By continuous i.v. infusion (preferred): *if ketotic*: start at about 6 U/h by pump; *if nonketotic*: about 3–4 U/h.

• Adjustments in these insulin doses may be required in some patients.

• Treatment is continued until blood glucose is 250 mg/dL; then the dose of insulin should be halved, and i.v. infusion of 10% dextrose commenced at 80 mL/h.

Continue i.v. insulin therapy until serum bicarbonate has returned to near normal levels.

Potassium

• The total body deficit of potassium is often ~1000 mEq.

• Infusion should be started when serum potassium is <5.0 mEq/L and urine output has been demonstrated.

• Potassium chloride, 20–80 mEq/h, well diluted in rehydration fluid, should be given.

• Treatment should be monitored by serum potassium measurement (and ECG, if hyperkalemic).

Sodium bicarbonate

• This is rarely of benefit. It may be given if pH is <7.1.

• Typical dose is sodium bicarbonate, 100 mL 8.4% over 30 minutes.

Other options

Anticoagulation: low-dose s.c. heparin, if no contraindications; consider full-dose i.v. heparin if serum osmolality >360 mOsmol/kg.

Antibiotics: broad spectrum if there is any suspicion of infection.

• Replacement of other electrolytes (magnesium, phosphate) is rarely required.

Complications of treatment

• Most complications are avoidable with meticulous care and attention to detail.

Hypokalemia or hyperkalemia.

Hypoglycemia.

Fluid overload, especially in elderly patients.

Cerebral edema.

Acute respiratory distress syndrome.

Treatment aims

To save the patient's life.

To rehydrate the patient.

To restore acid-base and electrolyte balance to normal.

To achieve euglycemia in 24–48 hours.

Prognosis

• Mortality remains at 5%–15% in diabetic ketoacidosis and 30%–50% in hyperosmolar coma, even in experienced units.

• In elderly patients, the cause of death is often the underlying precipitating disorder rather than the metabolic upset.

Follow-up and management

Response to treatment

• Response should be monitored at the bedside (pulse, blood pressure, respiratory rate every 30–60 minutes, capillary glucose hourly) and in the laboratory (glucose, sodium, potassium, bicarbonate, creatinine, pH on admission and at 2-hour intervals until clinically stable).

Later management

• Patients should be given fluids or a light diet when able to eat, but i.v. insulin should be continued.

• When patients can tolerate oral intake, they should be transferred to s.c. insulin regimen that includes long-acting insulin.

• A 1–3-hour overlap must be allowed before i.v. insulin is discontinued, to allow time for s.c. absorption.

Follow-up

• The events leading to admission should be reviewed in an effort to educate the patient and prevent further admissions; all patients should be taught "sick-day" rules, including advice on seeking professional help early.

• Patients presenting in hyperosmolar coma may not need long-term insulin, but continuing it for a few weeks is probably safer, before stopping under close supervision.

Key references

1. Siperstein MD: Diabetic ketoacidosis and hyperosmolar coma. *Endocrinol Metab Clin North Am* 1992, **21**:415–432.
2. Marshall SM: Hyperglycaemic emergencies. *Care Crit Ill*, 1993, **9**:220–223.
3. Berger W, Keller U: Treatment of diabetic ketoacidosis and non-ketotic hyperosmolar coma. *Clin Endocrinol Metab* 1991, **6**:1–22.

Hyperkalemia & hypokalemia

Diagnosis

Symptoms

• Often no symptoms are manifest.

Hyperkalemia

Skeletal muscle weakness.

Diarrhea.

Hypokalemia

Muscle weakness and fatigue.

Polyuria and polydipsia.

Palpitations.

Signs

Hyperkalemia

Skeletal muscle weakness.

Irregular pulse.

Ileus.

Bradycardia, heart block, cardiac arrest (asystolic).

Hypokalemia

Postural hypotension.

Ileus.

Skeletal muscle weakness: rarely, respiratory distress.

Cardiac arrhythmias: atrial and ventricular premature beats, atrial or ventricular tachycardia.

Investigations

• Markedly abnormal potassium levels should be repeated immediately with optimal venipuncture technique and rapid transfer to laboratory.

Renal function tests: blood urea nitrogen, creatinine.

Electrocardiography.

Acid–base analysis.

Magnesium, phosphate, and glucose measurements.

Urinary potassium and pH measurement.

Creatine kinase measurement.

Complications

Hyperkalemia

Sudden death: asystole.

Hypokalemia

Rhabdomyolysis on vigorous exertion (acute).

Growth retardation in children.

Nephrogenic diabetes insipidus.

Negative nitrogen balance.

Interstitial nephritis: renal impairment.

Glucose intolerance.

Myocardial fibrosis.

Differential diagnosis

Artifact of sampling technique (hyperkalemia).

Etiology

Hyperkalemia

• The most common cause is a combination of renal impairment (may be minimal or transient) with the following:

Excessive potassium intake: due to diet, salt substitutes, potassium penicillins, transfusion of stored blood.

Redistribution: due to acidosis, exercise, hyperkalemic familial periodic paralysis, hormonal deficiencies (insulin, aldosterone, cortisol), drugs (beta-blockers, alpha-antagonists), release from damaged tissues, hyperosmolality.

Impaired renal excretion: due to acute or chronic renal failure, potassium-conserving diuretics, inadequate mineralocorticosteroid hormones, angiotensin-converting enzyme inhibitors, NSAIDs, cyclosporine, pentamidine, type IV renal tubular acidosis.

Hypokalemia

Inadequate intake: due to diet.

Redistribution: due to anabolic states, correction of severe anemia, transfusion of washed or frozen erythrocytes, metabolic alkalosis, some myeloproliferative disorders, beta-agonists, correction of hyperglycemia, hypokalemic periodic paralysis.

Gut losses: due to vomiting or nasogastric aspiration, diarrhea, purgative abuse.

Urinary losses: due to diuretics, hyperaldosteronism, Bartter's syndrome, Cushing's syndrome, licorice abuse, excess adrenocorticotropic hormone, renal tubular acidosis, tubular toxins (e.g., cisplatin, amphotericin, aminoglycosides), urinary diversion into gut, magnesium depletion.

Epidemiology

• Hyperkalemia rarely occurs without renal impairment.

• Hypokalemia is more common, being associated with the use of common drugs (diuretics and purgatives) and as a common complication of diarrheal states.

Treatment

Diet and lifestyle

• Hyperkalemic patients with underlying chronic renal failure need dietary advice to restrict the daily potassium intake to 40–60 mEq/day; high-potassium foods include fruits, chocolate, nuts, and instant coffee.

• Hypokalemia can rarely be corrected by dietary means.

Pharmacological treatment

For hyperkalemia: moderate

• For moderate hyperkalemia with an acute rise in potassium to <6.5 mEq/L and normal ECG results, the following measures should be taken:

Intake of potassium decreased.

Offending drug removed.

Good urinary output ensured.

Plasma potassium concentration measured every 6 hours to ensure falling values.

For hyperkalemia: severe

• An acute rise in potassium to >6.5 mEq/L and abnormal ECG results or chronically raised potassium >8 mEq/L is a medical emergency.

• ECG monitoring is needed.

• Rapid correction is vital.

• Emergency dialysis is needed if the patient is oliguric and volume overloaded.

Standard dosage	*Acute therapies:* 10% calcium gluconate solution, 10 mL i.v. slowly (*see* Special points *below*). 50% glucose solution 50 mL, containing insulin, 10 U, i.v. *Longer-term therapies:* 8.4% sodium bicarbonate solution, 50 mL i.v. only if acidotic. Sodium polystyrene sulfonate, 15 g, and lactulose, 10 mL orally every 6 hours *or* sodium polystyrene sulfonate by rectal retention enema if no ileus present. Furosemide or bumetanide i.v. every 4–6 hours to achieve urine flow rate >50 mL/h.
Contraindications	None.
Special points	Patient must be checked for hypoglycemia after i.v. glucose and insulin. *Calcium gluconate:* a cardioprotective agent, does *not* lower plasma potassium concentration.
Main drug interactions	None.
Main side effects	None.

For hypokalemia

Standard dosage	Effervescent potassium chloride, 80–200 mEq orally daily. Potassium chloride, 60–120 mEq i.v. over 24 hours.
Contraindications	None.
Special points	Oral supplements should be used whenever possible. Intravenous repletion is potentially dangerous: 10 mEq/h is usually safe; higher rates may be used, but ECG monitoring is essential. Potassium as chloride should be used in patients with alkalosis to minimize continued urinary losses of potassium.
Main drug interactions	Hypokalemia exacerbates digoxin toxicity.
Main side effects	Late hyperkalemia due to delayed gastrointestinal absorption after oral potassium supplements.

Treatment aims

To restore acid–base balance and plasma potassium slowly over 24–72 hours.

Prognosis

• Prognosis depends on the underlying condition.

Follow-up and management

• If deviations are gross, frequent and repeated measurements of plasma potassium are essential for several days.

General references

Androgue HJ, Wesson DE: Potassium. In *Blackwell's Basics of Medicine*. Oxford: Blackwell Scientific Publications; 1994.

Jacobsen HR, Rector FC (eds.): Renal regulation of extracellular fluid composition. *Kidney Int* 1990, **38**:569–743.

Schrier RW (ed.): *Renal and Electrolyte Disorders*, edn 4. Boston: Little Brown & Co; 1992.

Tannen RL: Potassium metabolism. In *Current Nephrology*, vol 15. Edited by Gonick HC. St Louis: Mosby Year Book; 1992:109–148.

Hypernatremia & hyponatremia

Diagnosis

Symptoms

• Symptoms depend on absolute sodium level and rate of change.

Hypernatremia

Restlessness.

Irritability.

Lethargy, somnolence.

Hyponatremia

Lethargy.

Confusion and disorientation.

Anorexia.

Nausea.

Muscle cramps, weakness.

Signs

Hypernatremia

Increased reflexes.

Increased muscle tone, fasciculations.

Depressed consciousness.

Convulsions.

Altered consciousness, coma.

Hyponatremia

Decreased reflexes.

Hypothermia.

Pseudobulbar palsy.

Convulsions.

Cheyne–Stokes respiration.

Altered consciousness, coma.

Investigations

• Disorders of sodium concentration reflect abnormalities in water handling.

• Most cases of hyponatremia are due to the action of antidiuretic hormone (ADH) on the distal nephron causing free water retention.

• Changes in serum sodium concentration reflect alterations in the sodium : water ratio in the extracellular fluid and can occur with increased, normal, or decreased total body fluid volume.

Detection of edema, estimation of jugular venous pressure, tissue turgor, erect and supine pulse and blood pressure, peripheral perfusion, auscultation of lung bases, and patient weighing: vital for accurate documentation of volume status; edema always indicates raised total body sodium.

Simultaneous plasma and urine electrolytes, BUN, creatinine, urine and plasma osmolality, chest radiography, ECG, liver function tests, albumin, uric acid, glucose measurement, endocrine tests (thyroid and adrenal); echocardiography if cardiac disease suspected.

Complications

Hypernatremia

Seizures

Shrinkage of brain cells.

Rupture of cerebral veins.

Cerebral venous (sinus) thrombosis.

Intracranial hemorrhage.

Hyponatremia

Seizures

Cerebral edema.

Raised intracranial pressure.

Herniation of brain stem.

Central pontine myelinolysis: attributed to over-rapid correction; causes permanent residual neurological deficits; rare.

Hypernatremia and hyponatremia are associated with increased morbidity and mortality, which may reflect severity of underlying illness.

Differential diagnosis

Hyperlipidemia or hyperproteinemia: may cause pseudohyponatremia; serum osmolarity in these patients will be normal.

Hyperglycemia: also causes pseudohyponatremia. To estimate the decrease in serum sodium, divide serum glucose by 62.

Etiology

Causes of hypernatremia

Normal or slightly reduced fluid volume: diabetes insipidus, dry ventilation, hypodipsia, sweating.

Increased fluid volume (edema): excessive sodium intake, excessive adrenocortical hormones.

Decreased fluid volume (without free access to water): excessive loss of sodium in urine, excessive loss of gastrointestinal secretions, burns, sweating.

Causes of hyponatremia

Normal or slightly expanded fluid volume: excessive water intake, syndrome of inappropriate antidiuretic hormone secretion (SIADH), hypothyroidism, glucocorticoid deficiency.

Increased fluid volume (edema): acute or chronic renal failure, cardiac failure, cirrhosis with ascites, nephrotic syndrome, pregnancy.

Decreased fluid volume (with free access to water): excessive loss of sodium in urine, excessive loss of gastrointestinal secretions, burns, sweating, hydrochlorthigide.

Epidemiology

• Hypernatremia is common in the elderly and in immobile or unconscious patients, all of whom may lack access to water.

• Hyponatremia is common in hospitals because of inappropriate fluid replacement, usually with hypotonic solutions (or those containing dextrose or an osmole, which is metabolized rapidly, leaving free water).

Treatment

Diet and lifestyle

- Hypernatremia and hyponatremia usually develop in hospitals; thus, the primary underlying disease dominates the clinical picture.
- Alterations in sodium and fluid intake are needed for patients with changes in their extracellular fluid volume, *e.g.*, sodium restriction for those with edema.
- Compulsive water drinkers and drug abusers may need psychiatric consultation.
- Fluid restriction for SIADH.

Pharmacological treatment

Hypernatremia

- Extracellular fluid volume must first be defined and corrected; a decrease should be corrected by normal saline solution, an increase by diuretics or dialysis.
- Then the hypernatremia can be corrected *slowly* orally, per NG, or intravenously, including dextrose, dextrose with saline, or 0.9% saline solution, giving about half of the calculated volume replacement over the first 24 hours.
- If rapid correction required, correction should not exceed 1–2 mmol/L/h until symptoms resolve; then correct slowly over 24–48 h.
- Central venous pressure monitoring and urethral catheterization for monitoring urine output may be needed.

Hyponatremia

- For mild to moderate chronic dilutional hyponatremia, restriction of water intake alone may be sufficient.
- For edematous states and SIADH, loop diuretics (avoid thiazides) may need to be given in addition to water restriction.
- Patients with severe symptomatic hyponatremia may require administration of 3% hypertonic saline (without diuretics) solution infused slowly, to correct serum sodium concentrations—over-rapid correction may cause brain damage (hyponatremia should be corrected by 1.5–2 mEq/h if acute onset or ≤1 mEq/h if chronic). Serum sodium should be frequently monitored, and saline infusion discontinued when serum sodium reaches 120–125 mEq/L.
- Administration of sodium to edematous patients may precipitate cardiac failure; diuretics may be needed to normalize intravascular volume.
- In severe cases, central venous pressure monitoring and urethral catheterization to monitor urine output are needed.
- Resistant cases of hyponatremia in SIADH not responsive to fluid restriction may require declocycline (600–1200 mg/d).

Treatment aims

To correct extracellular fluid volume.

To correct serum sodium concentration.

To avoid morbidity secondary to rapid changes in serum sodium or ECFV.

Prognosis

- Prognosis depends on the underlying condition.
- Acute changes in onset or correction are more dangerous than slow changes.
- Very old or very young patients are most vulnerable.
- Permanent neurological deficits are common, especially if correction is over-rapid.

Follow-up and management

- Follow-up depends on the underlying condition.

General references

Fried LF, Palevsky PM: Hyponatremia and hypernatremia. *Med Clin North Am* 1997, **81**:585–609.

Lauriat SM: The hyponatremic patient: practical focus on therapy. *J Am Soc Nephrol* 1997, 1599–1607.

Palevsky PM: Hypernatremia. *Med Clin North Am* 1998, **18**:20–30.

Richardson RMA: Water metabolism. In *Current Nepphrology*, vol 15. Edited by Gonick HC. St Louis: Mosby Year Book; 1992:149–206.

Schrier RW: Body fluid volume regulation in health and disease: a unifying hypothesis. *Ann intern Med* 1990, **113**:155–159.

Spital A: Diuretic-induced hyponatremia. *Am J Nephrol* 1999, **19**:447–452.

Sterns Rh: Central nervous system complications of hyponatremia. In *International year Book of Nephrology*. Edited by Andreucci VE, Fine LG. Berlin: Springer-Verlag; 1992:55–74

Sodium. *Lancet* 1998, **22**:220–228.

Hyperprolactinemia

Diagnosis

Symptoms

• Symptoms can be subdivided into those directly related to hyperprolactinemia and those due to the mass effect of a pituitary macroadenoma (if present).

Hyperprolactinemia

Galactorrhea.

Amenorrhea, oligomenorrhea: in women.

Impotence: in men.

Infertility.

Reduced libido.

Macroadenoma

Headache.

Visual field defect: typically bitemporal hemianopia or diplopia.

Convulsions: temporal-lobe epilepsy due to local extension of tumor (rare).

Cerebrovascular accident: rare.

Signs

Macroadenoma

Hypopituitarism.

Optic atrophy: if tumor compressing optic nerve.

Loss of secondary sexual characteristics, postural hypotension, hypothyroidism, delayed or arrested puberty: signs of hypopituitarism.

Investigations [1,2]

Detailed drug history.

Serum prolactin measurement: thyroid-releasing hormone and other dynamic stimulation tests are of no value.

Thyroid function tests: hypothyroidism is a cause of raised serum prolactin.

Gonadotropin and gonadal steroids measurement: to determine if hypogonadism is present.

Pituitary MRI or CT: to identify tumor.

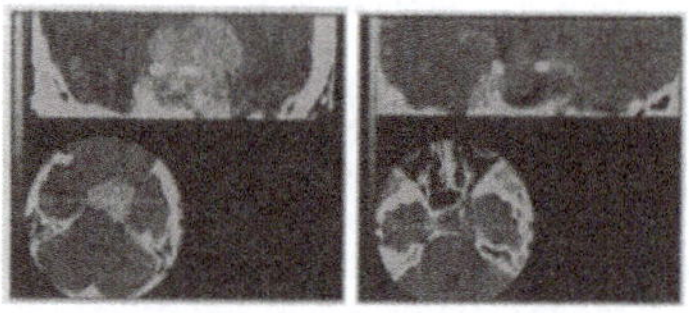

Axial and coronal view of large prolactinoma (*left*). Repeat scan (*right*) showing virtual disappearance of tumor on treatment by bromocriptine.

If macroadenoma is present

Visual field study.

Assess for possible adrenal insufficiency and/or hypothyroidism (*see* Hypopituitarism).

Dynamic pituitary function testing.

Complications

Hyperprolactinemia

Infertility, impotence.

Osteoporosis: due to hypogonadism.

Macroadenoma

Hydrocephalus.

Blindness.

Hypopituitarism.

Cranial nerve palsy.

Differential diagnosis

Prolactinoma: prolactin levels usually >150 mg/mL.

• Other causes of hyperprolactinemia (prolactin usually <150 ng/mL) include:

Hypothyroidism.

Medication (prolactin usually <150 ng/mL): substituted benzamides (metoclopropamide, sulpiride), phenothiazines, butyrophenones, reserpine, methyldopa, verapamil.

Compression of the pituitary stalk by other hypothalamic or pituitary tumors, thereby reducing transport of prolactin-inhibiting factors (primary dopamine) to the pituitary.

Stress: *e.g.*, venipuncture, epilepsy.

Breast stimulation.

Chest wall processes (tumor, herpes zoster).

Etiology [1,2]

• Prolactinomas are monoclonal tumors that secrete prolactin.

• Increased levels of estrogen (*e.g.*, oral contraceptives, pregnancy) may stimulate prolactinoma growth.

Epidemiology

• Prolactinomas occur much more often in women than in men.

Treatment

Diet and lifestyle

• Prolactinoma therapy will restore fertility to many women. Therefore, counseling regarding contraception is very important.

Pharmacological treatment [1–4]

Standard dosage Bromocriptine, 1.25 mg initially, in the middle of a snack last thing at night; dose titrated against serum prolactin. Cabergoline, 0.25 mg twice weekly, slowly increased to 1.0 mg twice weekly [5]. Recently approved for treatment of prolactinomas; major advantage is twice-weekly dosing.

Contraindications Toxemia of pregnancy, sensitivity to ergot alkaloid, history of psychosis.

Special points An alternative dopamine agonist in cases of bromocriptine or cabergoline intolerance or resistance is pergolide. However, pergolide is not specifically approved for the treatment of hyperprolactinemia.

Main drug interactions None.

Main side effects Gastrointestinal disturbance, particularly nausea; postural hypotension; first-dose hypotension (effect negated by drugs that raise prolactin concentration).

Special considerations

Oral contraceptive use

• Estrogens can stimulate prolactinoma growth. If oral contraceptives are used, prolactin levels should be monitored. If they rise, or patients develop symptoms of pituitary enlargement, then a pituitary MRI, visual fields, or both, should be obtained. Low-dose oral contraceptives (ethinyl estradiol, ≤30 μg daily) are preferred, and physicians should have a low threshold for discontinuing oral contraceptives if complications develop.

Pregnancy

• Neither prolactinoma nor bromocriptine therapy is an absolute contraindication to pregnancy. Prolactin rises normally during pregnancy, and may therefore be misleading in pregnant patients with pre-existing hyperprolactinemia. Instead, patients with prolactinomas should be followed closely for evidence of pituitary enlargement (*e.g.*, visual field abnormalities). Bromocriptine is not approved for use during pregnancy and should be discontinued if possible.

Treatment aims

To normalize serum prolactin concentration.
To retain normal pituitary function.

Other treatments [1,2]

Transsphenoidal surgery: typically reserved for patients who either fail therapy with dopamine agonists or have symptoms secondary to tumor mass. Resection of a microadenoma can be curative, and some authors believe this a viable alternative to long-term bromocriptine agonist therapy.
Pituitary radiotherapy: adjunct to surgery and medical therapy; associated with significant risk of long-term panhypopituitarism.

Prognosis

• 15%–20% of microprolactinomas resolve during long-term dopamine agonist treatment.
• 40% of patients with macroadenomas have normal serum prolactinomas after transsphenoidal hypophysectomy.

Follow-up and management

• Patients should be maintained on the minimum dose of bromocriptine necessary to normalize serum prolactin concentrations.
• Bromocriptine may be stopped every 2 years and serum prolactin concentration checked.
• Long-term follow-up is necessary.

Key references

1. Aron DC, Tyrrell JB, Wilson CB: Pituitary tumors: current concepts in diagnosis and management. *West J Med* 1995, **162**:340–352.
2. Cunnah D, Besser GM: Management of prolactinomas. *Clin Endocrinol* 1991, **34**:231–235.
3. Jones TH: The management of hyperprolactinemia. *Br J Hosp Med* 1995, **53**:374–378.
4. Faglia G: Should dopamine agonist treatment for prolactinomas be life-long? *Clin Endocrinol* 1991, **34**:173–174.
5. Webster J, *et al.*: A comparison of cabergoline and bromocriptine in the treatment of hyperprolactinemic amenorrhea. Cabergoline Comparative Study Group. *N Engl J Med* 1994, **331**:904–909.

Diagnosis

Symptoms

• Patients are usually symptomless; hypertension is discovered at opportunistic or organized screening visits or detected after a hypertensive complication has intervened (myocardial infarction, cardiovascular accident, peripheral vascular disease, heart failure).

• Patients should be asked about symptoms of underlying causes of hypertension, *e.g.*, flushing and palpitations with pheochromocytoma, also other endocrine causes.

Headaches: occasionally.

Poor vision, shortness of breath, angina: rare.

Signs

Uncomplicated mild hypertension

• No signs other than raised blood pressure are manifest.

Moderate to severe hypertension

Displaced forceful apex beat, fourth heart sound, left atrial lift: signs of cardiac hypertrophy.

Silver wire arterioles, arteriovenous nipping, hemorrhages, exudates, papilledema.

Hypertensive complications

Signs of heart failure, renal failure, peripheral vascular disease, strokes.

Underlying causes (much less common than essential hypertension)

Signs of Cushing's syndrome, renal artery stenosis, aortic coarctation, pheochromocytoma, acromegaly, Conn's syndrome.

Investigations

Blood pressure measurement: to confirm diagnosis; repeated over several visits or by ambulatory monitoring.

Chest radiography: for coarctation, *e.g.*, rib-notching and double aortic shadow.

Renal function and electrolyte analysis: to check for renal failure, low potassium in Conn's syndrome.

Urine microscopy: for hematuria, casts, proteinuria in nephritis.

24-hour urinary catecholamines, metanephrines, vanillylmandelic acid analysis: for pheochromocytoma.

Ultrasonography of kidneys: show small scarred kidneys of pyelonephritis or end-stage renovascular disease; obstructive nephropathy.

Nuclear renography or renal angiography: for renal artery stenosis.

Endocrine tests: for Cushing's syndrome, acromegaly, thyroid disease.

ECG or echocardiography: for left ventricular hypertrophy in patients with moderate to severe hypertension.

Microalbuminuria measurement: for kidney damage in patients with moderate to severe hypertension.

Complications

Atrial fibrillation, ischemic heart disease, heart failure.

Peripheral vascular disease.

Nephrosclerosis, renovascular disease, renal failure.

Transient ischemic attacks, cardiovascular accidents, encephalopathy.

Hemorrhage, infarction, papilledema, blindness.

Differential diagnosis

"White-coat" hypertension.

Pseudohypertension.

Etiology

• In most patients, no cause is found (essential hypertension).

• Underlying causes include the following:

Renal artery stenosis, nephritis, obstructive uropathy.

Coarctation.

Pheochromocytoma, Cushing's syndrome, Conn's syndrome, acromegaly, thyroid disease.

Cyclosporine, steroids, NSAIDs.

Pre-eclampsia, occasional autonomic neuropathy.

Epidemiology

• The frequency of hypertension depends on diagnostic cut-off levels of blood pressure: 10%–15% of the adult population have hypertension, increasing with age.

• Incidence and associations differ in non-white populations: *e.g.*, with insulin resistance in Asians, low-renin hypertension in Afro-Caribbeans.

Treatment

Diet and lifestyle

• Weight reduction if overweight.

• Reduce sodium intake to no more than 100 mmol/d (2.4 g sodium or 6 g sodium chloride).

• Maintain adequate intake of dietary potassium (approximately 90 mmol/d).

Maintain adequate intake of dietary calcium and magnesium.

Reduce intake of dietary saturated fat and cholesterol.

Limit alcohol intake to no more than 1 oz ethanol per day (1–2 drinks per day) or 0.5 oz ethanol per day for women and lower-weight people.

Increase aerobic physical activity (30–45 minutes most days of the week).

Pharmacological treatment

• Patients who have high-normal blood pressure as well as renal insufficiency, heart failure, or diabetes mellitus should be considered for prompt pharmacological therapy.

Initial therapy

• A low-dose diuretic (*e.g.*, 6.25 mg of hydrochlorothiazide) and/or a β-blocker should be chosen as initial therapy unless there are compelling or specific indications for another drug.

• In type I diabetes mellitus, start therapy with angiotensin-converting enzyme (ACE) inhibitor if proteinuria is present.

• In heart failure, start therapy with ACE inhibitor or diuretic.

• In myocardial infarction, start β-blocker therapy (non-ISA).

• In isolated systolic hypertension or in older patients, diuretics are preferred and long-acting dihydropyridine calcium antagonists may be considered.

Special points

• Low-dose diuretics with an ACE inhibitor and a nondihydropyridine calcium antagonist may reduce proteinuria more than either drug alone.

• Combinations of a dihydropyridine calcium antagonist and an ACE inhibitor induce less pedal edema than does the calcium antagonist alone.

• Immediate-release nifedipine has precipitated ischemic events and in large doses may increase coronary mortality in patients who have had a myocardial infarction. Therefore, this agent is best avoided.

• ACE inhibitors should be avoided in hypertension because of bilateral renal artery stenosis.

• Drugs with similar modes of action may provide additive effects, such as metolazone and a loop diuretic in renal failure.

• Angiotensin II receptor blockers should be used primarily in patients in whom ACE inhibitors are indicated but who cannot tolerate them.

• Neither sex nor age usually affects responsiveness to various agents.

• Direct-acting smooth-muscle vasodilators (*e.g.*, hydralazine hydrochloride, minoxidil), central α-agonists (*e.g.*, reserpine), and peripheral adrenergic antagonists are not well suited for initial monotherapy because they produce annoying adverse effects in many patients.

• In general, hypertension in African-American patients is more responsive to monotherapy with diuretics and calcium antagonists than to β-blockers or ACE inhibitors. However, if a β-blocker or ACE inhibitor is needed for other therapeutic benefits, differences in efficacy usually can be overcome with reduction of salt intake, higher doses of the drug, or addition of diuretic. Because of their greater prevalence of stage 3 hypertension, many African-American patients require multidrug therapy.

• If hypertension develops in a woman taking oral contraceptives, it is advisable to stop use.

Treatment aims

In uncomplicated hypertension, to achieve and maintain systolic blood pressure below 140 mm Hg and diastolic blood pressure below 90 mm Hg (lower if tolerated.)

In hypertensive patients with diabetes, renal failure, or heart failure, to achieve and maintain systolic blood pressure below 130 mm Hg and diastolic blood pressure below 85 mm Hg (lower if tolerated).

In hypertensive patients with renal failure and proteinuria (>1 g/24 hours), to achieve and maintain systolic blood pressure below 125 mm Hg and diastolic blood pressure below 75 mm Hg (lower if tolerated).

Prognosis

• Prognosis is excellent if blood pressure is controlled (almost always possible).

Follow-up and management

• Follow-up must be for life.

General references

The Sixth Report of the Joint National Committee on Prevention, Detection, Evaluation, and Treatment of High Blood Pressure. Bethesda, MD: U.S. Department of Health and Human Services, National Institutes of Health; 1997: NIH publication no. 98-4080.

Hyperthyroidism

Diagnosis

Symptoms

Weight loss, fatigue, sweating, heat intolerance, neck swelling.

Palpitations, shortness of breath.

Tremor, weakness, nervousness.

Increased frequency of bowel movements.

Staring, gritty eyes, swelling around eyes.

- Classic symptoms and signs may be absent in elderly patients.

Signs

Goiter: diffuse, with or without bruit, nodular, solitary nodule.

Fine tremor, proximal myopathy.

Lid retraction, lid lag, periorbital puffiness, chemosis, proptosis, corneal ulceration, ophthalmoplegia.

Sinus tachycardia, atrial fibrillation, cardiac failure.

Pretibial myxedema, palmar erythema, acropachy (finger clubbing).

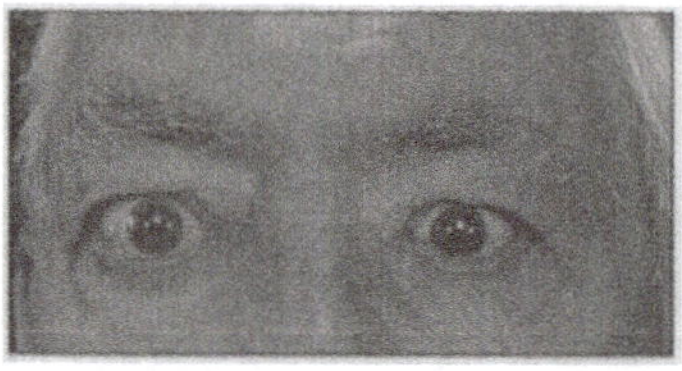

Periorbital edema, mild lid retraction and chemosis in a patient with Graves' ophthalmopathy. (*See Color Plate.*)

Investigations

Serum thyroid hormone measurements: free thyroxine (T_4) and total triiodothyronine (T_3) should be measured initially; T_3 may be elevated out of proportion to free T_4 in some patients (T_3-toxicosis).

Serum thyroid-stimulating hormone (TSH) measurement: undetectable in hyperthyroidism; normal value excludes primary hyperthyroidism.

Autoantibody tests: antithyroid peroxidase and antithyroglobulin antibodies are elevated in many forms of thyroid disease, including Graves' disease. Presence of anti-TSH receptor antibodies is diagnostic for Graves' disease.

Radioisotope scanning and uptake measurements: ^{99m}Tc scintigraphy distinguishes Graves' disease from toxic nodular goiter. Increased uptake of ^{131}I confirms hyperthyroidism, low uptake suggests thyroiditis.

Thyroid-releasing hormone stimulation test: rarely of use with advent of sensitive TSH assays.

Complications

Cardiac disease: especially atrial fibrillation and congestive cardiac failure (more common in elderly patients).

Reduced bone density and increased risk of osteoporotic fractures.

Graves' ophthalmopathy: may be progressive and occasionally sight-threatening because of corneal ulceration or optic nerve compression [1].

Differential diagnosis

Psychiatric disorders: e.g., anxiety.

Anemia.

Malignancy.

Pheochromocytoma.

Alcohol withdrawal.

Excess caffeine intake.

Etiology [2]

Common causes (95% of patients)

Graves' disease.

Toxic nodular goiter: single or multinodular.

Thyroiditis: subacute, silent, postpartum.

Uncommon causes

Exogenous iodide: kelp ingestion, amiodarone, radiographic contrast agents.

Factitious: ingestion of thyroid hormones.

Inappropriate secretion of TSH by pituitary: TSH-secreting tumor, thyroid hormone resistance syndromes.

Neonatal hyperthyroidism: baby born to mother with history of Graves' disease.

Epidemiology

- The prevalence of hyperthyroidism is ~20 in 1000 females and ~2 in 1000 males.
- Toxic nodular goiter is part of a spectrum of endemic or sporadic goiter, often found in patients with a long history of goiter; the peak incidence is at ~60 years.

Treatment

Diet and lifestyle

• Increased iodine intake may precipitate hyperthyroidism in patients with euthyroid goiter.
• Cigarette smoking significantly increases the risk of ophthalmopathy in Graves' disease.

Pharmacological treatment [2]

Beta-adrenergic blockers

• Beta-andergenic blockers are recommended for patients with moderate or severe symptoms until serum thyroid hormones have returned to normal; often they are the only treatment needed for thyroiditis.
• They provide quick symptomatic relief of tremor and palpitations resulting from sympathetic overactivity.

Standard dosage	Propranolol, 20–80 mg 3 times daily (higher dose may be needed because of increased first-pass metabolism). Atenolol, 50–100 mg daily.
Contraindications	Asthma, obstructive pulmonary disease; caution in heart failure, even if induced by hyperthyroidism.
Main drug interactions	*See Manufacturer's current prescribing information.*
Main side effects	*See Manufacturer's current prescribing information.*

Thionamides [3]

• Both thionamide and radioactive iodine are acceptable therapies for Graves' disease.
• Thionamides can be used as first-line treatment in patients with Graves' hyperthyroidism or as short-term treatment before radioiodine treatment.
• They produce biochemical improvement and symptomatic relief within 2 months in most patients; a full course of 18 months is important to allow remission of disease.

Standard dosage	Methimazole, 30 mg single daily dose at diagnosis, reduced to maintenance dose of 5–10 mg. Propylthiouracil, 100 mg 2–3 times daily at diagnosis, reduced to maintenance dose of 50–100 mg 1–2 times daily.
Contraindications	Thionamide-induced agranulocytosis, hepatitis, or other serious side effects.
Main drug interactions	No major interactions.
Main side effects	Agranulocytosis (rare; patients should stop a fever, sore throat, or other infection); hepatitis, cholestatic jaundice, lupus-like syndromes (rare but serious); skin rashes, nausea, arthralgia (common but not serious).

Radioiodine

• Radioiodine treatment must be done under specialist supervision.
• It is often used as first-line therapy for Graves' disease and is the treatment of choice for patients who fail thionamide therapy. It can be used in patients with small toxic adenomas (<3 cm) and in some patients with toxic multinodular goiter.

Standard dosage	Radioiodine single dose initially; second dose after 4–6 months if hyperthyroidism not cured; larger initial doses for elderly patients or those with severe disease to produce rapid effect and induce hypothyroidism.
Contraindications	Pregnancy (standard of care is to avoid pregnancy for 6 months following treatment), breast-feeding, hyperthyroidism secondary to thyroiditis; caution in patients with active ophthalmopathy.
Special points	Thionamides should be withdrawn at least 4 days before treatment. They can be restarted 4 days after treatment. Can exacerbate hyperthyroidism; rarely induce "thyroid storm."
Main drug interactions	None.
Main side effects	Hypothyroidism (>50% within 10 years of treatment), is often the intended outcome in patients with Graves' disease.

Alternative medicine

Recommended use: None.

Common use:kelp; bugle weed/Virginia (*Lycopus virginicus*); gypsy wart (*Lycopus europaeus*); cabbage juice; motherwort (*Leonurus cardicaca*).

Caution: None.

Treatment aims

To relieve symptoms.
To restore thyroxine, triiodothyronine, and TSH values to normal range.
To obtain long-term euthyroidism.

Other treatments

Partial thyroidectomy: for Graves' disease in patients with thyroid storm or large goiters causing compressive symptoms.
Surgery is used in some patients with toxic nodules.
• Patients should be rendered euthyroid before surgery by thionamides, beta-blocker, and possibly potassium iodide.

Prognosis

• Only 30% of patients with Graves' hyperthyroidism remain euthyroid in the long term after a course of thionamide; 15% become hypothyroid even without treatment.
• Medium-dosed radioiodine treatment and partial thyroidectomy are each associated with a 50% risk of permanent hypothyroidism; larger doses ablate the thyroid with rapid and permanent hypothyroidism.

Follow-up and management

• Serum-free thyroxine and thyroid-stimulating hormone concentration initially should be monitored every 4 weeks in patients on thionamides and every 3 months in those on maintenance doses.
• Thyroid function should be checked annually after resolution of disease.

Management of hyperthyroidism in pregnancy

• Radioactive iodine contraindicated during pregnancy; it can cause permanent destruction of fetal thyroid gland, resulting in neonatal hypothyroidism.
• Thionamides are the most appropriate agents; propythiouracil is preferred (crosses placenta less than methimazole, excreted less in breast milk).
• Dosage must be adjusted to maintain serum thyroxine at upper end of normal range (cause fetal goiter and hypothyroidism in high dose).
• Low doses needed in Graves' hyperthyroidism.
• Relapse is frequent after delivery.

Key references

1. Fells P: Thyroid-associated eye disease: clinical management. *Lancet* 1991, 338:29–32.
2. Franklyn JA: The management of hyperthyroidism. *N Engl J Med* 1994, 330:1731–1738.
3. Reinwein D, *et al.*: A prospective randomised trial of antithyroid drug dose in Graves' disease therapy. *J Clin Endocrinol Metab* 1993, **76**:1516–1521.

Hypertrophic cardiomyopathy

Diagnosis

Definition

The World Health Organization defined hypertrophic cardiomyopathy as left or right ventricular hypertrophy, which is usually asymmetric and involves the interventricular septum.

Symptoms

• Patients may be asymptomatic.

Severe cardiac failure: in infants.

Premature unexpected death: may be symptom in children or young adults.

Dyspnea on exertion: in ~50% of patients.

Chest pain: in ~50%; may be exertional or occur at rest.

Syncope: in 15%–25%.

Dizziness, palpitations.

Signs

• In patients without outflow tract gradient, abnormalities may be subtle.

Pulse

Rapid upstroke arterial pulse: best felt in carotid area.

Heart

Forceful left ventricular impulse: best appreciated on full held expiration in left lateral position.

Ejection systolic murmur: best heard at left sternal border; radiating toward aortic and mitral areas but not into neck.

Palpable atrial beat: reflecting forceful atrial systolic contraction.

Investigations

Two-dimensional echocardiography: to assess left ventricle structure and function, gradients, valvular regurgitation, and atrial dimensions. Classic findings include systolic anterior motion of mitral valve, asymmetric hypertrophy.

ECG: may be normal in < 5% of patients or show abnormalities reflecting left ventricular hypertrophy, atrial fibrillation, left axis deviation, right bundle branch block, and myocardial disarray; bizarre or abnormal findings in young patients should raise suspicion of hypertrophic cardiomyopathy, especially if a family member is affected.

Chest radiography: may be normal or show left or right atrial or left ventricular enlargement.

Treadmill exercise test with maximum oxygen ventilatory capacity: simple and noninvasive; provides useful functional information; maximum oxygen ventilatory capacity often moderately reduced; one-third of patients have abnormal blood pressure response, with drops of 25–150 mm Hg from peak systolic recordings; ST segment changes of > 2 mm documented in 25%, associated with symptoms of angina.

48-hour Holter monitoring: arrhythmias common during ECG monitoring; established atrial fibrillation in ~10% of patients, paroxysmal supraventricular arrhythmias in 30%, non-sustained ventricular tachycardia in 25%; ventricular tachycardia in 25%; ventricular tachycardia invariably asymptomatic during Holter monitoring, but most useful risk marker of sudden death in adults; sustained supraventricular arrhythmias often symptomatic and predispose to thromboembolic complications.

Thallium scintigraphy: fixed and reversible perfusion defects common, useful to assess ischemia.

Cardiac catheterization and left ventriculography: invasive evaluation not needed for diagnosis, but coronary arteriography often necessary in older patients with angina to exclude coronary artery disease; endomyocardial biopsy possibly necessary to exclude specific heart muscle disorder but has no other role in diagnosis because of patchy nature of myofiber disarray.

Complications

Sudden death; atrial fibrillation; infective endocarditis; systemic embolism.

Differential diagnosis

Aortic valve disease.

Systemic hypertension.

Etiology

• Hypertrophic cardiomyopathy is an autosomal dominant heart muscle disorder.

• Mutations in the gene encoding contractile proteins cause disease in 50–60% of patients.

• Due to mutations in the gene encoding for myofibrillary proteins; at least nine individual genes have been identified. β-heavy-chain myosin gene mutations are associated with left ventricular outflow obstruction, troponin T mutations are associated with modest left ventricular wall thickening, and mutations in myosin binding protein C are associated with onset in late adult life. Arginine gene mutations have a worse prognosis than leucine gene mutations.

Pathology

Macroscopic: asymmetric or symmetric increase in left ventricular wall thickness with a left ventricular cavity that is smaller.

Histologic: Myocyte disarray.

Pathophysiology

Systolic: hyperdynamic contraction; left ventricular outflow gradient (30%, associated mitral regurgitation).

Diastolic: impaired relaxation, impaired filling, decreased compliance.

Epidemiology

• The male:female ratio is equal, although the disease tends to affect younger men and older women.

• In children and adolescents, myocardial hypertrophy often occurs during growth spurts; a negative diagnosis made before adolescent growth has been completed must be tempered by the proviso of subsequent reassessment.

• Myocardial hypertrophy does not ordinarily progress after adolescent growth is completed.

• Sudden death can occur at any age, from childhood to 90 years, in persons who have been asymptomatic all their life. The annual mortality from sudden death is 3%–5% in adults and at least 6% in children and young adults.

• First-degree relatives of affected patients have a 50% chance of carrying the disease gene; they should be investigated by ECG and two-dimensional echocardiography.

Treatment

Diet and lifestyle

- Competitive exercise is not recommended in high-risk patients.
- Dehydration should be avoided.

Pharmacological treatment

- ***β-blockers:*** Symptomatic patients with obstructive cardiomyopathy should be given large doses of β-blockers: ~200 to 400 mg of propranolol per day or equivalent. Selective β-blockers lose their selectivity at high doses, so there is little to be gained by using them.
- ***Calcium-channel blockers:*** added to β-blockers to control symptoms. Verapamil in dosages of 240–320 mg/d may be used. These agents must be used cautiously in patients with large outflow tract obstruction because acute hemodynamic deterioration may result from peripheral vasodilatation.
- ***Anti-arrhythmics:*** Disopyramide may also be used but frequently causes urinary retention in men and causes dry mouth. It does not improve the diastolic dysfunction characteristic of the disorder in men. Amiodarone is used to control supraventricular and ventricular arrhythmias and may improve survival in adults with nonsustained ventricular tachycardia.

Nonpharmacological treatment

Surgical myomectomy

- In patients with left ventricular outflow tract obstruction, this alleviates symptoms and improves hemodynamics.
- Perioperative mortality is high, at 5%–10%.

Dual-chamber pacing

- Results in substantial reduction of gradient acutely and by a remodeling effect that further decreases the gradient long term.
- Ideal candidates are symptomatic, have resting obstruction, and are elderly.

Cardiac transplantation

- Transplantation is limited to patients who develop severe systolic dysfunction.

Treatment aims

To improve symptoms.

To prevent complications.

To prevent sudden death.

Prognosis

- Poor prognostic factors for sudden death include:

Nonsustained ventricular tachycardia (best predictor).

Family history of sudden death or syncope.

Recurrent syncope.

Abnormal blood pressure response to exercise.

Young age at presentation.

Male sex.

Follow-up and management

- Patients must be monitored for disease progression and risk of complications.
- All first-degree relatives should undergo screening with echocardiography, and younger affected members of the family should have genetic counseling if they plan to have a family.
- Antibiotics should be given prophylactically before medical and dental procedures to prevent infective endocarditis.

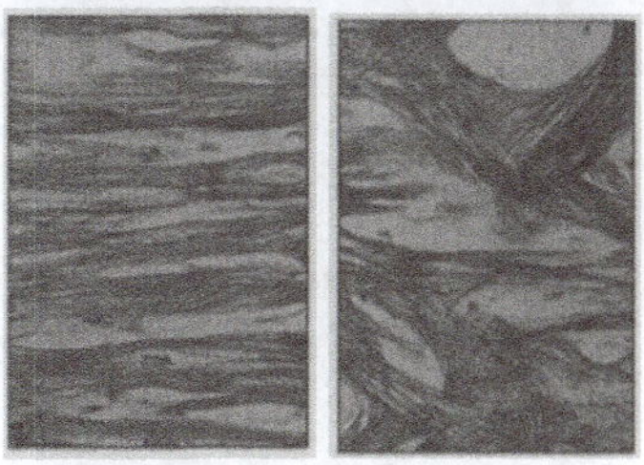

Myofibrillar stain from a normal person (*left*) and one with myocardial disarray (*right*). (See Color Plates.)

General references

Spirito P, *et al.*: The management of hypertrophic cardiomyopathy. *N Engl J Med* 1997, 336:775.

Watkins H: Sudden death in hypertrophic cardiomyopathy. *N Engl J Med* 2000, 342:422.

Hypocalcemia

Diagnosis

Symptoms

Paresthesia: especially around face, hands, and feet.

Tetany: causing painful cramps culminating in hands going into tetanic spasm position.

Seizures.

Bone pain: common in vitamin D deficiency.

Signs

- Mild hypocalcemia may be asymptomatic; signs are due to neuromuscular irritability.

Twitching of local facial muscles: after tapping over facial nerve in front of and below ear; Chvostek's sign (positive in some normal people, rarely in those with hypokalemia).

Development of tetanic spasm (Trousseau's sign): after inflation of a sphygmomanometer cuff on arm (a painful procedure and not recommended).

Proximal myopathy: common in vitamin D deficiency.

Obesity, "moon" face, shortened metacarpals and metatarsals: signs of pseudohypoparathyroidism.

Investigations [1]

Serum calcium measurement (total or ionized): low concentration.

Serum phosphorus measurement: low concentration in vitamin D deficiency, high in hypoparathyroidism, pseudohypoparathyroidism, and renal failure.

Serum creatinine measurement: raised concentration in renal failure.

Serum alkaline phosphatase measurement: often raised concentration in vitamin D deficiency.

Serum magnesium measurement: low concentration can cause hypocalcemia.

Serum parathyroid hormone measurement: raised concentration in vitamin D deficiency, pseudohypoparathyroidism, and renal failure; low concentration in patients with hypoparathyroidism.

Vitamin D level measurement.

Radiography: of wrists and knees in suspected rickets, chest and pelvis in suspected osteomalacia.

Complications

Epilepsy.

Cataracts and basal ganglia calcification: in longstanding hypocalcemia.

Differential diagnosis

Previous neck surgery.

Hypomagnesemia, especially if patient is an alcoholic, has extensive small-bowel disease or resection, or is on aminoglycoside drugs or cisplatinum.

Etiology [2]

Low plasma proteins (not true hypocalcemia as ionized calcium is normal).

Acute or chronic renal failure.

Vitamin D deficiency.

Hypoparathyroidism: usually after neck surgery, rarely idiopathic.

Pseudohypoparathyroidism.

Hypomagnesemia.

Severe acute pancreatitis.

Malabsorption.

Epidemiology

- Hypocalcemia is manifest most often at times of increased calcium shifts (*i.e.*, neonatal period, growth spurt, and pregnancy).

Treatment

Diet and lifestyle

• Patients should have an adequate calcium intake (800–2000 mg daily of elemental calcium).

• Vitamin D supplementation should be considered if exposure to sunlight is inadequate.

Pharmacological treatment [1]

For acute symptomatic hypocalcemia

Standard dosage	10% calcium gluconate, 10 mL i.v. slowly, followed by 50–100 mL i.v. in 1 L saline solution over 24 hours at a rate to relieve symptoms.
Contraindications	None.
Main drug interactions	None.
Main side effects	Tissue necrosis (if extravasation outside vein).

For hypoparathyroidism

Standard dosage	Calcitriol, 0.5–1.0 μg orally daily, plus adequate calcium intake.
Contraindications	None.
Special points	Regular serum calcium monitoring.
Main drug interactions	None.
Main side effects	Hypercalcemia.

For vitamin D deficiency

Standard dosage	Calciferol, 400–800 U orally daily, plus adequate calcium intake.
Contraindications	None.
Main drug interactions	None.
Main side effects	None at this dose range.

For renal failure

Standard dosage	Calcitriol, 0.5–1.0 μg orally daily, plus calcium intake as appropriate.
Contraindications	None.
Special points	Hyperphosphatemia should be controlled.
Main drug interactions	None.
Main side effects	Hypercalcemia.

For hypomagnesemic hypocalcemia

• Patients with severe, symptomatic hypomagnesemia are best treated initially by an i.v. preparation: magnesium sulfate, 5–10 mg 50% solution in 1 L 5% dextrose over 3–4 hours.

• Daily infusions may be needed until serum magnesium is maintained within the normal range.

• If magnesium losses continue (*e.g.*, short bowel syndrome), this can be treated by intermittent infusions or oral therapy (oral preparations may cause diarrhea).

Treatment aims

To correct hypocalcemia.

Prognosis

• Hypoparathyroidism usually needs life-long treatment.

• For vitamin D deficiency, treatment is needed throughout the period of increased vitamin D requirement.

Follow-up and management

• All patients on high doses of vitamin D need regular serum calcium measurements to prevent the occurrence of hypercalcemia.

Key references

1. Tohme JF, Bilezikian JP: Hypocalcemic emergencies. *Endocrinol Metab Clin North Am* 1993, **22**:363–375.

2. Rude RK: Hypocalcemia and hypoparathyroidism. *Curr Ther Endocrinol Metab* 1997, **6**:546–551.

Diagnosis

Symptoms

Sweating, shaking, anxiety, feeling hot, nausea, palpitations, tingling lips: due to sympathetic and adrenergic response to low blood glucose concentration (autonomic).
Dizziness, tiredness, confusion, difficulty speaking, inability to concentrate, headache: due to impaired cerebral cortical function resulting from low blood glucose level.
Hunger, weakness, blurred vision.
Headache, malaise, confusion: posthypoglycemic.
• Patients with recurrent hypoglycemic attacks often present with symptoms of decreased cognitive function or conscious level of which they have no subjective awareness.
Fasting hypoglycemia: a concerning symptom that requires a thorough medical evaluation.
"Reactive" hypoglycemia (following a meal): less likely to represent significant pathology.

Signs

Pallor, diaphoresis, tremor, tachycardia or occasionally bradycardia, increased pulse pressure, dilated pupils: autonomic.
Altered behavior, slurred speech, irritability, decreased level of consciousness, seizure, coma, transient focal neurological defects: neuroglycopenic.
• The formal diagnosis of hypoglycemia requires the following (Whipple's triad):
1. Symptoms consistant with neuroglycospenia.
2. Low blood glucose during symptoms.
3. Resolution of symptoms with correction of hypoglycemia.

Investigations [1]

For all cases

Blood glucose measurement: <40 mg/dL, in treated diabetic patients ≤60 mg/dL.
• Glucose tolerance tests are rarely of value in the evaluation of hypoglycemia.

For nondiabetic patients

Plasma insulin and C-peptide analysis.
Blood and urine screening: for sulfonylureas.
Blood urea nitrogen, creatine, liver function, insulin antibody tests.

For diabetic patients

Thyroid and adrenal function tests, gastric emptying studies, growth hormone measurement.

For suspected insulinoma

Fasting glucose, insulin, and C-peptide measurement: repeated during 72-hour fast or until hypoglycemia documented; high C-peptide and insulin suggest insulinoma, sulfonylureas, or insulin autoantibodies (rare); high insulin with low C-peptide indicates exogenous insulin.

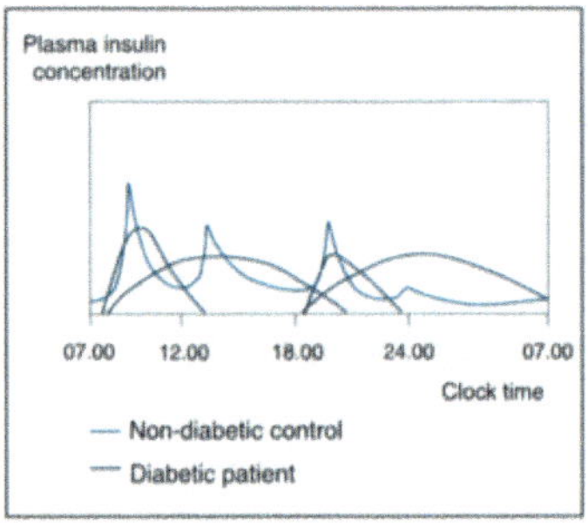

Plasma insulin concentrations over 24 hours from a patient on twice-daily injections of mixed exogenous insulins and an approximation of the plasma insulin profile of a nondiabetic person eating 3 meals daily, showing times of risk of hypoglycemia.

For noninsulinoma, nondiabetes-related hypoglycemia

08.00 hours cortisol and cosyntropin test, growth hormone, insulin-like growth factors, liver function tests.

For suspected "reactive" hypoglycemia

Home blood glucose monitoring: patients can be taught to perform home glucose monitoring during episodes for later laboratory estimates of blood glucose concentration.

Complications

Trauma: while patient is hypoglycemic.
Loss of subjective awareness of subsequent episodes.
Permanent neurological sequelae: usually only with large insulin overdosage.
Death.

Differential diagnosis

Acute
Other causes of coma or confusion, including the following:
Ketoacidosis, nonketotic hyperosmolar coma, intoxication or poisoning, uremia, epilepsy, stroke, intracranial hemorrhage, meningitis, head injury.

Recurrent
Epilepsy, arrhythmias, psychiatric disorder, pheochromocytoma.

Etiology [2]

Excess insulin action in diabetic patients [3]
Missed, small, or late meals, error in time or dose, exercise (effect may last several hours), alcohol (delayed effect), hypothyroidism, renal failure, gastroparesis: with pharmacological treatment of diabetes mellitus (insulin, sulfonylureas).
Vigorous insulin response to rapidly absorbed glucose or gastric surgery (dumping syndrome).
Insulinoma, nesidioblastosis.

Excess insulin action in nondiabetic patients
Tumors secreting insulin-like growth factor.
Surreptitious or malicious administration of insulin or sulfonylurea.

Increased insulin sensitivity
Cortisol deficiency.
Growth hormone deficiency.
Hypopituitarism and adrenal insufficiency (especially in children).

Defects of hepatic glucose production
Liver disease.
Alcohol toxicity.
Sepsis.
Congestive heart failure.
Glycogen storage diseases.
Ketotic hypoglycemia of childhood.
Prematurity.
Defective fatty acid oxidation.

Epidemiology

• 3% of the US population have diabetes mellitus.
• 10% of insulinomas are multiple, 10% are malignant, 9% are associated with multiple endocrine neoplasia.

Treatment

Diet and lifestyle

• In "reactive hypoglycemia," patients should eat small, regular meals with high complex carbohydrates and should avoid simple sugars.

• In childhood disorders of metabolism, frequent high-carbohydrate, low-fat meals should be eaten.

• In patients with diabetes, regular meals and snacks are essential, with patient-led dosage adjustments for certain situations, *e.g.*, excessive exercise.

Pharmacological treatment [1]

For conscious patients

Rapidly absorbed carbohydrates (20–30 g, *e.g.*, 4 glucose tablets, a glass of skim milk, or ½ glass orange juice), then snack.

For confused or unconscious patients

50% glucose, 50 mL, or 20% glucose, 100–150 mL i.v.

In children: 20% dextrose, 2.5 mL/kg.

In infants: 10% dextrose, 2.5 mL/kg.

• Extravasation of glucose must be avoided.

• If hypoglycemia is due to sulfonylurea treatment, massive insulin overdose, or unknown cause, the patient should be admitted to hospital for observation and treatment. Insulin overdoses should be treated with i.v. glucose, whereas sulfonylurea-induced hypoglycemia often responds well to octreotide therapy [4].

Alternatively, glucagon, 1 mg i.m., followed by 30 g complex carbohydrate orally on recovery.

• Glucagon's effect is transient (<60 minutes), and more definitive therapy should be instituted after initial recovery.

• Patients requiring glucagon at home should be seen promptly by a physician.

• Glucagon may not be effective in very undernourished or very alcohol-intoxicated patients.

Alternative medicine

Recommended use: none.

Common use: Siberian ginseng (*Panax ginseng*); Devils club (*Oplopanax horridus*); licorice (*Glycyrrhiza glabra*); burdock (*Arctium* spp.); dandelion (*Taraxacum officinale*); chromium.

Caution: licorice at high doses can cause hypertension and hypokalemia.

Treatment aims

To achieve recovery from acute event.

To prevent further episodes.

Other treatments

Surgery for insulinomas, tumors secreting insulin-like growth factor, nesidioblastosis.

Prognosis

• For diabetes, the prognosis is that of the underlying disease.

• For tumors secreting insulin-like growth factor, prognosis is poor.

Follow-up and management

Prevention of further episodes

• The diabetes regimen should be adjusted.

• Diazoxide can be given for insulinoma, after the diagnosis is established, pending definitive surgical management.

• Diet regimens should be followed for metabolic defects.

Key references

1. Service FJ: Hypoglycemic disorders. *N Engl J Med* 1995, **332**:1144–1152.
2. Amiel SA: Glucose counterregulation in health and disease: current concepts in hypoglycaemia recognition and response. *Q J Med* 1991, **293**:707–727.
3. Amiel SA: Hypoglycaemia in diabetes mellitus. *Med Int* 1993, **21**:279–280.
4. Boyle PJ, Justice K, Krentz AJ, *et al.*: Octreotide reverses hyperinsulinemia and prevents hypoglycemia induced by sulfonylurea overdoses. *J Clin Endocrinol Metab* 1993, **76**:752–756.

Hypopituitarism

Diagnosis

Symptoms

• Symptoms may be due to an underlying cause (*e.g.*, tumor) or to hormone deficiencies. Hormone deficiencies have a gradual onset if secondary to an expanding pituitary lesion.

Impotence or amenorrhea, decreased libido: due to deficiency of gonadotropins.

Poor growth and development, hypoglycemia: in children, due to deficiency of growth hormone.

Cold intolerance, weight gain, tiredness, lethargy: due to deficiency of thyroid-stimulating hormone.

Dizziness, nausea, vomiting: due to deficiency of corticotropic hormone.

Urinary frequency, nocturia: due to deficiency of vasopressin (unusual with pituitary tumors).

Headache or visual disturbance: due to macroadenoma.

Galactorrhea: due to prolactinoma or pituitary stalk compression by lesion (in contrast to other pituitary hormones, prolactin levels usually rise with pituitary enlargement).

Signs

Small soft testes, loss of pubic and axillary hair: due to deficiency of gonadotropins.
Short stature and rarely hyperglycemia: in children, due to deficiency of growth hormone.
Cool skin, absent or slow reflexes: due to deficiency of thyroid-stimulating hormone.
Visual field defect, diplopia or cranial nerve palsies, papilledema, CSF rhinorrhea: indicating macroadenoma.
Signs of secondary adrenal insufficiency.

Investigations

Cortisol measurement for adrenal axis: if 08.00 hours cortisol >20 μg/dL, significant deficiency improbable; if <2 μg/dL, corticotropic hormone (ACTH) deficiency very probable unless patient is taking steroids; intermediate values need cortrosyn stimulation test to assess adrenal function.
Thyroid tests: free thyroxine (T_4), thyroid-stimulating hormone (TSH); secondary hypothyroidism suggested by low free T_4 unaccompanied by raised TSH.
Sex hormone measurement for gonadal axis: *in men:* testosterone, follicle-stimulating hormone (FSH); gonadotropin deficiency suggested by low basal testosterone and no rise of FSH; *in women:* estradiol, FSH, progesterone on day 21 (normal concentration implies normal gonadal axis).
Prolactin test: on 2–3 occasions; hyperprolactinemia may suppress pulsatile gonadotropin secretion in either sex.
Growth hormone (GH) measurement: basal values usually undetectable and therefore unhelpful; insulin tolerance test sometimes used by specialists to assess GH reserve in children, but is usually unnecessary in adults [1].
Plasma and urine osmolality measurement for posterior pituitary: plasma osmolality >295 mOsm/L and urine : plasma osmolality ratio of <2 : 1 suggest diabetes insipidus.
Insulin tolerance test: to assess ACTH and GH reserve; must be done in a specialized unit; contraindicated in patients with ischemic heart disease, epilepsy, or unexplained blackouts; particular caution in children and elderly patients [2].
Releasing hormone tests: corticotropin-releasing, thyrotropin-releasing, and gonadotropin-releasing hormone tests only assess "readily releasable" pool of anterior pituitary hormones and cannot be used to diagnose normality of physiological secretion of the hormone.
MRI or CT of pituitary gland: to visualize macroadenomas and most microadenomas.

Complications

Expanding pituitary mass: with optic chiasm compression and invasion of local structures.
Hydrocephalus: with third ventricular compression by tumor.
Temporal-lobe epilepsy: with temporal extension of tumor (unusual).

Differential diagnosis

Primary adrenal or thyroid insufficiency.
Anorexia nervosa.

Etiology

Pituitary tumors: most common.
Iatrogenic disorders: previous surgery or radiotherapy [3].
Metastases: especially breast, lung.
Infectious disease: *e.g.*, tuberculosis.
Vascular disease: *e.g.*, Sheehan's syndrome, or pituitary apoplexy.
Severe exercise or malnutrition: may cause reversible loss of gonadotropin-releasing hormone release.

Epidemiology

• The incidence of panhypopituitarism is difficult to determine, but ~1 in 10 000 patients each year develops a pituitary tumor.

Treatment

Diet and lifestyle

• Patients need a steroid card, Medicalert bracelet or necklace, and emergency pack of parenteral hydrocortisone (for deficiencies of pituitary–adrenal axis).

Pharmacological treatment

For deficiencies of pituitary–adrenal axis

Standard dosage Hydrocortisone, 20 mg on waking, 5 mg with evening meal (variable).

Contraindications None.

Special points Response monitored by clinical assessment.
For mild cold or sore throat, no change in dosage; with moderate illness manifested primarily with fever, double hydrocortisone dose; with severe illness, especially vomiting or diarrhea, or for perioperative cover, parenteral treatment is needed (hydrocortisone, 100 mg i.m. every 8 hours).

Main drug interactions Estrogens increase cortisol-binding globulin and thus hydrocortisone requirements.

Main side effects Iatrogenic Cushing's syndrome due to over-replacement.

For thyroid deficiencies

Standard dosage Thyroxine, 100–150 µg daily (start with lower doses in the elderly and in patients with ischemic heart disease).

Contraindications None.

Special points Response monitored by clinical assessment and free T_4 levels.
TSH levels unreliable in patients with central hypothyroidism.
Rule out (or treat) adrenal insufficiency before beginning thyroxine therapy.

Main drug interactions Estrogens increase thyroid-binding globulin and raise total thyroxine requirements.

Main side effects None.

For growth hormone deficiencies [1]

• Children should be given growth hormone, 0.04 mg/kg daily.

• Growth hormone may be of some benefit in adults as it may improve psychological well-being and muscle strength and decrease adiposity. Expense remains a serious concern.

For deficiencies of pituitary–gonadal axis

Standard dosage *Men*: testosterone enanthate or cypionate, 200 mg i.m. every 2 weeks or 300 mg every 3 weeks; transdermal testosterone patch 2.5–5.0 mg daily.
Women: ethinyl estradiol, 30 µg daily, or conjugated equine estrogens, 0.125 mg daily. For intact uterus, medroxyprogesterone acetate, 5–10 mg for 10 days each month or 2.5–5.0 mg daily.

Contraindications Prostatic cancer, breast cancer.

Special points Response typically monitored by clinical findings (*e.g.*, erectile function or resolution of hot flashes).

Main drug interactions Estrogen increases many binding globulins and thus replacement hormone requirements.

Main side effects Aggression may occur with initial testosterone replacement (rare).

For posterior pituitary deficiencies

Standard dosage Desmopressin, 10–20 µg at night by intranasal spray; dose may also be needed in morning.

Contraindications None.

Special points Response monitored by plasma and urine osmolality.

Main drug interactions None.

Main side effects Dilutional hyponatremia due to over-replacement.

Treatment aims

To achieve clinical well-being.

To achieve normal target gland hormone concentrations.

To remove underlying cause.

Other treatments

• Surgery is indicated for the following:

Pituitary tumors that are growing or impinging on adjacent structures.

Visual field defects.

Cranial nerve palsies.

CSF rhinorrhea.

Prognosis

• Accurate and careful hormone replacement restores a normal life expectancy.

Follow-up and management

• Initial close supervision is necessary to ensure the correct dosage.

• Thereafter, patients should be reviewed every 6–12 months.

Key references

1. Cuneo RC, *et al.*: The growth hormone deficiency syndrome in adults. *Clin Endocrinol* 1992, **37**:387–397.
2. Jones SL, *et al.*: An audit of the insulin tolerance test in adult subjects in an acute investigation unit over one year. *Clin Endocrinol* 1994, **41**:123–128.
3. Littley MD, *et al.*: Hypopituitarism following external radiotherapy for pituitary tumors in adults. *Q J Med* 1989, **70**:145–160.

Hypothyroidism

Diagnosis

Symptoms [1]

Weight gain, fatigue, cold intolerance, neck swelling, hoarseness.

Angina, shortness of breath.

Aches and pains, depression, carpal tunnel syndrome.

Dry skin.

Menorrhagia, infertility, galactorrhea secondary to hyperprolactinemia.

Constipation.

Poor growth, mental retardation, delayed puberty: in children.

Signs

Bradycardia, pericardial effusion (rare), congestive heart failure.

Hoarseness, deafness, cerebellar ataxia, delayed relaxation of tendon reflexes, psychosis ("myxedema madness").

Anemia.

Goiter.

Dry skin, myxedema, vitiligo, yellowish discoloration, decreased sweating.

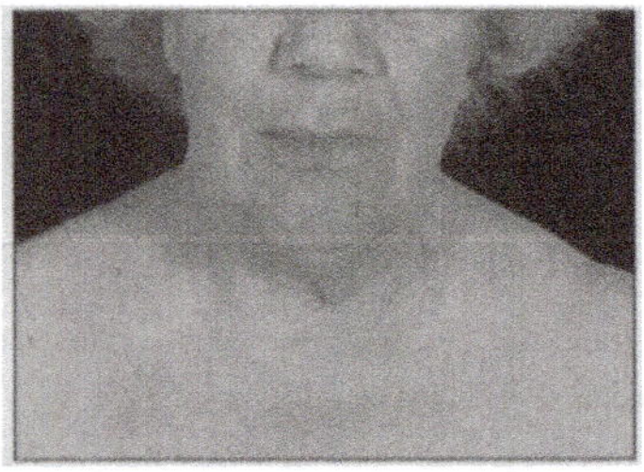

Hypothyroid appearance of an elderly patient with severe untreated Hashimoto's thyroiditis. (*See* Color Plate.)

Investigations [2]

Serum thyroid hormone measurement: reduction in free or total thyroxine (T_4) indicates severity of hypothyroidism; total triiodothyronine (T_3) usually normal except in severely ill patients, so measurement not helpful.

Serum thyroid-stimulating hormone (TSH) measurement: elevation indicates primary thyroid failure; raised TSH with normal thyroxine is termed "subclinical" hypothyroidism; TSH within or below normal range, with low serum thyroxine, suggests secondary hypothyroidism (hypothalamic/pituitary; same picture seen in "nonthyroidal" illness and treatment by certain drugs, *e.g.*, glucocorticoids).

Autoantibody measurement: antithyroid peroxidase and antithyroglobulin antibodies often present in high titer in Hashimoto's thyroiditis.

Complications

Hypothermia and coma: in severely ill patients, typically in the elderly in cold weather.

Hyperlipidemia and ischemic heart disease: associated with longstanding hypothyroidism.

Differential diagnosis

- Depressed patients often appear mildly hypothyroid and should be screened.

Menstrual disorders.
Weight change.
Anemia.
Unexplained heart failure.
Hyperlipidemia.
Unexplained ascites.
Primary amyloidosis.
Depression, psychosis.

Etiology [2]

Causes of primary thyroid failure

Autoimmune thyroiditis: Hashimoto's thyroiditis.
Previous treatment by radioiodine or thyroidectomy.
Idiopathic atrophy.
Iodine deficiency.
Antithyroid drugs or excess iodine.
Subacute or silent thyroiditis.
Poor compliance with thyroxine replacement.
Dyshormonogenesis, agenesis, infiltrative disease (uncommon).

Causes of secondary thyroid failure

Disease of pituitary or hypothalamus.

Epidemiology

- The prevalence of hypothyroidism is 5–15 in 100 females, ~1 in 100 males.
- In the United States, >90% of cases are due to autoimmune thyroiditis, idiopathic atrophy, or previous treatment for hyperthyroidism.

Congenital hypothyroidism

Prevalence: 1 in 5000 infants in the United States.

Detection: routine screening of all infants.

Possible causes: thyroid agenesis, ectopic or hypoplastic thyroid tissue, inherited disorders or hormonogenesis, transplacental passage of thyroid-stimulating hormone receptor blocking antibodies (such cases resolve spontaneously within a few months).

Iodine-deficient hypothyroidism

- Iodine deficiency is the major cause of hypothyroidism worldwide. It is typically found in mountainous regions.
- Iodine supplementation programs are effective in abolishing symptoms.

Treatment

Diet and lifestyle

• Long-term ingestion of iodine-containing compounds, *e.g.*, kelp preparations or expectorants, can result in hypothyroidism in adults.

Pharmacological treatment [3–5]

• Thyroxine for patients with symptomatic hypothyroidism; triiodothyronine is used occasionally in patients with myxedema coma to produce more rapid effect.

• Symptoms begin to resolve within 2-3 weeks of the beginning of treatment, but treatment at full dose for 8 weeks may be needed to restore serum thyroid-stimulating hormone to normal.

Standard dosage	Thyroxine, 100–150 µg daily as single dose. Triiodothyronine, 25 µg orally 2–3 times daily (rarely indicated).
Contraindications	Caution in severe ischemic heart disease (patient should be admitted to hospital and started on very low doses of thyroxine). Elderly patients with severe hypothyroidism should also be started on very low doses of thyronine (*e.g.*, 25 ug daily).
Main drug interactions	None.
Main side effects	Generally none; exacerbation of ischemic heart disease may follow initiation of treatment; can precipitate acute adrenal failure in patients with subclinical adrenal disease.

Alternative medicine

Recommended use: None.

Common use: kelp; mugwart (*Artemisia vulgaris*); St. John's wort (*Hypericum perforatum*); yellow dock (*Rumex crispus* and *R. obtusifolius*); vitamins A, C, and E; riboflavin, niacin, pyridoxine; zinc.

Caution: avoid the following foods, particularly if raw: turnips, cabbage, mustard, soybeans, peanuts, pine nuts, and millet.

Treatment aims

To relieve symptoms.

To restore serum thyroid-stimulating hormone and thyroxine to normal values.

Prognosis

• Life expectancy is not adversely affected by long-term thyroxine treatment.

• Thyroxine treatment (in doses that suppress serum thyroid-stimulating hormone) may reduce bone density. However, no increased risk of osteoporotic fractures has been observed.

• Up to 25% of patients prescribed thyroxine have biochemical evidence of undertreatment that may be associated with hyperlipidemia and increased risk of ischemic heart disease.

Follow-up and management

• Serum thyroid-stimulating hormone should be measured 6 weeks after starting treatment to check whether the dose needs to be increased, and should be measured annually in patients on established treatment.

• Treatment is generally lifelong, except in mild cases occurring within the first 6 months after radioiodine treatment, pregnancy, or partial thyroidectomy (possibly temporary) and in patients who are hypothyroid secondary to subacute or silent thyroiditis.

Key references

1. Anonymous: Hypothyroidism? *Lancet* 1990, **335**:1316.
2. Lazarus JH, Hall R (eds.): Hypothyroidism and goitre. *Ballières Clin Endocrinol Metab* 1988, **2**.
3. Toft AD: Thyroxine therapy. *N Engl J Med* 1994, **331**:174–180.
4. Utiger RD: Therapy of hypothyroidism. When are changes needed? *N Engl J Med* 1990, **323**:126–127.
5. Singer PA, *et al.*: Treatment guidelines for patients with hyperthyroidism and hypothyroidism. Standards of Care Committee, American Thyroid Association. *JAMA* 1995, **273**:808–812.

Infections in hematological malignancy

Diagnosis

Definition

• Infections in hematological malignancy are opportunistic infections that arise during the treatment of hematological malignancy due to the development of neutropenia. Patients are particularly vulnerable when the neutrophil count falls below 0.5×10^9/L.

Symptoms and signs

Fever: the only consistent indication of established infection.

Investigations [1]

• Full examination should always be made, including mouth, pharynx, genitalia, perianal region, central line, and other venous access device sites.

• Surveillance cultures can be predictive of infection, *e.g.*, with *Pseudomonas aeruginosa,* allowing planning of empirical treatment for individual patients and monitoring of prophylaxis, as well as facilitating infection control.

• Stool should be screened, *e.g.*, for parasites, if patient comes from a high-risk area.

Blood cultures: from central line and peripheral vein, for bacteria and fungi.

Hickman swab: if inflamed or cutaneous discharge.

Specimens from clinically suspicious sites.

Urinalysis and culture.

Chest radiography.

CT of thorax: invaluable in invasive aspergillosis.

Bronchoalveolar lavage: especially in bone-marrow transplant patients with dry cough or lesions seen on chest radiography early on.

Skin lesion aspiration: valuable in diagnosis of disseminated fungal infection.

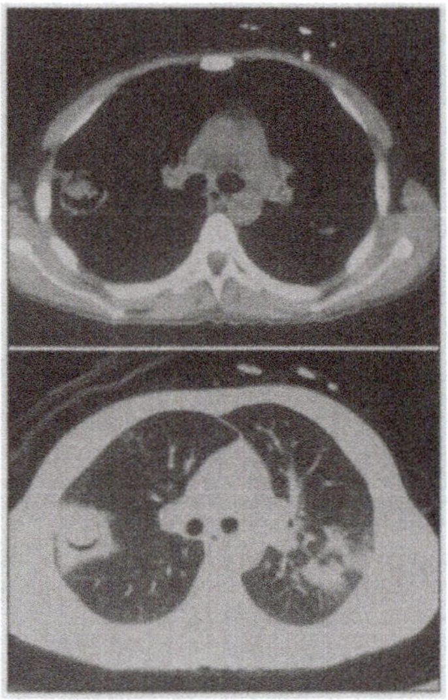

CT of lung with invasive aspergillosis. The mycotic lung sequestrum is usually pleural based and wedged shaped and often shows cavitation.

Complications

• Initially, complications may include those of septicemia, *e.g.*, adult tubular necrosis.

Increased risk of acute respiratory distress syndrome: in patients with *Streptococcus mitis* bacteremia.

Ecthyma gangrenosum in patients with local or disseminated *P. aeruginosa* infection.

Disseminated candidiasis: CT of liver or spleen can be helpful.

Pulmonary infarction or hemorrhage: especially in patients with invasive aspergillosis.

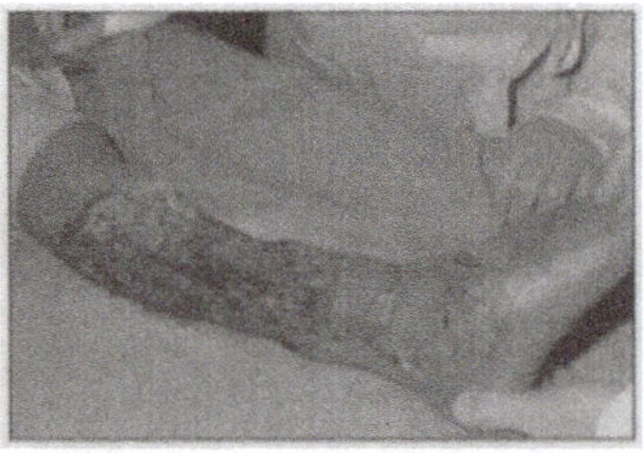

Extensive resection of necrotic tissue of the leg in a child with *Pseudomonas* septicaemia and ecthyma gangrenosum. (*See* Color Plate.)

Differential diagnosis

Reaction to transfusion of blood products.
Drug fever.
Graft-versus-host disease.
Fever associated with underlying disease.

Etiology

Causes of fever

Bacteremia in 20%–30% of patients.
Clinical or nonbacteremic microbiologically documented infection in 30%–40%.
Unexplained in 30%–40%.

Documented focus of infection

Lower respiratory tract (50%).
Upper respiratory tract (20%).
Skin and soft tissue, including perianal (20%–30%).
Urinary tract (<5%).

Predisposing factors for specific infections

Neutropenia: bacterial and fungal.
Lymphopenia: intracellular organisms, *e.g., Toxoplasma gondii, Pneumocystis carinii*, mycobacteria, herpesviruses.
Defects in humoral immunity and splenic hypofunction: encapsulated organisms.
Loss of physical barriers (mucosa, skin): bacteremia, fungemia.
Reservoir of infection (*e.g.*, bronchiectasis): *Pseudomonas* spp.
Geographical considerations: mycobacteria, malaria, strongyloides.

Sources of major pathogens

Staphylococci: skin commensal, cross-infection.
S. mitis: oral commensal.
Enterobacteriaceae: gut.
P. aeruginosa: environment, cross-infection.
Streptococcus pneumoniae: nasopharynx, cross-infection.
Mycobacterium tuberculosis: reactivation.
P. carinii: reactivation, possibly cross-infection.
T. gondii: reactivation, donor bone marrow.
Candida spp.: oropharynx or gut, cross-infection, parenteral feeding.
Aspergillus spp.: airborne (previous colonization).
Herpes simplex or varicella-zoster virus: reactivation (cross-infection).
Cytomegalovirus: reactivation, blood products.

Epidemiology

• ~1 febrile incident occurs per neutropenic episode (less with quinolone prophylaxis).

Treatment

Diet and lifestyle

• Neutropenic patients must eat a low-pathogen diet but maintain nutrition, *e.g.*, by parenteral route if needed.
• Patients should be given a dental review.
• Hygiene is important for patients and attendants, *e.g.*, hand-washing, cleaning of room and bedding, and i.v. catheter care.
• Water must be treated appropriately to prevent legionella infection.
• Patients must especially avoid exposure to measles and chickenpox; vaccination should be reviewed, but live vaccines must be avoided until immune recovery.

Pharmacological treatment [2–4]

Empirical treatment for pyrexia of unknown origin in neutropenia

• Patients with a temperature of 38.5°C or 38°C for 2 hours should receive prompt empirical antibiotic treatment: *e.g.*, ceftazidime, or ceftazidime and aminoglycoside, or antipseudomonal penicillin and aminoglycoside. If aminoglycoside was not part of the original regimen and fever persists beyond 24–72 hours or clinical deterioration is apparent, add aminoglycoside after reculturing of all potential infection sites. Regardless of initial antibiotic regimen, if fever persists, reculture and include vancomycin. Amphotericin B should be added if fever persists beyond 96 hours.

Standard dosage	Amphotericin B 1 mg/kg or AmBisome 3–5 mg/kg daily. Ceftazidine 2 g i.v. every 8 hours (adults). Gentamicin 1 mg/kg i.v. 3 times daily. Piperacillin 3–4 g i.v. every 4–6 hours. Vancomycin 500 mg i.v. every 6 hours or 1 g i.v. every 12 hours.
Contraindications	Hypersensitivity; caution in renal impairment; epilepsy, or known intracerebral lesion (imipenem).
Special points	Vancomycin and aminoglycoside dosages may need adjustment.
Main drug interactions	Ototoxicity when combined (uncommon with teicoplanin).
Main side effects	Nephrotoxicity (vancomycin, aminoglycosides, amphotericin). Ototoxicity (vancomycin, aminoglycosides).

Treatment of other specific infections

For most invasive fungal infection: amphotericin B, 0.5–1.5 mg/kg i.v. daily, possibly with 5-flucytosine, or liposomal amphotericin B 1–4 mg/kg daily.
For herpes simplex infection: acyclovir, 5 mg/kg every 8 hours for 7 days.
For varicella-zoster infection: acyclovir, 10 mg/kg every 8 hours for 7 days.
For cytomegalovirus infection: ganciclovir, 5 mg/kg i.v. every 12 hours for 2 weeks, maintained at 5 mg/kg daily for a further 2–3 weeks with immunoglobulin.
For *P. carinii* pneumonitis: co-trimoxazole, 120 mg/kg daily in divided doses, with steroids.

Prophylaxis [3]

For gram-negative bacteria: a 4-quinolone, *e.g.*, ciprofloxacin, 250–500 mg orally twice daily, with colistin, 1.5 MU orally.
For gram-positive bacteria: penicillin or macrolide antibiotic.
For mycobacteria (in cases of previous disease, family contact, endemic area): isoniazid 5 mg/kg daily or a 4-quinolone, *e.g.*, ciprofloxacin, 500 mg twice daily.
For legionella: a 4-quinolone, *e.g.*, ciprofloxacin, 500 mg twice daily.
For *Candida albicans* or *Cryptococcus neoformans*: fluconazole, 100–200 mg orally daily.
For *Candida glabrata*: amphotericin B suspension, 500 mg orally every 6 hours.
For aspergillosis: air filtration, itraconazole, or amphotericin B, 0.5–1 mg/kg i.v. daily.
For herpes simplex or varicella-zoster virus: acyclovir, 5 mg/kg every 8 hours.
For cytomegalovirus: possibly acyclovir, 10 mg/kg i.v. every 8 hours, ganciclovir (myelosuppression), or foscarnet.
For *P. carinii*: co-trimoxazole, 960 mg orally twice daily for 3 days weekly, or aerosolized pentamidine, 150 mg every 2 weeks.
For strongyloidiasis: thiabendazole, 25 mg/kg orally twice daily for 3 days.
For toxoplasmosis: pyrimethamine, 75 mg orally daily (loading dose, 100 mg), with folinic acid, 15 mg 3 times daily, and possibly sulfadiazine, 2 g i.v. or orally 3 times daily.

Treatment aims

To instigate antimicrobial therapy rapidly, using broad-spectrum cidal agents active against the most probable organisms.

Prognosis

• In patients with fever alone, mortality is <5%.
• In patients with fever and pulmonary infiltrates, mortality is 30%–60%.

Follow-up and management

• Subsequent management should take into account the following:
Initial empirical treatment: patients may need addition of a glycopeptide.
Underlying disease and treatment: *P. carinii* pneumonia and viral infection (especially cytomegalovirus) with lymphoid disease and bone-marrow transplantation.
Duration of neutropenia: invasive fungal infection increases with time.
Number of previous febrile episodes: increased risk of fungal infection with increased number.
History or evidence of latent infection: *e.g.*, invasive aspergillosis, tuberculosis.
Foreign travel, ethnic origin: e.g., risk of malaria, tuberculosis, strongyloidiasis.

Key references

1. Pizzo PA: Fever in immunocompromised patients. *N Engl J Med* 1999, **341**:893–900.
2. Freifeld AG, Walsh TJ, Pizzo PA: Clinical approaches to infections in the compromised host. In *Hematology: Basic Principles and Practice*, edn 3. Edited by Hoffman R, Benz EJ, Shattil SJ, *et al.* New York: Churchill Livingstone; 2000:1443–1500.
3. Prentice HG, Kibbler CC, MacWhinney PH: Antimicrobial prophylaxis and treatment after chemotherapy or marrow transplantation. In *Recent Advances in Hematology*, vol 6. Edited by Hoffbrand AV, Brenner M. London: Churchill Livingstone; 1991.
4. Ramphal R, Gucalp R, Rotstein C, *et al.*: Clinical experience with single agent and combination regimens in the management of infection in the febrile neutropenic patient. *Am J Med* 1996, **100(suppl)**:835–895.

Diagnosis

Symptoms

Dyspnea: on exertion, progressive.

Cough: usually unproductive and irritating.

Signs

Clubbing: in many patients.

Fine late inspiratory crackles: at lung base, later throughout lungs.

Cyanosis.

Late right ventricular heave, right ventricular gallop, loud pulmonary second sound, raised jugular venous pulse, peripheral edema: signs of cor pulmonale.

Hypoxemia: especially with exertion.

Investigations [1,3]

Chest radiography: shows small lung fields, irregular nodular or reticulonodular opacities, often maximal in lower zones (classic "ground-glass" appearance); honeycombing in end-stage patients; pulmonary artery enlargement; and cardiomegaly with cor pulmonale.

High-resolution CT: sensitive; may detect disease when chest radiograph normal; characteristically shows subpleural area of increased density, with central sparing; distortion of bronchi and cystic air spaces in advanced disease.

Pulmonary function tests: restrictive ventilatory defect, with low lung volumes, decreased lung compliance, and reduced carbon monoxide transfer.

Arterial blood gas analysis: may be normal in patients with mild disease; partial oxygen pressure typically falls on exercise. Severe hypoxia in severe disease.

Bronchoalveolar lavage: increased cell counts in bronchoalveolar fluid; cell differention may give diagnostic clues. Useful in eliminating infectious causes.

Lung biopsy: open lung biopsy gold standard but inappropriate in very ill or elderly patients; transbronchial, percutaneous, or needle biopsy produces smaller specimens, limiting histological analysis.

Hematology and biochemistry: usually not helpful; ESR may be raised; globulin or immunoglobulin (one or more classes) concentrations often raised; 30% of patients positive for rheumatoid or antinuclear antibody.

Complications [4]

Death: ~60% of patients die as direct consequence of fibrosing lung disease (some with terminal infection, others from respiratory failure).

Pulmonary hypertension, right heart failure: clinically evident in some patients.

Lung cancer: apparent excess in patients with interstitial fibrosis (smokers and non-smokers).

Differential diagnosis

- Many conditions have a tendency to develop into interstitial fibrosis.

Fibrogenic dust inhalation: *e.g.*, silica, asbestos.

Granulomas: due to extrinsic allergic alveolitis, berylliosis, sarcoidosis.

Chronic exudates: *e.g.*, chronic left ventricular failure, drugs, chronic renal failure.

Etiology

- The cause of many interstitial lung diseases is unknown.
- Interstitial fibrosis is characterized by an inflammatory exudate of the alveolar wall, with a tendency to form fibrosis.
- Interstitial fibrosis can occur alone or be associated with connective tissue disorders of unknown cause, *e.g.*, systemic sclerosis, SLE, rheumatoid arthritis, polymyositis.
- Certain drugs, *e.g.*, bleomycin, methotrexate, and amiodarone, can produce a picture similar to that of interstitial fibrosis.
- Certain viral agents, *e.g.*, influenza A2 virus, have been reported as inducing interstitial fibrosis.

Epidemiology

- Interstitial fibrosis is manifest mostly in middle age, often between 50–70 years of age.
- The prevalence is estimated to be 3–5 in 100 000 population.

Treatment

Diet and lifestyle

• Morbidity is increased, with progressive restriction of daily activities.

• Diet has no effect.

Pharmacological treatment [1–3]

• Treatment depends on diagnosis.

• The following treatments may be considered for idiopathic pulmonary fibrosis:

Corticosteroids

• 30%–50% of patients have some symptomatic benefit, at least short-term, from steroids; no more than 20% show objective radiographic or physiological improvement.

Standard dosage	Prednisone, 60 mg daily for 2–3 months; reduced slowly to maintenance dose if condition responsive.
Contraindications	Uncontrolled hypertension, diabetes mellitus, infection, severe osteoporosis.
Main drug interactions	None.
Main side effects	Weight gain, edema, bruising, purple striae in skin (especially of abdomen), moon face, osteoporosis, collapse of vertebrae, diabetes mellitus, hypertension, myopathy (especially proximal girdle muscles), hirsutism, menstrual disturbances, psychotic reactions, cataracts, withdrawal phenomena.

Cyclophosphamide

• Many patients fail to respond to high-dose steroids alone; in patients who continue to deteriorate, low-dose prednisone can be combined with cyclophosphamide, an immunosuppressant drug.

Standard dosage	Cyclophosphamide, 2 mg/kg daily with prednisone.
Contraindications	Severe renal impairment, porphyria.
Special points	Clinical improvement not expected within 2 months of starting treatment.
Main drug interactions	Muscle relaxants.
Main side effects	Hemorrhagic cystitis, bone-marrow suppression, alopecia.

Other drugs

• D-Penicillamine, azathioprine, colchicine, cyclosporin A, chlorambacil, and methotrexate have been tried in patients who were unresponsive to steroids.

Supportive treatment

Supplemental oxygen for patients with arterial oxygen tension of <55 mm Hg.

Diuretics for heart failure.

Opiates for suppression of cough and alleviation of breathlessness.

Pneumococcal and influenza vaccines: should be administered.

Treatment aims

To improve quality of life by preventing deterioration of lung function.

To relieve symptoms.

To give maximum supportive care, including counseling, when symptomatic relief not possible.

Other treatments

• Lung transplantation is indicated for patients with rapidly progressive disease and young patients who do not respond to conventional treatment.

Prognosis [5]

• Mortality within 5 years of diagnosis is 50%.

• Probable responders usually have a more cellular histological response.

• Improved survival may be achieved if the disease is detected early and more precise predictors of progression are developed to prevent high-risk patients, in whom more aggressive treatment would be justified.

• The 1-year survival rate after single-lung transplantation is 50%.

Follow-up and management

• The response should be assessed by clinical, subjective, and objective changes in chest radiography and pulmonary function tests.

Key references

1. American Thoracic Society: Idiopathic pulmonary fibrosis: diagnosis and treatment. International Consensus Statement. *Am J Respir Crit Care Med* 2000, **161**: 646–664.
2. Mason RJ, Schwarz MI, Hunninghake GW, Musson RA: NHLBI workshop summary. Pharmacological therapy for idiopathic pulmonary fibrosis: past, present, and future. *Am J Respir Crit Care Med* 1999, **160(5 pt 1)**:1771–1777
3. Schwarz MI, King TE Jr (eds.): *Interstitial Lung Disease*. St. Louis: Mosby-Yearbook, 1993.
4. Panos R, *et al.*: Clinical deterioration in patients with idiopathic pulmonary fibrosis: causes and assessment. *Am J Med* 1990, **88**:396–404.
5. Schwartz DA, *et al.*: Determinants of survival in idiopathic pulmonary fibrosis. *Am J Respir Crit Care Med* 1994, **149**:450–454.

Intracerebral hemorrhage

Diagnosis

Symptoms

Headache, nausea, vomiting, drowsiness: due to raised intracranial pressure.

Seizure: due to lobar hematoma, in 28%–30% of patients.

Diplopia, gaze impairment, hiccoughs, dysarthria, facial hyperesthesia: due to brain stem hematoma.

Signs

Confusion, coma, papilledema: due to raised intracranial pressure.

Hemiplegia, aphasia, homonymous visual-field defects: due to cortical or subcortical hematomas.

Vertical-gaze palsy, skew deviation of eyes, miotic unreactive pupils: due to thalamic hematoma.

III nerve palsy, skew deviation of eyes: due to midbrain hematoma.

Horizontal-gaze palsy, pin-point reactive pupil, hyperpyrexia: due to pontine hematoma.

Ipsilateral V–VII nerve palsy, ataxia or nystagmus: due to cerebellar hematoma.

Investigations [1]

• Laboratory tests are not diagnostic but may identify underlying abnormalities.

Hematology profile: to identify bleeding disorders.

Clotting profile: to identify disorders of coagulation.

ESR and antinuclear antibody measurement: to identify vasculitic disorders.

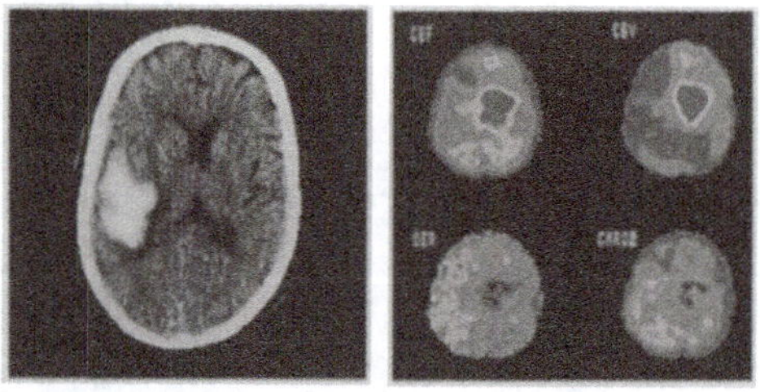

Intracerebral hemorrhage (*left*); fractional images of large arteriovenous malformation (*right*). (*See* Color Plate.)

CT of brain with bone windows: to identify skull fractures, hemorrhage, hydrocephalus, or edema; after 2 weeks, may be indistinguishable from infarct.

MRI of brain: examination of choice for cavernous angiomas; may help in identifying multiple lesions in patients with intracerebral metastasis.

Four-vessel angiography: to identify aneurysms (causing subarachnoid hemorrhage) or arteriovenous malformations; four-vessel because, in 20%–25% of patients, several aneurysms may be present.

Complications

Tentorial herniation: with large supratentorial hematoma; herniation from below may occur rarely with large brain stem or cerebellar hematoma.

Foramen magnum herniation: preterminal event with large hematoma.

Hydrocephalus: with ventricular extension of hemorrhage from extrinsic pressure on CSF pathways, especially at aqueduct level and in cerebellar, caudate (75%), and thalamic hemorrhages.

Hyperpyrexia: usually in preterminal pontine hemorrhage.

Seizures: subcortical hematoma, which isolates strip of cortex.

Rebleed and vasospasm: in subarachnoid hemorrhage, risk of bleeding again is 35% within 1 month, with 42% mortality; vasospasm causing cerebral ischemia occurs ~5 days after subarachnoid hemorrhage and may last ≥2 weeks.

Differential diagnosis

Hemorrhagic infarction: usually maximal neurodeficit from onset, raised intracranial pressure improbable, source of emboli present, CT showing mottled attenuation with minimal mass effect.

Subarachnoid hemorrhage: sudden (thunderclap) headache often preceded by warning (sentinel) headache (30%–60%), meningism with possible neck stiffness, photophobia, III (posterior communicating artery aneurysm) or VI nerve palsies, confusion and emotional lability (anterior communicating artery aneurysm).

Hemorrhage into brain tumor: papilledema, multiple-site hemorrhages, mass effect, noncontrasted CT showing high-density hemorrhage surrounding low-density center.

Etiology

Hypertensive intracerebral hemorrhage.

Vascular malformations.

Bleeding into intracranial tumor.

Anticoagulant treatment (8%–11% increased risk) and hemorrhagic disorders.

Sympathomimetic drugs (amphetamine, phenylpropanolamine).

Trauma.

Cerebral amyloid angiopathy (history of dementia in 10%–30%, rare before 55 years).

Granulomatous vasculitis of CNS.

Necrotizing systemic vasculitis.

Epidemiology [2]

• Intracerebral hemorrhage accounts for 10% of all strokes.

• Putaminal hemorrhage is the most usual variety of intracerebral hemorrhage (35%).

• Other common sites include the globus pallidus and pons.

Treatment

Diet and lifestyle

• No special precautions are necessary.

Pharmacological treatment

• Lack of prospective data on intracerebral hemorrhage treatment has led to most patients being treated nonsurgically.

For hypertension [3]

• Severe hypertension should be treated to maintain mean arterial pressure between 60 and 70 mm Hg.

• Intravenous beta-blockers with additional alpha-blocking action (labetalol) and diuretics are useful.

• Nitroprusside, hydralazine, and calcium antagonists should be avoided in the first week; these are cerebral vasodilators and may worsen intracerebral pressure.

Standard dosage	Labetalol, 2 mg/min i.v. infusion, 50–200 mg total.
Contraindications	Asthma, heart block.
Special points	Upright position must be avoided for 3 hours after infusion.
Main drug interactions	Antiarrhythmics.
Main side effects	Postural hypotension.

For seizures

• Routine prophylaxis is not justified.

• Tonic–clonic convulsions need urgent control.

Standard dosage	Diazepam, 10–20 mg i.v., and phenytoin, 1 g i.v. over 30–45 minutes, with cardiac monitoring.
Contraindications	None of importance.
Special points	May precipitate in 5% glucose solution.
Main drug interactions	None of importance.
Main side effects	Nausea, vomiting, mental confusion.

For coagulopathies

• Patients should be given fresh frozen plasma, vitamin K, or platelet infusion.

For raised intracerebral pressure

• If facilities permit, intracerebral pressure can be monitored, and cerebral perfusion pressure (blood pressure minus intracerebral pressure) can be measured.

• Current techniques for measuring intracerebral pressure are invasive and have a 2%–8% risk of intracranial infection.

• Intracerebral pressure should be maintained <20–25 mm Hg.

Standard dosage	Mannitol, 0.5 g/kg i.v. initially, with furosemide or subsequent albumin infusion.
Contraindications	Congestive cardiac failure, pulmonary edema.
Special points	Mannitol should not be used when serum osmolality is >320 mOsm/L.
Main drug interactions	None of importance.
Main side effects	Chills, fever.

• Hyperventilation is indicated to maintain arterial carbon dioxide concentration at 3.5 kPa; excessive hyperventilation may produce cerebral ischemia.

• Corticosteroids have no role in the management of raised intracerebral pressure caused by hemorrhage.

Treatment aims

To reverse neurodeficit.
To prevent complications.

Other treatments

• Direct evacuation of hematoma, ventricular drainage for hydrocephalus, or surgical obliteration for aneurysm is indicated for the following:
Cerebellar hemorrhage if signs of tegmental compression, hematoma 3 cm in diameter (on CT), hydrocephalus or obliteration of quadrigeminal cisterns.
Lobar hemorrhage (hematoma volume 20–40 mL), with progressive deterioration (100% mortality with medical treatment).
Acute hydrocephalus.
Subarachnoid hemorrhage: direct clipping aneurysms, thrombosis for giant aneurysms.
Hemorrhage from arteriovenous malformation: pre- and intraoperative embolization and staged resection.

Prognosis

• Large hematoma with progressive neurological deficits, coma at presentation, or ventricular extension has poor prognosis (overall mortality, 25%–60%).
• Large pontine hemorrhage is usually fatal within 24–48 hours.
• Caudate hemorrhage usually has a benign outcome despite ventricular extension and hydrocephalus.

Follow-up and management

• In patients needing anticoagulation after surgical treatment, aspirin can be started a few days after surgery, warfarin probably after 1 month unless mechanical valve necessitates earlier treatment.
• CT is mandatory if neurological deterioration occurs.

Key references

1. Kase CS: Intracerebral hemorrhage. In *Neurology in Clinical Practice*. Edited by Bradley WG, *et al*. Oxford: Butterworth–Heinemann; 1991:940–954.
2. Thompson DW, Furlam AJ: Clinical epidemiology of stroke. *Neurosurg Clin North Am* 1997, **8**:265–269.
3. Adans RF, Powers WJ: Management of hypertension in acute intracerebral hemorrhage. *Crit Care Clin* 1997, **13**:131–161.

Irritable bowel syndrome

Diagnosis

Symptoms

• Criteria for irritable bowel syndrome (IBS) are continuous or recurrent symptoms for at least 3 months consisting of abdominal pain and disturbed defecation (*i.e.*, at least two of the following: altered stool frequency, form, or passage; passage of mucus) [1].

Variants

Diarrhea-predominant IBS: frequent loose stools, often in the morning or after meals; mucus, urgency, or incontinence may be present.

Constipation-predominant IBS: small, hard stools that are difficult to pass; feeling of incomplete evacuation.

Pain/bloat–predominant IBS: often intermittent, crampy lower abdominal pain relieved by defecation or passage of flatus; associated with changes in stool consistency or frequency, bloating with visible abdominal distension may be major feature and is typically worse after meals or at the end of the day.

• Passage of blood, weight loss, new onset in older adult, or nocturnal symptoms that awaken the patient from sleep are "alarm symptoms" and suggest an alternative diagnosis.

Signs

Variable abdominal tenderness: often over palpable sigmoid colon; frequently present but nonspecific.

• Structural abnormalities such as a mass, ascites, or organomegaly are "alarm signs" that suggest an alternative diagnosis.

Investigations

• Irritable bowel disease is diagnosed on the basis of symptoms, signs, and the clinical course; diagnostic investigations should be aimed at excluding other competing diagnoses [2].

Colonic imaging: flexible sigmoidoscopy in young patients without "alarm" symptoms or signs. Increased pain with air insufflation during this procedure is more suggestive of IBS. In patients with "alarm" symptoms or signs and in those 40 years of age or older, barium enema or colonoscopy should also be performed to exclude cancer and inflammatory bowel disease. These studies should be normal in patients with IBS.

Colonic biopsy: may be useful in patients with diarrhea-predominant IBS to exclude microscopic colitis.

Stool studies: stool samples should be negative for fecal leukocytes, qualitative fat, bacterial pathogens, and parasites in patients with IBS.

Complete blood count: anemia or leukocytosis suggests an alternative diagnosis.

Urinalysis: normal in patients with IBS.

Liver chemistry tests: abnormal test results suggest an alternative diagnosis.

Thyroid function tests: for myxedema manifest as constipation, or thyrotoxicosis as diarrhea.

Assessment of mental health: a history of previous physical or sexual abuse is relatively common, particularly in women with functional abdominal symptoms; anxiety, depression, and personality disorders are frequently identified in these patients and adverse life events may precede symptoms.

Small bowel contrast studies, gastroscopy, abdominal ultrasonography or CT, duodenal or jejunal biopsy, or aspiration: only in selected cases to exclude Crohn's disease, peptic ulcer, biliary or pancreatic disease.

Plain abdominal radiography, colonic transit studies, full-thickness colonic biopsy, or defecography: of occasional use in patients with severe constipation to exclude megacolon, idiopathic slow-transit constipation, neuromuscular gut disorders, pelvic floor dysfuntion.

Complications

Major physical and psychological morbidity: this often leads to "doctor shopping" for a cure and, often, excessive testing.

Dependency on narcotics or benzodiazepines.

Differential diagnosis

Inflammatory bowel disease: Crohn's and ulcerative colitis.

Infections: *e.g.*, by *Giardia* spp.

Diverticular or celiac disease.

Colonic malignancy.

Lactose intolerance.

Gastric disorders: *e.g.*, peptic ulcer.

Pancreatic disorder: *e.g.*, chronic pancreatitis.

Biliary and liver disease: *e.g.*, gallstones.

Laxative abuse.

Etiology

Enhanced visceral sensitivity.

Abnormal central pain perception.

Abnormal gut motility.

Epidemiology

• Irritable bowel syndrome is common and occurs worldwide (10%–20% of population in industrialized countries).

• It occurs more frequently in women.

• Up to 50% of gastroenterological referrals are for IBS specialty.

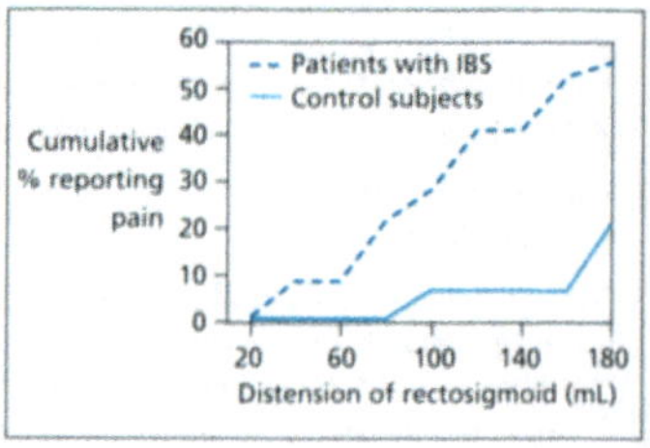

Irritable bowel syndrome. Heightened visceral sensitivity to balloon distention of the sigmoid colon in patients with irritable bowel syndrome (IBS) (*n*=25), using a latex balloon, compared with healthy persons (*n*=20). Visceral hypersensitivity is not caused by a nonspecific intolerance to pain, because pain tolerance to noxious stimuli such as arm immersion in ice-cold water is normal in patients with IBS [4].

Treatment

Diet and lifestyle

• A thorough explanation of the intermittent nature of the symptoms, despite therapy, must be stressed with the patient to achieve realistic expectations for future results.
• Patients should be encouraged to maintain a high-fiber diet and exercise regularly.
• A food-intake diary may identify certain foods that aggravate symptoms. A relationship of symptoms to ingestion of malabsorbed carbohydrates should be sought.

Pharmacological treatment

• Placebo response rates are high (range, 20%–70%).
• Few drugs seem to be of unequivocal benefit; many patients find drugs helpful in controlling symptoms, often preferring "as-required" medication to long-term usage [3].
• Treatment should be targeted to the predominant symptom.
• Avoid opiates and benzodiazepines because of potential for addiction.

Bulking agents

Standard dosage Bran ispaghula husk, or psyllium titrated to achieve ~1 bowel movement each day.
Milk of magnesia or Lactulose, 15 mL twice daily, increased as needed; stimulant laxatives are rarely needed.

Contraindications Intestinal obstruction, renal failure (milk of magnesia).

Special points Patients must take adequate fluid.

Main drug interactions None.

Main side effects Transient distension, flatulence, abdominal pain.

Antispasmodic drugs

Standard dosage *Dicyclomine:* orally, 10–40 mg up to four times daily, or *hyoscyamine,* 0.125 mg sublingually every 4 hours as needed or 0.375–0.5 mg sustained-release orally every 12 hours.

Contraindications Ileus, mechanical bowel obstruction, colitis, glaucoma, urinary outflow obstruction.

Special points Dosage times should be varied to suit the patient. Trials of sublingual hyoscyamine are useful in determining effectiveness because of rapid onset. Many patients have limited or poor symptom response to antispasmodic agents.

Main drug interactions Antacids may interfere with drug absorption; contraindicated in patients taking cisapride or procainamide

Main side effects Blurred vision, dry mouth, urinary hesitancy, drowsiness

Antidiarrheal drugs

Standard dosage Loperamide, 2–16 mg daily in divided doses or diphenoxylate and atropine, 2 tablets 3–4 times daily; dose adjusted to control symptoms.

Contraindications Intestinal obstruction, inflammatory bowel disease, fecal retention with overflow.

Special points Night-time dosage might prevent morning diarrhea.

Main drug interactions *Diphenoxylate/atropine:* anxiolytics and hypnotics.

Main side effects *Diphenoxylate/atropine:* constipation, dependence.

Other options

Polyethylene glycol 3350 may be used for refractory constipation, 17 g in 8 ounces water once or twice daily for short intervals.

For patients with predominant symptoms of pain, tricyclic antidepressants can be helpful but must be used cautiously because of side effects. Serotonin reuptake inhibitor antidepressants are likely to work as well, with fewer side effects. The 5-hydroxytryptamine-3 antagonists have proven efficacy for women with pain-predominant symptoms in the absence of constipation [3].

Alternative medicine

Recommended use: none.

Common use: enteric-coated peppermint oil; *Lactobacillus acidophilus*.

Caution: non-enteric-coated peppermint oil can cause gastroesophageal reflux.

Treatment aims

To reassure and educate patient regarding chronicity and intermittent nature of symptoms.

To control or cure the most intrusive symptom.

To treat associated psychological disorders [3].

Other treatments

• Behavioral therapy (hypnotherapy, psychotherapy, relaxation techniques) is effective for some intractable cases.
• Younger patients or those with identifiable psychological disease appear to benefit most.
• Behavioral therapy is relatively ineffective for older patients or patients with constant or chronic pain.

Prognosis

• This is a chronic relapsing condition.
• >75% of patients respond to treatment over 1 year.
• Response is better in men, patients with constipation-predominant IBS, and those with a short history or symptoms after acute diarrhea.

Follow-up and management

• Follow-up is not needed for mild or moderate cases.
• Regular, brief review of some moderate and severe cases may reduce inappropriate investigation and further referral.
• Patients must be monitored for change in symptoms; new or different symptoms should be investigated; persistent symptoms do not need further tests.

Key references

1. Drossman DA, Whitehead WE, Camilleri M: Irritable bowel syndrome: a technical review for practice guideline development. *Gastroenterology* 1997, **112**:2120–2137.
2. AGA Patient Care Committee: American Gastroenterological Association medical position statement: irritable bowel syndrome. *Gastroenterology* 1997, **112**:2118–2119.
3. Camilleri M: Therapeutic approach to the patient with irritable bowel syndrome. *Am J Med* 1999, **107**:27S–32S.
4. Whitehead WE, Engel BT, Schuster MM: Irritable bowel syndrome. *Dig Dis Sci* 1980, **25**:404–413.

Kaposi's sarcoma in AIDS

Diagnosis

Symptoms

Mucocutaneous
Generally asymptomatic, rarely painful or pruritic.

Lymphatic
Lymphadenopathy and edema.

Pulmonary
Dyspnea, cough.

Hemoptysis, chest pain (pleuritic or dull ache).

Gastrointestinal
Anorexia, abdominal pain, hematemesis, melena.

Signs

• Kaposi's sarcoma is a vascular neoplasm that can involve the skin, mucosa, or any organ system.

• Kaposi's sarcoma in AIDS differs from ordinary Kaposi's sarcoma in that patients present with multiple, widespread lesions.

• Visceral involvement occurs in 25% of patients with AIDS and Kaposi's sarcoma.

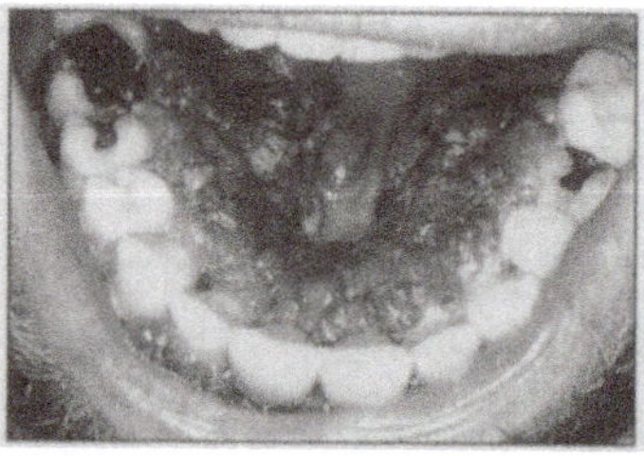

Oral Kaposi's sarcoma in HIV disease. (*See* Color Plate.)

Mucocutaneous
Violaceous macule, plaque, or nodule, surrounding edema.

Lymphatic
Firm or indurated lymphadenopathy.
Edema of dependent limbs.
Compression of adjacent structures.

Pulmonary
Pulmonary nodules or effusion.

Gastrointestinal
Palpable mass, tenderness.

Other signs
Organomegaly.

Investigations

General
Lymphocyte subset analysis: Kaposi's sarcoma usually occurs in patients with CD_4 cell count below 500/mm^3.
Complete blood count: to assess anemia; neutrophil and platelet count needed before chemotherapy.
Biopsy of involved organ: required for confirmation.

Serologic test: available to detect Kaposi's sarcoma–associated herpesvirus, but its sensitivity is insufficient for widespread use at this time.

Pulmonary
Chest radiography: to rule out infiltrates, nodules, or pleural effusion.
Fiberoptic bronchoscopy: for visualization and biopsy.

Gastrointestinal
Fiberoptic endoscopy or sigmoidoscopy: for visualization and biopsy.
Ultrasonography or CT: with guided biopsy, if disease is not seen by endoscopy.

Complications

Ulceration, infection, immobilization edema.

Respiratory failure.

Gastrointestinal obstruction, hemorrhage.

Differential diagnosis

Purpura, hematoma, angioma, nevus.

Bacillary angiomatosis, dermatofibroma, melanoma.

Etiology

Recent advances support a transmitted cofactor, human herpesvirus-8, also known as Kaposi's sarcoma–associated herpes virus.

• The following may have a role:

Genetic predisposition (elderly men from eastern Europe and Africa).

Immunosuppression.

HIV infection.

Growth factors and cytokines promoting growth of Kaposi's sarcoma.

Epidemiology

• Kaposi's sarcoma occurs in up to 48% of homosexual men with AIDS.

• It is increasing in heterosexual Africans with AIDS, in women who have acquired HIV from bisexual men, and in other risk groups.

• It is rare in children with AIDS.

• It is rarely seen in hemophiliac patients with AIDS.

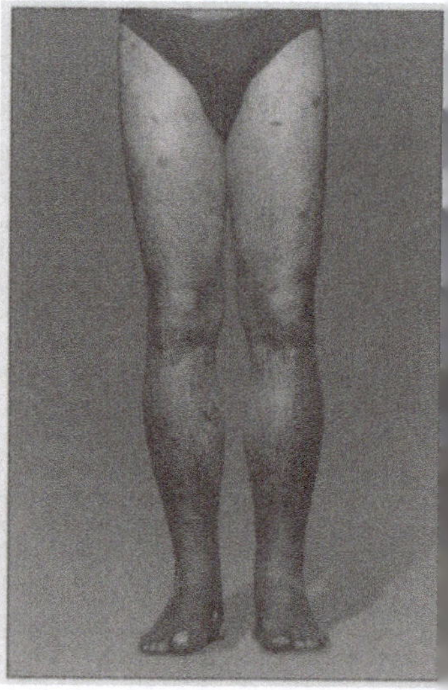

Generalized cutaneous Kaposi's sarcoma. (*See* Color Plate.)

Treatment

Diet and lifestyle

- Advise appropriate protection against sexually transmitted diseases.

Pharmacological treatment

- All treatment must be given under specialist supervision.

Topical therapy

Standard dosage Alitretinoin 0.1% gel, applied twice daily to cutaneous lesions.

Contraindications Pregnancy, not indicated when systemic anti-Kaposi's sarcoma therapy is required.

Special points Initial clinical trials showed response rates of 35%; response may be seen as early as 2–4 weeks, but most patients require longer application; application should continue as long as patient is still deriving benefit.

Main drug interactions DEET (N,N-dimethyl-m-toluamide, a common ingredient in insect repellents).

Main side effects Rash, burning/pain, pruritus, exfoliative dermatitis.

Intralesional chemotherapy

- Intralesional chemotherapy is indicated for limited mucocutaneous disease.

Standard dosage Bleomycin or vinblastine into lesion until blanching occurs.

Contraindications Infection at site.

Main drug interactions None of importance.

Main side effects Local pain and ulceration.

Interferon

- Interferons are indicated for good-prognosis Kaposi's sarcoma.

Standard dosage Interferon-α, 9 mu .i.m. or s.c. daily, possibly with zidovudine.

Contraindications Bone-marrow suppression, renal or hepatic impairment.

Special points Lesions may recur after treatment stops.

Main drug interactions None of importance.

Main side effects Influenza-like symptoms, neutropenia, anemia.

Liposomal anthracyclines

- The current standard treatment for advanced AIDS-related Kaposi's sarcoma.

Standard dosage Liposomal daunorubicin or doxorubicin, i.v. every 2 weeks.

Contraindications Pregnancy and lactation.

Special points Liposomes are stable, long-circulating carriers useful for delivering daunorubicin and doxorubicin to tumor sites with a lower toxicity than the free drug.

Main side effects Neutropenia, myocardial toxicity, mild anemia, alopecia.

Bleomycin and vincristine

- Indicated for patients with life-threatening or visceral disease.

Standard dosage Vincristine (or vinblastine if neuropathy develops) and bleomycin i.v. every 2 weeks, with hydrocortisone.

Contraindications Pregnancy and lactation (all), severe lung impairment (bleomycin); caution if patient has a neuropathy.

Main drug interactions Increased phenytoin concentrations.

Main side effects Neutropenia (all).
Bleomycin: rashes, increased skin pigmentation, Raynaud's phenomenon, hypersensitivity reaction, dose-related progressive pulmonary fibrosis.
Vincristine: alopecia, peripheral and autonomic neuropathy.
Vinblastine: myelotoxic, neurotoxic (less than vincristine).

Treatment aims

To achieve cosmetic improvement (limited disease).

To control new lesion development and to treat existing lesions (advancing disease).

To reduce tumor bulk and to treat pain, immobility, and infection (advanced disease).

Other treatments

- Isolated lesions can be excised to relieve symptoms.
- Radiation therapy provides good palliative results.

Prognosis

- Prognosis is extremely variable; survival has been shown to be extended in patients receiving highly active antiretroviral therapy.
- Death is often due to other AIDS-defining illnesses.
- Factors indicating poor prognosis include the following:

Previous opportunistic infections.

"B" symptoms.

Tumor-associated edema.

Nonnodal visceral Kaposi's sarcoma.

Follow-up and management

- Complete blood count must be monitored.
- Patients with limited disease must be followed up every 3 months.
- Patients with extensive disease must be followed up every 1–2 weeks.

General references

Boshoff C, Weiss RA: Kaposi's sarcoma-associated herpesvirus. *Adv Cancer Res* 1998, **75**:57–86.

Clearance given for Panretin gel. *Oncologist* 1999, **4**:187.

Gascon P, Schwartz RA: Kaposi's sarcoma. New treatment modalities. *Dermatol Clin* 2000, **18**:169–175.

Poignonec S, *et al.*: Intralesional bleomycin for acquired immunodeficiency syndrome-associated cutaneous Kaposi's sarcoma. *Arch Dermatol* 1995, **131**:228.

Yarchoan R: Therapy for Kaposi's sarcoma: recent advances and experimental approaches. *J Acquir Immune Defic Syndr* 1999, **21(1)**:S66–S73.

Knee injuries

Diagnosis

Symptoms

Pain: various locations—anterior, medial, lateral, posterior.

Locking.

Buckling/"giving-way."

Instability.

Popping.

Tearing.

Swelling.

Stiffness.

Limitation of flexion or extension.

Signs

Swelling (effusion, soft tissue).

Deformity.

Erythema.

Heat.

Muscular atrophy.

Tenderness to palpation (exact location).

Provocative maneuvers: Lachmann's test (best), Drawer sign, McMurray test, etc.

Investigations

Physical examination: of paramount importance; skillful examination by experienced musculoskeletal specialist may exceed the diagnostic accuracy of MRI, ultrasound, or arthrography.

Arthrocentesis.

Ultrasound.

Magnetic resonance imaging.

Arthrography.

Arthroscopy.

Complications

Atrophy.

Weakness.

Swelling.

Deformity.

Chronic pain.

Chronic arthritis.

Instability.

Locking.

Falling.

Gait disturbance.

Exercise limitation.

Chronic impairment.

Differential diagnosis

Hemarthrosis

Meniscal tears.

Ligamentous injuries.

Osteochondral fractures.

Patellar dislocation.

Locking

Bucket handle tear of meniscus.

Loose body.

Anterior cruciate ligament (ACL) tear.

Suprapatellar plica.

"Popping" noise

• ~70% of patients with ACL tear heard a "pop."

Immediate onset of effusion.

Unable to continue to participate in activity.

Timing of effusion

• Acute bleeding results in effusion within 1 hour of injury.

Ligamentous injuries.

Peripheral meniscal tears.

Osteochondral fractures.

• Late effusions (12–18 hours) are more typical for meniscal tears.

Etiology

Trauma of various types

Acute athletic injuries.

Chronic (repetitive, overuse).

Falling.

Multifactorial (*e.g.*, degenerative plus falling).

Mechanism of injury

• Internal or external rotation is most common.

• Contact is not required.

"Cutting" maneuvers.

Impact or collision.

Overuse.

Specific anatomical injuries

ACL tears.

Posterior cruciate ligament tears.

Meniscal tears.

Medical collateral ligament tears.

Sprains.

Patellar dislocation.

Fractures.

Proposed etiologies

Genetic predisposition.

"Q angle."

Inadequate pre-athletic competition conditioning.

Inadequate proprioceptive training.

Epidemiology

• Knee injuries are among the most common disabling injuries in all walks of life, especially among athletes (both casual/recreational and competitive/elite).

• Collision and contact sports are responsible for many knee injuries.

• An estimated 50% of high school football players will experience a knee injury per year.

Treatment

Diet and lifestyle

• Individualized treatment programs must consider patient preferences and activity expectations.

• Sports psychology strategies may be critical.

Pharmacological treatment

• Analgesic with acetaminophen, NSAIDs, codeine, and hydrocodone may be necessary.

• Attention to accurate diagnosis and early rehabilitation may help limit habituation.

Nonpharmacological treatment

• Conservative therapy involves the following:

RICE—*R*est, *I*ce, *C*ompression, *E*levation.

Early range-of-motion exercises.

Immobilization vs. ambulation.

Functional bracing.

Hamstring strengthening.

Rehabilitation: closed-chain kinetic exercises are best.

• Surgical therapy is another option.

• Other therapeutic options include arthroscopy and reconstructive surgery.

Treatment aims

To relieve pain.

To reduce swelling.

To restore full range of motion.

To prevent or reverse muscular atrophy.

To allow safe return to participation in previous activities.

Prognosis

• Prognosis varies widely depending on the specific structural injury and severity.

• ACL reconstruction may have a 50% failure rate.

• ACL-deficient knee may be complicated by degenerative changes in 40% of cases.

• Posterior cruciate ligament injury management is controversial: 5%–8% progress to arthritis; worse prognosis for combination injury; only moderate stability is currently achievable with surgery.

General references

Baker CL: *The Hughston Clinic Sports Medicine Book*. Baltimore: Williams and Wilkins; 1995.

Bergfeld JA: *Injuries of the Athlete's Knee*. Phoenix: American College of Rheumatology; 1996.

Birrer RB: *Sports Medicine for the Primary Care Physician*. Boca Raton, FL: CRC Press; 1994.

Garrick JG, Webb DR: *Sports Injuries: Diagnosis and Management*. Philadelphia: WB Saunders; 1990.

Mellion MB: *Sports Medicine Secrets*. Philadelphia: Hanley and Belfus; 1994.

Diagnosis

Symptoms and signs

- Any organ or tissue can be infected, so the clinical picture can vary enormously.
- The disease follows a biphasic course: the incubation period lasting 7–12 days (range, 2–20 days) is followed by the septicemic phase lasting 4–7 days, which precedes the immune phase lasting 4–30 days.

Anicteric leptospirosis

- This occurs in 90% of patients.
- Onset is abrupt.

Fever, headache, myalgia, malaise, prostration, with or without mental status changes.

Abdominal pain, nausea, vomiting, occasionally diarrhea.

Excruciating headache: usually heralds meningitis in immune stage.

Joint pains, myalgia, conjunctival suffusion, rashes, lymphadenopathy: common findings.

Lymphocytic meningitis: usually lasting a few days, never fatal.

Icteric leptospirosis (Weil's syndrome)

- This form occurs in 10% of patients.

Impaired renal and hepatic function: with anuria and deepening jaundice.

Hepatosplenomegaly, severe hemorrhages into skin, pleura, peritoneum, or gastrointestinal tract.

Vascular collapse and alterations in consciousness.

Myocarditis, hemorrhage, acute respiratory distress syndrome, multiorgan failure: causing death in 10%–20% of icteric patients.

Investigations

- Diagnosis is confirmed by isolation of the organism or detection of a rise in antibody titers.

Isolation: special media needed; organisms isolated from blood or CSF during septicemic phase and from urine during third week in untreated patients.

Serology: slide agglutination tests unreliable; antibodies appear in 6–12 days, reach maximum in 4 weeks, can be suppressed by antibiotic treatment; enzyme-linked immunosorbent assay IgM test detects antibodies from day 5 of illness; microagglutination test is specific and identifies infecting serotype.

Complete blood count and coagulation screen: to identify bleeding disorder and thrombocytopenia.

Liver function tests: usually normal except for raised bilirubin.

Serum creatinine measurement: to identify degree of renal impairment.

CSF analysis: to confirm lymphocytic meningitis.

Complications

Uveitis 6–12 weeks after original illness and chronic persistent leptospiruria: extremely rare.

Transplacental transmission, with fetal death and abortion: has occurred.

Differential diagnosis

Influenza-like illness, viral infections, aseptic meningitis, encephalitis.

Enteric-fever–like illness.

Infective hepatitis, other causes of jaundice.

Rickettsioses, brucellosis, malaria.

Septicemia, nephritis.

Leukemia, thrombocytopenic purpura, meningococcal disease.

Etiology

- In the United States, prevalent serotypes of pathogenic leptospires, *Leptospira interrogans*, are *icterohaemorrhagiae, australis, autumnalis,* and *canicola*.
- Wild and domestic animals, especially rats (*icterohaemorrhagiae*) and cattle.
- Contact of mucous membranes or abraded skin with infected animal tissue or urine or contaminated water or soil can lead to transmission.

Epidemiology

- People at risk include farmers, dairy-workers, abattoir workers, veterinarians, and those working or engaged in recreational pursuits on or in natural inland waters.

Treatment

Diet and lifestyle

• Rodents must be controlled in and around human habitations.

• Contamination of living, working, and recreational areas by infected urine should be prevented.

• Cuts should be covered by waterproof dressings and protective clothing worn.

• Immersion in natural inland waters should be avoided.

• Participants should shower after swimming, canoeing, windsurfing, or waterskiing.

• Safety cards should be issued to people at risk to show medical staff if illness occurs.

• Patients should be educated on modes of transmission and preventive measures.

• Domestic animals, especially cattle and dogs, should be immunized.

Pharmacological treatment

Antibiotics

• Antibiotics may influence the course of the disease only if given in the first week.

• Treatment may be needed for severe infections; efficacy unproven.

Standard dosage Penicillin G, 900 mg; ampicillin, 1 g; or erythromycin, 500 mg, all parenterally 4 times daily for 1 week.
Amoxicillin, 500 mg orally 3 times daily, or doxycycline, 100 mg twice daily for 1 week.

Contraindications Hypersensitivity; oral agents should be avoided in pregnancy, infancy, and childhood.

Special points *Penicillin:* can induce a short-lived exacerbation with pyrexia and hypotension: this Jarisch-Herxheimer reaction is regarded as a sign of leptospiral lysis.

Main drug interactions *Penicillins:* inactivate aminoglycoside in syringe.
Erythromycin: potentiates digoxin, warfarin, and carbamazepine.
Doxycycline: affects anticoagulant treatment.

Main side effects *Parenteral agents:* anaphylactic reaction, gastrointestinal reactions (rare).
Amoxicillin: erythematous rash in patients with glandular fever.
Doxycycline: photosensitivity (rare), permanent teeth discoloration.

For symptoms

Prompt correction of electrolyte imbalance.

Fresh blood, platelets, or clotting factors for hemorrhage.

Meperidine or morphine for severe pain.

Diazepam and phenytoin for seizures.

Steroids for thrombocytopenia.

Hemodialysis for renal failure.

Treatment aims

To alleviate symptoms.

Prognosis

• Most cases are mild and often undiagnosed; patients recover spontaneously.

• In Weil's syndrome with hepatorenal involvement, mortality is 10%–20%.

• No ill effects are seen after renal or hepatic involvement in surviving patients.

• Death without jaundice is extremely rare.

• Reinfection by a different serotype is possible.

Follow-up and management

• Supportive treatment includes analgesics, sedation, and antiemetics.

• Renal and cardiac function must be monitored daily.

General references

Ferguson IR: Leptospirosis surveillance: 1990–1992. *Commun Dis Rep* 1993, 3:R47–R48.

Ferguson IR: Leptospirosis update. *BMJ* 1991, **302**:128–129.

Hill MK, Sanders CV: Leptospiral pneumonia. *Semin Respir Infect* 1997, **12**:44–49.

Leukemia, acute lymphoblastic in adults

Diagnosis

Symptoms

• Usually, acute lymphoblastic leukemia (ALL) has a short history of 2–3 months.

Tiredness and dyspnea: due to anemia.

Recurrent infections: due to leukopenia.

Bruising and bleeding: due to thrombocytopenia.

Symptoms of hyperviscosity: if leukocyte count is very high (*e.g.*, $>200 \times 10^9$/L).

Joint and bone pain: less common than in children.

Signs

• Often, no physical signs are manifest.

Pallor.

Evidence of infection.

Purpura or bruising.

Lymphadenopathy or hepatosplenomegaly.

Investigations

General

Full blood count (with Romanowsky's or Wright-Giemsa stained film): diagnosis may be evident from careful morphological examination; leukemic blasts not always seen in peripheral blood; platelet count and hemoglobin may be low or normal.

Bone-marrow aspiration: blasts should be >30% to make the diagnosis.

Blood urea nitrogen, creatinine, electrolytes, calcium, phosphate, urate measurement: important initial investigations before starting treatment, particularly if leukocyte count is high.

Chest radiography: to look for mediastinal mass, seen in 70% of patients with T-cell acute lymphoblastic leukemia (ALL; high risk of tumor lysis syndrome if this is present).

Lumbar puncture with CSF cytology: important initial investigation to detect CNS involvement (unusual at presentation).

Special

• These tests help to confirm the diagnosis; confirming that blasts are lymphoid in origin is occasionally difficult on light microscopy.

• They also help to categorize the disease more fully, giving additional prognostic information.

Cytochemistry: helps to differentiate ALL from acute myeloblastic leukemia (*e.g.*, negative reaction with Sudan black).

Immunophenotyping: identifies origin of blast cell using panel of cell-surface "markers"; useful markers include TdT (all subtypes positive except B ALL), CD10 (identifies common ALL antigen), CD19 (positive in B-lineage ALL), CD2 (positive in T-lineage ALL).

Cytogenetics: direct examination of chromosomes at metaphase can identify translocations in ~70% of patients with ALL; this can identify poor-risk patients, *e.g.*, those with t(9,22) or Philadelphia-positive ALL, which has a bad prognosis; may provide a marker that can be used to detect early relapse.

Complications

• Most complications are related to bone-marrow failure (cytopenia) due to the disease or, more often, to the intensive treatment needed.

Differential diagnosis

Acute myeloid leukemia

Aplastic anemia: diagnosis of ALL might not be obvious initially if presenting leukocyte count is low and bone-marrow aspirate "dry."

Lymphoblastic lymphoma: predominantly lymphomatous presentation, with <25% blasts in bone marrow; distinction may be arbitrary in adults because treatment is often the same.

Etiology

• The cause of ALL is unknown; it is presumed to be due to genetic mutations, the risk of which is increased by DNA damage, *e.g.*, due to radiation or DNA repair defects.

• Victims of exposure to ionizing radiation have a higher incidence of leukemia, but this is more often myeloid than lymphoid in origin.

Epidemiology

• Acute lymphoblastic leukemia is uncommon in adults, particularly in those aged >30 years.

• Patients aged >15 years are defined as adults because they constitute a separate group with much poorer remission and survival rates.

Classification [1]

Morphological

• Based on appearance on light microscopy, the French–American–British (FAB) classifi-cation divides ALL into L1, L2, and L3.

• This has little correlation with prognosis or immunophenotype, except L3 morphology with B-cell ALL.

Immunological

• On the basis of expression of surface antigens by the blast cells, ALL is divided into T lineage (early T precursor and T cell ALL) and B lineage (early B precursor, common ALL, pre-B ALL, and B cell ALL).

Treatment

Diet and lifestyle

• Nutrition must be maintained.

• Psychological support should be provided to patients and their relatives, especially if a young family is involved; financial support should be considered if earnings are disrupted.

• Patients must take precautions against infection during neutropenia.

Pharmacological treatment [2,3]

Principles

• Treatment should be given under specialist supervision, within the context of a clinical trial if possible to allow adequate evaluation and the development of new treatments.

• Initial treatment involves several blocks of inpatient treatment.

Induction: remission (*i.e.*, <5% blasts in bone marrow) can be achieved in ~80% of adults, usually within 1 month of starting treatment; agents include steroids, vincristine, and anthracyclines.

Consolidation: usually follows quickly after induction, and new chemotherapeutic agents should be introduced; optimum duration and intensity of treatment have not yet been established.

CNS-directed treatment: often described as "CNS prophylaxis"; CNS leukemia occurs in ~37% of patients in hematological remission if no specific treatment directed at the CNS is given; possible treatments include cranial irradiation, intrathecal methotrexate, or high-dose i.v. methotrexate (which crosses the blood–brain barrier).

Maintenance therapy: continuous treatment for ~2 years improves outcome; usual treatment involves weekly methotrexate and 6-mercaptopurine, with monthly courses of vincristine and steroids.

Supportive treatment: particularly important in the early stages of treatment; includes allopurinol, adequate hydration, blood-product support, and timely use of antimicrobial treatment.

General complications of treatment

Myelosuppression (inevitable).

Hair loss.

Compromise or loss of fertility.

Infection, particularly during neutropenia: empirical treatment is often needed for bacterial, viral, or fungal infection.

Nausea and vomiting: may be easy to control.

Complications of specific drugs

Vincristine: extravasation injury, alopecia, muscle and jaw pain, urinary retention, dysphagia, peripheral neuropathy.

Prednisone: Cushing's syndrome and other steroidal side effects (including psychiatric).

L-Asparaginase: thrombotic episodes, pancreatitis, anaphylaxis.

Daunorubicin: extravasation injury, cardiomyopathy, bone-marrow suppression, vomiting, gut toxicity.

Cytarabine: gut and bone-marrow toxicity, erythema, cerebellar toxicity in high doses.

Thioguanine: hepatic and bone-marrow toxicity, rashes.

VP16 epipodophyllotoxin: gut and bone-marrow toxicity.

Methotrexate: renal, hepatic, and gut dysfunction; bone-marrow suppression; mucositis (depending on dose and mode of treatment); affects intellect.

Mercaptopurine: bone-marrow suppression, rashes, hepatic dysfunction.

Treatment aims

To maximize chance of cure, with minimal toxicity.

Other treatments [3,4]

Allogeneic bone-marrow transplantation

• Adults should receive allograft in first complete remission if they have a matched sibling donor and are aged 20–50 years; this is particularly indicated in Philadelphia-positive disease (incurable by drugs alone).

Autologous bone-marrow transplantation

• The role is less well established; by definition, it is available to more patients but will probably be less effective because of lack of "graft-versus-leukemia effect."

Prognosis

• Despite best available treatment, overall survival in adult disease is poorer than in childhood disease; studies indicate a 5-year leukemia-free survival of 20%–35% in unselected patients.

• Poor prognostic factors include increasing age, high leukocyte count at presentation (>30 × 10^9/L), t(9,22), and failure to reach complete remission after 1 month of treatment.

Follow-up and management

• After discharge the patient must be seen regularly for full blood count; if patient is receiving maintenance therapy, the dose may need adjustment.

• Prophylactic is usually given during this time.

Relapsed disease

• ~70% of patients relapse; the risk varies from 40% for young adults to >80% for patients aged >50 years.

• Treatment depends on age, duration of initial remission, and previous treatment.

• Relapsed disease is not curable by conventional chemotherapy.

Key references

1. Bain BJ: *Leukaemia Diagnosis: A Guide to the FAB Classification.* London: Gower Medical Publishing; 1990.
2. Copelan EA, McGuire EA: The biology and treatment of acute lymphoblastic leukemia in adults. *Blood* 1995, **85**:1151–1168.
3. Pui CH, Evans WE: Acute lymphoblastic leukemia. *N Engl J Med* 1998, **339**:605–615.
4. Bruserud O (ed.): Lymphoblastic leukemia. *Leukemia* 1997, **11(suppl 4)**:1395–1597.

Leukemia, acute lymphoblastic in children

Diagnosis

Symptoms

• A constellation of symptoms is seen, many nonspecific and related to bone-marrow failure.

Easy bruising, bone pain, fevers, pallor, lethargy, anorexia, malaise: due to bone-marrow failure.

Abdominal distention: due to hepatosplenomegaly.

Shortness of breath, facial swelling: due to mediastinal mass; unusual.

Headache, vomiting: due to CNS disease; unusual.

Overt bleeding: due to bone-marrow failure; unusual.

Signs

Pyrexia, mucosal bleeding, skin purpura, pallor, congestive heart failure (rare): due to bone-marrow failure.

Hepatosplenomegaly, lymphadenopathy, upper trunk and facial edema with distended superficial veins, skin infiltrates, testicular enlargement: due to leukemic "mass."

Cranial nerve palsies (III, V, VI, VII), papilledema, fundal hemorrhages, leukemic infiltrates: due to CNS disease (rare).

Investigations

Full blood count: shows pancytopenia, normal counts, or isolated raised leukocyte count.

Blood film: shows possible presence of leukemic blasts.

Bone-marrow morphology: confirms diagnosis in conjunction with cytochemistry and immunophenotyping (mature B cell varieties treated on lymphoma-type protocols).

Chest radiography: for mediastinal mass.

Lumbar puncture: for CNS disease.

Blood urea nitrogen, creatine, electrolytes, and urate analysis.

Liver function tests: for liver failure (rare).

Complications

Early

• Early complications are usually related to drug side effects or further bone-marrow suppression.

Tumor lysis syndrome, associated with hyperkalemia, hyperuricemia, hyperphosphatemia, renal dysfunction.

Infection of all types.

Bleeding.

Anemia.

Vomiting, hair loss, peripheral neuropathy and myopathy, mucositis.

Late

Learning difficulties: *e.g.*, problems with short-term memory or concentration; due to cranial radiation.

Cardiotoxicity: due to anthracycline treatment.

Cataracts, sterility, growth and hormone problems: due to cyclophosphamide treatment and total body irradiation for bone-marrow transplantation.

Secondary malignancies: due to epipodophyllotoxins.

Differential diagnosis

Lymphadenopathy

Infections: *e.g.*, infectious mononucleosis.

Lymphomas or other tumors.

Hepatosplenomegaly

Leishmaniasis.

Macrophage, metabolic, storage, or autoimmune disorders.

Lymphomas.

Bone-marrow failure

Aplastic anemia.

Myelodysplasia.

Macrophage disorders.

Autoimmune disorders.

Bone-marrow tumor: *e.g.*, neuroblastoma.

Infections: *e.g.*, tuberculosis, visceral leishmaniasis.

Etiology [1]

• The cause is unknown but is presumed to be a genetic mutation.

• Increased risk is associated with the following:

Down syndrome.

Fanconi's anemia.

Bloom syndrome.

Ataxia telangiectasia and various immunodeficiency disorders.

• The effects of irradiation or electromagnetic fields are unconfirmed.

Epidemiology [1]

• Acute lymphoblastic leukemia is the most common malignant disease of childhood.

• A peak incidence at 2–5 years accounts for 20% of all leukemia.

• Slightly more boys than girls are affected.

• 85% of childhood leukemia is acute lymphoblastic.

Treatment

Diet and lifestyle

- Specialist support is needed for children and their families, including siblings, both in the hospital during treatment and after discharge.
- Maintenance of nutrition is important.

Pharmacological treatment

- Treatment should be given under specialist supervision, in the context of a clinical trial if possible to allow adequate evaluation and the development of new treatments.

Treatment choice [2–6]

For high-risk patients (slow remitters, near haploid, Philadelphia-chromosome positive, older boys with high leukocyte counts, usually $>100 \times 10^9$/L): transplantation in first remission.

For patients at high risk of CNS disease relapse (leukocyte count $>50 \times 10^9$/L): cranial irradiation or high-dose i.v. methotrexate or cytosine arabinoside or triple-drug therapy.

For lower-risk patients (leukocyte count $<50 \times 10^9$/L): continuing intrathecal or high-dose methotrexate or cytosine arabinoside.

For patients with CNS disease at diagnosis: craniospinal or cranial irradiation and continuing intrathecal methotrexate.

For infants <6 months: intensive multiagent treatment.

Principles

Induction: usually vincristine, asparaginase, steroids; remission in 97% of patients.

Consolidation: intensive treatment with some different drugs from induction course to eradicate "resistant clones."

CNS-directed treatment: to eradicate disease in CNS sanctuary site.

Consolidation: as for second step; two or three consolidations may be needed.

Continuation of treatment up to 2 years: to eradicate minimal residue disease.

Complications of specific drugs

Vincristine: extravasation injury, alopecia, muscle and jaw pain, urinary retention, dysphagia, peripheral neuropathy.

Prednisone: Cushing's syndrome and other steroidal side effects (including psychiatric).

L-Asparaginase: thrombotic episodes, pancreatitis, anaphylaxis.

Daunorubicin: extravasation injury, cardiomyopathy, bone-marrow suppression, vomiting, gut toxicity.

Cytarabine: gut and bone-marrow toxicity, erythema, cerebellar toxicity in high doses.

Thioguanine: hepatic and bone-marrow toxicity, rashes.

VP16 epipodophyllotoxin: gut and bone-marrow toxicity.

Methotrexate: renal, hepatic, and gut dysfunction, bone-marrow suppression, mucositis (depending on dose and mode of treatment); affects intellect.

Mercaptopurine: bone-marrow suppression, rashes, hepatic dysfunction.

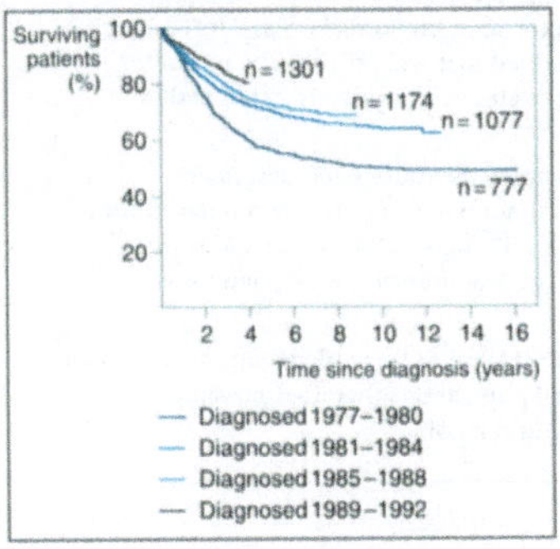

Survival rates of patients with acute lymphoblastic leukemia 1977–1992.

Treatment aims

To cure patient at least cost (toxicity of specific drugs and complications).

Other treatments

Transplantation.

Cranial irradiation.

See Pharmacological treatment *for indications.*

Prognosis

- Adverse prognostic features include failure to remit after 1 month of treatment, Philadelphia-chromosome positive, near haploid, older age, male sex, high leukocyte count, infants aged <6 months.

Follow-up and management

- Patients receiving continuation treatment should be followed up every 1–2 weeks, depending on blood count.
- After completion of treatment, all patients should be followed indefinitely; for the first 6 years, they must be checked carefully for signs of relapse (organomegaly, testicular swelling, low blood count, blasts on film) and endocrine, growth, intellectual, and cardiac late effects.
- Prophylactic co-trimoxazole should be given for pneumocystis.
- Advice should be given on returning to school and when normal childhood immunization can be given.

Key references

1. Greaves MF: Speculations on the cause of childhood acute lymphoblastic leukemia. *Leukemia* 1988, 2:120–125.
2. Chessell JM: Treatment of childhood acute lymphoblastic leukemia: present issues and future prospects. *Blood Rev* 1992, 6:193–203.
3. Eden OB, *et al.*: Report to the MRC: results of MRC UKALL VIII. *Br J Haematol* 1990, **78**:187–196.
4. Hann IM: CNS directed therapy in childhood. *Br J Haematol* 1992, **82**:2–5.
5. Hann IM, *et al.*: UKCCSG MACHO chemotherapy for B stages IV NHL & B-ALL. *Br J Haematol* 1990, **76**:359–364.
6. Pinkel D, Woo S: Prevention and treatment of meningeal leukemia in children. *Blood* 1994: **84**:355–366.

Diagnosis

Symptoms

• Some patients are symptom-free.

Lethargy, irritability, fatigue, reduced exercise tolerance: symptoms of anemia.

Infection: due to leukopenia.

Spontaneous bleeding or bruising: symptom of thrombocytopenia.

Signs

Pallor, infections, bruises, petechiae.

Lymphadenopathy or hepatosplenomegaly: occasionally.

Gum hypertrophy, skin infiltration: features of monocytic leukemia.

Hemorrhagic manifestations: feature of promyelocytic leukemia.

Investigations

Complete blood count: often shows reduced hemoglobin; thrombocytopenia frequent; leukocyte count $>100 \times 10^9$/L unusual, associated with poor response to treatment; presentation with count $<3.0 \times 10^9$/L common; differential leukocyte count usually abnormal, with neutropenia and presence of "blast cells" (large cells, ~1.5–2 times diameter of erythrocytes; usually have large nuclear:cytoplasmic ratio [less common with acute myeloid leukemia]; nucleus may contain at least one nucleolus [usually large single nucleus in monoblast]; blasts may show features of maturation, *e.g.*, cytoplasmic granulation, Auer rods, or monocytic features); numerical thrombocytopenia confirmed morphologically.

Bone-marrow analysis: increased proportion of blast cells; conventionally, >30% of bone-marrow cellularity to distinguish from the blastic forms of myelodysplasia.

Cytochemistry: useful to confirm myeloid or monocytic origin of blast cells; Sudan black, chloroacetate esterase, or myeloperoxidase stains.

Immunophenotyping: most reliable method of determining hematopoietic lineage of origin; expression of CD33 or CD15 indicates some myeloid maturation; CD34 and HLA DR earlier nonlymphoid markers, providing important objective methods for distinguishing myeloid from lymphoid leukemia; antigens are expressed on normal cells, but "leukemia-specific" or aberrant phenotypes have been identified that will probably be useful for monitoring remission status when normal antigens are inappropriately expressed on leukemic cells.

Cytogenetics: many structural chromosome abnormalities have been described; relationship between prognosis and cytogenetic abnormality, *e.g.*, better prognosis with French-American-British (FAB) M3 (usually has 15:17 translocation), some M2s (8:21 translocation), and inverted 16; worse prognosis with abnormalities or deletions of chromosomes 5 and 7.

Molecular genetics: molecular probes for the 15:17 and 8:21 translocations now available; polymerase chain reaction detection of minor cell populations therefore possible; such technology will be important in assessing quality of remission.

Complications

Overwhelming infection.

Bleeding: especially intracranial in promyelocytic leukemia.

Differential diagnosis

Any cause of pancytopenia.

Etiology

• The risk is increased in the following:

Radiation exposure.

Chemotherapy for cancer, *e.g.*, Hodgkin's disease.

Chronic myeloproliferative disorders or myelodysplasia.

Epidemiology

• Acute myeloid leukemia is the most common form in adults.

• The median age of presentation is ~60 years.

• The male:female ratio is equal.

• The prevalence increases with age (*e.g.*, 1 in 10^5 in children, up to 3 in 10^5 in patients aged >70 years).

Classification

• Based on morphological appearance, acute myeloid leukemia is divided into FAB types M0–7.

• The M3 type (promyelocytic) has a high chance of remission and a lower risk of relapse.

• Although valuable in standardizing terminology, this classification has limited prognostic power.

Treatment

Diet and lifestyle

• Nutrition must be maintained.

• Psychological support should be provided to patients and their relatives, especially if a young family is involved; financial support should be considered if earnings are disrupted.

• Patients must take precautions against infection during neutropenia.

Pharmacological treatment

Supportive

• Infection can be prevented by expert nursing care; isolation in a single room with air filtration; mouth care; vigilance of temperature, mucous membranes, perineum, and central-line site.

• Infection can be treated, after appropriate bacteriological, fungal, and viral samples have been taken, by rapid introduction of i.v. antibiotics (usually aminoglycoside and ceftazidime or penicillin with anti-pseudomonal activity).

• If a response occurs within 48 hours, treatment should be continued for 3–5 days; in cases of no or incomplete response and no bacteriological guidance, vancomycin should be added; if further failure, i.v. amphotericin should be added. (*See* Infections in hematological malignancy *for details.*)

For coagulopathy

• Coagulation factor deficiency should be corrected by appropriate blood products or vitamin K supplements.

• Severe coagulopathy, including disseminated intravascular coagulation, can be a dominant feature in promyelocytic leukemia (FAB M3), needing specific attention.

• All-*trans*-retinoic acid (ATRA) can be effective in correcting the defect (usually within 2–3 days).

• Blood-product support is essential, but fibrinolytic inhibition (tranexamic acid) and heparin have become less widely used.

Chemotherapy [1–3]

• Treatment should be given under specialist supervision.

• If induction of remission and consolidation phases are sufficiently intense, maintenance should be of no benefit.

• Drugs include anthracyclines, cytosine arabinoside, thioguanine, and etoposide; side effects include cardiotoxicity.

• Intensive supportive care is needed during remission induction, but most patients achieve complete remission with one course.

• An extra course may be needed for less intensive approaches, and more supportive care may be needed overall in all patient groups.

Treatment aims

To restore normal bone-marrow function.
To establish prolonged remission or cure.

Other treatments [4]

Allogeneic bone-marrow transplantation

• The risk of relapse is reduced from 60% to 15%.

• Treatment-related mortality of 30% is due to toxicity, infection, pneumonitis, and graft-versus-host disease.

• Treatment may result in infertility and late cataracts (in 10%–15% of patients).

• Allogeneic transplantation is available only to 10%–15% of patients.

Autologous bone-marrow transplantation

• Autologous transplantation is indicated for patients aged <55 years without a sibling donor.

Advantages: less toxicity, no graft-versus-host disease, available to more patients, low procedure-related mortality (6%–8%).

Disadvantages: potential for the harvested marrow to be contaminated, lack of graft-versus-leukemia effect.

Prognosis [1–3]

• Current schedules achieve remission in 80% of patients aged <55 years (range, 90% in children to 70% in those in fifth decade); in older patients, remission rates of 60% should be achieved.

• 30%–40% of patients aged <55 years treated by chemotherapy alone and 20% of older patients remain in remission at 5 years.

• Allogeneic bone-marrow transplantation cures 50%–60% of recipients; autologous transplantation cures 45%–55% of recipients.

• Treatment failure >5 years is rare after bone-marrow transplantation but occurs in chemotherapy patients, although at a much lower rate than in the first 2–3 years.

Follow-up and management

• 2–3 weeks after recovery from hypoplasia induced by chemotherapy, the bone marrow should be checked for remission status.

Key references

1. Burnett AK, Lowenberg B: Treatment options for remission in acute myeloid leukemia. In *Hematological Oncology*, vol 1. Cambridge: Cambridge University Press; 1991.
2. Foon KA, Gale RP: Therapy for acute myelogenous leukemia. *Blood Rev* 1992, **6**:15–25.
3. Zittoun RA, Mondelli F, Willemze R, *et al.*: Autologous or allogeneic bone marrow trans-plantation compared with intensive chemo-therapy in acute myelogenous leukemia. *N Engl J Med* 1995, **332**: 217–223.
4. Edenfield WJ, Gore SD: Stage-specific application of allogeneic and autologous marrow transplantation in the management of acute myeloid leukemia. *Semin Oncol* 1999, **26**:21–34.

Leukemia, chronic lymphocytic

Diagnosis

Symptoms

• 70% of patients are asymptomatic, the diagnosis being made on incidental blood count.

Enlarged lymph nodes or discomfort in left upper quadrant of abdomen: in 20%.

Symptoms of anemia: uncommon.

Bruising or bleeding: rare.

Weight loss, fever unassociated with infection, night sweats: "B" symptoms; very unusual and often signal transformation to high-grade lymphoma.

Signs

Lymphadenopathy in cervical, axillary, or inguinal regions: in 30% of patients.

Mild to moderate splenomegaly: in 10%.

Hepatomegaly: rare.

Anemia: unusual.

Purpura: rare.

Investigations [1]

Complete blood count: shows lymphocytosis $>5 \times 10^9$/L, mature monomorphic small lymphocytes with smear cells.

Lymphocyte marker analysis: shows sparse surface immunoglobulin of a single light chain (κ or λ): $CD5^+$, $CD19^+$, $CD20^+$, $CD23^+$, $CD37^+$, $CD3^-$, $CD10^-$, $CD22^-$.

Serum immunoglobulin measurement: reduced concentration in all classes; IgM paraprotein in 5% of patients.

Direct antiglobulin test: positive in 10%.

Bone-marrow trephine analysis: interstitial, nodular, or diffuse infiltration by small lymphocytes.

Karyotyping: trisomy 12 in 30%, deletion 13q14 in 25%.

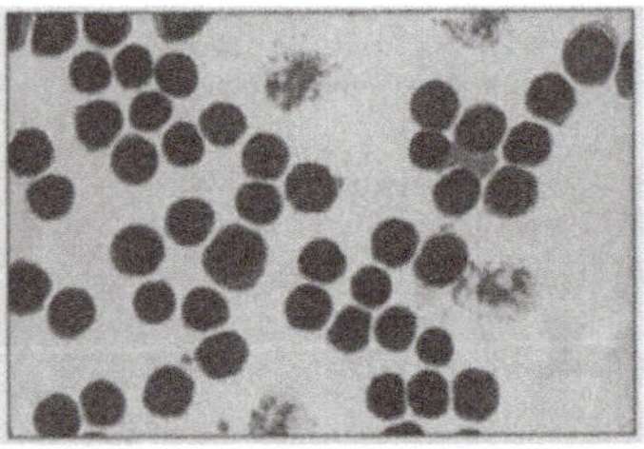

Leukapheresis specimen from chronic lymphocytic leukemia with Romanowsky's stain, showing small monomorphic lymphocytes with occasional prolymphocytes and smear cells. (*See* Color Plate.)

Complications

Autoimmune hemolytic anemia: in 10% of patients, more in stage C.

Autoimmune thrombocytopenia, neutropenia, pure erythrocyte aplasia: in <2%.

Infection: due to hypogammaglobulinemia in a few patients.

Shingles: in 25%.

Transformation to prolymphocytic leukemia or high-grade lymphoma: in 10% and 2% (Richter's syndrome), respectively.

Pneumococcal pneumonia.

Differential diagnosis

Prolymphocytic leukemia.

Hairy cell leukemia.

Splenic lymphoma with villous lymphocytes.

Large granular lymphocytic leukemia.

Sézary syndrome and adult T-cell lymphoma/leukemia.

Follicle center cell lymphoma and mantle cell lymphoma.

Etiology

• The cause is unknown.

• No association has been found with radiation or retroviruses.

Epidemiology

• Chronic lymphocytic leukemia is the most common leukemia in western Europe and North America.

• It is increasingly common with age, the median age at presentation being 69 years.

• The male : female ratio is 2 : 1, but, because women live longer, in the elderly population, ~50% of patients are female.

• A slight familial tendency has been found.

Staging

Rai (United States)

Stage 0: lymphocytosis alone.

Stage I: with lymphadenopathy.

Stage II: with spleno- or hepatomegaly.

Stage III: with anemia; hemoglobin <110 g/L.

Stage IV: with thrombocytopenia; platelets $<100 \times 10^9$/L.

Binet (Europe) [2]

Stage A: no anemia or thrombocytopenia; <3 lymphoid areas* enlarged.

Stage B: no anemia or thrombocytopenia; 3 or more lymphoid areas* enlarged.

Stage C: hemoglobin <100 g/L or platelets $<100 \times 10^9$/dL.

*Cervical, axillary, or inguinal lymph nodes; spleen; and liver.

Treatment

Diet and lifestyle

• Patients should be encouraged to lead a normal life.

Pharmacological treatment

• All treatment should be given under specialist supervision.

• Stage A patients should not receive chemotherapy.

Alkylating agents

• Chlorambucil is the mainstay of treatment.

• The response rate is 50%.

Standard dosage	Chlorambucil, continuous oral dose or intermittently every 4 weeks. Cyclophosphamide, orally or i.v. every 2–3 weeks.
Contraindications	None.
Main drug interactions	None established.
Main side effects	Nausea and bone-marrow suppression, drug rash (in 5% of patients on chlorambucil), alopecia (cyclophosphamide).

Nucleoside analogues

• Fludarabine is a purine analogue that produces responses in up to 50% of patients resistant to chlorambucil.

• 2-Chlorodeoxyadenosine is a similar agent.

Standard dosage	Fludarabine, i.v. daily for 5 days every 28 days.
Contraindications	None.
Special points	Less bone-marrow suppression than chlorambucil, but profound T lymphocytopenia, which predisposes to infection by viruses, fungi, or protozoa.
Main drug interactions	None established.
Main side effects	Bone-marrow suppression, immunosuppression.

Other options

Prednisone: for patients with autoimmune complications; effects a redistribution of lymphocytes from tissue to blood and may be useful in thrombocytopenic patients beginning treatment with alkylating agents.

CHOP chemotherapy (cyclophosphamide, doxorubicin, vincristine, prednisone): may be more effective than chlorambucil in stage C cases.

Immunoglobulin replacement therapy: for patients with recurrent infections whose serum immunoglobulin concentration is <4 g/L.

Under investigation

Bone-marrow transplantation: for younger patients with HLA matched sibling donor [3].

Treatment aims

To relieve symptoms.

To prolong life in stage B or C patients.

Other treatments

• Leukapheresis may be used to prevent or treat hyperleukocytosis in patients with very high leukocyte counts (>500 × 10^9/L) or to control the leukocyte count in drug-resistant patients.

Prognosis [4]

• Stage A patients have the same prognosis as age- and sex-matched controls.

• Median survivals achieved with chlorambucil are 12 years for stage A, 5 years for stage B, and 2 years for stage C patients.

Follow-up and management

• Patients should be observed to determine whether the disease is progressive; patients whose disease is static and who are asymptomatic may safely be observed.

• Progressive disease should be treated by chlorambucil.

• All patients need long-term follow-up, the frequency being determined by the pace of the disease.

Key references

1. Pangalis GA, Angelopoulou MK, Vassilakopoulos TP, *et al.*: B-chronic lymphocytic leukemia, small lymphocytic lymphoma, and lymphoplasmacytic lymphoma, including Waldenström's macroglobulinemia: a clinical, morphologic, and biologic spectrum of similar disorders. *Semin Hematol* 1999, **36**:104–114.
2. Boussiotis VA, Freedman AS, Nadler LM: Bone marrow transplantation for low-grade lymphoma and chronic lymphocytic leukemia. *Semin Hematol* 1999, **36**:209–216.
3. Binet JL: Treatment of chronic lymphocytic leukaemia. *Clin Haematol* 1993, **6**:867–878.
4. Mauro FR, Foa R, Giannarelli, *et al.*: Clinical characteristics and outcome of young chronic lymphocytic leukemia patients: a single institution study of 204 cases. *Blood* 1999, **94**:448–454.
5. Meinhardt G, Wendtner CM, Hallek M: Molecular pathogenesis of chronic lymphocytic leukemia: factors and signaling pathways regulating cell growth and survival. *J Mol Med* 1999, **77**:282–293.

Leukemia, hairy cell

Diagnosis

Symptoms

• 25% of patients are asymptomatic.

Fatigue, weight loss, weakness: in 25%.

Bruising or infections: in 25%.

Abdominal fullness or discomfort: in 25%.

Signs

Moderate to massive splenomegaly: in 75% of patients.

Lymphadenopathy: rarely.

Hepatomegaly: occasionally.

Signs of infection, bleeding, or bruising.

Investigations

Complete blood count: shows normochromic, normocytic anemia, neutropenia, monocytopenia, thrombocytopenia, "hairy" leukocytosis. Hairy cells are large lymphocytes with open nucleus, with loose, lacy chromatin and one or two distinct nucleoli; the cytoplasm is pale blue-grey, with fine, hair-like projections; usually few are found in blood, but they number >10 × 10^9/L in 10% of patients.

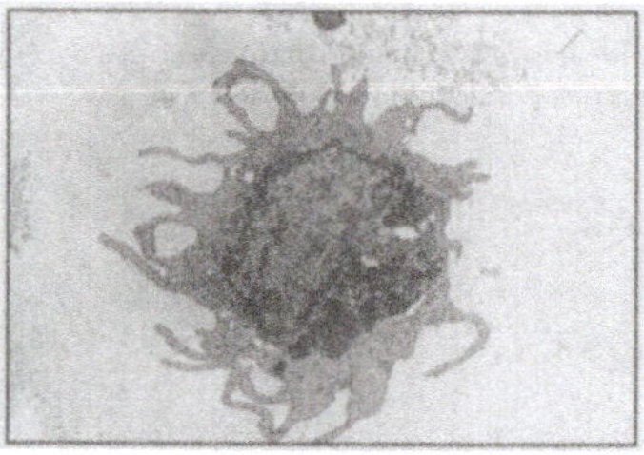

Hairy cell on transmission electron microscopy.

Bone-marrow trephine: shows diffuse or patchy infiltration of leukemic cells, characteristic pale halos of cytoplasm surrounding monotonous, bland nuclei.

Cell marker analysis: moderately positive for surface immunoglobulin of a single light chain class; $CD11c^+$, $CD19^+$, $CD20^+$, $CD25^+$, $CD37^+$, $CD3^-$, $CD15^-$, $CD10^-$; tartrate-resistant acid phosphatase positive.

Complications

Infections: neutropenia and monocytopenia render patients susceptible to infection, so both bacterial and more atypical infections are seen; fungal, protozoan, and mycobacterial organisms are implicated.

Vasculitis: microscopic polyarteritis in 5% of patients.

Differential diagnosis

Tumors with similar "hairy" cytoplasmic projections: *e.g.*, splenic lymphoma with villous lymphocytes, hairy cell variant, and monocytoid B-cell lymphoma (may be distinguished by careful morphological examination and cell markers).

Other causes of isolated splenomegaly with hypersplenism.

Etiology

• The cause is unknown, although in one case of the rare T-cell hairy cell leukemia, the human T-cell lymphotrophic virus II retrovirus was isolated.

Epidemiology

• This is a rare leukemia, with an incidence of 1 in 500 000 population.

• The male : female ratio is 4 : 1.

• The median age at presentation is 55 years (range, 20–90 years).

Treatment

Diet and lifestyle

• Patients should be encouraged to live as normal a life as possible.

Pharmacological treatment [1]

• Treatment should be given under specialist supervision.

2-Chlorodeoxyadenosine

Standard dosage	0.1 mg/kg/day by continuous infusion for 7 days.
Main side effects	Fever and infection during the first month following therapy, decline in the neutrophil and platelet counts, which generally reverses by the end of the fourth week.

• This is currently the drug of choice in the United States.

• It may be capable of producing long-term complete remissions [2].

• Side effects include myelotoxicity (intense hematological support needed early in treatment to prevent death from hemorrhage or infection), and the risk of fungal, viral, or protozoan infection due to $CD4^+$ T-cell suppression (similar to effects seen with 2′deoxycoformycin).

Additional agents

α-Interferon

Standard dosage	α-Interferon, 3 MU 3 times weekly usually for 2 years, is effective in 80% of patients.
Contraindications	Hypersensitivity, severe renal failure, hepatic or myeloid dysfunction.
Special points	Early in treatment, cytopenias may be exacerbated, with risk of hemorrhage or infection. Antibodies to α-interferon occur in 50% of patients but only occasionally cause treatment failure.
Main drug interactions	No information available.
Main side effects	Mild influenza-like symptoms (improve with time).

2′Deoxycoformycin

• This inhibitor of adenosine deaminase produces a higher rate of complete remissions than interferon (up to 80%); early studies suggest that most remissions are prolonged beyond 4 years.

Standard dosage	2′Deoxycoformycin, 4 mg/m² weekly for 3 weeks, then on alternate weeks for 6 weeks.
Contraindications	Low glomerular filtration rate; caution in renal dysfunction.
Main drug interactions	No information available.
Main side effects	Risk of fungal, viral, or protozoan infections due to $CD4^+$ T-cell suppression.

Treatment aims

To allow patient to lead symptom-free life.

To attempt, particularly in younger patients, long-term remission, albeit at some early risk from increased pancytopenia.

Other treatments

• Splenectomy was the mainstay of treatment before effective drugs were available; it is still used in patients with the following:

Important splenomegaly and cytopenias.

Relatively little bone-marrow involvement.

Intolerance of pharmaceutical intervention.

Laparotomy for other reasons.

Prognosis

• With modern treatment, most patients have a normal lifespan.

• Only a few patients achieve complete remission after interferon treatment, but most achieve sufficient hematological improvement to make their disease of no consequence to them.

• Relapse occurs progressively 1–2 years off treatment with interferon [2].

• Progression-free survival 83% for 4 years for patients with complete remission.

Follow-up and management

• All patients should be followed up indefinitely.

• Treatment should be reintroduced if symptoms or blood count warrants it.

Key reference

1. Pettitt AR, Zuzel M, Cawley JC: Hairy-cell leukaemia: biology and management. *Br J Haematol* 1999, **106**:2–8.
2. Tallman MS, Peterson LC, Hakimian D, *et al.*: Treatment of hairy-cell leukemia: current views. *Semin Hematol* 1999, **36**:155–163.

Liver failure, fulminant

Diagnosis

Symptoms

(*See* Hepatic encephalopathy for *grading scheme*.)

Lethargy, nausea, vomiting: prodromal symptoms of viral hepatitis.

Abdominal pain, hematemesis: common after acetaminophen overdose.

Drowsiness or confusion: in grades 1 and 2 encephalopathy.

Restlessness, agitation: possibly aggressive; in grade 3.

Unresponsiveness: in grade 4.

Signs

Jaundice: common but not always manifest at presentation.

Encephalopathy of varying severity: asterixis, fetor hepaticus late features.

Liver size: typically normal, although hepatomegaly may be seen in severe hepatitis, Budd–Chiari syndrome.

Ascites: late finding.

Systemic hypertension, decerebrate posturing, hyperventilation: indicating cerebral edema.

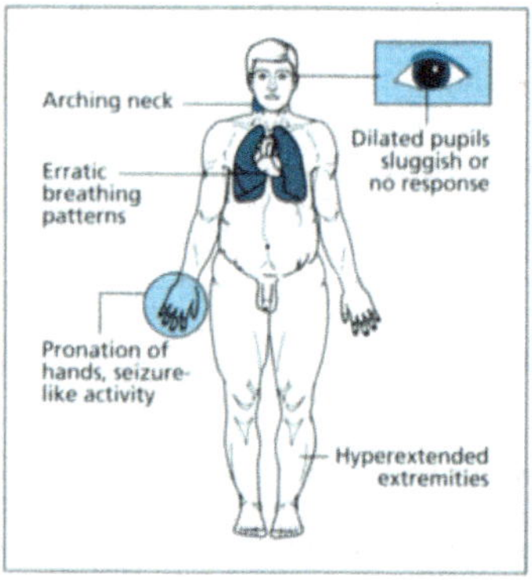

Physical findings in patients with fulminant liver failure.

Investigations

History: of toxin (amanita mushrooms, carbon tetrachloride) or drug exposure (*e.g.*, acetaminophen, isoniazid, NSAIDs).

Prothrombin time or INR measurement: prolongation (in the absence of disseminated intravascular coagulation or vitamin K deficiency) indicates severe hepatic dysfunction.

Hemoglobin measurement: hemolytic anemia suggests Wilson's disease.

Serum bilirubin measurement: prognostic significance in non-acetaminophen-induced cases.

Serum creatinine measurement: urea underestimates renal impairment; prognostic significance in acetaminophen-induced cases.

Glucose measurement: hypoglycemia indicates poor prognosis.

Acetaminophen measurement.

Hepatitis A serology: to detect IgM anti-hepatitis A virus.

Hepatitis B and D serology: to detect IgM anti-core, hepatitis B surface antigen, anti-hepatitis D virus (only in patients with positive hepatitis B surface antigen and risk factors such as illicit intravenous drug use).

Hepatitis C antibody: often negative in fulminant non-A, non-B viral hepatitis.

Ceruloplasmin and 24-hour urinary copper excretion: low and high, respectively, in Wilson's disease.

Cytomegalovirus, Epstein-Barr serology: particularly important in immunosuppressed or pregnant patients.

Ultrasonography: to assess liver size and texture; doppler studies to assess hepatic vasculature.

Complications

• All of the following are late complications, mainly occurring in patients with advanced encephalopathy.

Hypoglycemia.	**Cerebral edema [1].**	**Respiratory failure.**
Renal failure.	**Bleeding, infection.**	**Hypotension.**

Differential diagnosis

Acute decompensation of chronic liver disease.

Reye's syndrome.

Other metabolic encephalopathy.

Intracranial lesions, bleeding central nervous system infections.

Etiology

Acetaminophen ingestion.

Hepatitis A, B, B/D, or E virus infection, seronegative hepatitis (non-A, non-B, non-C), halothane hepatitis, idiosyncratic drug reactions.

Pregnancy-related, Budd–Chiari syndrome, autoimmune liver disease, malignancy, mushroom poisoning [2,3].

Epidemiology

• Fulminant liver failure complicates 0.1%–4.7% of hospitalized patients with viral hepatitis, depending on the cause.

Classification

Fulminant liver failure

Acute liver failure with encephalopathy in a patient presumed to have a normal liver within 8 weeks of the onset of illness.

Hyperacute liver failure

Encephalopathy within 7 days of onset of jaundice, characterized by high incidence of cerebral edema; despite this, many patients survive with medical management.

Subacute liver failure [1]

Encephalopathy 8–12 weeks after onset of jaundice, low incidence of cerebral edema and less severe prolongation of prothrombin times, but poor prognosis [4,5].

Treatment

Diet and lifestyle

- Referral to a liver transplant center is required.
- Parenteral or enteral nutritional support is usually needed.

Pharmacological treatment

(*See also* Hepatic encephalopathy.)

N-acetylcysteine

- Administration should begin as soon as possible and optimally within 12 hours of ingestion of acetaminophen [6].
- Most patients with liver failure from acetaminophen will not benefit from N-acetylcysteine.

Standard dosage *N*-acetylcysteine, 140 mg/kg loading dose, followed by maintenance dose of 70 mg/kg orally every 4 hours (for 17 doses).

Contraindications Hypersensitivity.

Main drug interactions None.

Main side effects Occasional hypersensitivity reactions; watch for vomiting and aspiration.

Gastric protection

- H_2 antagonists or sucralfate reduce the incidence of gastrointestinal bleeding.

Standard dosage Ranitidine, 50 mg i.v. every 8 hours.
Sucralfate, 1 g orally 6-hourly every 6 hours.

Contraindications Hypersensitivity.

Main drug interactions None relevant.

Main side effects *Ranitidine:* thrombocytopenia.

Lactulose

- This is often ineffective and recommended only in patients with grade 1 or 2 encephalopathy.

Standard dosage Lactulose, 30 mL every 8 hours; doses titrated to three bowel movements daily.

Contraindications Gastrointestinal obstruction.

Main drug interactions None relevant.

Main side effects Nausea, flatulence, abdominal discomfort.

King's College criteria for liver transplantation in fulminant liver failure

PT >100 seconds (irrespective of grade of encephalopathy) or any of the following criteria:

- Age <10 or >40 years
- Period of jaundice to encephalopathy >7 days
- PT >50
- Bilirubin >17 mg/dL
- Etiology: viral hepatitis, halothane, drug reaction, Wilson's disease

For acetaminophen-induced liver failure

pH <7.3 (irrespective of grade of encephalopathy) or all three of the following:

- Grade III-IV encephalopathy
- PT >100
- Serum creatinine >3.4 mg/dL

Treatment aims

To anticipate and treat complications.

Other treatments

- Liver transplantation must be considered early in patients with progressive fulminant hepatitis (see table) [7].

Prognosis

- Most patients who do not progress beyond grade 2 encephalopathy survive.
- Survivors make complete recoveries; progression to chronic liver disease is unusual.

Follow-up and management

- Long-term medical follow-up is rarely needed, except in liver-graft recipients.
- Psychiatric and social support is important in overdose cases.

Key references

1. Blei AT, *et al.*: Complications of intracranial pressure monitoring in fulminant hepatic failure. *Lancet* 1993, **341**:157–158.
2. Riordan SM, Williams R: Treatment of hepatic encephalopathy. *N Engl J Med* 1997, **337**:473–479.
3. Fingerote RJ: Fulminant hepatic failure. *Am J Gastroenterol* 1993, **88**:1000–1010.
4. O'Grady JG, Schalm SW, Williams R: Acute liver failure: redefining the syndromes. *Lancet* 1993, **342**:273–275.
5. Devlin J: Pretransplantation clinical status and outcome of emergency transplantation for acute liver failure. *Hepatology* 1995, **21**:1018–1024.
6. Harrison PM, *et al.*: Improvement by *N*-acetylcysteine of hemodynamics and oxygen transport in fulminant hepatic failure. *N Engl J Med* 1991, **324**:1853–1857.
7. Lee WM: Management of acute liver failure. *Semin Liver Dis* 1996, **16**:369–378.

Low back pain

Diagnosis

Symptoms

Back pain: acute, <7 days' duration; chronic, >30 days' duration.

"Hip pain" (buttock).

Morning stiffness.

Leg pain.

Limitation of motion.

Functional impairment.

Signs

Loss of lumbar lordosis.

Muscle spasm: visible, palpable.

Thoracolumbar scoliosis.

Pelvic tilt.

Antalgic gait.

"Foot drop" gait.

"Listing gait."

Limitation of lumbar motion: flexion, extension, lateral bending.

Soft-tissue tenderness.

Straight leg raising test.

Great toe extension weakness.

Ankle dorsiflexion weakness.

Diminished ankle strength reflexes.

Sensory deficit.

Calf wasting.

Sciatica.

Normal hip range of motion and examination results.

Investigations

Complete blood count, alkaline phosphatase, prostate-specific antigen.

Plain radiographs.

CT/MRI imaging.

Electromyography.

Serum protein electrophoresis.

Myelography.

Cybex muscle strength testing.

Complications

Sensory deficit.

Motor deficit.

Gait disturbance.

Work impairment.

Narcotic dependence.

Foot drop.

Bowel/bladder incontinence.

Paresis.

Atrophy.

Differential diagnosis

Osteoarthritis.

Herniated nucleus pulposus.

Infection (osteomyelitis).

Seronegative spondyloarthropathy (ankylosing spondylitis).

Compression fracture.

Spinal stenosis.

Neoplasm.

Radiculopathy.

Etiology

Muscle spasm.

Herniated nucleus pulposus.

Spondylolisthesis.

Bony spurring.

Spinal stenosis.

Degenerative disk disease.

Infection (vertebral body or disk).

Seronegative spondyloarthropathy.

Ankylosing spondylitis.

Psoriatic arthritis.

Reiter's syndrome.

Enteropathic arthritis.

Epidemiology

- 25% of patients are 30–50 years of age.
- The most common cause of disability in people aged <45 years.
- 60% of patients have recurrence within 1 year.
- Low back pain accounts for ~10% of family practice visits annually.
- Risk factors for low back pain include occupation, anxiety, depression, pregnancy, and cigarette smoking.
- Back pain is among the top 10 most common symptoms seen by internists.
- Back pain is the second most common reason for surgery in the United States.
- Costs are estimated at $25 billion in direct medical care costs annually (1995).
- Associated costs are >$40 billion (includes lost productivity, compensation, litigation).

Treatment

Diet and lifestyle

• Patients should discontinue smoking.

• Weight reduction and a regular exercise regimen are important in the treatment of low back pain.

• Patient education and participation in their own rehabilitation is important in maintaining back health and preventing back pain recurrence ("back school").

• Job modification may be necessary.

• Physiatry referral may be helpful.

Pharmacological treatment

NSAIDs: ibuprofen, 400–800 mg 4 times daily; piroxicam, 20 mg daily.

• NSAIDs are of modest benefit.

• Analgesics and narcotics are best avoided or used only in short-term strategy.

• The use of muscle relaxants is controversial.

Nonpharmacological treatment

Chronic pain management techniques, visual imagery, meditation, relaxation techniques.

Electrical stimulation.

Transcutaneous electrical nerve stimulation unit: controversial.

Physical therapy (ultrasound, massage).

Extension exercises.

Flexion exercises.

Activity restriction.

Alternative medicine

Recommended use: none.

Common use: meadowsweet (*Filipendula ulmaria*); kava kava (*Piper methysticum*); valarian (*Valarian officinalis*); Jamaican dogwood (*Piscidia erythrina*); true unicorn root (*Aletris farinosa*).

Caution: kava kava use may have adverse environmental effects.

Treatment aims

To restore range of motion.

To improve comfort.

To improve sleep.

To improve function.

Prognosis

• Prognosis is highly variable.

• 90% of back pain sufferers experience recurrences.

Follow-up and management

• A multidisciplinary approach may be very helpful.

General references

Borenstein DG: Chronic low back pain. *Rheum Dis Clin North Am* 1996, **22**:439–456.

Cavanaugh JM, Ozaktay AC, Yamashita T, *et al.*: Mechanisms of low back pain: a neurophysiologic and neuroanatomic study. *Clin Orthop* 1997, **335**:166–180.

Lower gastrointestinal tract bleeding

Diagnosis

Symptoms

Visible red blood per rectum (*i.e.,* hematochezia).

Rectal urgency.

Orthostatic light-headedness.

Abdominal pain: relief most common with defecation.

Burning perianal pain with defecation: suggests a perianal fissure.

- Black stool (*i.e.*, melanoma) suggests upper gastrointestinal bleeding.

Signs

Perianal inflammation: friable hemorrhoid; sentinel tag in midline with underlying fissure.

Hematochezia (occasionally melena).

Tachycardia, orthostatic hypotension: indicates significant blood loss.

Occult blood in stool.

Pallor: in patients with anemia.

Investigations

Complete blood count: to determine the presence of anemia.

Patients with acute blood loss will initially have normal or "baseline" hemoglobin levels that decrease with the compensatory shift of fluid into the vascular compartment.

Microcytic anemia suggests iron deficiency and chronic ongoing loss. Thalassemia or nongastrointestinal blood loss (*e.g.*, menstruation) should also be considered.

- Iron deficiency requires a thorough evaluation of the lower gastrointestinal mucosa (*i.e.*, colonoscopy) and, if normal, studies of the small bowel or upper gastrointestinal tract in patients with upper gastrointestinal symptoms or weight loss.

Colonic imaging: usually required to exclude the presence of malignancy; lower gastrointestinal bleeding in the setting of clinical infection in patients <50 years of age can usually be managed without colonic imaging; however, careful observation for inflammatory bowel disease is warranted and a high suspicion for pseudomembranous colitis maintained.
Anoscopy: to evaluate symptoms of perianal bleeding (*i.e.*, blood only on the toilet paper or surface of formed stool) in relatively young patients without a family history of gastrointestinal malignancies if a bleeding source is readily identified (*e.g.*, fissure, hemorrhoid).
Colonscopy: to evalute patients >50 years of age with lower gastrointestinal bleeding, or if hemoglobin decreases; signs and symptoms of obvious perianal disease alone in patients with no family history for gastrointestinal cancer may be evaluated with flexible sigmoidoscopy alone with close clinical follow-up.
Air contrast barium enemas: relatively poor sensitivity for etiologies of lower gastrointestinal bleeding, particularly of the rectosigmoid and perianal regions.

Upper gastrointestinal tract studies: endoscopy, small bowel barium radiography, enteroscopy should be considered in patients with occult bleeding and anemia. Arteriovenous malformations are the most common cause of occult gastrointestinal bleeding, and this diagnosis is often rendered presumptively when other diseases of the proximal gastrointestinal tract have been excluded.

Stool studies: for *Clostridium difficile* and *Entamoeba histolytica*, infectious causes of lower gastrointestinal bleeding that respond to antibiotics (*e.g.*, metronidazole, 500 mg every 8 hours), that may be lethal if missed; other infectious causes should be considered in patients with dysentery (*see* Infectious diarrhea).

Nuclear medicine scans: tagged erythrocyte scans for patients with unexplained recurrent blood loss; Meckel's scan for patients with possible Meckel's diverticulum [1].

Mesenteric angiography: usually for patients with active bleeding (usually verified by a tagged erythrocyte nuclear medicine scan) when embolic therapy or a focused surgical resection is being considered.

Complications

Exsanguination.
Cardiac or cerebrovascular ischemia.
Metabolic acidosis.
Prerenal insufficiency.

Etiology

Slow or brisk bleeding most commonly from the colon but occasionally from the small intestine.

Epidemiology

More common in the elderly.

Differential diagnosis

Diverticular bleeding.
Arteriovenous malformations/angio-dysplasia.
Hemorrhoids.
Perianal fissure.
Inflammatory bowel disease (ulcerative colitis > Crohn's disease; acute self-limited colitis).
Infectious colitis/enteritis (*e.g., E. histolytica, Campylobacter jejuni, Shigella* spp., *Salmonella* spp., *Escherichia coli, C. difficile.*)
Ischemic colitis, radiation colitis.
Colonic malignancies (e.g., adenocarcinoma, lymphoma, carcinoid).
NSAID enteropathy.
Upper gastrointestinal bleeding with rapid transit.
Meckel's diverticulum.

Treatment

Diet and lifestyle

- Patients should seek medical advice promptly.
- Patients must maintain proper hydration.
- Patients should refrain from inhibitors of platelet function (*i.e.*, aspirin, other NSAIDs).
- High-fiber diet and sitz baths are recommended for patients with perianal disease (*i.e.*, fissures, hemorrhoids).

Pharmacological treatment

- *See* Anal fissure, Hemorrhoidal disease, Diverticular disease of the colon, Colorectal cancer, *and* Inflammatory bowel disease.

Iron replacement

- Patients with gastrointestinal blood loss and iron deficiency anemia typically benefit from iron replacement therapy, *e.g.*, ferrous sulfate.

Standard dosage	325 mg 3 times daily on an empty stomach.
Contraindications	Hypersensitivity.
Main drug interactions	Antacids, tetracycline impair the absorption of iron and should not be taken within 2 hours.
Main side effects	Nausea, abdominal discomfort, and constipation; parenteral iron therapy may be required if side effects of oral iron are intolerable.
Special points	Inform patient that iron supplements will result in black stool that may be confused with (or mask) gastrointestinal bleeding; iron supplements compromise visualization of the mucosa during colonoscopy and as such should be discontinued at least 5 days before the procedure.

- Intra-arterial vasopressin via selective catheterization of the bleeding vessel may be effective in the control of bleeding from diverticula or angiodysplasia.
- Chronic anemia from angiodysplasia despite the use of iron supplements may respond to daily estrogen-progesterone therapy (*e.g.*, ormonovum = 1 mg norethindrone + 0.05 mg mestranol); use with caution in men or patients with cardiovascular disease.

Treatment aims

To identify source of bleeding.

To treat underlying disease process to achieve cessation of bleeding.

To prevent complications from anemia or hypovolemia.

Other treatment options

Therapeutic colonoscopy or enteroscopy with cautery of identified bleeding sites.

Angiographic embolization of bleeding vessels [2].

Surgical resection of bleeding site (identified by endoscopy, radionuclide scans, or angiography).

Prognosis

Highly dependent on the source of bleeding and degree of blood loss [4].

Follow-up and management

Highly dependent on the source of bleeding; an explanation for gastrointestinal blood loss must always be sought.

Key references

1. Saeed ZA, Woods KL: Gastrointestinal bleeding. *Curr Pract Med* 1998, **1**:785–796.
2. Barkin JS, Ross BS: Medical therapy for chronic gastrointestinal tract bleeding of obscure origin. *Am J Gastroenterol* 1998, **93**:1250–1254.
3. Gostout CJ: The role of endoscopy in managing acute lower gastrointestinal bleeding. *N Engl J Med* 2000, **342**:125–127.
4. Moreno P, *et al.*: Efficacy and safety of an early discharge protocol in low-risk patients with upper gastrointestinal bleeding. *Am J Med* 1998, **105**:176–181.

Diagnosis

Symptoms

Cough, hemoptysis, breathlessness, hoarseness.

Chest pain, lymphadenopathy.

Weight loss, general malaise.

Intellectual impairment, headache, focal neuropathy, tremor.

Signs

- Signs are not always manifest.

Lung nodule or mass.

Lobar or lung collapse, consolidation, pleural effusion, monophonic wheeze.

Cervical lymphadenopathy, hepatomegaly, local chest-wall tenderness, Horner syndrome, neurological deficit.

Finger clubbing, cerebellar degeneration, peripheral neuropathy.

Investigations [1]

For diagnosis

Chest radiography: shows mass, collapse, distal infection, abscess, adenopathy, metastases.

Sputum cytology: shows malignant cells.

Bronchoscopy: tumor often is directly visible; operability can be assessed, and samples can be obtained for cytology and histology.

Pleural aspiration and biopsy: primary test if effusion present; malignant cells indicate inoperable tumor.

For staging

Bronchoscopy: to assess presence of central disease.

CT of thorax (including adrenal glands): to assess presence of hilar or mediastinal adenopathy, as well involvement of adrenal glands (metastatic site).

Mediastinoscopy: to evaluate lymphadenopathy.

Biochemistry: may indicate bone or liver involvement; sodium and calcium disturbance may occur without metastasis.

Liver ultrasonography: disease often spreads to liver.

CT of brain: disease often spreads to brain.

Pulmonary function tests: to assess ability to tolerate lung resection.

Complications

Lobar collapse, obstruction of superior vena cava.

Pneumonia, abscess.

Pain, pleural effusion.

Pericardial effusion, direct invasion.

Metastases: especially bone, brain, liver, adrenal glands.

Local neurological invasion, neuropathies.

Cushing's syndrome, inappropriate antidiuretic hormone secretion, hypercalcemia.

Recurrent venous thrombosis.

Clubbing, hypertrophic osteoarthropathy.

Differential diagnosis

Simple pneumonia.

Benign tumor or cysts.

Tuberculosis.

Pulmonary metastases.

Other causes of lung abscess.

Other causes of pleural effusion.

Etiology [2]

- Causes include the following:

Cigarette smoking: lung cancer was rare in the 19th century, and its increase is closely linked to the increasing popularity of cigarettes in the 20th century.

Atmospheric pollution: increased rates in urban areas.

Radioactivity: radon, uranium.

Manufacturing: chromate, asbestos, nickel, arsenic, hematite.

Epidemiology

- Lung cancer is the most common fatal cancer in men and women in the United States.
- The rate of lung cancer mortality is increasing.

Treatment

Diet and lifestyle

- Anorexia is a common feature; no specific diet is needed.
- Patients should be encouraged to be active.
- Most patients stop smoking after diagnosis, but this does not alter prognosis significantly.

Pharmacological treatment [3–6]

- Chemotherapy is the treatment of choice for small-cell cancer; various regimens are available.
- No satisfactory regimen has yet been found for large-cell tumors (*i.e.*, adenocarcinoma, squamous-cell or anaplastic tumors).
- The local oncology service should be consulted.

Nonpharmacological treatment [3,4]

Surgical resection

- Surgical resection is possible in only a few patients.
- It is limited by the frequent involvement of mediastinal nodes and central structures.
- Adequate lung function is needed (forced expiratory volume in 1 second >1.2 L for lobectomy, >1.5 L for pneumonectomy).
- Surgical resection is rarely appropriate for small-cell lung cancer (usually has extensive central disease, even if endoscopically resectable).

Radiation therapy [4,7]

- Palliative radiation therapy is useful in the management of hemoptysis and bony deposits.
- Radiation therapy can achieve local control of primary tumor and may improve survival.
- "Local" (endobronchial) radiation therapy, a novel experimental treatment, has yet to show any superiority to palliative external-beam radiation therapy.

Endobronchial laser resection [8]

- This is a palliative procedure for tracheal or main bronchus disease.
- It is available in only a few specialist centers.

Treatment aims

To identify patients who can be treated surgically.

To identify patients with small-cell cancer and treat them by chemotherapy.

To provide palliative treatment, guided by symptoms, to the remaining patients.

Prognosis

- Prognosis is generally poor unless the tumor is resectable.
- When disease is technically resectable, the 5-year survival rate is ~28%.

Follow-up and management

- Surgical cure is possible in 5%–10% of patients.
- In patients who are inoperable, the main goal is palliation.
- Local symptoms are usually best treated by radiation therapy.

Key references

1. Lillington G: Management of solitary pulmonary nodules. *Dis Mon* 1991, **37**:279–318.
2. Sethi T: Science, medicine, and the future: lung cancer. *BMJ* 1997, **314**:652–655.
3. Murren J, Buzaid A: Chemotherapy and radiation for the treatment of non–small-cell lung cancer. *Clin Chest Med* 1993, **14**:161–200.
4. Adjei AA, Marks RS, Bonner JA: Current guidelines for the management of small cell lung cancer. *Mayo Clin Proc* 1999, **74**:809–816.
5. Burn PA, Corney DN: Overview of Chemotherapy for small cell lung cancer. *Semin Oncol* 1997, **24**:S7–S74.
6. Ardizzoni A, Grossi F, Meazza R, Ferrini S: New perspectives for the pharmacological and biological therapy of small cell lung cancer. *Crit Rev Oncol Hematol* 1999, **31**:135–145.
7. Hazuka MB, Bunn PA: Controversies in the nonsurgical treatment of stage III non–small-cell lung cancer. *Am Rev Resp Dis* 1992, **145**:967–977.
8. Pierce RJ: Lasers, brachytherapy and stents—keeping airways open. *Resp Med* 1991, **85**:263–265.

Diagnosis

Symptoms

• Patients may be asymptomatic.

Acute disease

• Symptoms occur 3–32 days after tick bite.

Influenza-like illness: malaise, pyrexia, myalgia, arthralgia, sore throat.

Rash.

Stiff neck.

Photophobia.

Chronic disease

• Symptoms occur weeks or months later.

Headache, stiff neck, photophobia, confusion, concentration and memory impairment, pain in extremities.

Chest pain.

Joint pain and swelling.

Abdominal pain, tenderness, diarrhea.

Rashes.

Signs

Acute disease

Pyrexia, tender muscles or joints, inflamed throat.

Erythema chronicum migrans: characteristic rash (~5 cm), red macule or papule at site of tick bite, enlarges peripherally with central clearing over several weeks; metastatic lesions may develop; can last months.

Lymphadenopathy.

Meningism.

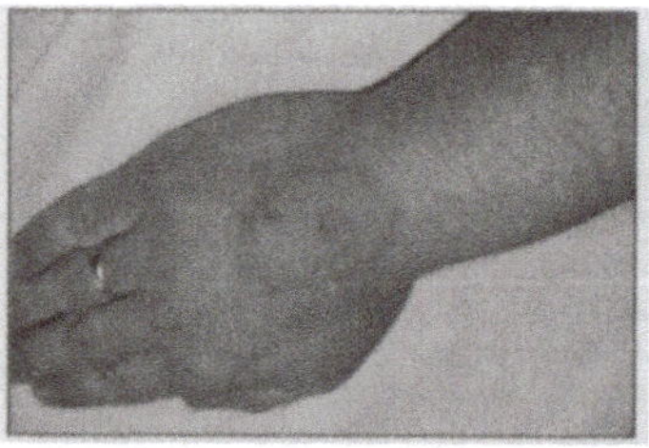

Erythema chronicum migrans. (*See* Color Plate.)

Chronic disease

Meningitis, encephalitis, cranial neuritis (especially Bell's palsy), radiculoneuritis, peripheral neuropathies.

Atrioventricular block, myopericarditis.

Arthritis.

Hepatomegaly, splenomegaly.

Acrodermatitis chronica atrophicans: vivid red lesions becoming sclerotic or atrophic.

Acrodermatitis chronicum atrophicans.

Investigations

Microscopy, histopathology, and culture: lack sensitivity and not widely available but may be diagnostic.

Serological tests: widely available but not diagnostic (support clinical diagnosis); IgM tests positive 3–6 weeks after infection, may persist for many months, but may not be reproducible; IgG tests positive 6–8 weeks after infection, may remain positive for years, but more reproducible so are mainstay of diagnosis; immunofluorescence tests and enzyme-linked immunosorbent assays most widely available.

• False-negative antibody results may occur early in illness, with antibiotic treatment, or due to immune complexes; a negative antibody test does not exclude the diagnosis. False-positive results are due to other spirochete infections, other infections, or the test; Western blotting may distinguish true- from false-positive results.

Complications

CNS abnormalities.

Cardiac conduction disturbances.

Oligoarthitis.

Differential diagnosis

Erythema chronicum migrans

Erythema marginatum.

Erythema multiforme rheumaticum.

Granuloma annulare.

Lymphadenopathy

Infectious mononucleosis.

Cytomegalovirus.

Toxoplasmosis.

Neurological symptoms

Infectious diseases.

Toxoplasmosis.

Guillain–Barré syndrome.

Multiple sclerosis.

Cardiac symptoms

Infectious diseases.

Chronic heart disease.

Digitalis use.

Arthritis

Rheumatoid arthritis.

Reactive arthritis.

Other dermatological symptoms

Erythema nodosum.

Circulatory insufficiencies.

Lymphoma.

Etiology

• Infection is transmitted by tick bites, usually *Ixodes scapularis* in the United States.

• The causative organism is *Borrelia burgdorferi*, a spirochete.

Epidemiology

• Lyme disease is found in the United States, Europe, Russia, China, Japan, and Australia.

• Occurrence parallels distribution and infection in ticks (0%–25%).

• In forested areas, 5%–10% of the population has antibodies.

• Infection peaks in June and July.

• It is found in patients of all ages but especially in the most active and those exposed to ticks.

Treatment

Diet and lifestyle

• No special precautions are necessary.

Pharmacological treatment

Criteria for treatment

• The risk depends on infected tick attachment: <24 hours, little risk; 48 hours, 50% risk; 72 hours, almost certain infection.

• Infection occurs in ~10% of people bitten by infected ticks, so empirical treatment is not justified in areas where infected ticks are rare.

• Erythema chronicum migrans must be treated; acute disease with positive serology and chronic disease when other causes are excluded warrant treatment.

• Treatment should be considered in anxious patients with possible infection but without high expectation of success.

• Asymptomatic individuals with positive serology probably should not be treated.

For acute disease or Bell's palsy

Standard dosage Doxycycline, 200 mg orally daily for 14 days.
Amoxicillin, 500 mg 3 times daily for 14 days.

Contraindications *Doxycycline:* pregnancy, lactation, children aged <12 years, systemic lupus erythematosus, porphyria.
Amoxicillin: penicillin hypersensitivity.

Main drug interactions *Doxycycline:* anticoagulants, antiepileptics, oral contraceptives.
Amoxicillin: anticoagulants, oral contraceptives.

Main side effects *Doxycycline:* nausea, vomiting, diarrhea, headache.
Amoxicillin: nausea, diarrhea, rashes.

• Erythromycin and clarithromycin are less effective but can be used in penicillin-sensitive children.

For chronic disease

• Chronic disease may be cardiac, neurological, or rheumatological.

Standard dosage Ceftriaxone, 2 g i.v. or i.m. daily for 14–21 days.
Penicillin G, 3 g i.v. 4 times daily for 14–21 days.

Contraindications *Ceftriaxone:* hypersensitivity to cephalosporin.
Penicillin: hypersensitivity.

Main drug interactions *Ceftriaxone:* anticoagulants, probenecid.
Penicillin: anticoagulants, oral contraceptives.

Main side effects *Ceftriaxone:* gastrointestinal symptoms, allergic reactions, rashes, hematological disturbance, liver dysfunction.
Penicillin: sensitivity reactions, especially urticaria, angioedema, anaphylaxis.

Alternative medicine

Recommended use: none.

Common use: thyme (*Thymus vulgaris*); garlic (*Allium sativa*); echinacea (*Echinacea purpura* and *E. angustifolia*); licorice (*Glycyrrhiza glabra*).

Caution: licorice at high doses can cause hypertension and hypokalemia.

Treatment aims

To kill organism.

To prevent disease progression.

To alleviate symptoms.

Prognosis

• Despite antibiotic treatment, symptoms recur in 50% of patients, although severity and duration are greatly reduced; occasionally, recurrent symptoms may last several years.

• Acute Lyme disease and carditis have good prognosis.

• Cranial nerve palsies and meningitis have good prognosis; radiculoneuritis, peripheral neuropathy, encephalitis, and encephalomyelitis usually have a favorable outcome, but a tendency toward chronic or recurrent disease is seen.

• Arthritis often resolves, but response may be slow, often needing further treatment.

• In chronic disease, recurrence is not usual.

Follow-up and management

• Patients may need careful monitoring for months or years, depending on the severity of the symptoms.

General references

Halperin JJ (ed.): Lyme disease. *Semin Neurol* 1997, **17**:1–77.

Hofmann H: Lyme borreliosis: problems of serological diagnosis. *Infection* 1996, **24**:470–472.

Lutwick LI: Postexposure prophylaxis. *Infect Dis Clin North Am* 1996, **10**:899–915.

Magid D, *et al.*: Prevention of Lyme disease after tick bites. *N Engl J Med* 1992, **327**:534–541.

Nagi KS, Joshi R, Thakur RK: Cardiac manifestations of Lyme disease: a review. *Can J Cardiol* 1996, **12**:503–506.

Rahn DW, Malawista SE: Recommendations for diagnosis and treatment. *Ann Intern Med* 1991, **114**:472–481.

Weber K, Pfister H: Clinical management of Lyme borreliosis. 1994, **343**:1017–1020.

Measles

Diagnosis

Symptoms

Fever: for 3–4 days.
Rash.
Systemic upset; "misery."
Unproductive cough.
Catarrh.
Conjunctivitis.

Signs

Prodromal period before rash

Fever.

Enanthema, Koplik's spots: pathognomic small greyish-white spots on reddened mucous membranes, notably the buccal mucosa.

Rash: maculopapular, blotchy, not itchy; starts on face and behind ears; spreads downward over a few days; lasts ~5 days; almost invariably stains (persisting discoloration that does not blanch on pressure) from erythrocyte leakage during active rash.

Associated with development of rash

Reddened throat.
Bronchitic cough.
Conjunctivitis.
Lymph-node enlargement.

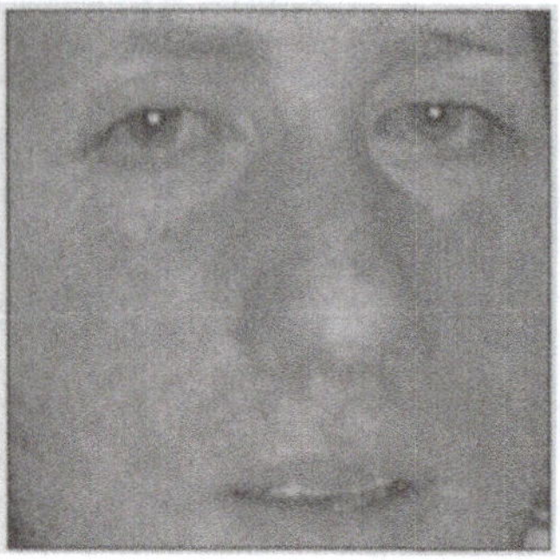

Blotchy rash of measles and conjunctivitis. (*See* Color Plate.)

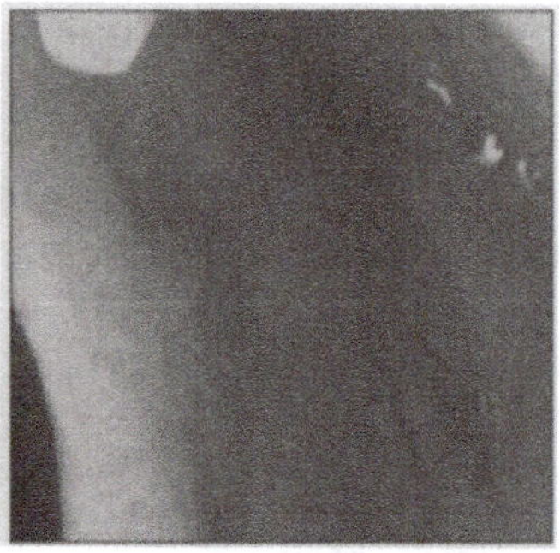

Koplik's spots in measles. (*See* Color Plate.)

Investigations

- The clinical picture is usually diagnostic.

Throat swab or nasopharyngeal aspirate: measles virus may be grown (technically difficult).
Immunofluorescent staining of throat secretions: may identify measles virus.
Serology: measles-specific IgM may be present in blood early in illness.
Paired sera examination: may show diagnostic rises in antibody (about fourfold).

Complications

- Complications are more severe in old or very young patients.

Measles bronchiolitis: when rash heaviest on trunk.
Secondary bacterial pneumonia and otitis media: in ~15%, especially children.
Febrile convulsions: in children, especially during prodrome.
Post–acute measles encephalitis: immune-mediated, at about day 6 of illness.
Subacute sclerosing panencephalitis: caused by persisting measles virus infection in nervous system, usually fatal; develops several years after acute infection.
Gastroenteritis: in malnourished children can lead to kwashiorkor and acute vitamin A deficiency.
Thrombocytopenia.
Giant-cell pneumonia or measles encephalitis: progressive in immunocompromised patient.

Differential diagnosis

Drug rashes: do not usually evolve from above downward, may be itchy, only occasionally stain, often not associated with fever.

Rubella: patients not usually ill, rash not usually blotchy.

Adenovirus or enterovirus infection.

- Koplik's spots are not a feature in any of the above.

Etiology

- Measles is caused by measles virus, an RNA virus.
- Transmission is by respiratory droplets.

Epidemiology

- Measles occurs worldwide.

Infectivity

- Measles is highly infectious: patients are infectious for about 4 days before the rash and until the rash has stained.
- Active infection without illness and a rash is extremely rare.
- Immunity after an attack is for life.
- Maternally derived antibodies protect babies for about the first 6 months of life.
- There is no infective carrier state.

Mean incubation period

To febrile illness: 10 days.

To rash: 14 days.

Treatment

Diet and lifestyle

• Patients should be isolated during the period of infectivity, which usually lasts from the onset of symptoms until the rash has stained.

Pharmacological treatment

Symptomatic

Analgesics, *e.g.*, acetaminophen.

Antibacterial drugs for bacterial complications.

Prophylactic

Vaccination by live virus preparation in second year of life as MMR: may cause mild measles-like illness.

Pooled human immunoglobulin: protective if given shortly after exposure.

• Vaccination and pooled human immunoglobulin can be given together if vaccination of vulnerable patients (*e.g.*, those with cystic fibrosis) is desired.

• Vitamin A deficiency (clinical or subclinical) increases the severity, complications, and risk of death from measles.

• In countries where the measles fatality rate is 1% or more, vitamin A should be given in all cases; elsewhere, it should be given in severe cases.

Treatment aims

To relieve symptoms.

To treat complications promptly.

Prognosis

• Most patients make a full recovery and are immune thereafter.

Follow-up and management

• No follow-up is necessary.

General references

de Quadros CA, Olive JM, Hersh BS, *et al.*: Measles elimination in the Americas: evolving strategies. *JAMA* 1996, **275**:224–229.

Hutchins S, Markowitz L, Atkinson W, *et al.*: Measles outbreaks in the United States, 1987 through 1990. *Pediatr Infect Dis J* 1996, **15**:31–38.

Lutwick LI: Postexposure prophylaxis. *Infect Dis Clin North Am* 1996, **10**:899–915.

Makhene MK, Diaz PS: Clinical presentations and complications of suspected measles in hospitalized children. *Pediatr Infect Dis J* 1993, **12**:836–840.

Melanoma

Diagnosis

Symptoms

• Patient concern about the presence of a changing pigmented lesion, usually different in appearance from other pigmented lesions present on the patient's skin.

Signs

• Cutaneous lesions are found most frequently on the lower extremities in women and on the back in men.

• Early lesions demonstrate the ABCDs:

Asymmetry.

Border irregularity.

Color variation.

Diameter >6 mm.

• Skin findings of intermediate-thickness and thick melanomas typically include variation in color, an irregular raised surface, an irregular border with indentations, and ulceration of the surface epithelium. These lesions also tend to change in appearance (size, configuration, color) over time.

A typical cutaneous melanoma lesion demonstrating characteristic asymmetry; irregular, scalloped border; variation in color. Diameter > 6 mm. (See Color Plate.)

Investigations

Full-thickness (to subcutaneous tissue) excisional, incisional, or punch biopsy of the cutaneous lesion(s).

Excision of assessable enlarged lymph nodes: to evaluate for metastatic disease.

Liver function serologies: to evaluate for evidence of metastatic disease.

• For patients with resected stage III disease and those with symptoms, signs, or laboratory findings consistent with metastatic disease, a careful physical examination, chest radiography, and CT of the abdomen (with or without pelvis and with or without chest) should be performed.

Growth pattern classification of melanomas

Superficial (radial) spreading.	Nodular.
Lentigo maligna.	Acral lentiginous.
Unclassified.	Desmoplastic variant (rare).

Staging system

The Clarke microstaging method categorizes melanomas by the relative depth of invasion into the dermal layers and subcutaneous fat (levels II, III, IV, or V).

The Breslow microstaging method measures the nodule thickness of the lesion (vertical height).

American Joint Committee on Cancer Staging System

Correlates microstaging criteria of disease with metastatic risk and prognosis.

Stage IA: localized melanoma <0.75 mm or level II (T1N0M0).

Stage IB: localized melanoma 0.76–1.5 mm or level III (T2N0M0).

Stage IIA: localized melanoma >1.5–4 mm or level IV (T3N0M0).

Stage IIB: localized melanoma >4 mm or level V (T4N0M0).

Stage III: limited nodule metastases involving only one regional lymph node basin or fewer than five in-transit metastases without nodal metastases (any T,N1,M0).

Stage IV: distant metastases (any T, any N, M1).

Differential diagnosis

Melanocytic lesions

Nevomelanocytic nevi (benign moles).

Blue nevi.

Lentigo.

Nonmelanocytic lesions

Seborrheic keratoses.

Pigmented basal cell carcinomas.

Pyogenic granuloma.

Thrombosed hemangioma.

Kaposi's sarcoma.

Etiology

The cause of melanoma is unknown.

Intermittent exposure to ultraviolet B radiation (*e.g.*, sunlight), and its associated genetic effects, is implicated in the etiology of melanoma.

Many chromosomal abnormalities have been identified in melanoma.

Epidemiology

Worldwide, there is an increasing incidence in persons with light-colored skin.

In the United States, the incidence is approximately 12 per 100 000.

Risk factors

Number of common nevi >2 mm.

Freckling.

Number of atypical nevi >5 mm.

History of severe blistering sunburn.

Propensity to sunburn.

Previous nonmelanocytic skin cancer.

Time spent outdoors from ages 10–24 years.

Family history of melanoma.

Previous dysplastic nevi.

Fair complexion and light-colored skin.

Changing mole.

History of active lentigenes.

Treatment

Diet and lifestyle

• No special diet is necessary.

• Emphasize the importance of sun avoidance and sun protection. Sun protection includes the use of protective clothing and daily sunscreens, preferably of broad-spectrum ultraviolet A plus ultraviolet B with sun protection factor of 15 or higher.

Surgical treatment

Local control of primary cutaneous lesion.

Wide local surgical excision is the treatment of choice. Modification of the surgical approach is often necessary for melanomas located on digits, sole of the foot, ears, or face.

Size of margin of normal-appearing skin excised with lesion depends on the subtype of melanoma.

Local recurrences

• Local recurrence is defined as any melanoma lesion that occurs within 5 cm of the scar of a previously excised melanoma.

Choice of therapy depends on location and characteristics of recurrent tumor(s) and includes:

Surgical excision.

Isolated limb perfusion with regional chemotherapy (*e.g.*, melphalan/interferona/tumor necrosis factor combination), and hyperthermia.

External-beam radiation therapy.

In-transit metastases

• In-transit metastases are defined as melanoma located between the primary lesion site and the first draining, regional lymph node region.

• Choice of therapeutic approach depends on site, number, extent, and characteristics of the metastases.

Therapeutic options

Surgical excision.

Isolated limb perfusion with chemotherapy and/or immune modulator therapy.

Regional chemotherapy infusion (intra-arterial).

Radiation therapy.

Intralesional immunotherapy (*e.g.*, bacille Calmette-Guérin).

Systemic chemotherapy.

Electroporation.

Distant metastases

Melanoma can metastasize to almost every major organ and tissue.

Poor prognosis.

Treatment options include:

No treatment.

Surgical excision: can often provide the quickest and longest-lasting palliation.

Radiation therapy: for localized management.

Systemic chemotherapy: because of the limited utility of current regimens, enrollment in clinical trials is encouraged.

Treatment aims

To achieve cure with the best cosmetic result.

Other treatments

The role of adjuvant chemotherapy and/or radiation therapy in patients at high risk for recurrent disease is unclear.

Therapeutic approaches with tumor vaccines and gene therapy modulation of the immune response to melanomas are being investigated in clinical trials.

Prognosis

The risk of recurrent disease and death persists well beyond 10 years after initial diagnosis and treatment.

Local recurrences are associated with an increased risk of metastatic disease. In patients with local recurrences, the median survival is 3 years and the 10-year survival rate is 20%.

Follow-up and management

Lifetime, regular, periodic (at least annually) follow-up is recommended for all patients. More frequent, closer follow-up should be provided for patients with a higher risk of recurrence and those with active disease.

Patients should be instructed in self-skin examinations.

Key references

1. Gilchrist BA, Eller MS, Geller AC, Yaar M: The pathogenesis of melanoma induced by ultraviolet radiation. *N Engl J Med* 1999, **340**:1341–1348.
2. Garcia ED, Santolaya R, Requena T: Treatment of malignant melanoma. *Ann Pharmacother* 1999, **33**:730–738.

General references

Barnhill RL, Mihm MC Jr, Fitzpatrick TB, Sober AJ: Neoplasms: malignant melanoma. In *Dermatology in General Medicine*, edn 4. Edited by Fitzpatrick TB, Eisen AZ, Wolff K, *et al.* New York: McGraw-Hill; 1993:1078–1115.

Balch CM, Reintgen DS, Kirkwood JM, *et al.*: Cutaneous melanoma. In *Cancer: Principles and Practice of Oncology*, edn 5. Edited by DeVita VT Jr, Hellman S, Rosenberg SA. Philadelphia: Lippincott-Raven; 1997:1947-94.

Meningitis, bacterial

Diagnosis

Symptoms

Headache.
Neck and back pain and stiffness.
Vomiting.
Photophobia.
Fever.
Altered level of consciousness.
Seizures.

• Atypical clinical manifestations may occur in very young, elderly, or immunocompromised patients (highest-risk groups).

Signs

Nuchal rigidity: on flexion only, not on lateral rotation.

"Meningeal cry": high-pitched, in infants.

Kernig's sign: pain and hamstring spasm on passive knee extension with hip flexed.

Brudzinski's sign: spontaneous knee and hip flexion on attempted neck flexion.

Cranial nerve palsies and other focal signs.

Deteriorating level of consciousness: in up to 25% of patients.

Papilledema, bulging fontanelle in infants: indicating raised intracranial pressure.

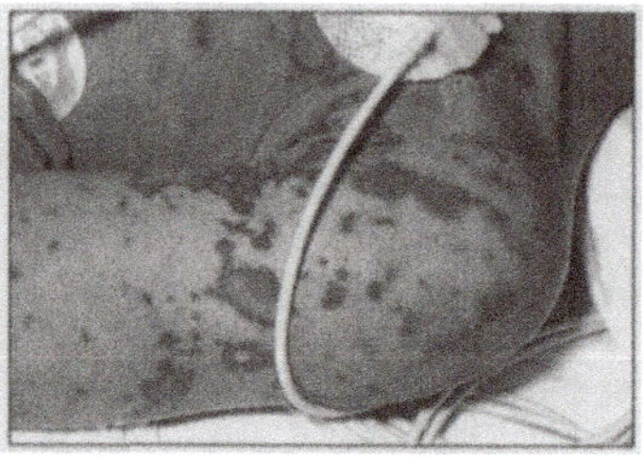

Purpuric rash of meningococcal meningitis. (*See* Color Plate.)

Fever, tachycardia, shock, evidence of primary source of infection: *e.g.*, pneumonia, endocarditis, sinusitis, otitis media.

Rash: in ~50% of patients with meningococcal infections, sometimes briefly erythematous before becoming petechial or purpuric.

Investigations

Lumbar puncture: in untreated acute bacterial meningitis, reveals turbid CSF under raised pressure, neutrophilic pleocytosis (hundreds or thousands of cells/µL), protein concentration usually >1 g/L, glucose concentration low. Specific tests for causative organisms include Gram stain, culture, sensitivity testing, fungal and tubercular microscopy and culture, and bacterial antigen immunoassay. Contraindications include papilledema, deteriorating level of consciousness, and focal neurological signs; prepuncture cranial CT is needed in such patients to exclude mass lesion.

Complete blood count: to detect neutrophil leukocytosis.

Coagulation screen and fibrin degradation product analysis: for disseminated intravascular coagulation.

Electrolyte analysis: to detect hyponatremia.

Blood culture: may be positive when CSF sterile.

Chest and skull (sinus) radiography: to identify primary source of infection.

Complications

Seizures, focal CNS signs, raised intracranial pressure, subdural effusion, cerebral or subdural abscess formation, hydrocephalus (obstructive or communicating).

Septic shock, disseminated intravascular coagulation with adrenal hemorrhage: Waterhouse-Friderichsen's syndrome, complication of meningococcal meningitis.

Inappropriate antidiuretic hormone secretion: in <10% of patients.

Arthritis: septic or immune complex, in <10% of meningococcal infections.

Behavioral disturbances, mental retardation, hearing loss, epilepsy, cranial nerve palsies, visual and motor deficits: long-term complications (more usual in *Streptococcus pneumoniae* infections; <30% of patients).

Differential diagnosis

• Few patients, even with severe headache and fever, have meningitis.

Viral meningitis, especially enteroviruses, mumps.

Intercurrent infections, especially influenza A and B with meningismus.

Cranial infections: cerebral abscess, sinusitis, throat infections.

Noninfective meningitis: subarachnoid hemorrhage, leukemic infiltration, Mollaret's meningitis (recurrent fever, meningeal signs, and CSF pleocytosis).

Autoimmune diseases, vasculitis.

Chemical meningitis, e.g., intrathecal drugs.

Etiology

• 70%–90% of cases of bacterial meningitis are due to one of three organisms:

Neisseria meningitidis.

Haemophilus influenzae (type b).

Streptococcus pneumoniae.

• Other organisms found in specific at-risk groups include the following:

Enterobacteriaceae, group B streptococci in neonates.

Listeria monocytogenes in neonates and immunocompromised patients.

Mycobacterium tuberculosis in patients from developing countries and immunocompromised patients.

Staphylococci in patients with head trauma or neurosurgical shunts.

Epidemiology

• The incidence of bacterial meningitis is ~5–10 in 100 000 annually in developed countries.

• The three common organisms have characteristic patterns of occurrence: *N. meningitidis* in epidemics, *H. influenzae* in children aged <5 years, *S. pneumoniae* in patients aged >40 years (especially alcoholic, splenectomized, and sickle-cell anemic patients).

Treatment

Diet and lifestyle

• No special precautions are necessary.

Pharmacological treatment

General management

• Bacterial meningitis may prove fatal within hours; successful treatment depends on early diagnosis and i.v. administration of appropriate antibiotics in appropriate doses; agents that penetrate CSF and cover likely pathogens should be used (*e.g.*, ampicillin and ceftriaxone).

• If lumbar puncture is delayed by the need for prepuncture CT, antibiotic treatment should be started before the scan, after blood cultures.

• Treatment should ideally be bactericidal with a high therapeutic ratio, the drug penetrating the CSF in adequate concentrations; very high i.v. doses may be needed despite damage to the blood–brain barrier in meningitis.

• Adjunctive corticosteroids are indicated when bacterial organisms are present on Gram stain or in the setting of increased intracranial pressure.

Against *N. meningitidis, S. pneumoniae*, and *H. influenzae*

Standard dosage	*Adults:* ceftriaxone, 2 g every 12 hours for 10 days.
Contraindications	Cephalosporin hypersensitivity; caution in renal impairment, history of allergy.
Special points	Other options include cefotaxime, ceftriaxone, and chloramphenicol.
Main drug interactions	None.
Main side effects	Sensitivity reactions.

Against penicillin-susceptible pneumococcus or established meningococcus

Standard dosage	*Adults:* penicillin G, 14.4 g (24 MU) i.v. daily in divided doses (usually 4 MU initially, then 2 MU every 2 hours; can be relaxed to every 4 or 6 hours regimen with evidence of clinical improvement, usually within 48–72 hours); treatment should continue for 7 days after the patient has become afebrile. *Children and infants:* penicillin G, 100–300 mg/kg daily depending on age, according to manufacturer's current prescribing information.
Contraindications	Penicillin hypersensitivity; caution in renal impairment, history of allergy.
Special points	Other options include cefotaxime, ceftriaxone, and chloramphenicol.
Main drug interactions	None.
Main side effects	Sensitivity reactions.

Prevention

• Chemoprophylaxis (using rifampicin or ciprofloxacin) is indicated for household contacts and index patients before hospital discharge.

• Immunization against *H. influenzae* infection (using *H. influenzae* type b vaccine) is recommended routinely for children at the ages of 2, 3, and 4 months.

Treatment aims

To secure survival and prevent persistent neurological complications.

To reduce the of recurrence by treating any predisposing cause.

To prevent spread to close contacts.

Prognosis

• Mortality is ~10% overall, 5%–10% from *H. influenzae* infection, 5%–10% from *N. meningitidis* infection, and 10%–30% from *S. pneumoniae* infection.

• Long-term sequelae are 9%–22%, 4%–6%, and 14%–40%, respectively.

Follow-up and management

• Repeat lumbar puncture to monitor treatment is not necessary if the patient is improving.

• Bacteriological relapse needs immediate reinstitution of treatment.

• Adults should be reviewed at 3 months, children at 6–12 months, and neonates for longer to detect any long-term sequelae.

Causes of treatment failure

Wrong diagnosis: *e.g.*, tuberculosis, abscess.

Wrong drug: poor CSF penetration, antimicrobial resistance.

Wrong route: intraventricular instillation needed for ventriculitis with "resistant" infections.

Poor-risk patient: extremes of age, immunocompromise.

Unrecognized complication: treatable raised intracranial pressure, abscess or ventriculitis, subdural effusion or abscess (treatable); vasculitis, cerebritis (less treatable).

Shock.

General references

Miller LG, Choi C: Meningitis in older patients: how to diagnose and treat a deadly infection. *Geriatrics* 1997, **52**:43–55.

Quagliarello V, Scheld WM: Bacterial meningitis: Pathogenesis, pathophysiology and progress. *N Engl J Med* 1992, **327**:864–872.

Segreti J, Harris AA: Acute bacterial meningitis. *Infect Dis Clin North Am* 1996, **10**:797–809.

Tunkel AR, Wispelwey B, Scheld M: Bacterial meningitis: recent advances in pathophysiology and treatment. *Ann Intern Med* 1990, **112**:610–623.

Meningitis, cryptococcal in AIDS

Diagnosis

Symptoms

• Symptoms are usually chronic, usually <3 weeks, but can be acute.

Immunosuppression: with CD4 counts $<100 \times 10^6$/L.

Headache: in 81% of patients.

Fever: in 77%.

Nausea or vomiting: in 44%.

Photophobia: in 27%.

Seizures: in 5%; can be the presenting feature.

Signs

• No signs are reported in >50% of patients.

Abnormal mental status: in 28%. Nuchal rigidity uncommon.

Focal neurological signs and papilledema: rare; may be present if the patient has cryptococcomas.

Extraneural involvement: in 20%, with pulmonary infiltrates, skin lesions, and prostatic involvement.

Investigations

• Cryptococcal antigen in blood is positive in 90% of patients.

CT or MRI: should be performed before lumbar puncture to exclude a mass lesion if focal neurological signs are present; usually shows no abnormality or cerebral atrophy; communicating hydrocephalus infrequent; low-density lesions, scattered and symmetrical, sometimes seen, attributed to cryptococci.

CSF analysis: to establish diagnosis; usually shows minimum pleocytosis (<20 leukocytes) and raised protein; glucose may be low. The CSF may be entirely normal; India-ink preparation may show cryptococci; cryptococcal antigen (>1:16) positive in 95% of patients.

Other investigations: cryptococcus can be cultured from other sites (sputum, blood, bone marrow). Abnormal liver function, low albumin concentration, or hyponatremia in 20%; lymphopenia common in peripheral blood.

Complications

Death: during the acute illness despite treatment; increased intracranial pressure or progression of the meningitis with seizures, cranial nerve palsies, stupor, and coma.

Cerebral cryptococcomas: may occur.

Poor prognostic factors

Abnormal mental status.

High CSF cryptococcal antigen.

Cryptococcemia.

Low CSF leukocyte count.

Differential diagnosis

Viral and tuberculous meningitis.

Cerebral toxoplasmosis.

Cerebral lymphoma.

Benign headaches (migraine, tension, depression).

Meningitis due to hysteria.

Etiology

• Cryptococcus is a yeast present in high quantities in the environment.

• Infection is acquired by inhalation.

• The spread to the CNS is hematogenous.

Epidemiology

• Most cases of cryptococcal meningitis are AIDS-related.

• Cryptococcal meningitis is found in 2%–12% of AIDS patients in different clinical series.

• It is the most frequent cause of meningitis.

Treatment

Diet and lifestyle

- No special precautions are necessary.

Pharmacological treatment

Initial treatment

- The established initial treatment is by amphotericin B and flucytosine.
- Treatment of the first episode fails in 20%–40% of patients.

Standard dosage	Amphotericin B, 0.7 mg/kg i.v. daily. Usual course is 7–14 days.
Contraindications	Renal failure, pregnancy, breast-feeding, old age.
Special points	Hepatic and renal function, blood count, electrolytes, and drug concentrations must be monitored.
Main drug interactions	*Amphotericin B:* increased risk of nephrotoxicity with cyclosporine, aminoglycosides; antagonizes miconazole.
Main side effects	*Amphotericin B:* nausea, vomiting, fever, nephrotoxicity. *Flucytosine:* diarrhea, bone-marrow suppression.

Adjunctive 5-fluorocytosine

- This agent may improve the outcome when added to amphotericin.

Standard dosage	5F-C, 100 mg/kg daily.
Contraindications	Hepatitis, vomiting.
Main drug interactions	None.
Main side effects	Vomiting, hepatitis, bone-marrow suppression. Serum levels should be monitored.

Maintenance treatment

- ~50% of HIV-seropositive patients with cryptococcal meningitis relapse without maintenance treatment.
- The relapse rate can be markedly reduced with fluconazole.

Standard dosage	Fluconazole, 200 mg orally daily for life.
Contraindications	Possibly breast-feeding, pregnancy, children.
Special points	May be considered for initial treatment i.v. or orally at 400 mg daily only in mildly ill patients who are not obtunded and have low cryptococcal antigen. Itraconazole is a useful alternative.
Main drug interactions	Enhances warfarin, phenytoin, theophylline, cyclosporine, sulfonylureas; reduces rifampin.
Main side effects	Diarrhea, bone-marrow suppression.

Treatment aims

To eradicate cryptococcal infection.

Prognosis

- Improved on HAART-treated patients.

Follow-up and management

- Patients should be closely followed, particularly for the first year when relapses are more common.

General references

Chuck SL, Sande MA: Infections with *Cryptococcus neoformans* in the acquired immunodeficiency syndrome. *N Engl J Med* 1989, **321**:794–799.

Sharkey PK, Graybill JR, Johnson ES, *et al.*: Amphotericin B lipid complex compared with amphotericin B in the treatment of cryptococcal meningitis in patients with AIDS. *Clin Infect Dis* 1996, **22**:315–321.

van der Horst CM, Saag MS, Cloud GA, *et al.*: Treatment of cryptococcal meningitis associated with the acquired immunodeficiency syndrome. *N Engl J Med* 1997, **337**:15–21.

Weinke T, *et al.*: Cryptococcosis in AIDS patients: observations concerning CNS involvement. *J Neurol* 1989, **236**:38–42.

Menopause & hypoestrogenism

Diagnosis

Symptoms [1]

• Symptoms are primarily due to estrogen deficiency.

Shortened, irregular, or absent menstrual periods: menstrual cycle normally shortens during the perimenopause due to a reduced follicular phase.

Vasomotor symptoms ("hot flashes"): affect about half of all women in the first 2 years of menopause; sudden onset of vasodilation, heat, and perspiration in the upper body; typically lasts several minutes; can be debilitating, but symptoms decrease with time in most women.

Vaginal atrophy and dyspareunia.

Urethral syndrome: symptoms of urinary tract infection without evidence of infection (controversy exists as to whether these symptoms are secondary to estrogen deficiency, aging, or both).

Fractures: due to loss of bone mineral density (*see* Osteoporosis *for further details*).

Psychological symptoms: incidence of depression does not increase during menopause, but, stress associated with menopause may exacerbate underlying problems.

Signs

• Symptoms predominate over signs in most women.

Genitourinary complications: pale, atrophic, friable vaginal mucosa; vagina, cervix, and uterus may decrease in size; increased incidence of cystoceles and rectoceles (may be related to aging).

Investigations

• Menopause and hypoestrogenism are primarily clinical diagnoses.

Serum estradiol levels: <20 pg/mL (in the setting of an elevated follicle-stimulating hormone) is consistent with ovarian failure.

Follicle-stimulating hormone levels: elevated in ovarian failure; may be low or normal with other causes of hypogonadism.

Bone densitometry: useful in women at risk of osteoporosis; some women find this information helpful in deciding whether to begin hormone replacement therapy.

Lipid panel: loss of cardiovascular protective effects of estrogen at menopause increases the importance of diagnosing and treating hyperlipidemia.

Complications

Premenopausal hypogonadism

Failure to achieve predicted peak bone mass: increases risk of subsequent osteoporosis and fractures.

Early loss of cardioprotective effects of estrogen.

Infertility.

Menopause

• Most complications are related to symptoms and signs discussed above, including osteoporotic fractures and coronary artery disease.

Differential diagnosis

Other causes of amenorrhea, including pregnancy, anatomical abnormalities, prior hysterectomy, polycystic ovarian syndrome, adrenal disorders, eating disorders. (Note: not all cases of amenorrhea are due to hypoestrogenism.)

Other causes of sweating and flushing, such as hyperthyroidism and carcinoid.

Etiology

• Most common cause of female hypogonadism is menopause.

• Other etiologies include oophorectomy, athletic amenorrhea [2], hyperprolactinemia, premature ovarian failure (often autoimmune), hypopituitarism, Turner's syndrome, thyroid dysfunction, uremia, chemotherapy (alkylating agents), idiopathic.

Epidemiology

• 50% of postmenopausal women will die of cardiovascular disease.

• In a large retrospective study, postmenopausal women with one or more cardiac risk factors had longer life expectancies on estrogen replacement therapy [3].

• ~75% of women started on estrogen replacement therapy will not be refilling their prescriptions 1 year later.

Treatment

Diet and lifestyle

• Weight-bearing exercise, healthy diet, smoking cessation, and adequate intake of calcium and vitamin D is important in preventing bone loss in the postmenopausal patient.

• Women with athletic amenorrhea should be encouraged to alter their exercise and diet to facilitate the return of normal menses, or offered oral contraceptive therapy.

• Physicians should inquire about eating disorders in young, thin, amenorrheic women.

Pharmacological treatment

Estrogen replacement therapy (ERT)

• Estrogen replacement remains the therapy of choice when suitable due to its beneficial effects on menopausal symptoms, bone density, and overall mortality; may also decrease the incidence, but not progression, of senile dementia.

• ERT, in retrospective studies, has been associated with a decreased risk of cardiac and overall mortality. However, a recent prospective study suggests that this may not be true after a recent myocardial infarction [4]. The same study also showed a small increased risk of venous thromboembolism among patients on a typical postmenopausal estrogen replacement regimen.

• ERT, again in retrospective studies, has been shown to decrease osteoporotic fractures at spine and hip. Prospective studies examining this issue are in progress.

Standard dosage	*Anovulatory premenopausal women*: low-dose oral contraceptives, containing <35 µg/d of ethinyl estradiol. *Postmenopausal women*: ethinyl estradiol, 5–10 µg daily; Estrace, 1–2 mg/d; Ogen, 0.625 daily; Premarin, 0.625–0.9 mg/d; estrogen patches.
Contraindications	Patients with estrogen-responsive tumors or strong family history of breast cancer, pregnancy, abnormal vaginal bleeding, history of thromboembolic disease.
Special points	If the uterus is present, progestational therapy is required to reduce the incidence of endometrial cancer. Can be given as a cyclic regimen (medroxyprogesterone, 10 mg/d for 10 days of each month) or continuously (medroxyprogesterone, 2.5–5.0 mg/d). Estrogen patches avoid first-pass metabolism through the liver, and may be useful in women with a history of thromboembolic disease who wish to be on estrogen.
Main drug interactions	May increase requirements for thyroxine in women on thyroid hormone replacement.
Main side effects	Breast swelling and tenderness, weight gain.

Several combination estrogen-progestin products are available, including:
Prempro: Premarin 0.625 mg with either 2.5 mg or 5.0 mg of medroxyprogesterone.
FemHRT: Ethinyl estradiol 5 µg with norethidrone acetate 1 mg.
Prefest: Alternating 3-day cycles of estradiol 1 mg followed by a combined tablet containing both estradiol 1 mg and norgestimate 0.09 mg.

Raloxifene

• Raloxifene is an estrogen-like molecule with estrogen-like activity on bone density and lipids, but antiestrogen activity at breast and uterus. Prospective studies show it to decrease vertebral osteoporotic fractures and reduce the incidence of breast cancer (over a 4-year trial) [5].

Standard dosage	Raloxifene (Evista) 60 mg daily.
Contraindications	Patients with history of thromboembolic disease. Abnormal vaginal bleeding, pregnancy. *See* manufacturer's prescribing information.
Special point	No need for concomitant therapy with progestins (as with ERT).
Main drug interactions	*See* manufacturer's prescribing information.
Side effects	May cause hot flashes and leg cramps.

Nonhormonal therapies for vasomotor symptoms [5]

Clonidine: dosages range from 50–400 µg/d. Increased incidence of side effects at higher doses (insomnia, orthostatic hypotension).
Medroxyprogesterone: 20–40 mg/d. Effective at treating hot flashes but with detrimental effects on lipids.
• If indicated, patients should also be treated for osteoporosis and hyperlipidemia.

Treatment aims

Menopause
To alleviate or reduce symptoms of estrogen deficiency.
To maintain a favorable lipid profile.
To prevent the rapid loss of bone mass associated with menopause.
Premenopause
To restore normal estradiol levels, either by the resumption of normal menses or by ERT.

Prognosis

• Menopause is a normal part of the aging process and does not have a specific prognosis.
• The deleterious effects of estrogen deficiency (in premenopausal and postmenopausal women) can be effectively treated, with good prognoses.

Follow-up and management

• Estrogen doses may be titrated upward in women with persistent vasomotor symptoms.
• All women should be encouraged to have regular Papanicolaou smears and, if indicated, mammograms. This is particularly important in postmenopausal women on ERT.
• Patients should receive ongoing assessment of bone density and lipid profile, as clinically indicated.

Key references

1. Greendale GA, Sowers M: The menopause transition. *Endocrinol Metab Clin North Am* 1997, **26**:261–277.
2. Hergenroeder AC: Bone mineralization, hypothalamic amenorrhea, and sex steroid therapy in female adolescents and young adults. *J Pediatrics* 1995, **126**:683–689.
3. Grodstein F, Stampfer MJ, Colditz GA, *et al.*: Postmenopausal hormone therapy and mortality. *N Engl J Med* 1997, **336**:1769–1775.
4. Hulley S, Grady D, Bush T, *et al.*, for the Heart and Estrogen/Progestin Replacement Study (HERS) Research Group. Randomized trial of estrogen plus progestin for secondary prevention of coronary heart disease in postmenopausal women. *JAMA* 1998, **280**:605–613.
5. Cummings SR, Eckert S, Krueger KA, *et al*: The effect of raloxifene on risk of breast cancer in postmenopausal women: results from the MORE randomized trial. *JAMA* 1999, **281**:2189–2197.

Migraine

Diagnosis

Definition

Migraine with aura (classic migraine): characterized by aura followed by episodic unilateral throbbing headache, with nausea, photophobia, and phonophobia; auras usually last 10–20 minutes but can persist for up to 1 hour; laterality of neurological disturbance not related to side of ensuing headache.

Migraine without aura (common migraine): characterized by episodic unilateral or bilateral headache, gastrointestinal upset, photo- or phonophobia, but no aura.

• Migraine headaches are paroxysmal, lasting from a few hours up to 3 days, but with periods of complete relief between attacks.

Cluster headache: 90% of sufferers men; paroxysmal very severe unilateral periorbital pain lasting 0.5–2 hours, once or twice daily (often at night) for weeks, with months or years of relief between bouts; usually associated with Horner's syndrome, lacrimation, and nasal stuffiness ipsilateral to pain.

Ophthalmoplegic migraine: recurrent attacks of III or VI cranial nerve palsies associated with headache; resolution of deficit may be delayed by several days.

Retinal migraine: monocular visual loss involving scotoma or altitudinal defect followed by headache.

Hemiplegic migraine: recurrent attacks of hemiparesis of rapid onset followed by headache; weakness may last hours.

• Migraine variants are diagnoses of exclusion; other more serious causes of the clinical picture (*e.g.*, stroke, aneurysmal leak, transient ischemic attack) must be excluded, especially if the pain is severe, before the diagnosis is accepted.

Symptoms

• The aura of classic migraine may be visual (in 50% of patients) or sensory (in 30%) or occasionally may involve dysphasia or motor deficit.

Visual auras: teichopsia, fortification spectra, fragmentation, scotoma, homonymous hemianopia.

Transient tingling or numbness: sensory symptoms; upper limbs more frequently involved than lower limbs.

Signs

• Common migraine may have no signs.

• The scotomas, hemianopia, and sensorimotor phenomena of classic migraine may be detected if the aura is still present at the time of examination.

• Prolonged deficit requires exclusion of other causes.

Investigations [1,2]

• Investigation is not needed if the diagnosis of migraine is well founded; it is needed when the diagnosis is in doubt and in patients with residual neurological deficit after migraine.

• Investigation including the following is aimed at excluding alternative diagnoses:

ESR measurement: for temporal arteritis.

Radiography, MRI: for cervical spondylosis.

CT or MRI: for tumor, vascular malformation, hydrocephalus.

CSF analysis: for subarachnoid bleeding, arteritis.

Angiography: for aneurysmal bleeding.

Complications

Complicated migraine: rarely, residua from migraine auras continue as permanent deficits or stroke.

Dehydration.

Migrainous infarction: rare, usually posterior parietal or occipital.

Differential diagnosis

Tension headache: continuous dull, pressure-like pain over vertex or around head; lasts weeks to years; nausea occasional, vomiting rare; may coexist with migraine to produce pattern of constant headache with episodic exacerbations.

Temporal arteritis: in patients usually aged >65 years with unilateral temporal pain and tenderness; visual disturbances may occur before blindness; high ESR.

Local disease: *e.g.*, glaucoma, sinusitis, nasopharyngeal lesions, vascular abnormalities.

Tumor: cerebral tumors usually manifest with epilepsy, focal neurological deficits, clouded consciousness, and rarely headache, although this may develop later.

Hemorrhage: abrupt onset of severe headache, usually occipital and associated with neck stiffness and photophobia; aneurysms may produce pressure effects; no history of recurrent similar headaches.

Arteriopathies: SLE may manifest with migraine; polyarteritis nodosa may produce headache and transient neurological deficits.

Etiology

• Migraine is probably due to a combination of genetic predisposition and environmental triggers (*e.g.*, stress, certain foods) causing changes in neurotransmitter release (5-HT), with alteration in cerebral blood flow and pain in the distribution of the trigeminal nerve.

Epidemiology [3]

• The prevalence is ~5% in men and 12%–15% in women, although some investigators have quoted prevalence rates as high as 60%–70%.

• The incidence increases from puberty to young adulthood; onset >50 years is unusual.

Treatment

Diet and lifestyle

• Dietary precipitants, *e.g.*, chocolate, cheese, coffee, red wine, should be avoided.

• Stress is a common precipitant of migraine: appropriate measures may reduce the frequency of attacks.

• Avoid oral contraceptives; contraindicated in migraine with focal neurological deficits.

Pharmacological treatment

• Many patients treat attacks satisfactorily with rest, darkness, and simple analgesics, including naproxen, Midrin, ketorolac.

For migraine with and without aura: acute

• Patients with gastrointestinal disturbance and more severe headache may benefit from a combination of analgesic and antiemetic; the antiemetic not only reduces vomiting but increases gastric emptying, thereby improving absorption of the analgesic.

• Severe attacks unresponsive to this treatment may be treated by sumatriptan or ergotamine.

Standard dosage Sumatriptan, 25–100 mg orally at onset or 6 mg s.c. by autoinjector. Ergotamine in varying doses according to route.

Contraindications *Sumatriptan:* patients aged >65 years or with history of coronary disease; to be avoided in children or hemiplegic migraine.
Ergotamine: vascular disease, active infection, hemiplegic migraine.

Special points *Sumatriptan:* effective in 60% at 2 hours and 80% at 4 hours.
Ergotamine: maximum dose of preparation must not be exceeded because of risk of vasospasm.

Main drug interactions *Sumatriptan:* ergotamine, monoamine oxidase inhibitors, lithium.
Ergotamine: beta-blockers, methysergide, and sumatriptan all increase risk of vasospasm.

Main side effects *Sumatriptan:* chest pain or tightness, light-headedness, transient pain at site of injection.
Ergotamine: nausea, vomiting, headache (possibly due to overuse), tingling, chest tightness.
Zolmitriptan: under development.

For common and classic migraine: prophylactic [4]

• Beta-blockers or 5-HT antagonists should be considered for ≥2 attacks a month; 6–12 months' effective treatment may allow withdrawal at original frequency.

Standard dosage Propranolol, 60–160 mg long-acting daily (or nadolol or metaprolol). Tricyclic antidepressants: amitriptyline, nortriptyline.

Contraindications *Beta-blockers:* asthma, cardiac failure, heart block.

Main drug interactions *See manufacturer's current prescribing information.*

Main side effects *Beta-blockers:* bradycardia, heart failure, bronchospasm, fatigue, depression.
Tricyclic antidepressants: dry mouth, orthostasis, fatigue, weight gain.

• Other agents that may be helpful include nonsteroidals (naproxen sodium, ketorolac tromethamine), valproic acid, calcium-channel blockers, or methysergide.

For cluster headache: acute

Sumatriptan or ergotamine.
Oxygen (>40%), if not contraindicated.
Prednisolone, 60 mg (occasionally helpful).

For cluster headache: prophylactic

Short-term sumatriptan or ergotamine before predicted onset of attack.
Lithium and methysergide in refractory patients: regular monitoring of lithium concentrations and checking of thyroid function needed; methysergide used intermittently (no longer than 6 months) to reduce risk of retroperitoneal fibrosis.

Alternative medicine

Recommended use: feverfew (*Tanacetum parthenium*).
Common use: ginger (*Zingiber officinale*); cayenne pepper (*Capsicum frutescens*); garlic (*Allium sativa*); kava kava (*Piper methysticum*); valerian (*Valerian officinalis*); biofeedback; acupressure.
Caution: kava kava may have adverse environmental effects.

Treatment aims

To provide adequate relief from symptoms.
To adjust treatment appropriately to severity and frequency of attacks.
To minimize effect of migraine on work and leisure activities.

Prognosis

• Most patients respond well to acute or prophylactic treatment, or both.
• The frequency of migraine often declines with age but only occasionally does migraine disappear.

Follow-up and management

• Regular follow-up in hospital is not required for uncomplicated migraine.
• GPs should assess the response to treatment until appropriate and successful treatment is established.
• Prophylactics should be continued for 6–12 months before withdrawal.

Key references

1. Dalessio DJ: Diagnosing the severe headache. *Neurology* 1994, **44(suppl 3)**:S6–S12.
2. Pryse-Phillips WE, Dodick DW, Edmeads GW, *et al.*: Guidelines for the diagnosis and management of migraine in clinical practice. *Can Med Assoc J* 1997, **156**:1273–1287.
3. Baumel B: Migraine. *Neurology* 1994, **44 (suppl 3)**:S13–S17.
4. Tfelt-Hansen P: Prophylactic pharmacotherapy of migraine: some practical guidelines. *Neurol Clin* 1997, **15**:153–165.

Mitral regurgitation

Diagnosis

Symptoms

Asymptomatic or mild symptoms: often.

Dyspnea: due to pulmonary congestion.

Fatigue: due to low cardiac output.

Palpitation: due to atrial fibrillation.

Fluid retention: in late-stage disease.

Signs

Pulse

Irregular pulse: if patient is in atrial fibrillation.

Low-amplitude pulse pressure.

Raised venous pressure.

Heart

Parasternal heave: right ventricular hypertrophy and systolic left atrial expansion.

Laterally displaced and hyperdynamic apical impulse.

Pansystolic murmur.

Third heart sound.

Loud pulmonary second sound: if patient has pulmonary hypertension.

Investigations

ECG: shows broad bifid P wave (P mitrale), atrial fibrillation.

Chest radiography: shows pulmonary congestion, left atrial enlargement, cardiac enlargement, pulmonary artery enlargement (if severe and long-standing).

Echocardiography and Doppler ultrasonography: large left atrium, large left ventricle, increased fractional shortening, regurgitant jet (Doppler), leaflet prolapse (floppy valve or flail leaflet). The echocardiogram provides baselines estimation of left ventricle and left atrial volume, an estimation of left ventricular ejection fraction, and approximation of the severity of regurgitation. It can be helpful to determine the anatomic cause of mitral regurgitation (MR). In the presence of even mild tricuspid regurgitation, pulmonary artery pressure can be estimated. Currently, echocardiography provides only a semiquantitative estimate of the severity of mitral regurgitation.

Transesophageal echocardiography: may give better visualization of valve prolapse. It is useful intraoperatively to establish the anatomic basis for MR and to guide repair. It is also useful in patients for whom transthoracic echocardiography provides nondiagnostic images.

Cardiac catheterization: large V waves in wedge trace, angiographic evidence of mitral regurgitation. Coronary angiography is indicated when coronary artery disease is suspected. Left ventriculography and hemodynamic measurements are indicated when noninvasive tests are inconclusive regarding the severity of MR, left ventricular function, or the need for surgery.

Complications

Systemic embolism.

Pulmonary hypertension, right heart failure.

Endocarditis.

Differential diagnosis

Tricuspid regurgitation: the murmur is better heard in inspiration, whereas the murmur of MR is better heard in expiration.

Hypertrophic cardiomyopathy: ECG and echocardiographic evidence of left ventricular hypertrophy.

Etiology

Nonischemic MR

Rheumatic heart disease.

Mitral valve prolapse.

Infective endocarditis.

Collagen vascular disease.

Anorectic drugs.

Ruptured chordae tendineae.

Ischemic MR

Coronary artery disease.

Epidemiology

- The increasing availability of echocardiography may result in more patients with mitral regurgitation being found.

Treatment

Diet and lifestyle

• Asymptomatic patients with mitral regurgitation in sinus rhythm who have normal left ventricular size may exercise without restriction.

• In mildly symptomatic patients and those with left ventricular dilatation or atrial fibrillation, exercise should be limited to activities with low to moderate dynamic and low to moderate static cardiovascular demands.

Pharmacological treatment

• In the asymptomatic patient with chronic MR, there is no generally accepted medical therapy. Although the use of vasodilators may appear intuitively logical for the same reasons that they are effective in acute MR and chronic atrial regurgitation, no large long-term studies indicate that they are beneficial. In the absence of systemic hypertension, vasodilating drugs in asymptomatic patients with preserved left ventricular function have no known indication.

• However, in patients with MR resulting from increased preload (*i.e.*, coronary artery disease or dilated cardiomyopathy), preload reduction may be beneficial. In a small series of patients with chronic MR in New York Heart Association functional class I–III, 1 year of quinapril therapy reduced left ventricular volumes and mass and improved functional class.

• If atrial fibrillation develops, heart rate should be controlled with digitalis, rate-lowering calcium-channel blockers, β-blockers, or, rarely, amiodarone.

• Although the risk of embolism with the combination of MR and atrial fibrillation was formerly considered similar to that of mitral stenosis and atrial fibrillation, more recent studies suggest that embolic risk may be less in MR. It is recommended that the international normalized ratio be maintained at 2–3 in this population.

Nonpharmacological: surgery

Indications

Symptomatic patients with normal left ventricular function: surgery most appropriate when patients with MR develop symptoms but have preserved left ventricular function (ejection fraction >0.60 and end-systolic dimension < 45 mm).

Symptomatic patients with evidence of left ventricular dysfunction: ejection fraction >0.60 and end-systolic dimension < 45 mm. However, the surgical candidacy of symptomatic patient with MR and far-advanced left ventricular dysfunction is a dilemma.

Asymptomatic patients with normal left ventricular function: in patients with newly acquired severe MR and in those with chronic MR with recent onset of episodic or chronic atrial fibrillation in whom the likelihood of successful valve repair is high. Operative mortality increases with age (> 75 years), especially if mitral valve replacement must be performed or if the patient has concomitant coronary artery disease. Therefore, patients ≥ 75 years should be considered only when symptomatic.

Three types of surgery

Mitral valve repair: the operation of choice when the valve is suitable for repair and appropriate surgical skill and expertise are available. This procedure preserves the native valve and thus avoids anticoagulation except in atrial fibrillation.

Mitral valve replacement with preservation of mitral valve apparatus: leads to better left ventricular function and survival than in patients whose apparatus is removed.

Mitral valve replacement with removal of mitral apparatus: rarely performed and only when the native valve and apparatus are distorted so that the mitral apparatus cannot be spared.

Ischemic mitral regurgitation.

• The outlook for the patient with ischemic MR is substantially worse than that for regurgitation from other causes. A worse prognosis accrues from the fact that ischemic MR is usually caused by left ventricular dysfunction resulting from myocardial infarction.

• Unlike nonischemic MR, in which mitral repair is clearly the operation of choice, the best operation for ischemic MR is controversial. In one recent report, mitral valve replacement had a better outcome than repair, especially when annular dilatation rather than chordal or papillary muscle rupture was the cause of MR.

Treatment aims

To achieve normal functional capacity.

To perform surgical repair prior to development of left ventricular dysfunction owing to chronic volume overload.

Prognosis

• Prognosis is good unless pulmonary artery pressures have been chronically high or left ventricle is severely impaired.

• Prognosis for the patient with ischemic MR is substantially worse than that for patients with regurgitation from other causes.

• Elderly patients with MR fare more poorly with valve surgery than do their counterparts with aortic stenosis.

Follow-up management

• After surgery, follow-up is essential to detect late surgical failure and assess left ventricular function.

General references

Bonow RO, *et al.*: ACC/AHA guidelines for the management of patients with valvular heart disease: executive summary. A report of the American College of Cardiology/ American Heart Association Task Force on Practice Guidelines (Committee on Management of Patients with Valvular Heart Disease). *Circulation* 1998, **98:** 1949–1984.

Carabello BA: Valvular heart disease. *N Engl J Med* 1997, **337:**32–41.

Mitral stenosis

Diagnosis

Symptoms

Fatigue: insidious onset; due to low cardiac output [1].

Dyspnea, orthopnea: due to pulmonary congestion.

Palpitation: due to atrial fibrillation.

Signs

Irregular pulse: in atrial fibrillation.

Loud (palpable) first heart sound.

Opening snap: if valve is mobile.

Mitral diastolic murmur: long if severe.

Raised venous pressure.

Parasternal heave: right ventricular hypertrophy.

Loud pulmonary second sound.

Investigations

ECG: shows broad bifid P wave (P mitrale), usually atrial fibrillation if disease advanced.

Chest radiography: shows left atrial enlargement, pulmonary congestion, prominent pulmonary arteries (in pulmonary hypertensive patients).

Echocardiography and Doppler ultrasonography: show thickened mitral valve with reduced movement, large left atrium, reduced left ventricular filling rate, reduced mitral valve area.

Cardiac catheterization: shows raised right heart pressures and an end-diastolic gradient from pulmonary artery wedge pressure (or left atrium if transseptal puncture done) to left ventricle.

Complications

Systemic embolism: from left atrium.

Pulmonary hypertension, right heart failure.

Endocarditis: unusual.

Differential diagnosis

Left atrial myxoma: physical signs may be identical (echocardiography confirms diagnosis).

Etiology

Rheumatic disease.

Congenital abnormality (rare).

Epidemiology

- The occurrence of mitral stenosis is decreasing in developed countries as a result of the declining incidence of rheumatic fever.

Treatment

Diet and lifestyle

• Patients should avoid being overweight, give up smoking, and maintain normal activities, if possible.

Pharmacological treatment

Digoxin

• If the patient is in atrial fibrillation, digoxin is indicated for control of ventricular rate.

Standard dosage	Digoxin, 0.5 mg loading dose, repeated after 8 hours; maintenance dose usually 0.25 mg daily, adjusted according to serum digoxin concentration.
Contraindications	Caution in patients who are elderly, relatively small, or renally impaired (reduced dosage).
Main drug interactions	Diuretic-induced hypokalemia enhances effect of digoxin.
Main side effects	Nausea, vomiting, diarrhea, yellow discoloration to vision (xanthopsia), bradycardia.

Diuretics

• Diuretics are indicated for dyspnea or fluid retention.

Standard dosage	Furosemide, 20–80 mg daily with potassium supplements or potassium-sparing agent (particularly if patient is also taking digoxin).
Contraindications	None.
Special points	May precipitate attacks of gout in susceptible patients and may interfere with diabetic control.
Main drug interactions	Digoxin.
Main side effects	Hypokalemia, dehydration.

Anticoagulants

• Anticoagulants are mandatory if the degree of stenosis is high, even if the patient is still in sinus rhythm.

Standard dosage	Warfarin, 10 mg daily for 3 days; maintenance dose depends on regular checks of INR.
Contraindications	Bleeding tendency.
Main drug interactions	Any drug that displaces warfarin from protein-binding sites or increases liver enzyme activity may cause alteration in INR and thus necessitate dose adjustment.
Main side effects	Increased bleeding tendency.

Beta-adrenergic blockers

• For patients in atrial fibrillation who have effort-related tachycardia despite digitalis, beta-blockers are helpful in reducing tendency to extreme tachycardia.

Standard dosage	Atenolol, 25–100 mg daily, or metoprolol, 50–100 mg daily to control heart rate.
Contraindications	Asthma, heart failure, bradycardia, heart block.
Main drug interactions	Bradycardia when combined with digitalis or calcium channel blockers. Low doses are usually the rule when used with digitalis.

Treatment aims

To achieve normal exercise capability and normal functional capacity.

Other treatments

Balloon valvuloplasty if valve is mobile and not heavily calcified [2].

Surgical valvotomy or replacement.

Prognosis

• The prognosis is good unless pulmonary hypertension is chronic.

Follow-up and management

• Restenosis may occur after valvotomy or valvuloplasty.

• Drug treatment may become inadequate and indicate intervention eventually.

• Patients should have prophylactic treatment against endocarditis (*see* Endocarditis *for details*).

Key references

1. Wood P: An appreciation of mitral stenosis. *BMJ* 1954, **1**:1051–1055.
2. Abascal VM, *et al.*: Echocardiographic evaluation of mitral valve structure and function after percutaneous mitral valvuloplasty. *J Am Coll Cardiol* 1988, **12**:606–615.

Motor neuron disease

Diagnosis

Definition

• Motor neuron disease is one of many motor neuron disorders. The term covers amyotrophic lateral sclerosis (the most common form), progressive muscular atrophy, and progressive bulbar palsy (thought to be variants of the same disorder).
• The disorder is progressive and is characterized by degeneration of cortical, brain stem, and spinal-cord motor neurons.

Symptoms [1]

Cramps or fasciculations: may precede other symptoms by months.
Asymmetrical painless weakness or wasting of proximal or distal upper limb muscles: presenting symptom in 40%–60% of patients with upper limb involvement and 20% with lower limb involvement (unilateral foot drop common).
Dysarthria: presenting complaint in 25%–30%, usually followed by limb involvement; 70%–80% presenting with limb involvement develop dysarthria, culminating in anarthria.
Dysphagia: accompanying dysarthria.
Shortness of breath: usually due to diaphragmatic weakness.
Minor sensory symptoms: occasionally.
Changes in character and behavior: in 5%–10%.
Frontal-lobe dementia: rarely.

Signs

Typical disease

Fasciculations, wasting, depressed reflexes: lower motor neuron signs.
Spasticity, slowing of alternating movements, brisk tendon reflexes, Babinski responses: upper motor neuron signs.

• Typical motor neuron disease has lower and upper motor neuron signs in several regions (cranial nerves, arms, legs), with evidence of disease progression.
• Signs are usually asymmetrical in the early stages, with no evidence of sensory signs or bladder or bowel involvement.

Bulbar involvement

Emotional lability, with inappropriate laughter and crying, brisk jaw jerk, spasticity of facial muscles, spastic dysarthria, dysphagia, spasticity of tongue: indicating upper motor neuron involvement (pseudobulbar palsy).
Wasting of facial and jaw muscles, fasciculation and wasting of tongue, nasal speech, dysphagia, bovine cough: indicating lower motor neuron involvement (bulbar palsy).

Investigations

• Laboratory results are usually normal (creatine kinase activity may be 2–3 times normal).

Electromyography: shows widespread anterior horn cell damage; nerve conduction studies usually normal; electrophysiology supports clinical diagnosis and excludes root and plexus lesions or motor neuropathy; characteristic abnormalities include fibrillation potentials and positive sharp waves, fasciculations, abnormal motor units of increased amplitude and duration.
MRI or myelography: may be needed to exclude spinal cord or root compression; MRI may show altered signal in posterior limb of internal capsule in region of degenerating corticospinal tract fibers.
Muscle biopsy: sometimes needed to exclude other diagnoses in atypical cases; confirms denervation, with small angular fibers and prominent fiber type grouping.

Complications

Depression: social and emotional isolation, especially in patients with severe dysarthria.
Dysphagia: leading to weight loss, malnutrition, dehydration, and aspiration.
Bronchopulmonary infections: related to aspiration and ventilatory muscle weakness.
Venous thrombosis and pulmonary embolism.
Constipation: due to pelvic and abdominal wall weakness and poor fluid intake.
Ventilatory failure: usual cause of death.

Differential diagnosis

Myasthenia gravis with bulbar onset.
Postpoliomyelitis muscular atrophy syndrome.
Cervical myelopathy.
Intramedullary spinal cord lesions.
Motor neuronopathy.
Late-onset spinal muscular atrophy.
Kennedy's syndrome.
Late-onset hexosaminidase A deficiency.

Etiology [2,3]

• 5%–10% of patients have a family history suggesting autosomal-dominant inheritance.
• Point mutations of the gene encoding Cu/Zn superoxide dismutase on chromosome 21q are present in 10%–20% of families.
• X-linked bulbospinal neuronopathy (Kennedy's syndrome) is caused by a mutation of the gene encoding the androgen receptor.
• The cause of sporadic motor neuron disease is unknown; free radical damage and excitotoxicity have been implicated.

Epidemiology

• The incidence of motor neuron disease in Europe and North America is 2 in 100 000.
• The prevalence is 3–6 in 100 000.
• The male : female ratio is 1.5:1.
• The peak onset in sporadic disease is at 60 years, about a decade earlier in familial disease.
• The incidence may be increasing, especially in older age groups.

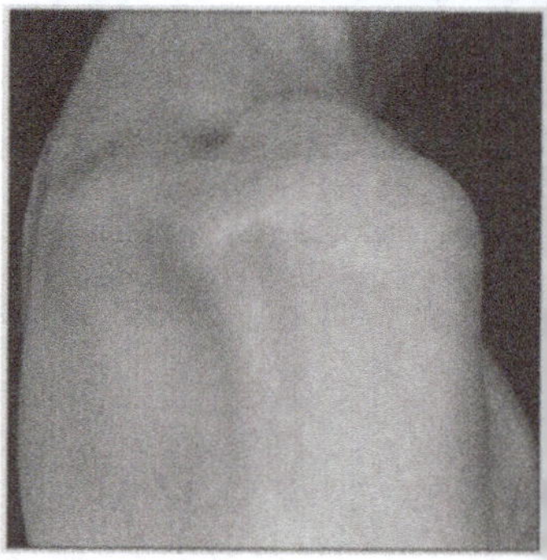

Marked muscle wasting around the shoulder girdle in a patient with motor neuron disease. (*See* Color Plate.)

Treatment

Diet and lifestyle

• Dietary advice is needed for patients with dysphagia and those who are being treated by percutaneous endoscopic gastrostomy.

Pharmacological treatment

Symptomatic medications

Glycopyrrolate, hyoscine (orally or transdermal patches), amitriptyline for drooling.

Quinine for cramps.

Baclofen, tizanidine, diazepam for spasticity.

Amitriptyline, dothiepin, fluoxetine for depression and emotional lability.

Fibercon, Colace, Mylanta, glycerine suppositories for constipation (with increased fluid intake).

Opiates, diazepam for symptomatic relief of anxiety related to dyspnea.

• The antiglutamate agent riluzole prolongs survival modestly.

To slow progression and prolong survival

• Riluzole's action is through inhibition of glutamate release [4].

Standard dosage	Riluzole, 100 mg/day orally. Gabapentin, 800 mg 3 times daily orally.
Contraindications	*Riluzole:* hepatic dysfunction, pregnancy. *Gabapentin:* pregnancy.
Special points	*Riluzole:* check liver function monthly for 3 months then every 3 months. *Gabapentin:* approved for epilepsy; early trials in ALS show a trend toward slower progression of weakness.
Main side effects	*Riluzole:* asthenia, nausea, dizziness, elevated hepatic enzymes. *Gabapentin:* tremor, dizziness, sedation.

•Other drug trials with insulin-like growth factor 1 show some promise.

Nonpharmacological treatment

Physical therapy.

Counseling for depression.

Percutaneous endoscopic gastrostomy for dysphagia (best considered early).

Radiotherapy to the parotid glands for excess saliva.

Assisted ventilation for respiratory failure: techniques available include nasal intermittent positive airway pressure ventilation, a rocking bed, a cuirasse, or, in exceptional circumstances, a tracheostomy and intermittent positive pressure ventilation.

Treatment aims

To maintain patient's independence and quality of life.

To alleviate symptoms.

Prognosis

• 80%–90% of patients develop upper and lower motor neuron signs at some stage.

• 10% show only lower motor neuron signs (progressive muscular atrophy).

• The median survival is 4 years (2 years for bulbar onset).

• 5%–10% of patients survive for 5 years or more; a few live for 15 years or more.

• Patients with only lower motor neuron signs tend to have a better prognosis than those with typical motor neuron disease.

Follow-up and management

• A multidisciplinary neuro-care team approach is recommended; the team comprises neurologist, physical therapist, occupational therapist, speech therapist, dietitian, social worker, and other relevant health care workers. Each patient may be allocated a "key worker" to integrate the activities of the team.

• Communication and other aids should be provided, and the home adapted.

• Patients might require referral to a hospice.

Patient support

Amyotrophic Lateral Sclerosis Association, 21021 Ventura Blvd., Suite 321 Woodland Hills, CA 91364; phone (818) 340-7500 or (800) 782-4747.

Key references

1. Miller RG, Sufit R: New approaches to the treatment of ALS. *Neurology* 1997, **48(suppl 4)**:S28–S32.
2. Leigh PN, Ray-Chaudhuri K: Motor neurone disease. *J Neurol Neurosurg Psychiatry* 1994, **57**:886–896.
3. Rosen DR, *et al.*: Mutations in the Cu/Zn superoxide gene are associated with familial amyotrophic lateral sclerosis. *Nature* 1993, **362**:59–62.
4. Miller RG, *et al.*: Clinical trials of riluzole in patients with ALS. ALS/Riluzole Study Group II. *Neurology* 1996, **47(suppl 2)**: S86–S90.

Diagnosis

Symptoms

• Up to 10% of patients are asymptomatic.

Anorexia, weight loss.
Bone pain, back pain, pathological fracture.
Anemia, purpura, infection: symptoms of bone-marrow failure.
Polyuria, nocturia, pruritus: symptoms of renal failure.
Abdominal pain, anorexia, polyuria, polydipsia, constipation: symptoms of hypercalcemia.
Infection: due to hypogammaglobulinemia.
Visual symptoms, confusion, dyspnea, bleeding manifestations, polyneuropathy: symptoms of hyperviscosity.
Cardiac failure and edema: due to increased plasma oncotic pressure or viscosity.

Signs

Anemia, purpura.
Bony tenderness: over sites of lytic deposits.
Infections: especially skin, respiratory tract, and urinary tract.
Skin and soft-tissue deposits: particularly in IgD myeloma.
Proteinuria.
Peripheral neuropathy: due to paraprotein deposition.
Hepatosplenomegaly and lymphadenopathy: rare; suggest an IgM paraprotein or amyloidosis.

• Diagnosis requires the presence of >10% abnormal plasma cells in bone marrow and one of the following: bone lesions, serum paraprotein, and urine paraprotein.

Investigations [1]

Complete blood count: to check for anemia or bone-marrow failure.
ESR measurement: characteristically raised, often exceeds 100 mm/h.
Complete biochemical screening: including creatinine, creatinine clearance, serum calcium (alkaline phosphatase usually normal), albumin.
Skeletal survey: preferred to isotope bone scan, to show osteolytic lesions, vertebral collapse or osteoporosis.
Serum protein electrophoresis, immunoelectrophoresis, serum and urine analysis: to measure immunoglobulin concentrations, paraprotein quantification, and urinary Bence Jones protein.
β_2-Microglobulin and CRP measurement: to assess prognosis.
Bone-marrow aspiration and trephine biopsy: to show infiltration by malignant plasma cells and to assess normal bone-marrow reserve.
Microbiological cultures: if signs of infection.
Plasma cell labeling index, immunophenotype analysis, cytogenetic and DNA studies: if available, for further characterization of disease and prognosis.
MRI: a sensitive indicator of skeletal disease, especially good for detecting deposits around spine.

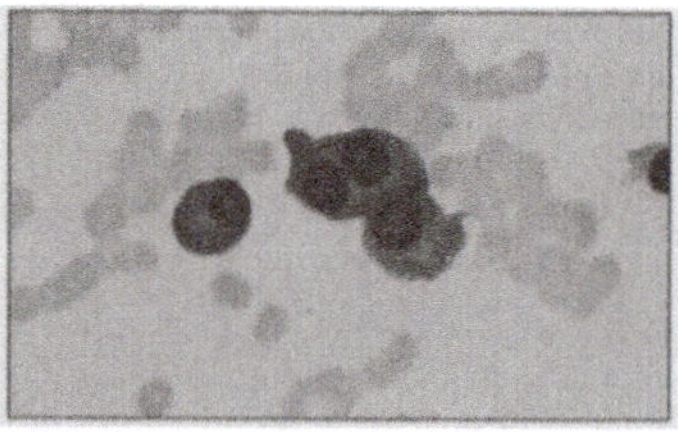

Plasma cells infiltrating bone marrow. (*See* Color Plate.)

Complications

Renal failure, hypercalcemia, hyperviscosity syndrome.

Infection: most common cause of death.

Pathological fracture and spinal-cord compression.

Polyneuropathy, cardiac and renal failure, macroglossia, skin infiltration: in 5%–10% of patients, caused by amyloidosis.

Differential diagnosis

Metastatic carcinoma: hypercalcemia, lytic lesions, but normal alkaline phosphatase differentiates.

Polymyalgia rheumatica, temporal arteritis: anemia, high ESR, but no paraprotein.

Other causes of renal failure.

Benign monoclonal gammopathy: but paraprotein is <30 g/L, with normal concentrations of other immunoglobulins, anemia, renal failure, lytic lesions all absent, little or no Bence Jones proteinuria and no progression on follow-up.

Solitary plasmacytoma, primary amyloidosis, other lymphoproliferative disorders (*e.g.*, Waldenström's macroglobulinemia, non-Hodgkin's lymphoma).

Etiology [1,2]

• The cause is largely unknown, but risk factors include the following: ionizing radiation, organic chemical exposure, chronic antigenic stimulation, chronic inflammatory disease.

• Genetic predisposition: acquired genetic mutations to oncogenes may promote tumor growth, and certain cytokines (*e.g.*, interleukin-6) may function as growth factors.

• Human herpesvirus-8 (HHV-8) may have a role in disease pathogenesis.

Epidemiology [1]

• Multiple myeloma forms ~1% of all malignancies, 10%–15% of all hematological malignancies.

• The median age at diagnosis is 71 years.

• The disease occurs more often in blacks.

• The male:female ratio is ~5:3.

Staging [1]

Stage I: hemoglobin >10 g/dL, normal calcium, normal skeletal survey or solitary plasmacytoma, low paraprotein (IgG <50 g/L, IgA <30 g/L, urinary Bence Jones protein <4 g/24 h).

Stage II: neither stage I nor stage III.

Stage III: hemoglobin <8.5 g/dL, hypercalcemia, advanced skeletal disease, high paraprotein (IgG >70 g/L, IgA >50 g/L, urinary Bence Jones protein >12 g/24 h).

Subclassification: A, normal creatinine; B, raised creatinine.

Treatment

Diet and lifestyle

- Patients may need a diet appropriate for the degree of renal failure.
- Cooked food is needed for severely neutropenic patients.
- Patients should avoid bone damage, *e.g.*, heavy lifting.

Pharmacological treatment

Supportive treatment

- Careful supportive care is important, *e.g.*, the following:

Hydration and promotion of diuresis in renal failure and before chemotherapy.

Appropriate antibiotics or antifungal agents.

Adequate analgesia.

Blood component support.

Treatment of hypercalcemia (*e.g.*, bisphosphonates): pamidronate may also reduce progression of bone disease and relieve pain.

Chemotherapy [3,4]

- Oral chemotherapy is the simplest protocol and involves melphalan and prednisone for 4–7 days every 4–6 weeks.
- Intravenous combination chemotherapy generally leads to a more rapid response, with higher complete remission rates, but the survival advantage over melphalan and prednisone is marginal and probably occurs only in patients aged <70 years. Current regimens include the following:

ABCM (doxorubicin, BCNU, cyclophosphamide, melphalan).
VBMCP (vincristine, BCNU, melphalan, cyclophosphamide, prednisone).
VAD (vincristine, doxorubicin by continuous i.v. infusion over 4 days with oral dexamethasone; standard for relapsed patients, also has a place in induction).

- α-Interferon, s.c. 3 times weekly, may improve combination therapy response rates and may prolong remission ("plateau" phase) and overall survival.
- Relapsed patients can be given cyclophosphamide orally or i.v. weekly, high-dose steroids (dexamethasone or methylprednisolone), and melphalan, single i.v. dose (high or intermediate).
- VAD gives responses in up to 40% of patients, and cyclosporine (to block multiple drug resistance) combined with VAD may be even more effective. High-dose cyclophosphamide with etoposide and granulocyte-macrophage colony-stimulating factor is valuable in VAD-resistant myeloma.
- Thalidomide may be useful in previously treated patients whose condition has relapsed.

Complications of treatment

- Chemotherapy is immunosuppressive and myelotoxic.
- Growth factor support (granulocyte and granulocyte-macrophage colony-stimulating factor) elevates the leukocyte count to reduce infective complications due to leukopenia, but also causes bone pain.
- Recombinant erythropoietin reduces red blood cell transfusion requirement, particularly in renal failure.
- VAD and cyclophosphamide are preferred in renal failure because they are metabolized primarily by the liver.
- Antibacterial and antifungal prophylaxis with blood component support (principally platelets) is needed for myeloablative and intensive chemotherapy regimens.
- Hair loss, nausea, vomiting, mucositis (i.v. melphalan); bone demineralization (prednisone); and fatigue, fever, and anorexia (α-interferon) also occur.
- NSAIDs may accelerate renal failure if used for pain relief.

Treatment aims

To achieve normal immunoglobulin and blood counts and to relieve bone pain.

Other treatments [5]

- Indicated for primary nonresponders, relapsed patients, or those with local complications:

Radiation therapy: relieves pain from lytic lesions; systemic activity against tumor but often leads to prolonged pancytopenia.
Internal fixation of pathological fractures.
Allogeneic bone-marrow transplantation: after conditioning by high-dose cyclophosphamide and total-body radiation therapy; for patients aged <50 years with histocompatible sibling.
Autologous bone-marrow transplantation or peripheral blood stem cell infusion: intensive treatment for patients aged <60 years, after high-dose chemotherapy.
Plasma exchange: for hyperviscosity syndrome.
Dialysis.

Prognosis

- In untreated patients, the median survival is <1 year; with treatment, it rises to 3–4 years.
- β_2-Microglobulin concentrations correlate with prognosis (<6 mg/L good, 6–12 mg/L intermediate, >12 mg/L poor prognosis).
- Raised CRP, poor response to treatment, age >75, skin or soft-tissue involvement, and advanced stage indicate poor prognosis.
- Disappearance of paraprotein and restoration of normal immunoglobulin or normal blood counts with stable paraprotein are achieved after 4–6 cycles of chemotherapy in >85% of patients.

Follow-up and management

- Complete blood count, renal function, β_2-microglobulin and serum and urine paraprotein concentrations should be assessed regularly (every 1–2 months) to monitor the disease and the effects of treatment.
- Patients should be checked for opportunistic infection and new skeletal abnormalities.

Key references

1. Barlogie B, ed: Multiple myeloma. *Hematol Oncol Clin North Am* 1992, **6**:211–484.
2. Lokhorst HM, Sonneveld P, Verdonck LF: Intensive treatment for multiple myeloma: where do we stand? *Br J Haematol* 1999, **106**:18–27.
3. Alexanian R, Dimopoulos M: The treatment of multiple myeloma. *N Engl J Med* 1994, **330**:484–489.
4. Bataille R: New insights in the clinical biology of multiple myeloma. *Semin Hematol* 1997, **34**:23–28.
5. Vescio RA, Berenson JR: The role of human herpesvirus-8 (HHV-8) in multiple myeloma pathogenesis. *Curr Top Microbiol Immunol* 1999; **246**:403–409.

Multiple sclerosis

Diagnosis

Symptoms

Relapsing and remitting

• 90% of patients initially have relapses and remissions of neurological disturbance attributable to CNS white matter lesions, including the following:

Visual loss.
Diplopia.
Vertigo.
Numbness.
Weakness.
Incoordination.
Paresthesia.
Urinary urgency/incontinence.
Pain.
Impotence.

Progressive

• Progressive disease takes two forms.

Primary, in 10%: progressive from onset without remission.

Secondary, in 50%: progressive after an initially relapsing and remitting course.

Signs

• Signs are variable but include the following:

Optic atrophy.

Ophthalmoplegia.

Nystagmus.

Weakness: hemiparesis or paraparesis.

Sensory loss.

Spasticity.

Investigations

• The diagnosis is primarily clinical and depends on the demonstration of two or more necessarily separate CNS lesions in a patient with a history of two characteristic episodes.

• Investigations provide invaluable support, but none of the abnormalities is specific to multiple sclerosis.

Evoked potentials: especially visual and somatosensory, to detect subclinical involvement and provide evidence for demyelination.

MRI: to detect subclinical involvement and the characteristic pattern of lesions.

CSF analysis: for electrophoresis to show oligoclonal IgG, present in 90% of patients; CSF can be useful in making the diagnosis in patients with only a single clear flare of disease.

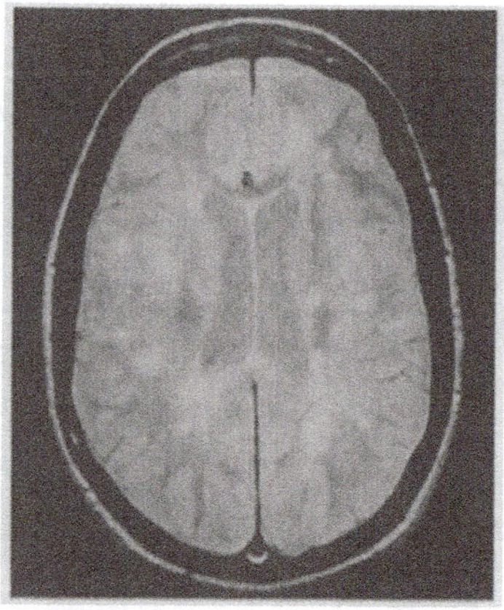

T_2-weighted MRI showing areas of abnormal signal in the cerebral hemispheres in a patient with multiple sclerosis.

Complications

Visual loss, paresis, tremor, incontinence: due to persistent neurological deficit.

Significant cognitive impairment: may occur late.

Differential diagnosis

Relapsing and remitting

Collagen vascular disease.

Neurosarcoidosis.

Lyme disease.

Progressive

Compression: *e.g.*, tumor, craniocervical anomaly.

Spinocerebellar degeneration.

Motor neuron disease.

Leukodystrophy.

Etiology [1]

Genetic predisposition: HLA association, but probably additional factors.

Extrinsic factor: probably infective, possibly viral.

Epidemiology [2]

• 60 in 100 000 population in the United States are affected by multiple sclerosis.

• 20% of patients have an affected relative.

• Multiple sclerosis is diagnosed in patients aged <10 years or >40 years in only 13% of cases.

Treatment

Diet and lifestyle

• Patients should be assessed for functional limitations to determine appropriate modifications in lifestyle (neurorehabilitation, physical therapy, occupational therapy).

• Exposure to heat or fever worsens the motor symptoms temporarily.

Pharmacological treatment [3]

For symptoms

Standard dosage	*For spasticity:* baclofen initially, 5 mg 3 times daily; maximum 100 mg daily. *For urinary frequency, urgency, and incontinence:* oxybutynin, 5 mg 2–3 times daily.
Contraindications	*Baclofen:* peptic ulceration. *Oxybutynin:* bladder outflow obstruction, glaucoma.
Main drug interactions	*Baclofen:* muscle relaxants. *Oxybutynin:* antimuscarinics.
Main side effects	*Baclofen:* weakness, sedation enhanced by alcohol. *Oxybutynin:* antimuscarinic effects.

• For impotence, patients should be referred to a urologist.

For relapse

• Steroids are indicated when functional impairment is significant.

Standard dosage	Methylprednisolone, 1 g in 250 mL normal saline solution i.v. over 30 minutes daily for 3 days, often followed by oral taper.
Contraindications	Hypertension, diabetes, peptic ulceration, systemic infection, history of tuberculosis, osteoporosis, history of psychiatric disorder.
Special points	Frequent use should be avoided.
Main drug interactions	Other drugs causing hypokalemia, drugs inducing liver enzymes.
Main side effects	Fluid retention, hypokalemia, depression, psychosis, hypertension, glucose intolerance, peptic ulceration, osteoporosis.

For prophylaxis

Standard dosage	Interferon-β 1b, 8 million IU s.c. every other day or interferon-β 1a, weekly i.m., or copaxone 20 mg daily s.c. to reduce relapses in some patients with relapsing-remitting disease.
Contraindications	Hypersensitivity.
Main side effects	Fatigue, malaise, flu-like symptoms, injection site reactions, sometimes depression with interferon-β 1b.

• Several agents (*e.g.*, linomide, oral myelin) have recently failed trails, whereas others are still under investigation.

• In chronic progressive multiple sclerosis, there are no clearly proven agents; interferons-β are in trials. Interferons seem to reduce MRI burden of disease in even secondary progressive disease.

Alternative medicine

Recommended use: none.

Common use: ginkgo biloba; thiamine; evening primrose (*Oenothera biennis*).

Caution: none.

Treatment aims

To alleviate symptoms.

To control relapse.

To modify course.

Prognosis

• Prognosis is very variable, ranging from death in a few months to survival without disability for 50 years.

• At least one-third of patients have little disability after 15 years.

Follow-up and management

• Follow-up depends on the condition of the patient.

• In complete remission, regular follow-up is not needed.

• When significant disability is present, assessment in a comprehensive neurological rehabilitation clinic is useful as the condition changes.

Patient support

National Multiple Sclerosis Society, 733 3rd Ave., New York, NY 10017-3240; phone (212) 986-3240 or (800) FIGHT-MS

Key references

1. Sowcer S, Goodfellow PN, Compston A: The genetic analysis of multiple sclerosis. *Trends Genet* 1997, **13**:234–239.
2. Matthews WB, *et al.* (eds.): *McAlpine's Multiple Sclerosis*. Edinburgh: Churchill Livingstone; 1991.
3. McDonald WI: New treatments for multiple sclerosis. *BMJ* 1995, **310**:345–346.

Myasthenia gravis

Diagnosis

Symptoms

Painless muscle weakness increasing with exercise ("fatigue").

Drooping eyelids (one or both) and double vision.

• Weakness may characteristically also affect smiling, swallowing, chewing, speaking, neck muscles, arm elevation, elbow extension, hand movements, walking, and breathing.

• Symptoms are worst at the end of the day.

Signs

Fatiguable ptosis.

Variable limitation of eye movement.

Impaired eye closure.

Transverse smile.

Nasal speech.

Fatiguable weakness of affected muscles.

Wasting: rare.

Hypoactive tendon reflexes.

Investigations

Serum acetylcholine receptor (AChR) antibody analysis: raised titer specific for myasthenia gravis.

Edrophonium (Tensilon) test: double-blind test showing transient improvement.

Clinical electrophysiology: increased decrement to repetitive motor nerve stimulation; increased jitter on single fiber study.

CT of chest: for thymoma, lung tumor.

Striated muscle antibody analysis: positive in 90% of patients with thymoma, 50% of patients with generalized myasthenia gravis.

Complications

Myasthenic crisis: acute respiratory or bulbar symptoms.

Cholinergic crisis: due to excess anticholinesterase treatment; causing hypersalivation, lacrimation, increased sweating, vomiting, and miosis; can also cause weakness and respiratory failure.

Local or pleural spread of thymoma.

Differential diagnosis

Lambert–Eaton myasthenic syndrome.

Congenital myasthenia gravis.

Chronic fatigue syndrome.

Etiology

• Antibodies to muscle AChRs cause receptor loss.

• Immune response genes influence susceptibility.

• Penicillamine may induce AChR antibodies and typical myasthenia gravis.

• Placental transfer of AChR antibodies causes neonatal myasthenia gravis in the offspring of 12% of mothers with the disease [1].

• "Seronegative" myasthenia gravis is antibody-mediated: the antigenic target is not known.

Epidemiology

• The prevalence is 8–9 in 100 000 people.

• The annual incidence is 0.4 in 100 000.

• All races are susceptible; restricted ocular myasthenia gravis is more frequent in Asian patients.

• The disease is manifest from infancy to extreme old age.

Clinical classification

• The clinical subgroup influences treatment selection; typical features are shown below.

Early onset (50%)

Symptom distribution: generalized.
Age at onset: <40 years.
Thymus pathology: hyperplasia.
AChR antibody titer: high.

Late onset (25%)

Symptom distribution: generalized or ocular.
Age at onset: >40 years.
Thymus pathology: atrophy/normal.
AChR antibody titer: low.

Seronegative (15%)

Symptom distribution: ocular or generalized.
Age of onset: any.
Thymus pathology: atrophy/normal.
AChR antibody titer: absent.

Thymoma (10%)

Symptom distribution: generalized.
Age at onset: any.
Thymus pathology: thymoma.
AChR antibody titer: intermediate.
Increased frequency of striated muscle antibody.

Treatment

Diet and lifestyle

- No special precautions are necessary.
- Elevated body temperature can worsen weakness.

Pharmacological treatment [2,3]

Management strategy

- The following treatments are helpful, usually in this order:

Anticholinesterase for immediate symptom control.
Plasma exchange in some cases (*see* Other treatments).
Thymectomy in some patients (*see* Other treatments).
Prednisone.
Azathioprine.
Intravenous immunoglobulin.
Other immunosuppressive treatment (cyclosporine, cyclophosphamide).

Drugs to be avoided

Antiarrhythmics (quinidine), antibacterials (aminoglycosides, clindamycin, lincomycin, and polymyxins), antimalarials (chloroquine), beta-blockers (propranolol), lithium, muscle relaxants.

Anticholinesterase

- This relieves symptoms.

Standard dosage	Pyridostigmine, 30–120 mg 5 times daily. Glycopyrrolate, 1 mg up to 3 times daily, if necessary, to control adverse gastrointestinal effects.
Contraindications	Intestinal or urinary obstruction.
Main drug interactions	*See* Drugs to be avoided.
Main side effects	Diarrhea, abdominal cramps, increased salivation, nausea and vomiting.

Prednisone

- For generalized disease of moderate severity unresponsive to other treatments (inpatients).

Standard dosage	*Outpatients:* prednisone, 5-mg single dose on alternate days, increased by 5 mg at weekly intervals to controlling dose or 0.75–1 mg/kg/day, whichever is lower. *Inpatients:* prednisone, or solumedrol burst, usually with simultaneous plasmaphoresis. In both groups, dose should be tapered by 5 mg/month when remission is established and adjusted to define effective minimal dose.
Contraindications	Osteoporosis, diabetes.
Main drug interactions	Antibacterials, *e.g.*, rifampicin, antiepileptics.
Main side effects	Initial exacerbation of myasthenic symptoms, adrenal suppression, diabetes, osteoporosis, avascular necrosis of femoral head, mental disturbance, weight gain, cushingoid features, cataracts.

Azathioprine

- Azathioprine is indicated in combination with prednisone for generalized moderate or severe disease; often takes months to be effective.

Standard dosage	Azathioprine, 2.5 mg/kg/day orally.
Contraindications	Myelosuppression.
Special points	Full blood count and liver function tests weekly for 8 weeks, every 1–3 months thereafter.
Main drug interactions	Allopurinol enhances toxic effect.
Main side effects	Myelosuppression, hepatotoxicity, gastrointestinal symptoms, rashes, B-cell lymphoma (very rare).

Treatment aims

To allow patient to recover strength.

Other treatments

Plasma exchange

- Plasma exchange is indicated for the following:

Symptomatic control in severe cases.
Myasthenic crisis.
Preparation for thymectomy.
After thymectomy while awaiting response.
Recurrently, in severe myasthenia gravis, while awaiting response to immunosuppressive drug therapy.

Thymectomy (by median sternotomy)

- Thymectomy is indicated for the following:

Thymoma (because of risk of local spread).
Early-onset generalized myasthenia gravis (outcome in subsequent 1–2 years 25% remission, 50% improvement, 25% neutral).

Prognosis

- Most patients achieve substantial improvement or full recovery.

Follow-up and management

- In patients treated by immunosuppressive drugs, continuing low-dose treatment and regular follow-up is usually needed to maintain disease control.

Key references

1. Shillito P, Vincent A, Newsom-Davis J: Congenital myasthenic syndromes. *J Neuromusc Dis* 1993, **3**:183–190.
2. Verma P, Oger J: Treatment of acquired autoimmune myasthenia gravis. *Can J Neurol Sci* 1992, **19**:360–375.
3. Younger DS: Advances in the diagnosis, pathogenesis, and treatment of myasthenia gravis. *Neurology* 1997, **48(suppl 5)**:S1–S81.

Mycobacterium avium complex infection in AIDS

Diagnosis

Symptoms

• Symptoms of disseminated *Mycobacterium avium* or *M. intracellulare* infection may be difficult to distinguish from those of other opportunistic infections associated with HIV infection.

• Disseminated infection may be asymptomatic.

Systemic

Fever: with or without sweats.

Anorexia and malaise.

Weight loss: often associated with anemia and neutropenia.

Gastrointestinal

Chronic diarrhea and abdominal pain: resulting from *M. avium-intracellulare* invasion of the colon or small bowel or bulky retroperitoneal lymph nodes infected by *M. avium-intracellulare.*

Signs

Weight loss, oral candidiasis: evidence of underlying HIV infection and other HIV-associated complications.

Weight loss, anemia, hepato(spleno)megaly: indicating disseminated disease.

Localized or cutaneous abscesses, endophthalmitis, arthritis, lymphadenopathy.

Investigations

Blood culture: using lysis/centrifugation or radiometric technique, yield increased (from 60% to almost 100%); 5–50 days needed for blood cultures to become positive.

Biopsy: diagnosis of disseminated *M. avium-intracellulare* infection made by isolation or culture from any normally sterile site (blood, bone-marrow, lymph-node, and liver biopsy best); negative blood cultures unusual with positive histology from lymph-node, liver, or bone-marrow biopsy; stains may show acid-fast bacilli before blood cultures become positive, thus suggesting diagnosis.

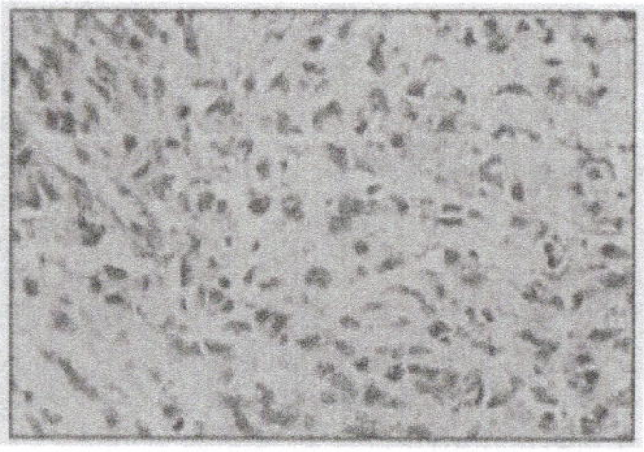

Lymph-node biopsy. Numerous clumps of acid-fast bacilli are seen within the tissue. There is no granulamatous response. Magnification × 400. (*See* Color Plate.)

• Isolation of *M. avium-intracellulare* from sputum and bronchoalveolar lavage or stool usually represents colonization rather than infection.

Complications

None.

Differential diagnosis

Progression of HIV or other systemic opportunistic infection.

Etiology

• *M. avium* complex, cause widely disseminated infection in AIDS patients.

• Disseminated infection occurs exclusively in patients with advanced HIV disease and CD4 counts <75 × 10^6/L.

• The source of invasion in AIDS patients may be gastrointestinal; large numbers of mycobacteria within macrophages of the small bowel lamina propria suggest that the bowel is the portal of entry.

Epidemiology

• *M. avium-intracellulare* is ubiquitous in the environment, being found in water, soil, animals, and dairy products.

Pathogenesis and pathology

• Almost all AIDS patients with disseminated *M. avium-intracellulare* have positive blood cultures (in contrast to those with stool, urine, or respiratory secretion colonization).

• Histology of involved organs reveals absent or poorly formed granulomata and mycobacteria within macrophages. Little tissue destruction is seen, despite heavy mycobacterial load.

Treatment

Diet and lifestyle

• No special precautions are necessary.

Pharmacological treatment

• More than 50% of strains can be inhibited by achievable concentrations of amikacin, azithromycin, ciprofloxacin, clarithromycin, clofazimine, cycloserine, ethambutol, ethionamide, or rifabutin.

• Treatment with clarithromycin and ethambutol with or without rifampin is recommended.

• Additional agents may be used if the standard two- or three-drug regimens have failed or have resulted in toxicities.

Standard dosage

Ethambutol, 15 mg/kg orally once daily, with clarithromycin monitoring therapy with the use of susceptibility testing, 500–1000 mg orally twice daily.

Ciprofloxacin, 500 mg orally twice daily, rifubutin 150 mg daily may be added. Ciprofloxacin and rifabutin are used in case of toxicities or failure.

Amikacin, 7.5 mg/kg i.v. once daily, may be added for patients with refractory fever or anorexia. Treatment is given for 2–4 weeks.

Contraindications

Previous drug hypersensitivity.

Rifabutin: jaundice, porphyria.

Ethambutol: renal impairment, optic neuritis.

Clarithromycin: porphyria, hepatic or renal failure.

Main drug interactions

Rifabutin: induces hepatic microsome enzyme activity and so increases metabolism of azole drugs; interacts with fluconazole or clarithromycin to produce uveitis in 30% of patients if >300 mg of rifabutin are given daily. Levels are increased in patients receiving protease-inhibitor agents.

If steroids are given with an antibacterial regimen containing rifampin or rifabutin, the dose should be doubled to take into account the hepatic microsome-inducing effects of the drugs.

Main side effects

Rifabutin: nausea and vomiting, diarrhea, anorexia; body fluids become orange-red.

Ethambutol: optic neuritis, red-green color blindness, peripheral neuritis.

Ciprofloxacin: nausea and vomiting, abdominal pain, diarrhea, headache, photosensitivity, arthralgia, myalgia.

Clarithromycin: nausea and vomiting, abdominal pain, diarrhea.

Treatment aims

To reduce mycobacteremia or fever and transfusion requirements.

• Cure is not achievable.

Prognosis

• Survival in AIDS patients with disseminated *M. avium-intracellulare* infection has been extended in patients receiving HAART.

•The presence of *M. avium-intracellulare* in gastrointestinal secretions predicts the subsequent development of disseminated infection.

Follow-up and management

• Treatment is for life.

General references

Fordham von Reyu C, Arbeit RD, Tostesum AN, *et al.*: The international epidemiology of disseminated *Mycobacterium avium* complex infection in AIDS. *AIDS* 1996, **10**:1025–1032.

Jacobson MA: Mycobacterial disease. In *The Medical Management of AIDS*, edn 3. Edited by Sande MA, Volberding PA. Philadelphia: WB Saunders; 1992:284–296.

Masur H: Recommendations on prophylaxis and therapy for disseminated *Mycobacterium avium* complex disease in patients infected with the human immuno-deficiency virus. *N Engl J Med* 1993, **329**:898-904.

Diagnosis

Symptoms

• Chronic myeloid leukemia is usually manifest in chronic phase; it transforms spontaneously to an accelerated phase and then to an acute blastic phase normally within 3–6 years of diagnosis (range, 0–10 years).

• Polycythemia vera, essential thrombocythemia, and primary myelofibrosis are manifest more insidiously and evolve more slowly.

• Symptoms are an incidental finding in many patients.

Abdominal pain and distention: due to splenomegaly and may also be due to renal occlusive disease in polycythemia vera.

Spontaneous bleeding: including hematuria, bruising, visual disturbances.

Sweats, weight loss.

Priapism: in chronic myeloid leukemia.

Pruritus: in chronic myeloid leukemia.

Symptoms of hyperviscosity syndrome: in polycythemia vera.

Gout.

Peptic ulceration and hypertension: in polycythemia vera.

Signs

Splenomegaly.

Ecchymoses, retinal hemorrhages.

Weight loss.

Hepatomegaly: occasionally.

Investigations

Complete blood count: raised leukocyte count (20 to >500 × 10^9/L); increased numbers of blasts, promyelocytes, neutrophils, eosinophils, basophils; low neutrophil alkaline phosphatase content in chronic myeloid leukemia; variable anemia; thrombocytosis, especially in essential thrombocythemia; raised hemoglobin, packed-cell volume, and erythrocyte mass in polycythemia vera.

Bone-marrow analysis: hypercellular, loss of fat spaces; increased megakaryocyte count, especially in essential thrombocythemia; variable amounts of fibrosis in chronic myeloid leukemia; increased reticulin and collagen in myelofibrosis; in chronic myeloid leukemia, all dividing cells have a Philadelphia chromosomal translocation, designated t (9;22)(q34;q11), bringing into apposition parts of the *bcr* gene normally on chromosome 22q with the bulk of the *abl* proto-oncogene normally present on chromosome 9q.

Biochemistry: uric acid raised, especially in myelofibrosis; increased vitamin B_{12} and vitamin B_{12}-binding protein.

Complications

"Blast" transformation: in chronic myeloid leukemia; blast cells may be myeloid or lymphoid.

Changes between groups: *e.g.*, polycythemia vera to myelofibrosis.

Vascular or thrombotic complications: in polycythemia vera.

Gout: especially in myelofibrosis.

Renal tubular obstruction.

Splenic infarction: in chronic myeloid leukemia.

Retinal hemorrhages: in chronic myeloid leukemia.

Gonadal failure: due to busulfan.

Differential diagnosis

Leukocytosis

Infections.

Allergic conditions.

Bone-marrow invasion by cancer.

Splenomegaly

Malaria, visceral leishmaniasis.

Acute leukemia, lymphoma.

Gaucher's disease.

Thalassemia syndromes.

Portal hypertension.

Etiology [1–3]

• Causes include the following:

Acquired abnormality in hematopoietic stem cells: such stem cells and their progeny carry a Philadelphia chromosome (22q-) with the *bcr/abl* chimeric gene in chronic myeloid leukemia.

Idiopathic disease.

Association with previous radiation exposure occasionally in chronic myeloid leukemia.

Epidemiology

• Chronic myeloid leukemia occurs in ~1 in 100 000 annually worldwide.

Treatment

Diet and lifestyle

• Patients may live normal lives during the chronic phase of chronic myeloid leukemia.

Pharmacological treatment [1,2,4,5]

• Drug treatment is indicated for polycythemia vera (hydroxyurea, radioactive phosphorus [^{32}P]), myelofibrosis (hydroxyurea, busulfan), and essential (primary) thrombocythemia (hydroxyurea, busulfan, Anagrelide [imidazole-2,1-b, quinazolin-2-1] ^{32}P, supportive measures, *e.g.*, dipyridamole, aspirin).

• α-Interferon (given daily or on alternate days by injection) controls hematological features in 70%–80% of patients with CML and induces some degree of Philadelphia chromosome negativity in the bonemarrow in 10%–20%; it is the drug of first choice.

• Hydroxyurea is easier to tolerate.

• Busulfan should not be used in patients aged <50 years but can be used for older patients or those who cannot take hydroxyurea.

• Investigational studies with BCR-ABL protein tyrosine kinase inhibitors may be a promising new approach to therapy for chronic myeloid leukemia.

Nonpharmacological treatment

Bone-marrow transplantation [1,2,6]

• Transplantation is the only potentially curative therapy for chronic myeloid leukemia. If applicable, it should be done within 1 year of diagnosis.

• Allogeneic bone-marrow transplantation is indicated for patients aged <55 years with HLA-identical siblings (~15% of all patients).

Other treatments

Polycythemia vera: venesection.

Myelofibrosis: splenic irradiation, splenectomy (in selected patients).

Treatment aims

To cure the patient.

To prolong life without cure.

To prevent or alleviate symptoms.

To maintain leukocyte count in normal range.

To re-establish Philadelphia chromosome-negativity with interferon treatment.

Prognosis

• The median duration of chronic phase CML is 4 years and of survival with conventional treatment is 4.3 years.

• A few patients survive >10 years in chronic phase.

• The 5-year disease-free survival after bone-marrow transplantation is about 65%; most of these patients are cured; the procedure-related mortality is 15%–20%, and the relapse rate 10%–15%.

Follow-up and management

• Regular follow-up is needed if the patient is receiving chemotherapy or interferon.

• Bone marrow must be checked annually for progressive fibrosis or cytogenetic evolution.

• Patients should have the usual follow-up for bone-marrow transplantation.

Key references

1. Sawyers CL: Chronic myeloid leukemia. *N Engl J Med* 1999, **340**:1330–1340.
2. Faderl S, Talpaz M, Estrov Z, Kantarjian HM: Chronic myelogenous leukemia: biology and therapy. *Ann Intern Med* 1999, **131**:207–219.
3. Tefferi A. Pathogenetic mechanisms in chronic myeloproliferative disorders: polycythemia vera, essential thrombocythemia, agnogenic myeloid metaplasia, and chronic myelogenous leukemia. *Semin Hematol* 1999, **36(Suppl 2)**:3–8.
4. Kantarjian HM, *et al.*: Chronic myelogenous leukemia: a concise update. *Blood* 1993, **82**:691–703.
5. Bentley MA, Taylor KM, Wright SJ: Essential thrombocythaemia. *Med J Austral* 1999, **171**:210–213.
6. Soutar RL, King DJ: Bone-marrow transplantation. *BMJ* 1995, **310**:31–36.

Myocardial infarction

Diagnosis

Symptoms

Chest pain: typically precordial, often with radiation to left arm, throat, lower jaw, epigastrium, or back; usually severe; crushing or vice-like pain often described as indigestion-like, may be relieved by belching.

Breathlessness: common, often without cardiac failure.

Malaise, nausea, vomiting, syncope, apprehension, sweating.

- Many patients die from sudden cardiac death.

Signs

- Few cardiovascular signs may be apparent on acute presentation.

General

Malaise, pallor, sweating, restlessness.

Pyrexia: usually developing the day after infarction.

Pulse

Raised jugular venous pressure: only with significant right ventricular failure.

Unexpectedly slow or rapid pulse.

Heart

Third or fourth heart sounds, dyskinetic apical impulse: indicating significant myocardial dysfunction.

New murmurs or pericardial rub: may be heard in patients with complications.

Lungs

Chest crackles: may indicate left ventricular failure.

- The emergency department acute myocardial infarction protocol should yield a targeted clinical examination and a 12-lead electrogram within 10 minutes.

Investigations

12-lead ECG: often sufficient to establish diagnosis; adjunctive tests may be necessary for confirmation if infarction is minor or if ECG shows pre-existing abnormalities, *e.g.*, previous infarction, conduction abnormalities (especially left bundle branch block). ECG should be obtained and interpreted within 10 minutes of arrival in the emergency department in all patients with suspected acute ischemic-type chest discomfort.

Chest radiography: to check for pulmonary congestion.

Cardiac enzyme evaluation: creatine kinase, aspartate transaminase, and lactate dehydrogenase rise characteristically after myocardial infarction; creatine kinase MB cardiospecific isoenzyme may be helpful with skeletal damage. Troponin I or T also are routinely used.

Echocardiography: to assess wall motion abnormalities, ventricular septal defect, regurgitation, and mural thrombus.

Complications

Left ventricular failure.

Cardiogenic shock.

Bradyarrhythmias.

Tachyarrhythmias.

Cardiac rupture.

Pericarditis.

Acute ventricular septal defect.

Acute mitral regurgitation.

Systemic emboli.

Aneurysm formation.

Dressler's syndrome.

Differential diagnosis

Angina without infarction.

Pericarditis.

Esophageal or gastrointestinal pain.

Aortic dissection.

Pulmonary embolus.

Musculoskeletal or nonspecific chest pain.

Etiology

Causes

Thrombotic occlusion of a coronary artery, related to rupture of an atherosclerotic plaque and subsequent intraluminal hemorrhage.

Risk factors

Smoking.

Increasing age.

Family history.

Hypertension.

Diabetes mellitus.

Lack of exercise.

Male gender.

Hyperlipidemia.

Thrombotic tendency (fibrinogen).

Obesity.

Surgical menopause at young age.

Epidemiology

- 10–17 in 1000 men aged 40–69 years sustain myocardial infarctions.
- In the United States >500 000 myocardial infarctions occur per year.

Treatment

Diet and lifestyle

• Patients must quit smoking, reduce weight, exercise egularly, and eat low-fat, low-cholesterol diet.

Pharmacological treatment

ST-segment elevation and myocardial infarction

Oxygen; analgesia; aspirin; nitrates; β-blockers.

Thrombolysis: indicated in all patients with ST-segment elevation, symptoms that developed ≥12 h before presentation, and age <75 years or in those with bundle-branch block and history suggesting myocardial infarction. Should be avoided when time to therapy is >24 hours and when there is ST-segment depression only.

Angiotensin-converting enzyme (ACE) inhibitors: should be administered: patients within 24 hours of a suspected acute myocardial infarction with ST-segment elevation in ≥2 anterior precordial leads or with clinical heart failure in the absence of hypotension or known contraindications to ACE inhibitors; patients with myocardial infarction and left ventricular ejection fraction <40% or patients with clinical heart failure on the basis of systolic pump dysfunction during and after convalescence from acute myocardial infarction.

Heparin: indicated i.v. in patients undergoing percutaneous or surgical revascularization and patients undergoing reperfusion therapy with alteplase and treated with nonselective thrombolytic agents who are at high risk for systemic emboli; should be withheld for 6 h, partial thromboplastin time should be measured before initiation of therapy.

Calcium-channel blockers: not usually indicated in acute myocardial infarction. Short-acting nifedipine should be avoided; occurrence of reflex sympathetic activation, tachycardia, and hypotension associated with its use. Verapamil and diltiazem may be useful in rate control when β-blockers are contraindicated; should be avoided in patients with left ventricular dysfunction or congestive heart failure.

Nonpharmacological treatment

Primary coronary angioplasty:

May be more effective than thrombolytic therapy in establishing antegrade coronary flow and relieving fixed coronary obstruction. Indicated:

As alternative to thrombolytic therapy in patients with acute myocardial infarction and ST-segment elevation of new or presumed left bundle-branch block who can undergo angioplasty of the infarct-related artery within 12 hours of onset of symptoms or beyond 12 hours if ischemic symptoms persist, if performed within 90 minutes after admission.

In patients who are within 36 hours of an acute ST-segment elevation/Q-wave or new left bundle-branch myocardial infarction who develop cardiogenic shock, are <75 years of age, and who can undergo revascularization within 18 hours of onset of shock.

Urgent coronary artery bypass graft surgery:

Indicated for patients with coronary anatomy suitable for surgery in whom angioplasty has failed and in whom pain or hemodynamic instability persists.

Acute myocardial infarction with persistent or recurrent ischemia refractory to medical therapy in patients with coronary anatomy suitable for surgery who are not candidates for catheter intervention. Is indicated at the time of surgical repair of post-infarction ventricular septal defect or mitral valve insufficiency.

Secondary prevention

Management of lipids:

• American Heart Association (AHA) step II diet, should be instituted in all patients after recovery from acute myocardial infarction.

• Patients with low-density lipoprotein (LDL) cholesterol levels 125 mg/dL despite AHA step II diet should be prescribed drug therapy to reduce LDL cholesterol level to 100 mg/dL.

• Patients with normal plasma cholesterol levels who have high-density lipoprotein cholesterol level ≤35 mg/dL should be prescribed nonpharmacological therapy designed to raise it.

ACE inhibitors: captopril is indicated for all patients with left ventricular ejection fraction < 40% or myocardial infarction complicated by congestive heart failure. Low-dose ramipril (2.5–5 mg) is indicated in all patients.

β-blockers: initiate within few days of acute myocardial infarction and continue indefinitely.

Long-term anticoagulation: indicated in all patients with persistent atrial fibrillation or patients with left ventricular thrombus.

Treatment aims

To relieve pain and other symptoms.

To salvage threatened myocardium by opening occluded cornary artery.

To prevent and treat complications.

Other treatments

Early coronary angiography for patients with:

• Electrical or hemodynamic instability.

• Stuttering course, recurrent ischemic symptoms, or significant ischemia on pre-discharge stress test.

Prognosis

• In-hospital mortality after acute myocardial infarction is ~10%; subsequent mortality is higher than for age-matched control populations [5].

• Mortality is falling because of therapeutic advances and changes in the natural history.

• Poor prognosis is indicated by advanced age, severe left ventricular dysfunction, and multivessel coronary disease.

• Coronary artery bypass grafting may improve prognosis in some high-risk groups.

• Coronary angioplasty is treatment of choice in cardiogenic shock.

Follow-up and management

• Risk factors, e.g., hyperlipidemia, hypertension, or diabetes, should be controlled.

• Exercise testing is needed to check for residual ischemia, followed by coronary angiography if the test is positive.

General references

Ryan TJ, *et al.*: 1999 update: ACC/AHA guidelines for the management of patients with acute myocardial infarction: executive summary and recommendations: a report of the American College of Cardiology/ American Heart Association Task Force on Practice Guidelines (Committee on Management of Acute Myocardial Infarction). *Circulation* 1999, **100:** 1016–1030.

Myositis, inflammatory

Diagnosis

Symptoms

Weakness: principally affecting proximal muscles in arms and legs; 15%–30% of these patients have associated arthralgias, Raynaud's phenomenon, or myalgia; painless weakness is common [1].

Unusual, severe manifestations: interstitial lung disease, pulmonary hypertension, ventilatory failure, heart block or arrhythmias, dysphagia [2].

Skin rashes.

• Patients with dermatomyositis, especially men aged >45 years, may have an accompanying tumor, causing various symptoms, *e.g.*, weight loss [3].

Signs

Muscle wasting: principally of proximal muscles.

Loss of muscle reflexes: in late-stage disease.

Heliotrope rash: lilac discoloration around eyelids.

Gottron's papules: small raised reddish plaques over knuckles.

Erythematous rash: over face, upper chest, and arms, usually on extensor surfaces.

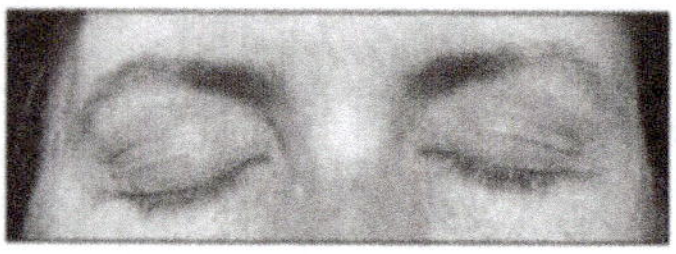

Classic heliotrope rash on the eyelids of a patient with dermatomyositis. (*See* Color Plate.)

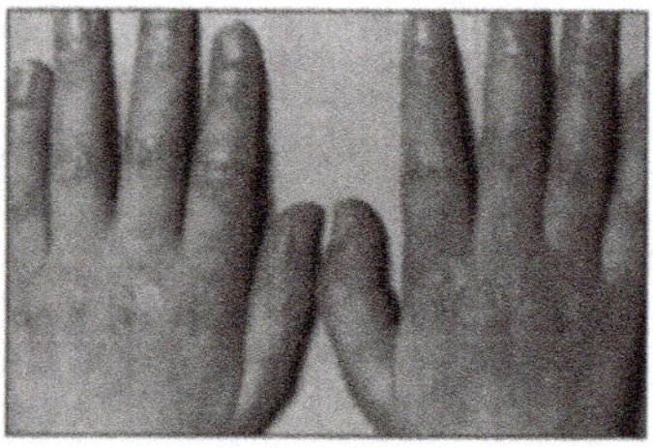

Gottron's papules. (*See* Color Plate.)

Investigations

Key investigations

Creatine kinase, aldolase measurement: concentration 5–30 times upper limit of normal but not disease-specific; concentrations higher in many patients with muscular dystrophy [4] and hypothyroidism.

Electromyography: to check for insertional irritability and small polyphasic potentials.

Muscle biopsy: needle or open surgical technique; classic changes are inflammation, with mononuclear cell infiltrate composed mainly of lymphocytes (some macrophages and plasma cells), with muscle-fiber necrosis, and, in chronic cases, replacement of muscle fibers by fat and fibrous tissue; changes often patchy, and up to 20% of patients may have relatively normal appearance. Important to rule out metabolic myopathy, inclusion body myositis through use of histochemical muscle enzyme staining, electron-microscopy.

Other investigations

Measurement of other enzymes: *e.g.*, transaminase concentrations may be raised [4].

24-hour urine creatine excretion measurement: may be high; more sensitive but less specific than raised creatine kinase.

Myoglobin measurement: appears to reflect disease activity.

Autoantibody analysis: weak positive antinuclear antibody reaction in 60%–80% of patients with myositis; antibodies to transfer RNA synthetase enzymes have been found to be virtually disease-specific, notably the anti-Jo-1 antibody.

Thyroid stimulating hormone (TSH).

Complications

Interstitial lung fibrosis, arthritis, Raynaud's phenomenon: in patients with Jo-1 antibody.

Cardiac or respiratory failure: rare; caused by rapidly progressive myositis.

Underlying neoplasm: muscle disease often intractable until tumor identified and treated.

Recurrent falls and danger of major internal trauma: caused by an unusual, steroid-resistant form of myositis, associated with inclusion bodies.

Differential diagnosis

Hypothyroidism.
Inclusion body myositis [1].
Metabolic myopathies (*e.g.*, McArdle's disease).
Drug-induced inflammatory disease (including D-penicillamine).
Muscular dystrophy.
Rhabdomyolysis.
Osteomalacia.

Etiology

• Inflammatory muscle diseases are part of the family of autoimmune rheumatic diseases.
• Causes include the following:
Hormonal component.
Immunogenetic predisposition: HLA B8 and DR3 associated with myositis, principally in whites; DR3 linked to Jo-1 antibody.
Environmental factors: increased risk of developing myositis at different times of year found in one study.
Viruses, *e.g.*, picornaviruses and retroviruses: may be triggering factors; link between myositis and HIV has been suggested.

Epidemiology

• The annual incidence of myositis is 5 in one million population.
• The prevalence is 5–8 in 100 000.
• The female:male ratio is 2–3 : 1 overall and 9 : 1 in patients with an associated autoimmune rheumatic disease.

Factors suggesting malignancy [1,3]

Dermatomyositis in male patients.
Age >45 years.
Weight loss.
Poorer than expected response to treatment.
Absence of autoantibodies.
Unexplained historical, physical, or laboratory abnormalities.

Dermatomyositis or polymyositis? [1]

Dermatomyositis
Onset: childhood to old age.
Skin rash, microvascular injury.
Perifascicular atrophy common.
Endomysial infiltration less common.
Surrounded and invaded fibers less than in polymyositis.
Anti-Jo-1 in 5%, other antisynthetases at least as much as in polymyositis.

Polymyositis
Onset: adulthood.
No skin rash or microvascular injury.
Perifascicular atrophy uncommon.
Endomysial infiltration common.
Surrounded and invaded fibers frequent.
Anti Jo-1 in 30%.

Treatment

Diet and lifestyle

• Exercise and activity are limited during the inflammatory period. Rehabilitative efforts must be limited until muscle enzymes return to nearly normal.

• No special diet is necessary.

Pharmacological treatment

Corticosteroids

• After the diagnosis has been established, treatment should be initiated quickly [1,2,5,6].

Standard dosage	Prednisone, 1 mg/kg daily initially (usually 60–80 mg); continued until creatine kinase returned to near normal (usually 1–3 months); then reduced to 5–10 mg daily over following 3 months.
Contraindications	Severe osteoporosis.
Main drug interactions	None.
Main side effects	Osteoporosis, increased risk of infection, diabetes, hypertension.

Other immunosuppressants

• These are indicated in patients who have not shown a response to high-dose steroids after 1 month or who cannot tolerate them [5].

Standard dosage	Azathioprine, 2–3 mg/kg. Methotrexate, up to 15 mg weekly.
Contraindications	*Methotrexate:* abnormal liver function, major renal disease, porphyria.
Main drug interactions	*Methotrexate:* many analgesics and antibacterials.
Main side effects	Bone-marrow suppression, liver damage.

Other options [6]

• Oral or occasionally i.v. cyclophosphamide has been used in severely affected patients, occasionally combined with steroids and methotrexate or azathioprine.

• Reports of the use of cyclosporine in myositis are conflicting, and it is not widely used in this disease.

• Intravenous gammaglobulin may be used.

Nonpharmacological treatment

Plasmapheresis.

Total lymph-node irradiation and thoracic duct drainage in severe cases.

Physical therapy and hydrotherapy.

Treatment aims

To control disease as soon as possible.

To maintain reasonable degree of mobility.

To reduce treatment to smallest dose needed after 3–4 months of aggressive therapy to avoid side effects (e.g., intercurrent infection or osteoporosis).

Prognosis

• ~20% of patients recover fully.

• 10%–20% die as a direct result of the disease or as a consequence of its treatment.

• Most patients are left with some muscle weakness.

• Patients who respond most slowly to initial treatment have the poorest prognosis.

Follow-up and management

• Patients must be followed for several years.

• Regular clinical examination, creatine kinase measurement, and formal muscle strength testing are needed.

• Physical therapy and hydrotherapy help to keep the range of joint movement normal and to maintain muscle power.

Key references

1. Dalakas MC: Polymyositis, dermatomyositis, and inclusion-body myositis. *N Engl J Med* 1992, **325**:1487–1498.
2. Targoff IN: Polymyositis and dermatomyositis: adult onset. In *Textbook of Rheumatology*. Edited by Maddison P, *et al.* Oxford: Oxford University Press; 1993:794–821.
3. Sigurgeirsson B, *et al.*: Risk of cancer in patients with dermatomyositis or polymyositis. *N Engl J Med* 1992, **326**:363–367.
4. Bohlmeyer TJ, *et al.*: Evaluation of laboratory tests as a guide to diagnosis and therapy of myositis. *Rheum Dis Clin North Am* 1994, **20**:845–856.
5. Joffe MM, *et al.*: Drug therapy of the idiopathic inflammatory myopathies: predictors of response to prednisone, azathioprine and methotrexate in a comparison of their efficacy. *Am J Med* 1993, **94**:379–387.
6. Villalba L, Adams EM: Update on therapy for refractory dermatomyositis and polymyositis. *Curr Opin Rheumatol* 1996, **8**:544–551.

Nasal polyposis

Diagnosis

Symptoms

Nasal obstruction.

Hyposmia and/or hypogeusia.

Dry mouth.

Snoring.

Signs

Glistening, yellow-tan mass in middle meatus or nasal cavity.

Pharyngeal mass (choanal polyp).

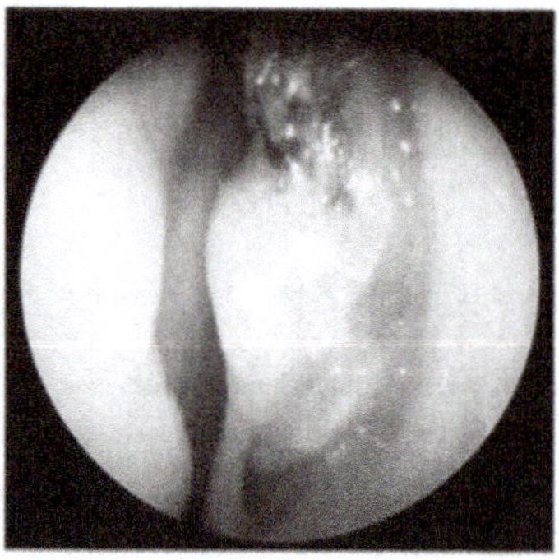

Nasal polyp. (*See* Color Plate.)

Investigations

CT: to rule out invasive process, tumor, fungal disease, encephalocele and to define potential extent of associated rhinosinusitis.

MRI: rarely indicated except for instances of tumors or encephaloceles to define soft-tissue involvement. Otherwise MRI shows bony architecture of sinuses poorly and is overly sensitive to mucosal changes.

Sweat chloride: in some young patients with polyposis to rule out cystic fibrosis.

Allergy skin testing: to help avoid allergens, to find therapy for environmental allergies.

Complications

Chronic rhinosinusitis due to sinus obstruction, poor mucociliary clearance.

Sleep apnea secondary to obstruction.

Broadening of nasal bones.

Exacerbation of asthma: especially in triad asthma patients.

Aspirin hypersensitivity triad (polyposis, asthma, aspirin intolerance)

• Typical onset is after age 20 years.

• Common first symptom is profuse watery rhinorrhea.

• Patients then develop nasal congestion, hyposmia indicative of hyperplasia of the mucosa.

• Polyps typically develop early in disease.

• Aspirin sensitivity may develop years later.

• Aspirin intolerance is characterized by profuse rhinorrhea, rash, abdominal complaints, followed by asthma attack, which is typically severe.

• Patients will have cross-sensitivity to all NSAIDs, which should be avoided. Acetaminophen in routine doses is rarely problematic.

• Patients typically have chronic purulent sinusitis, which exacerbates the asthma.

• In patients refractory to steroid and antibiotic therapy, surgery is indicated.

Differential diagnosis

Nasal tumor: must be suspected in unilateral nasal mass or if bony erosion on CT scan. Inverted papilloma most common tumor; has high recurrence rate and 5%–10% chance of malignant degeneration.

Encephalocele: must be ruled out in patients with unilateral nasal polyps, meningitis and polyps, or unilateral clear rhinorrhea and polyps.

Turbinate hypertrophy.

Etiology and associated conditions

Triad asthma (aspirin sensitivity, asthma, nasal polyps).

Allergic rhinitis.

Chronic sinusitis (bacterial or fungal).

Cystic fibrosis.

Kartagener's syndrome.

Mucosal diseases (Wegener's disease, sarcoidosis, Churg-Strauss syndrome, Young's syndrome).

Epidemiology

• Nasal polyps occur in 7% of asthmatics, 36% of patients with aspirin intolerance, and 90% of patients with asthma and sinusitis; 70% of patients with polyps have associated asthma.

Treatment

Diet and lifestyle

• Patients should avoid allergens, irritants, and smoke.

• Saline irrigations with Ocean Spray or similar saline sprays are recommended.

• Bulb syringe saline irrigations (1 teaspoon salt in 2 cups water mixed daily) are recommended for patients with stasis of secretions and bacterial crusting or suprainfections (most patients).

Pharmacological treatment

Prednisone

Standard dosage 40–60 mg daily divided twice daily with rapid taper over 7–12 days.

Contraindications Caution should be used in patients with diabetes, hypertension, peptic ulcer disease, history of tuberculosis, other infections that may be masked.

Special points Steroids will be most effective for watery, acutely inflamed polyps than for more mature fibrotic polyps; polyps will typically return with repeated infectious, inflammatory or allergic exacerbations; surgery may be indicated for patients with recurrent symptomatic polyps after steroids.

Main side effects Cushingoid features, osteoporosis, easy bruisability, weight gain, growth retardation in children, hypertension, aseptic necrosis of bone, glucose intolerance, hyperlipidemia, cataracts, gastritis.

Topical nasal steroid sprays

Special points Used for daily maintenance therapy; patients must be sure to aim toward turbinate, not septum, to avoid atrophy of mucosa, dryness, crusting, bleeding, and subsequent septal perforation; adrenal suppression rare except for dexamethasone preparations.

Contraindications Atrophic rhinitis, epistaxis, septal perforation.

Treatment aims

To minimize symptoms of obstruction and hyposmia.

To prevent or minimize the occurrence of sinusitis.

Other treatments

Antibiotics for 3–6 weeks if associated purulent sinusitis (see Sinusitis).

Antihistamine–decongestants as needed.

• Endoscopic sinus surgery is effective for symptomatic polyps after medical therapy; typically performed for nasal obstruction and/or chronic rhinosinusitis; prognosis is excellent, although polyps will eventually return in many patients; short course of moderate-dose steroids postoperatively assists with healing.

• Allergy testing and possibly immunotherapy are indicated for patients with severe seasonal or perennial allergic rhinitis not responsive to avoidance therapy, steroid sprays, and antihistamine therapy.

Prognosis

• If polyps are large and mature, steroid therapy will not cause complete involution of polypoid disease and recurrence is eventually likely. Many will benefit from surgical removal.

• Endoscopic sinus surgery will typically yield longer symptom-free periods than will medical treatment, but polyps will recur in many patients.

• After medical or surgical therapy, aspirin-sensitive patients will typically have substantial improvement in nasal and asthma symptoms but tend to have recurrent polyps sooner than patients without aspirin sensitivity.

Follow-up and management

• Follow-up should be as needed based on patient symptoms and the frequency and severity of complications such as sinusitis.

• Consider a referral to an otolaryngologist if surgical treatment is needed.

• Watch for symptoms of aspirin sensitivity; the triad of polyposis, asthma, and aspirin intolerance may develop late in the course of the disease.

General references

Holmberg K, Karlsson G: Nasal polyps: medical or surgical management? *Clin Exp Allergy* 1996, **26(3)**:23–30

Lumry WR, Curd JG, Zeiger RS, *et al.*: Aspirin sensitive rhinosinusitis: the clinical syndrome and effects of aspirin administration. *J Allergy Clin Immunol* 1987, **80**:788–790.

Settipane GA, Settipane RA: Nasal polyposis: clinical spectrum and treatment approaches. In *Diseases of the Sinuses*. Edited by Gershwin ME. Totowa, NJ: Humana Press; 1995.

Diagnosis

Symptoms and signs

Acute interstitial nephritis

• This is usually manifest as acute (usually reversible) nonoliguric renal failure.

• The clinical picture may be dominated by the disease process for which an offending drug was administered or by features of extrarenal infection.

Fever, skin rash, and eosinophilia: in cases associated with beta-lactam antibiotics (the most common medication other than NSAIDs causing acute interstitial nephritis).

• NSAIDs are typically not associated with a hypersensitivity syndrome, but instead present with acute renal failure and often nephrotic range proteinuria.

Arthralgias and lymphadenopathy.

Anterior uveitis and granulomatous infiltration of other organs: in a small group of patients with idiopathic disease.

Many patients have no specific symptoms or signs.

Chronic interstitial nephritis

• This usually manifests insidiously as chronic (irreversible) renal failure.

• The clinical picture may be dominated by features of an underlying disease process or by the condition for which analgesics were taken.

• No specific features allow differentiation from other causes of chronic renal failure.

• May be accompanied by papillary necrosis.

Investigations

Complete blood count: with differential for eosinophilia in acute interstitial nephritis.

Blood urea nitrogen, creatinine clearance, 24-hour urinary protein excretion measurement: to quantify renal function.

Blood cultures and other specific serological tests: if systemic infection, connective tissue disease, or vasculitis suspected.

Urinalysis: culture of midstream urine to look for casts and pyuria.

Urine test for eosinophils.

Urinary Bence Jones protein and serum protein electrophoresis: to screen for myeloma.

Ultrasonography of urinary tract and plain abdominal radiography: in all patients.

Renal biopsy: may be indicated in selected patients.

Complications

Acute interstitial nephritis

• The major complications are those of acute renal failure.

Chronic interstitial nephritis

• The major complications are those of chronic renal failure.

Salt wasting, renal tubular acidosis, occasionally Fanconi's syndrome.

Symptomatic anemia inappropriate to level of renal function: in patients with analgesic nephropathy.

Differential diagnosis

Acute interstitial nephritis

Other causes of acute renal impairment, especially rapidly progressive glomerulonephritis (either idiopathic or associated with systemic vasculitis).

Chronic interstitial nephritis

All other causes of chronic renal failure.

Etiology

Causes of acute interstitial nephritis

Drug hypersensitivity: beta-lactam antibiotics (*e.g.*, methicillin, ampicillin), other antibiotics (*e.g.*, sulfonamides, rifampicin), NSAIDs (*e.g.*, fenoprofen, indomethacin), diuretics (*e.g.*, thiazides, furosemide), and many other miscellaneous drugs (*e.g.*, phenindione, phenytoin, allopurinol).

Infections: complicating urinary tract infection (especially in diabetic patients) or extrarenal infection (*e.g.*, with streptococci, legionella, brucella, tuberculosis, leptospira, mycoplasma, *Toxoplasma* spp., infectious mononucleosis, hantavirus).

Immunological disorders: interstitial lesions sometimes overshadow glomerular (*e.g.*, lupus polyarteritis nodosa).

Idiopathic.

Causes of chronic interstitial nephritis

Toxic and metabolic: analgesics, lithium, cis-platinum, lead, cadmium, hypercalcemia.

Granulomatous: sarcoidosis, tuberculosis, drugs.

Immunological: associated with primary glomerular disease, Sjögren's syndrome, vasculitis, transplant rejection, rheumatoid arthritis.

Miscellaneous: reflux nephropathy, post-obstructive, myeloma, sickle cell disease, radiation nephritis, Balkan nephropathy, hereditary.

Causes of papillary necrosis

Analgesic nephropathy, sickle cell disease, diabetes mellitus, obstruction with infection, tuberculosis, cryoglobulinemia.

Epidemiology

• Renal biopsy studies suggest that acute interstitial nephritis accounts for 10% of cases of acute renal failure.

• 5%–10% of patients being treated for end-stage renal failure have chronic interstitial nephritis.

Treatment

Diet and lifestyle

• Patients who habitually abuse analgesics may benefit from psychological support and counseling.

• Occupational health measures have helped to limit industrial exposure to heavy metals.

• Patients with chronic renal failure have accelerated atherogenesis; smoking should be discouraged, and a diet low in saturated fat recommended.

• Patients with drug-related acute interstitial nephritis should be advised never to take the same or a related drug in the future.

Pharmacological treatment

• Patients may present with features of severe uremia and need stabilization by urgent dialysis before definitive investigation and treatment can safely be carried out.

For acute interstitial nephritis

Drug-associated: withdrawal of offending drug; prednisolone, 40 mg daily, with rapid tapering according to response, may hasten resolution.

Infection-associated: antibiotic treatment tailored to causative organism; steroids not indicated at least until infection is controlled.

Idiopathic disease associated with uveitis: steroids as for drug-associated disease dramatically improve renal and ocular lesions.

For chronic interstitial nephritis

Toxin-induced: withdrawal of causative agents.

Reflux nephropathy: childhood urinary tract infection must be eradicated by appropriate antibiotics; this should be followed by long-term low-dose chemoprophylaxis until reflux is resolved or renal growth complete. Surgical remediation should be considered in patients with severe reflux.

Sarcoidosis: long-term steroid treatment, using minimum dose to maintain stable renal function (*see* Sarcoidosis *for details*).

Tuberculosis: antituberculous chemotherapy; concurrent use of low-dose steroids may limit renal scarring (*see* Tuberculosis, extrapulmonary *for details*).

Myeloma: referral to hematologist or oncologist recommended for institution of appropriate treatment regimen; hypovolemia must be avoided; allopurinol to prevent acute urate nephropathy (*see* Multiple myeloma *for details*).

Keep blood pressure <130/80 mm Hg if possible. Angiotensin-converting enzyme inhibitors may be beneficial.

For analgesic nephropathy

Withdrawal of offending drugs.

Provision of psychological support.

Monitoring and treatment of the following:
Hypertension: antihypertensive agents (diuretics often inappropriate). Maintain blood pressure <130/80 mm Hg if possible.
Salt wasting: oral sodium salts prevent volume depletion.
Renal tubular acidosis: oral sodium salts prevent volume depletion.
Inappropriate anemia (gastrointestinal blood loss): misoprostol, iron supplements.
Early renal osteodystrophy: alpha calcidol and calcium carbonate.
Frequent urinary tract infection: prolonged treatment for upper tract infections.
Obstruction due to sloughed papillae: nephrostomy or double-J stents.
Increased incidence of urothelial tumors: regular urine cytology.
Increased atheromatous renovascular disease.

Treatment aims

Acute interstitial nephritis
To provide dialysis support if needed, pending restoration of normal renal function.

Chronic interstitial nephritis
To stabilize renal function.

To reduce rate of progression and complications of chronic renal failure.

To institute renal replacement therapy when necessary.

Prognosis

Acute interstitial nephritis
• Normal renal function is recovered in many patients by prompt treatment.

Chronic interstitial nephritis
• Withdrawal of offending toxins or specific treatment (when possible) may stabilize or improve renal function (occasionally).
• When renal damage has been severe (serum creatinine, >300 μmol/L), progression to end-stage renal disease is probable; even in chronic glomerular disease, the degree of interstitial damage is the major correlate of progression.

Follow-up and management

Acute interstitial nephritis
• When recovery of renal function is incomplete, long-term follow-up is needed.

Chronic interstitial nephritis
• Long-term follow-up is needed.
• Control of hypertension slows progression.
• Patients with salt wasting (5%–10%) need supplements of sodium chloride or bicarbonate.
• Phosphate binders (e.g., calcium carbonate) help prevent secondary hyperparathyroidism; hypercalcemia must be avoided.
• Preparations for renal replacement therapy should be made in good time.

General references

Bennett WM, Henrich WL, Stoff JS: The renal effects of nonsteroidal anti-inflammatory drugs: summary and recommendations. *Am J Kidney Dis* 1996, **28(suppl 1)**:S56–S62.

Delzell E, Shapiro S: A review of epidemiologic studies of nonnarcotic analgesis and chronic renal disease. *Medicine* 1998, **77**: 102–121.

Dillons MJ, Goonasekera CD: Reflux nephropathy. *J Am Soc Nephrol* 1998, **12**:2377–2383.

Michel DM, Kelly CJ: Acute interstitial nephritis. *J Am Soc Nephrol* 1998, **9**: 506–515.

Diagnosis

Definition

• Acute herpetic neuralgia merges into postherpetic neuralgia. The most widely accepted definition seems to be persistent pain 1 month after skin eruption.

Symptoms

• Pain may precede the eruption by days to weeks and may persist months to long-term. It may be continuous, paroxysmal, or lancinating and is generally dermatomal.

Signs

Depigmented scars.

Sensory: Local decreased sensation over scars; hyperalgesia and allodynia in other areas of dermatome.

Weakness: Very rare, if virus spreads to other parts of CNS segment.

Investigations

• No investigation is needed in most patients.

• In younger patients, shingles, either isolated or with generalized zoster, may be a symptom of immunosuppression, particularly associated with lymphoma or leukemia; HIV and cancer are also associated. Appropriate investigation of patients at risk is needed.

Complications

Depression: common, sometimes severe.

Weakness in a limb: when an appropriate dermatome is affected.

Differential diagnosis

Other causes of sensory ganglion and root disease, including diabetes, Sjögren's disease.

Etiology

• Reactivation of dormant herpes varicella zoster virus in dorsal root ganglion causes acute shingles.

• Corticosteroid treatment for an unrelated condition sometimes precipitates shingles.

• Histopathology in postherpetic neuralgia shows damage to peripheral nerve, dorsal root ganglion, sensory root, and dorsal horn atrophy [1].

Epidemiology

• The female:male ratio is 3:2.

• The overall incidence of postherpetic neuralgia at 1 year is 3%–10% of all patients with acute shingles.

• The most common sites are the mid-thoracic dermatomes and the ophthalmic division of the trigeminal nerve: it may occur in any dermatome.

• Postherpetic neuralgia becomes more common with increasing age.

Treatment

Diet and lifestyle

• No special precautions are necessary.

Pharmacological treatment

• Prednisone bursts and antiviral therapy (acyclovir, 800 mg 5 times daily, or famciclovir, 750 mg 3 times daily for 7 days) lessen acute pain.

• Some studies do report a decrease in incidence in postherpetic neuralgia after acute treatment with antivirals, but this remains controversial.

Local

• Possibilities for local treatment must always be exhausted because simple measures may give partial relief and avoid the side effects so often seen with systemic drug treatment in this mainly elderly patient population.

• Treatments include the following:

Local anesthetic ointment (5% lidocaine) 3 times daily: sometimes effective.

Capsaicin, 0.075% ointment 3 times daily: causes initial burning but helps a few patients significantly [2].

Systemic

Standard dosage	Amitriptyline or nortriptyline, 10–25 mg at night, gradually increased, as tolerated.
Contraindications	Recent myocardial infarction, heart block, mania, porphyria.
Special points	Up to maximum tolerated doses have been consistently shown in controlled trials to provide partial relief of postherpetic neuralgia.
Main drug interactions	Sedation enhanced by other sedatives.
Main side effects	Drowsiness, constipation, urinary hesitancy, dry mouth, blurred vision, postural hypotension, tachycardia, sweating, tremor.

• Anticonvulsants may be useful for lancinating pain, and opioids may be helpful in refractory cases.

Alternative medicine

Recommended use: cayenne pepper (*Capsicum frutescens*).

Common use: rosemary (*Rosmarinus officinalis*); lavender (*Lavandula* spp.); St. John's wort (*Hypericum perforatum*).

Caution: the above are used topically as creams or ointments.

Treatment aims

To relieve pain.

Other treatments

Local measures

• Cold packs applied for 15–20 minutes several times daily may produce partial analgesia, sometimes lasting a few hours after a single application.

• Transcutaneous electrical nerve stimulation and biofeedback may each be helpful in some patients.

• Local anesthetic, peripheral nerve or root blocks, and sympathetic blocks (occasionally) may temporarily relieve postherpetic neuralgia but has no long-term benefit.

Psychological measures

• Counseling by a clinical psychologist about coping strategies may help some patients.

Prognosis

• Most patients with troublesome postherpetic neuralgia at 1 year have the condition lifelong, although some patients slowly improve over long periods.

• After acute shingles, persistent, trouble-some neuralgia gradually decreases over months.

Follow-up and management

• ~50% of patients with postherpetic neuralgia benefit from regular long-term follow-up; the role of a sympathetic doctor who is prepared to listen should not be underestimated, even when all treatment options have apparently been exhausted.

• Many patients can be discharged from follow-up when treatment leads to partial relief of pain.

Key references

1. Bennett GJ: Hypotheses on the pathogenesis of herpes zoster associated pain. *Ann Neurol* 1994, **35(suppl)**:S38–S41.
2. Kost RG, Straus SE: Drug therapy: postherpetic neuralgia. *N Engl J Med* 1996, **335**:32–43.

Neuralgia, trigeminal

Diagnosis

Symptoms

Pain: unilateral shooting, shock-like, usually along zygomatic arch; rare in ophthalmic division; paroxysmal, lasting <1 minute but may occur frequently; occurs spontaneously but often triggered by innocuous facial or oral stimulation, *e.g.*, wind, touching face, washing or shaving, brushing teeth, eating, talking, and drinking; bouts last weeks to months, with remissions of months to years; may become chronic in some patients; rarely develops on contralateral side; in chronic trigeminal neuralgia, some patients complain of background aching pain.

Signs

- Idiopathic trigeminal neuralgia has no signs.

Trigeminal sensory impairment: caused by a compressive lesion of the trigeminal root; such lesions may rarely lead to trigeminal neuralgia.

Investigations

- Investigation is not usually needed.

CT or MRI: in patients being considered for surgical treatment (V nerve decompression) or in whom sensory impairment is present.

Complications

Depression.

Differential diagnosis

- No other facial pain has the same stereotyped paroxysmal nature.
- Migrainous neuralgia, atypical facial pain, or ophthalmic postherpetic neuralgia.

Etiology

- The mechanisms of this unique paroxysmal neuropathic pain are poorly understood but involve peripheral and central factors.
- The following may play a role:

Mild compression of the trigeminal root by a blood vessel, usually an ectatic superior cerebellar artery, in chronic sufferers.

Minor degenerative changes in nerve ganglion or root.

Epidemiology

- The female:male ratio is 3:1.
- Onset usually occurs after the age of 50 years.
- The disease is associated with multiple sclerosis, but most young patients (age <50 years) with trigeminal neuralgia do not develop multiple sclerosis.

Treatment

Diet and lifestyle

- No special precautions are necessary.
- Soft foods helpful during flares.

Pharmacological treatment

Carbamazepine

- Carbamazepine is the drug of choice.

Standard dosage	Carbamazepine, 100 mg twice daily initially, increased to a dose that controls pain or to maximum tolerated dose.
Contraindications	Hypersensitivity.
Special points	Blood level monitoring often helpful.
Main drug interactions	Sedation enhanced by other sedatives.
Main side effects	Drowsiness, nausea, ataxia, hypersensitivity rash, neutropenia.

Other drugs

- Phenytoin, tricyclic antidepressants, and baclofen are also often helpful.

Treatment aims

To alleviate pain until onset of remission.

Other treatments

Surgery

- Surgery is indicated for patients who have unremitting pain or who are unresponsive to or intolerant of medical treatment.

Controlled thermocoagulation gangliolysis

- This is a minimally invasive procedure.
- It is effective, usually giving pain relief of at least 1–2 years, with low risk.
- It can be repeated if necessary.
- Morbidity includes facial sensory impairment; in rare instances, this is severe enough to lead to anesthesia dolorosa and neuroparalytic keratitis.

Microvascular decompression

- This is effective, often permanently.
- Morbidity is the same as for thermocoagulation but also includes deafness and brain stem damage (rare).

Prognosis

- Some patients have bouts lasting weeks, with remissions of years.
- Some develop chronic trigeminal neuralgia.

Follow-up and management

- Frequent follow-up is needed until the pain is controlled.
- Withdrawal of treatment must be supervised to assess whether remission has occurred.

General references

Gonda JJ, Brown JA: Atypical facial pain and other pain syndromes: differential diagnosis and treatment. *Neurosurg Clin North Am* 1997, **8**:87–100.

Loeser JD: Tic douloureux and atypical face pain. In *Textbook of Pain*, edn 3. Edited by Wall PD, Melzack R. Edinburgh: Churchill Livingstone; 1994:699–710.

Neuropathy, peripheral

Diagnosis

Symptoms

General

Distal numbness.

Paresthesia, burning, lancinating pain.

Progressive distal weakness and wasting.

Foot and hand deformities, neuropathic ulcer, neuropathic arthropathy.

Of autonomic neuropathy

Impotence, orthostatic hypotension, dry eyes or mouth, urinary or fecal incontinence, nausea and vomiting, constipation or diarrhea.

Signs

General

Stocking-glove sensory loss.

Muscle weakness and wasting.

Reduced or absent tendon reflexes.

Sensory ataxia, neuropathic tremor.

Nerve thickening.

Of autonomic neuropathy

Anhidrosis, unreactive or asymmetric pupils, postural hypotension (fall of 30 mm Hg in systolic and 15 mm Hg in diastolic pressure).

Investigations

All patients

Complete blood count.

ESR measurement.

Glucose tolerance test: if random and fasting samples give equivocal results.

Liver and renal function tests.

Measurement of thyroid-stimulating hormone, vitamin B_{12} (folate), serum protein electrophoresis, autoantibodies.

Urinalysis: for glucose, Bence Jones protein, porphyrins.

CSF analysis: elevated protein concentration in inflammatory neuropathies.

Nerve conduction studies: diagnosis confirmed by slowing of motor or sensory conduction velocities (moderate in axonal type, marked in demyelinating type) and reduction in sensory action potential amplitude (small in axonal neuropathy).

Electromyography: characteristic pattern in denervated muscle.

Sometimes indicated

DNA analysis: for hereditary demyelinating neuropathies; chromosome 17 duplication in a subgroup of patients with HMSN type 1 (HMSN 1A); chromosome 17 deletion associated with hereditary liability to pressure palsies (tomaculous neuropathy).

Sensory threshold recording: thermal (useful in patients with small-fiber neuropathy).

Imaging: screening for malignancy in patients with suspected paraneoplastic neuropathy; skeletal survey for suspected myeloma; chest radiography for suspected sarcoidosis.

Nerve biopsy: done in operating room under strict aseptic conditions using local anesthetic; fascicular biopsy limits degree of sensory loss; full thickness biopsy indicated for suspected vasculitis; used to discover cause of progressive neuropathy not revealed by detailed investigation or to confirm presence of vasculitis, leprous neuropathy, or inflammatory infiltrates; sensory nerves (sural, superficial peroneal, superficial radial) usually undergo biopsy.

Bone-marrow biopsy: for myeloma.

Formal autonomic function tests, endoscopy, colonoscopy, barium studies, urodynamic studies: for autonomic neuropathy.

Complications

Burns, cuts, bruising, neuropathic ulcers: unnoticed when sensory loss is severe.

Distal weakness.

Differential diagnosis

- The differential diagnosis depends on the cause.

Combined systems degeneration.

Polyradiculopathy.

Etiology

Causes of sensory polyneuropathy

Diabetes, uremia, hypothyroidism.

Amyloidosis.

Paraneoplastic, paraproteinemic.

Thallium, isoniazid, vincristine, cisplatin, metronidazole.

Sjögren's syndrome.

Leprosy.

HIV, Lyme borreliosis infection.

Hereditary sensory and autonomic neuropathies.

Fabry's disease.

Vitamin B_{12} deficiency.

Causes of sensorimotor polyneuropathy

Hereditary motor and sensory neuropathies.

Alcohol.

Acute or chronic inflammatory demyelinating polyradiculoneuropathy.

Vasculitis.

Paraproteinemic, paraneoplastic.

Diabetes, uremia, hypothyroidism, acromegaly.

Sarcoidosis.

Arsenic.

Causes of motor neuropathies

Acute or chronic inflammatory demyelinating polyradiculoneuropathy.

Porphyria, diphtheria, lead.

Hereditary motor neuropathies [1].

Causes of focal and multifocal neuropathies

Entrapment and compression syndromes [2].

Polyarteritis nodosa, connective tissue disorders.

Wegener's granulomatosis.

Lymphomatous and carcinomatous infiltration, neurofibromatosis.

Tuberculoid leprosy, herpes zoster, HIV, Lyme borreliosis.

Sarcoidosis: especially facial nerve.

Hereditary liability to pressure palsies.

Multifocal motor neuropathy with conduction block.

Epidemiology

- The epidemiology depends on the cause, but most common causes overall are diabetic, hereditary, and alcoholic.

Treatment

Diet and lifestyle

- Patients with alcoholic neuropathy should abstain from drinking alcohol.
- Postural hypotension can be improved by wearing support stockings.
- Examine feet daily, use night light, remove obstacles to reduce foot injury.

Pharmacological treatment

For focal and multifocal neuropathies

For vasculitis: prednisone, 60 mg daily orally; azathioprine or cytoxan can be introduced to enable dose of steroids to be reduced; degree of immunosuppression and duration of treatment depend on clinical response.

For protection against peptic ulceration: H_2 antagonists.

For alcoholic neuropathy: vitamin B supplements.

For herpes zoster infection: acyclovir, 800 mg orally 5 times daily for 1 week.

- Leprosy should be treated under specialist supervision.

For autonomic neuropathy

For postural hypotension: fludrocortisone, 100–400 mg, or ephedrine, 15–60 mg daily.

For gastroparesis: erythromycin, 125 mg daily; cisapride, 10 mg 3 times daily; domperidone, 10–20 mg 3 times daily; or metoclopramide, up to 10 mg 3 times daily.

For diarrhea: diphenoxylate (Lomotil), loperamide (Imodium), codeine phosphate.

For impotence: penile intracavernous papaverine injection.

For painful neuropathy

- Treatment is extremely difficult and often unsatisfactory.

Regular simple analgesic, *e.g.*, acetaminophen, 1 g 4 times daily.

For burning diffuse pain and paresthesia: amitriptyline, 25–75 mg at night; gabapentin, 300–600 mg 3 times daily.

For shooting pain: carbamazepine, 100 mg at night, increasing slowly to 600 mg daily in divided doses; mexiletine, 100–400 mg daily may be worth trying.

For postherpetic neuralgia or diabetes: topical capsaicin, 0.075% after lesions have healed.

For chronic inflammatory demyelinating polyradiculoneuropathy

For acute disorder: *see* Guillain–Barré syndrome.

For mild to moderate disease: prednisone, 60 mg/day, tapering as possible; azathioprine may be added for steroid-sparing effect.

For progressive disease or relapses: i.v. plasmapheresis or immunoglobulin, 0.4 g/kg/day for 5 days and possible replacement of azathioprine with either cyclosporine titrated to leukocytes or cyclophosphamide [3].

Treatment aims

- Treatment aims depend on the type of neuropathy.

To treat underlying illness.

To treat dysesthesias or pain, orthostasis.

Other treatments

For focal and multifocal neuropathies

Conservative: wrist and foot support, elbow pad.

Surgical decompression:

Median and ulnar nerve entrapment with evidence of wasting or weakness of denervated muscles.

For persistent sensory symptoms when conservative measures have failed.

For chronic inflammatory demyelinating polyradiculoneuropathy

Plasma exchange for progressive neuropathy unresponsive to immunoglobulin.

Prognosis

- Prognosis depends on the underlying cause of the neuropathy.

Follow-up and management

- Regular follow-up is needed to assess progression.
- Patients requiring immunosuppression need frequent follow-up.

Key references

1. Lupski JR, *et al.*: DNA duplication associated with Charcot–Marie–Tooth disease type 1A. *Cell* 1991, **66**:219–232.
2. Chance PF, *et al.*: DNA deletion associated with hereditary neuropathy with liability to pressure palsies. *Cell* 1993, **72**:143–151.
3. van Doorn PA, *et al.*: High dose intravenous immunoglobulin treatment in chronic inflammatory demyelinating neuropathy: a double blind, placebo controlled, crossover study. *Neurology* 1990, **40**:212–214.

General references

Dyck PJ, Thomas PK: *Peripheral Neuropathy*, edn 3. Philadelphia: WB Saunders; 1993.

Wokke JH, van Dijk GW: Sensory neuropathies including painful and toxic neuropathies. *J Neurol* 1997, **244**:209–221.

Non-Hodgkin's lymphoma

Diagnosis

Symptoms

Lymph node in neck, axilla, or groin, noticed by patient as unexplained "lump": the most common presenting symptom.

• The disease may be seen in multiple sites at presentation.

• Systemic symptoms (*e.g.*, the "B" symptoms of Hodgkin's disease) are less common than in Hodgkin's disease.

• Symptoms may relate to the anatomical site of disease, *e.g.*, superior vena cava obstruction due to mediastinal nodes or to primary lymphomas at extranodal sites (*e.g.*, CNS, gastrointestinal tract).

• Primary extranodal non-Hodgkin's lymphoma occurs much more often than extranodal Hodgkin's disease.

Signs

Palpable lymphadenopathy: careful examination of all nodal areas is essential.

Hepatomegaly and splenomegaly: possibly.

Signs of other organ involvement: *e.g.*, pleural effusion as a result of pulmonary parenchymal involvement, skin involvement (rarely).

Investigations

• Initially, investigations must be directed at confirming the diagnosis.

• A good sample of tissue that has not been placed in formalin is needed.

• The diagnosis may be apparent on routine staining with hematoxylin-eosin or Giemsa.

• Immunohistochemistry, especially markers for T and B lymphocytes and leukocyte common antigen, is vital in subclassification and may help to distinguish undifferentiated lymphomas from carcinoma.

• Subsequent investigations must be systematic and thorough to enable accurate localization of disease and if possible to estimate disease volume.

Complete blood count: usually normal.

Urine and electrolyte analysis: as a baseline.

Liver function tests: may be abnormal if liver is involved.

Lactate dehydrogenase measurement: useful marker of disease bulk and activity.

Chest radiography: to rule out hilar or mediastinal nodes or intrapulmonary disease.

CT of chest, abdomen, and pelvis: to rule out node or organ involvement.

Bone-marrow examination: trephine is particularly important.

Examination of postnasal space and tonsillar fossa.

Lumbar puncture with cytology: in high-grade disease only.

Complications

Recurrent or atypical infections.

Autoimmune hemolysis and thrombocytopenia.

Bone-marrow failure.

Gastrointestinal bleeding or perforation: obstructive jaundice.

Differential diagnosis

Other causes of lymphadenopathy: *e.g.*, Hodgkin's disease.

Infective causes: *e.g.*, toxoplasmosis, glandular fever, Epstein–Barr virus.

Etiology

• The cause is unknown, but the following may have a role:

Epstein–Barr virus: associated with endemic Burkitt's lymphoma in Africa.

Adult T-cell leukemia–lymphoma: associated in all cases with human T-cell lymphotropic virus type I.

HIV infection: particularly primary CNS non-Hodgkin's lymphoma (rare in other settings).

•*Helicobacter pylori:* associated with some mucosa-associated lymphoid tissue lymphomas.

Epidemiology

• The median age of onset is 50 years.

• Intermediate- or high-grade disease is more common in younger patients.

Classification [1]

• Non-Hodgkin's lymphomas constitute a diverse group of disorders arising from different cell types, usually T and B lymphocytes; the wide spectrum of disease biology is reflected by the varying clinical presentations, responses to treatment, and overall outcomes.

• Various schemes for classification have been proposed and developed; the most useful are those that can be used to predict clinical behavior and prognosis.

• Classifications include the following:

Rappaport.

Lukes-Collins.

Lennert: the Kiel classification.

The Working Formulation (used here): an international attempt to provide a translation from one classification to another, now widely used in its own right; non-Hodgkin's lymphoma is divided into low, intermediate, and high grades, each having different treatment and prognosis.

Staging

• Patients may be staged I–IV according to the Ann Arbor system originally developed for Hodgkin's disease (see Hodgkin's disease).

• Staging is less useful than for Hodgkin's disease because, with the exception of stage I disease, all patients with non-Hodgkin's lymphoma should receive chemotherapy.

Treatment

Diet and lifestyle

• Many patients maintain a fairly normal lifestyle during treatment, but some are unwell and need multiple hospital admissions.

Pharmacological treatment [2]

• Treatment should take place in the context of a clinical study whenever possible.

• It should be given by a hematologist or oncologist.

For intermediate-grade non-Hodgkin's lymphoma

• Treatment should begin as soon as investigation is completed.

• These lymphomas are usually sensitive to many chemotherapy drugs, and many effective combination regimens may be curative.

• Stage I disease may be treated successfully by radiation therapy alone, but localized disease is very unusual in non-Hodgkin's lymphoma.

• The standard treatment is by CHOP (cyclophosphamide, doxorubicin, vincristine, prednisone), usually given on a monthly cycle for 6 months; other regimens that include additional drugs are given more intensively, reducing total time taken for treatment, but none has been shown to be superior to CHOP [3].

• Allopurinol, 300 mg daily, should be given for at least the first month.

• Main side effects include hair loss, nausea (often preventable), and myelosuppression (for which dose reductions may be needed during subsequent cycles).

For low-grade non-Hodgkin's lymphoma

• These lymphomas are also sensitive to chemotherapy, but, although they usually do not behave aggressively clinically, they are usually considered incurable by standard treatment.

• A conservative approach is often advocated, particularly in elderly asymptomatic patients, because early treatment has no survival advantage.

• 50% of patients may avoid treatment for up to 3 years.

• In truly localized low-grade disease, radiation therapy may give long-term remission.

• Patients may respond well to treatment and often may have considerable periods when no treatment is needed.

• Initial treatment is usually by oral chlorambucil, best used cyclically rather than continually.

• Combination chemotherapy, *e.g.*, cyclophosphamide with prednisone, vincristine, and possibly an anthracycline, is sometimes used but has no proven advantage over chlorambucil initially.

• The new agents fludarabine and 2-chlorodeoxyadenosine may be of value in relapsed disease [4].

• α-Interferon has just been licensed for low-grade disease, but its indications and benefits are not yet clear.

• Monoclonal antibody therapy for lymphomas is currently a promising new therapy for low-grade lymphomas, available under research protocol in some centers [5].

• Main side effects of chlorambucil include myelosuppression and mild nausea.

For high-grade non-Hodgkin's lymphoma

• Lymphoblastic and Burkitt's lymphomas are very aggressive clinically and often manifest with widespread disease, including bonemarrow and CNS involvement; they need intensive leukemia-style treatment, usually involving very myelosuppressive inpatient regimens and CNS-directed prophylaxis.

For mucosa-associated lymphoid tissue non-Hodgkin's lymphoma

•Treatment with an anti-*H. pylori* antibiotic regimen may result in complete remission in some patients (primarily for those with gastric disease).

Other treatments [6]

• High-dose treatment and autologous bone-marrow transplantation are indicated for the following: Intermediate grade: age <60 years, relapsed disease still sensitive to chemotherapy. Low grade: criteria difficult to define because long-term follow-up is needed to assess benefit because of the indolent nature of the disease.

• Allogeneic transplantation may have a role for young patients with high-grade disease.

Treatment aims

To cure patient, with minimum toxicity.

To palliate if cure is not possible.

Prognosis

Low grade

• At 5 years, ~70% of patients are still alive, but few are in complete remission; most patients eventually die of their disease.

• In many patients, the disease ultimately transforms to high grade and becomes refractory to chemotherapy.

Intermediate and high grades

• The complete remission rate is ~85% in patients with limited disease, ~55% with extensive disease.

• Overall disease-free survival is ~40% and depends on several factors; poor prognostic factors include stage III or IV disease, high lactate dehydrogenase concentration, failure to attain complete remission on first-line treatment, and older age.

Follow-up and management

• During treatment, regular follow-up is needed, including examination and full blood count before each course of chemotherapy; toxicity must be monitored, and complications treated.

• After treatment is completed, full restaging should take place: if the patient is in complete remission, regular follow-up should be continued to detect early relapse.

Key references

1. Falzon M, Isaacson PG: Histological classification of the non-Hodgkin's lymphoma. *Blood Rev* 1990, **4**:111–115.
2. Vose JM: Current approaches to the management of non-Hodgkin's lymphoma. *Semin Oncol* 1998, **25**:483–491.
3. Armitage JO: The place of third generation regimens in the treatment of adult aggressive non-Hodgkin's lymphoma. *Ann Oncol* 1991, **2(suppl 1)**:37–41.
4. Cheson B: New chemotherapeutic agents in the treatment of low grade non-Hodgkin's lymphomas. *Semin Oncol* 1993, **20**:96–110.
5. Renner C, *et al.*: Monoclonal antibodies in the treatment of non-Hodgkin's lymphoma: recent results and future prospects. *Leukemia* 1997, **11(suppl 2)**:S555–S559.
6. Shipp MA, Abeloff MD, Antman KH, *et al.*: International consensus conference on high-dose therapy with hematopoietic stem cell transplantation in aggressive non-Hodgkin's lymphomas: report of the jury. *J Clin Oncol* 1999, **17**:423–429.

Nonulcer dyspepsia

Diagnosis

Definition [1,2]

Discomfort ("indigestion," pain, or nausea) located in the upper abdomen and frequently is related to meals.

Symptoms of a chronic or recurrent nature occurring over at least a 3-month period.

Not attributed to identifiable disease by usual testing; thus, the condition is considered "functional."

Frequent aerophagia and subsequent belching are typical subconscious mechanisms by which patients respond to their symptoms; they are rarely the primary cause of discomfort.

Symptoms are atypical of gastroesophageal reflux or biliary colic; a history of nonsteroidal antiinflammatory drug (NSAID) use or "alarm symptoms" (*i.e.*, dysphagia, unexplained weight loss, acute onset in older patients, blood loss) suggests an alternative diagnosis

Signs [3]

Physical examination results are typically normal, although some patients have the nonspecific finding of epigastric tenderness.

Evidence of weight loss, epigastric mass, organomegaly, and adenopathy all suggest an alternative diagnosis.

Investigations

Nonulcer dyspepsia is a diagnosis based on a compatible history and normal examination after appropriate testing has been done to exclude competing diagnoses.

Dyspepsia in a patient younger than 45 years of age can often be treated empirically with focused testing. In select patients, consider the following:

Testing for *Helicobacter pylori* infection: most experts conclude that *H. pylori* is not a cause of nonulcer dyspepsia in the absence of ulcer disease; however, it is an early diagnostic test in patients with dyspepsia because it directs empirical therapy. Biopsies at the time of endoscopy are the gold standard; ***H. pylori* breath testing** (after ingestion of radiolabeled urea) is most accurate for active infection; serology is least expensive but of more limited sensitivity and specificity.

Complete blood count, liver chemistries, urinalysis, amylase: if abnormal, consider other diagnosis.

Serum glucose, creatinine, electrolytes, calcium, thyroid function: measure if clinical suspicion warrants or if empirical treatment is inadequate; any abnormalities suggest other diagnoses.

Stomach imaging: barium upper gastrointestinal imaging is relatively inexpensive and more accessible to primary care physicians; endoscopy is more specific and sensitive for minor mucosal disease and allows biopsies to be obtained.

Abdominal ultrasonography: important in patients suspected of having disease of the liver, biliary tract, or pancreatic disease by history, examination, or screening laboratory studies.

Gastric emptying study: normal in most patients with nonulcer dyspepsia; useful in a select group of patients with prominent anorexia, nausea, or vomiting in whom prokinetic agents are contemplated after other conditions have been excluded.

24-hour pH probe: rarely required but done to evaluate patients in whom gastroesophageal reflux is manifesting atypically as dyspepsia.

Complications

Extensive time and resources expended by patients seeking symptom control.

Depression, anxiety: particularly common when patients are worried about an undiagnosed serious disease

Differential diagnosis

Peptic ulcer disease.
NSAID gastropathy.
Gastric cancer.
Reflux esophagitis.
Gallstone disease.
Hepatobiliary cancer.
Pancreatitis.
Pancreatic cancer.
Crohn's disease.
Lactose intolerance.
Irritable bowel syndrome.
Medication side effect.
Renal disease.
Hypothyroidism.
Mesenteric ischemia.
Colorectal cancer.

Etiology

Unknown: probably a combination of disturbed sensory and motor function.

Shared etiologies: overlap with irritable bowel syndrome.

Psychosocial factors often contribute to how symptoms are interpreted and to treatment success.

Epidemiology

Prevalence of dyspepsia worldwide is 10%–40%, but prevalence and incidence of nonulcer dyspepsia are unknown.

Fewer than 50% of patients in western countries with dyspepsia seek medical attention.

Treatment [2,4]

Diet and lifestyle

Dietary components unique to each patient may aggravate symptoms; patients should be urged to keep a diary to identify patterns with foods that are more consistently associated with symptoms.

Aggravation of symptoms with coffee and spicy foods most common.

Attention to psychosocial components may be required to restore a patient's compensatory mechanism for dealing with chronic symptoms.

Pharmacological treatment

No single group of medications has been found to be consistently efficacious in patients with nonulcer dyspepsia; a prominent placebo effect is seen with most agents.

Medications should be used sparingly when their benefit-risk ratio is favorable and of proven benefit to patients.

Acid antisecretory agents: patients do not have abnormal amounts of acid but may respond to low-dose acid reduction therapy (*see* antisecretory drug regimens in Esophageal reflux).

Regimens for *H. pylori* eradication: if patients are infected, most experts advise treating the infection (*see* eradication regimens for *H. pylori* in Duodenal ulcer disease), but symptomatic response in patients with nonulcer dyspepsia is unlikely to differ from placebo effect.

Prokinetic agents: side effects usually do not justify their use (*i.e.*, metoclopramide: CNS/extrapyramidal effects, particularly in the elderly; cisapride: associated with multiple drug-drug interactions placing patients at risk for cardiac arrhythmias and sudden death and is contraindicated in patients with heart disease or with prolonged QT intervals on electrocardiography [the latter should be monitored shortly after initiating drug therapy]).

Antidepressants: as in irritable bowel syndrome, patients with predominant symptoms of pain may improve with antidepressant therapy; tricyclic antidepressants (*e.g.*, amitriptyline, 25–50 mg at night) may be helpful in a subset of patients but must be used cautiously because of side effects. Serotonin reuptake inhibitor antidepressants (*e.g.*, fluoxetine, 20 mg daily) are likely to work as well and have fewer side effects.

Avoid opiate analgesic or benzodiazepine medications because of potential for addiction in patients with chronic symptoms.

Treatment aims

Reassure patients about the absence of a serious, progressive underlying disease.

Improve symptoms.

Assist the patient with chronic pain management skills.

Other treatment options

Educate patients with a careful explanation of this common condition, reassure them that it is not "just in their head," and exclude serious underlying diseases; these steps are more important than any other treatment.

Prognosis

Symptoms tend to be intermittent, with a variable pattern in most patients; patients usually can identify methods or agents that can provide at least some relief most of the time.

Follow-up and management

Patients must be educated about the recurrent nature of their symptoms; they should expect to focus more on managing their symptoms than on curing their disease. Unless this point is fully understood, patients will frequently seek advice from multiple caregivers, hoping to find someone who can make the "right diagnosis" and bring about a total cure.

Key references

1. McQuaid K: Dyspepsia. In: *Sleisenger & Fordtran's Gastrointestinal and Liver Disease*. Edited by Feldman M, Scharschmidt BF, Sleisenger MH. Philadelphia: WB Saunders; 105–117.
2. American Gastroenterological Association Position Statement. Evaluation of dyspepsia. *Gastroenterology* 1998, **114**:579–581.
3. Talley NJ, *et al.*: AGA Technical Review. Evaluation of dyspepsia. *Gastroenterology* 1998, 114:582–595.
4. Pandolfino JE, Howden CW, Kahrilas PJ: Motility-modifying agents and management of disorders of gastrointestinal motility. *Gastroenterology* 2000, **118**:S32–S47

Osteoarthritis

Diagnosis

Symptoms

• Many patients are asymptomatic.

• Women have more symptoms than men.

• Symptoms occur more frequently in large, weight-bearing joints.

• They are often phasic and are not always progressive; muscle weakness and psychological status are often better predictors of symptoms or functional impairment than structural damage [1].

Pain: typically on use.

Stiffness after inactivity: "gelling" phenomenon common.

Functional impairment: particularly of gait; a major problem.

Signs

• Signs are often discordant with symptoms.

Bony swelling, deformity, crepitus, restriction of movement: bony swelling may be marked in interphalangeal joints (Heberden's and Bouchard's nodes).

Joint-line tenderness.

Local heat, effusion: occasional inflammatory features, particularly in crystal-related osteoarthritis or developing finger nodes.

Investigations

• Osteoarthritis is principally a clinical diagnosis. Often occuring in middle-aged or elderly patients, the question is not usually whether it is present but whether it is the cause of current symptoms; only clinical examination can answer this.

General

Radiography: may show structural change, *e.g.*, loss of joint space (cartilage), osteophytosis, sclerosis, cysts, osteochondral bodies.

Premature osteoarthritis

• Onset occurs before the age of 55 years [1].

Ferritin measurement: for hemochromatosis.

Calcium, phosphate, alkaline phosphatase measurement: for hyperparathyroidism.

Urine homogentisic acid measurement: if ochronosis suspected.

Lateral spine radiography: for spondyloepiphyseal dysphasia.

Pituitary studies: if acromegaly suspected.

Acute flare

Synovial fluid examination: for sepsis and crystals.

"Locking" of knee

• *See* Knee injuries *for details.*

Arthroscopy or MRI: for loose bodies (osteochondral), meniscal lesions.

Complications

Acute crystal synovitis: mainly calcium pyrophosphate crystals.

Septic arthritis.

Loose-body formation.

Avascular necrosis.

Differential diagnosis

• Periarticular lesions may coexist and may be the prime source of symptoms.

Polyarticular osteoarthritis
Inflammatory arthropathies.
Gout.

Poor bone response and destruction
Charcot's arthropathy.
Sepsis.

Acute crystal-related oligoarthritic osteoarthritis
Sepsis.
Gout.
Inflammatory arthropathy.

Etiology

• Osteoarthritis probably has many causes; recognized factors include the following:
Obesity.
Age.
Occupational trauma.
Genetics: nodal osteoarthritis, (spondylo-) epiphyseal dysplasia, type II collagen abnormalities.
Metabolic or endocrine disorders: hemochromatosis, hyperparathyroidism, ochronosis, acromegaly [1].
Previous joint disease or damage.

Epidemiology

• Osteoarthritis is strongly age-related.

• It is the most common cause of locomotor disability.

• Nodal osteoarthritis may manifest with florid polyarticular disease and Heberden's nodes in menopausal women.

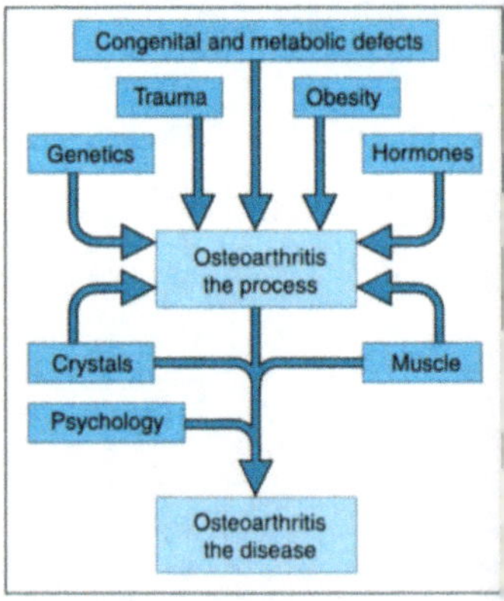

Factors leading to progression of osteoarthritis.

Treatment

Diet and lifestyle

• Patients should be encouraged to take control of the condition.
• Physical activity should be encouraged, *e.g.*, aerobic fitness and muscle strengthening.
• Biomechanical factors, *e.g.*, obesity, varus knee deformity, should be tried (wedge insoles, shock-absorbing footwear, use of cane).
• Caloric reduction may improve osteoarthritis of the hip or knee.

Pharmacological treatment [2]

Topical antirheumatics

• These include NSAIDs and capsaicin ointment.
• Their role is controversial, but they are probably effective.
• Contraindications include sensitive or broken skin.

Analgesics

• These are often sufficient [2].
• Compound preparations with opiates may only increase adverse effects, without improving symptom control.

Standard dosage	Acetaminophen, 1 or 2 650-mg tablets orally every 6–8 hours, as required [2].
Contraindications	Liver disease.
Main drug interactions	None.
Main side effects	Rare, except in overdosage when hepatic failure may ensue.

NSAIDs

• NSAIDs may be tried [1,3,4].
• Use should be regularly reviewed.
• **COX-2 inhibitors:** Celecoxib 100 mg orally twice daily; contraindicated with sulfa allergy. Rofecoxib 12.5 to 25 mg orally.

Three times less likely to result in NSAID gastropathy. No effect on platelet activity.

Standard dosage	Depends on agent; lowest dose needed for benefit.
Contraindications	Active peptic ulceration, hypersensitivity, renal impairment (relative).
Special points	Patients show marked variation in response to different drugs.
Main drug interactions	Warfarin.
Main side effects	Gastrointestinal ulceration, anemia, renal dysfunction, skin rashes.

Intra-articular steroids

• **Hyaluronic acid intra-arterial injection:** long-term results similar to ibuprofen and intra-arterial steroids; expensive series of three injections of 15 days.
• Local corticosteroids are indicated for short-term relief of inflammatory episodes or coexistent periarticular lesions.

Standard dosage	Depends on agent and joint; in large joints, generally no more than every 3 months; in small joints, yearly.
Contraindications	Septic arthritis, hypersensitivity (rare).
Special points	Longer-acting steroids provide more benefit.
Main drug interactions	None.
Main side effects	Occasional facial flushing, deterioration of diabetic control.

Nonpharmacological treatment

• Arthroplasty is particularly helpful for patients with disease of hips, knees. Indications include exercise/activity limitation, sleep disturbance, poor quality of life secondary to joint pain.
• Physical therapy (heat, cold, range-of-motion exercises, joint protection, pacing of activities, splinting, assistive devices) may be more helpful than medication.

Alternative medicine

Recommended use: glucosamine sulfate.
Common use: chondroitin sulfate; alfalfa (*Medicago sativa*); yucca leaves (*Yucca* spp.); Devil's claw (*Harpagophytum procumbens*); boswellia serrata.
Caution: chondroitin sulfate is poorly absorbed.

Treatment aims

To relieve pain.
To maintain functional ability.

Other treatments

Arthroplasty: for patients with persistent pain or marked functional impairment.

Prognosis

• Many patients show phasic symptoms, and some improve with time.
• Symptoms may remain static for years.

Follow-up and management

• Follow-up is usually in a primary care setting.
• The aims are to determine the need for further intervention as a result of deterioration in symptoms or function and to monitor treatment, particularly by NSAIDs, to assess the need for continued use and the development of adverse effects.

Key references

1. Brandt K: The pathogenesis of osteoarthritis. *Rheumatol Rev* 1991, **1**:3–11.
2. Bradley JD, *et al.*: Comparison of an anti-inflammatory dose of ibuprofen, an analgesic dose of ibuprofen, and acetaminophen in the treatment of osteoarthritis of the knee. *N Engl J Med* 1991, **325**:87–91.
3. Brandt KD: NSAIDs in the treatment of osteoarthritis. Friends or foes? *Bull Rheum Dis* 1993, **42**:1–4.
4. Kraus VB: Pathogenesis and treatment of osteoarthritis. *Med Clin North Am* 1997, **81**:85–112.

Diagnosis

Symptoms

• Most patients are asymptomatic.

Loss of height.

Fractures with minimal trauma: especially Colles', vertebral, hip, and rib fractures.

Kyphosis.

Symptoms of menopause in women, hypogonadism in men.

Signs

• There are few other specific signs for osteoporosis: *see* Symptoms.

Inadequate calcium intake.

Early menopause, including surgical.

Longstanding amenorrhea or oligomenorrhea.

Signs of Cushing's syndrome (endogenous or exogenous).

Investigations

Bone densitometry: several methods are available; dual emission x-ray absorptiometry (DEXA) of the hip and spine is the test of choice.

Gonadal function: Follicle-stimulating hormone and estradiol in women, follicle-stimulating hormone and testosterone in men.

Chemistry panel (including liver function tests), thyroid function tests, serum protein electrophoresis, urinalysis, urinary calcium, intact parathyroid hormone, vitamin D level analysis: to rule out secondary causes of osteoporosis.

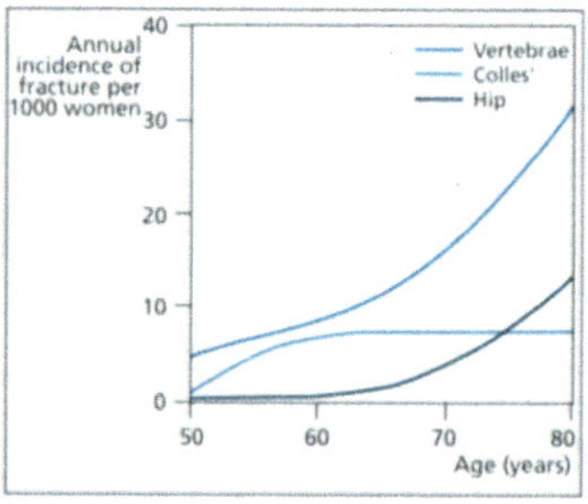

Incidence rates for vertebral, Colles', and hip fractures in women.

Glucocorticoids [1], dilantin, phenobarbitol, heparin, gonadotropin-releasing hormone analog: to identify medications associated with bone loss.

Tests for other illnesses associated with bone loss: *see* Etiology.

Complications

Fractures in the elderly: associated with significant mortality and frequent nursing home placement.

Fractures in younger patients: can cause significant pain and loss of mobility.

Loss of height.

Differential diagnosis

Metastatic disease.

Fracture in otherwise normal bone.

Etiology

Most common: postmenopausal women, older women and men, anovulatory postmenopausal women (*e.g.*, competitive athletes), hypogonadal men.

Less common: Cushing's syndrome, thyrotoxicosis, liver disease, rheumatoid arthritis, alcoholism.

Epidemiology

• Health care costs resulting from osteoporotic fractures exceed $13 billion annually.

• One-third of women >65 years of age will have one or more vertebral fractures.

• One-third of women >80 years of age will have a hip fracture.

• 25% of all hip fractures occur in men.

Other information

• DEXA scores are reported as T-scores and Z-scores. T-scores compare bone mass with that of young persons (matched for gender) and are reported in standard deviations above or below the mean. Z-scores compare bone mass of persons of the same age and gender. T-scores are more predictive of fracture risk.

• Osteopenia is defined as a T-score of -1.0 to -2.5. Osteoporosis is defined as a T-score of >-2.5.

Treatment

Diet and lifestyle

- Patients should be encouraged to intake 1000–1500 mg of elemental calcium through diet (preferably) or calcium supplementation.
- Fall hazards should be removed from the home.
- Patients should be encouraged to perform weight-bearing exercises.

Pharmacological treatment [2]

Calcium

- Calcium supplementation is recommended for all patients (*see* Diet and lifestyle *for guidelines*).

Standard dosage	Calcium carbonate, 40% elemental calcium by weight (1250-mg tablet contains 500 mg calcium). Calcium citrate, 21% elemental calcium by weight (950-mg tablet contains 200 mg calcium).
Special points	Supplements should be taken with meals to enhance absorption and reduce the incidence of nephrolithiasis.

Vitamin D_3

- Vitamin D_3 is recommended for all patients.

Standard dosage	400–800 U daily.
Special points	Most multivitamins contain 400 U; activated forms of vitamin D (*e.g.*, calcitriol and dihydrotachysterol) are rarely required.

Estrogen replacement therapy

See Menopause and hypoestrogenism *for further details.*

Androgen replacement therapy

Standard dosage	*Hypogonadal men*: testosterone enanthate, 200 mg i.m. every 2 weeks; Testosterone patches (2.5–5 mg daily).
Contraindications	Prostatic disease.
Special points	Rule out prostate cancer in men aged >50 years before beginning testosterone therapy; no evidence that testosterone therapy improves bone mass in eugonadal men.
Main side effects	Increased libido; priapism with initial dose (very rare).

Nasal calcitonin (Miacalcin)

Standard dosage	One squirt (200 IU) daily, alternating nostrils.
Special points	*Pros*: reduces vertebral fractures, excellent safety profile, easy administration; may reduce pain associated with vertebral compression fractures. *Cons*: only modest increases in bone density; minimal data on fracture prevention.

Biophosphonates [3]

Standard dosage	Alendronate 10 mg daily. Risedronate 5 mg daily. Correct administration is critical because alendronate is poorly absorbed and can cause esophagitis: take on an empty stomach with a full glass of water; must then remain upright and take nothing by mouth for 30 minutes.
Contraindications	Esophogeal lesions, including dysmotility; inability to take biphosphonates as described above.
Special points	*Pros*: gives greater increases in bone density than estrogen or calcitonin; reduces hip and vertebral fractures in well-controlled prospective trials. *Cons*: effectiveness frequently limited by difficulties in administration; not suitable for bedridden patients.

Treatment aims

To prevent fractures.

To increase bone density or prevent further bone loss.

To optimize functional status.

Other treatments

Etidronate: can be used intermittently to prevent glucocorticoid-induced bone loss.

Prognosis

- Osteoporosis, especially in the elderly, is not usually curable. However, therapy can result in significant decreases in subsequent fractures and associated morbidity and mortality.

Follow-up and management

- DEXA bone densitometry should be done every 2 years to assess response to therapy.
- Urinary markers of bone resorption are available for monitoring response to antiresorptive therapy. However, no consensus yet exists on their routine use.
- Biochemical markers should not be used to diagnose osteoporosis.

Key references

1. Canalis E. Clinical review 83: mechanisms of glucocorticoid action in bone: implications to glucocorticoid-induced osteoporosis. *J Clin Endocrinol Metab* 1996, **81**:3441–3447.
2. Kleerekoper M: Extensive personal experience: the clinical evaluation and management of osteoporosis. *J Clin Endocrinol Metab* 1995, **80**:757–763.
3. Black DM, Cummings SR, Karpf DB, *et al.*: Randomised trial of effect of alendronate on risk of fracture in women with existing vertebral fractures. *Lancet* 1996, **348**: 1535–1541.

Ovarian failure

Diagnosis

Symptoms [1]

Primary or secondary amenorrhea: erratic menstruation or oligomenorrhea in earliest phases.

Delayed puberty.

Primary or secondary infertility.

Hot flashes, vaginal dryness and dyspareunia, thin skin, and scalp hair loss: symptoms of estrogen deficiency.

Signs [1]

• Few signs are manifest, particularly shortly after onset of amenorrhea.

Incomplete pubertal maturation: indicating primary amenorrhea.

Atrophic vaginal mucosa.

Short stature, webbed neck: if secondary to Turner's syndrome.

Investigations

For the disorder

Serum follicle-stimulating hormone (FSH) measurement: persistently raised concentration (>40 IU/L); in women with possible incipient ovarian failure (erratic cycles and moderately raised serum FSH [10–40 IU/L]), care must be taken to ensure sampling was not done during a preovulatory gonadotropin surge (risk of false-positive results) [2].

• Absence of menstrual bleeding following progesterone therapy (progesterone-induced withdrawal bleeding) suggests an anovoluntary state. This is *not* an indication of ovarian failure, but is consistent with the diagnosis.

For the underlying cause

Autoimmune profile: including antiovarian antibodies.

Chromosome analysis: to check for aneuploidy (45XO, 47XXX, 46XY).

Laparoscopy: if streak ovaries present, possibility of conception is ruled out; if ovaries "normal," then biopsy unhelpful because conception has been reported in women with no follicles on histology.

For assessment of bone state

Radiography for bone age: if delayed in girls with primary amenorrhea, ultralow-dose estrogen should be used to achieve maximum height (ethinyl estradiol, 2 μg daily).

Bone densiometry: to assess degree of bone loss [3].

Complications

Infertility: usually permanent, but spontaneous pregnancies have been reported.

Osteoporosis or atraumatic fractures: resulting from estrogen deficiency [3].

Cardiovascular disease: effect of estrogen deficiency on lipid state.

Gonadal neoplasia: in women with gonadal dysgenesis and 46XY karyotype.

Differential diagnosis

Gonadotropin-secreting pituitary adenomas (with elevated FSH) are rare; the distinguishing feature is estrogenization.

Spurious elevation of FSH.

Polycystic ovarian syndrome.

Etiology

Autoimmune: antiovarian antibodies.

Idiopathic premature menopause.

Gonadal dysgenesis: *e.g.*, Turner's syndrome, pure gonadal dysgenesis.

Infection: mumps.

Irradiation or chemotherapy.

Extensive ovarian surgery: for endometriosis or recurrent cysts.

Treated galactosemia.

17α-hydroxylase deficiency (non-salt-wasting congenital adrenal hyperplasia).

Epidemiology

• The lifetime risk (before age 40 years) is 0.6%.

• ~5% of cases of anovulation, 10% of amenorrhea, and 2% of oligomenorrhea are due to ovarian failure.

Treatment

Diet and lifestyle

• Advice about increasing dietary calcium and the risk of atraumatic fractures should be given to women with long-standing untreated amenorrhea.

• Women not wishing to conceive should be warned of the small risk of conception.

Pharmacological treatment

• Sex-steroid therapy alleviates symptoms of estrogen deficiency and prevents osteoporosis and cardiovascular disease.

• Estrogen is the active agent; progestogens are used to prevent endometrial neoplasia.

• Standard hormone replacement preparations are not contraceptive; women who wish to avoid the small risk of conception should use low-dose combined oral contraceptive.

Standard dosage	Depends on patient's needs.
Contraindications	Undiagnosed abnormal menstruation.
Main drug interactions	Anticonvulsants, warfarin.
Main side effects	*Estrogen:* nausea (avoided by slow introduction). *Progestogen:* premenstrual symptoms.

Treatment aims

To avoid general health risks.
To achieve conception.

Other treatments

For infertility [4]

• Ovarian failure represents end-organ failure for which the chances of resumption of ovulation (spontaneous or induced) are small and difficult to predict.

• Several methods of inducing ovulation have been described, but, for most women, in-vitro fertilization with donated oocytes offers the best chance of pregnancy.

Prognosis [4]

• The results from one trial of estrogen and human menopausal gonadotropin treatment in 91 women with hypergonadotropic amenorrhea are as follows:
34 patients ovulated.
19 conceptions.
10 miscarriages (53% of conceptions).
1 stillbirth.
8 live births.

Key references

1. Rebar RW, *et al.*: Clinical features of young women with hypergonadotrophic amenorrhea. *Fertil Steril* 1990, **53**:804–810.
2. Cahill DJ, *et al.*: Spurious elevation of follicle-stimulating hormone. *Acta Obstet Gynecol Scand* 1992, **71**:388–389.
3. Davies MC, *et al.*: Bone mineral loss in young women with amenorrhea. *BMJ* 1990, **301**:790–793.
4. Check JH, *et al.*: Ovulation induction and pregnancies in 100 consecutive women with hypergonadotrophic amenorrhea. *Fertil Steril* 1990, **53**:811–817.

Pancreatic cancer

Diagnosis

Symptoms

Weight loss: in 90% of patients.

Pain: in 80%.

Anorexia: in 60%.

Lethargy: in 40%.

Diabetes mellitus: in 15%.

Acute pancreatitis: atypical for patients to present with or develop acute pancreatitis (i.e., <5%)

Signs

Jaundice: in 85% of patients, often painless.

Cachexia: in 70%.

Hepatomegaly: in 60%.

Palpable gallbladder: Courvoisier's sign in 40%.

Epigastric mass: in 15%.

Ascites: in 10%.

Abdominal tenderness: in 5%.

Trousseau's syndrome: migratory thrombophlebitis in <1%.

Virchow's node: firm fixed node in left supraclavicular fossa in <1%.

Splenic-vein thrombosis: gastric fundus varices in <1%.

Investigations

Liver chemistry tests: to confirm "obstructive" jaundice; alkaline phosphatase often elevated and albumin low.

Clotting studies: prothrombin time may be prolonged but should correct after vitamin K, 10 mg i.m.

Complete blood count: to detect anemia or leukemoid reaction.

Serum marker analysis: *e.g.*, CA-19-9 (sensitivity 80%; specificity 90%); may be influenced by jaundice and have poor sensitivity for "early" pancreatic cancer [3].

Ultrasonography: to confirm dilated bile ducts and to localize disease (75% accuracy); increased detection of small tumors and better staging with endoscopic ultrasonography (90% accuracy).

Contrast-enhanced CT: 80%–90% accuracy [2].

Percutaneous biopsy: 80%–93% accuracy; should not be used in patients with potentially resectable tumors.

Endoscopic retrograde cholangiopancreatography: 90%–95% accuracy; brush or pancreatic juice cytology positive in 60%–70% of cases [1].

Laparoscopy: Often performed just before laparotomy to resect localized disease; resection for cure is typically abandoned if metastatic lesions are found at laparoscopyto detect small metastatic lesions otherwise missed [3].

Complications

Massive gastrointestinal hemorrhage: fair; caused by erosion into duodenum.

Gastric outlet obstructions/gastroparesis: common.

Pruritus: in 40%.

Acute cholangitis: in 2%.

Deep vein thrombosis: in 1%.

Differential diagnosis [4]

Obstructive jaundice

Bile-duct stones, ampullary tumor, tumors of the biliary tract, benign bile duct strictures, metastatic disease, duodenal cancer.

Hepatic jaundice

Chronic hepatitis, sclerosing cholangitis, congestive heart failure.

Cachexia

Gastric, colorectal, or ovarian cancer.

Other pancreatic disease

Chronic pancreatitis (may coexist), non-functioning endocrine tumors, metastases to pancreas.

Etiology

- The cause is largely unknown, but the following may have a role:

Smoking: relative risk, ~2.0 (compared with relative risk of lung cancer, ~20).

Diets high in total or animal fat.

Genetic predisposition (rare): familial colonic and pancreatic cancer, hereditary chronic pancreatitis, familial adenomatous polyposis, Peutz–Jeghers disease, von Hippel–Lindau disease, Lynch II, ataxic telangiectasia.

Long-standing chronic pancreatitis.

Epidemiology

- The incidence varies widely according to country and ethnicity, the highest incidences being in central and northern Europe, North America, and Australasia.
- The incidence standardized by age is 8–11 in 100 000 women and 10–12.5 in 100 000 men.
- Pancreatic cancer occurs less in premenopausal women, but the difference between men and women decreases with age.
- The mean age of presentation is 67 years for women and 63 years for men.

Pathology

- 70%–80% of pancreatic cancers arise in the head of the gland, the rest in the body or tail or diffusely located; <6% are multicentric.

Duct cell origin: 95%.

Acinar cell origin: 2%.

Uncertain histogenesis: 2%.

Nonepithelial tumors: 1%.

Treatment

Diet and lifestyle

• Abnormal gastric emptying results in malnourishment and dehydration in most patients.
• Parenteral nutrition does not alter the course of unresectable disease.

Pharmacological treatment

Before surgery or endoscopy

• The following are needed initially before resection or relief of jaundice:
Correction of anemia, optimization of nutritional status.
Vitamin K, 10 mg i.m. daily for 3 days if prothrombin time is prolonged.
Crystalloid solution, 1–2 L i.v. for at least 24 hours before any procedure.
For any procedure requiring instrumentation of the biliary tract.
Palliative chemotherapy for unresectable disease.
Chemotherapy offers very modest benefits in survival and variable impact on quality of life.
When used, regimens using 5-fluorouracil or gemcitabine are most common [6,7].
Radiation may enhance the value of chemotherapy.

For pain

• In many patients, the disease is so advanced that conservative management is most appropriate (*i.e.*, pain relief and palliative care).
• NSAIDs may precipitate acute renal failure, gastropathy.
• Patients can be given morphine slow-release orally, i.v., or by epidural infusion using a portable pump; this may cause constipation, nausea, and drowsiness.
• Metoclopramide hydrochloride (10 mg every 8 hours oral or i.v.) may be used for nausea, although benefits are often limited.

Chemotherapy [5]

• Gemcitabine has been shown to produce clinical benefit, improved survival, and increased time to disease progression in patients with locally advanced or metastatic disease.

Standard dosage	1000 mg/m i.v. infused over 3 minutes weekly.
Contraindications	Known hypersensitivity to gemcitabine; pregnancy.
Main drug interactions	None of significance.
Special points	Prolongation of infusion over 60 minutes may increase toxicity.
Main side effects	Myelosuppression, nausea, vomiting, elevated hepatic transaminases.

Nonpharmacological treatment

• Treatment choice for jaundice depends on age, tumor burden, and local expertise.
• In-hospital mortality figures are comparable for the different techniques, although endoscopic methods are probably superior.
• Potential surgical candidates must be appropriately staged, with the help of a radiologist and surgeon.

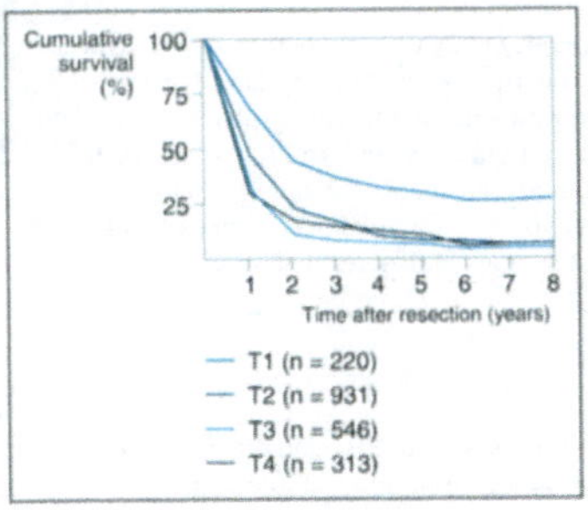

Survival rates after resection for pancreatic cancer stages T1–T4, based on data from the Japanese Pancreatic Cancer Registry.

Surgical resection

• Resection is possible in 10%–15% of patients, with a hospital mortality of 3%–10% [6].

Endoscopic stents

• Stents are most useful in patients with symptoms caused by biliary tract obstruction.
• Expandable metal stents need fewer changes and are recommended for patients with an expected better survival rate [7].

Percutaneous internal stenting

• The complication rate is higher than for endoscopic stents.

Surgical bypass

• Duodenal bypass may be used to avoid obstruction from growth into duodenum.

Treatment aims

To relieve jaundice, duodenal obstruction, weight loss, and pain.

Prognosis

• Cure is rarely possible, but a drainage procedure often results in the best palliation.
• After palliative treatment, mean survival is 3-6 months.
• After resection, mean survival is 12–18 months, and the 5-year survival rate is 5%–15%; the survival rate may be increased by adjuvant radiochemotherapy.

Follow-up and management

• Patients who have had resection may be suitable for postoperative adjuvant external beam radiotherapy followed by chemotherapy for 6–24 months.
• After palliative treatment, stents may need to be changed, gastric bypass may be needed for duodenal obstruction, and patients may need pain control.
• Localized recurrence may be worth re-resecting in some patients.

Key references

1. Zerby AL III, Lee MJ, Brugge WR, Mueller PR: Endoscopic sonography of the upper gastrointestinal tract and pancreas. *AJR Am J Roentgenol* 1996, **166**:45–50.
2. Raptopoulos V, Steer ML, Sheiman RG, *et al.*: The use of helical CT and CT angiography to predict vascular involvement from pancreatic cancer: correlation with findings at surgery. *AJR Am J Roentgencol* 1997, **168**:971–977.
3. Gattani AM, Mandeli J, Bruckner HW: Tumor markers in patients with pancreatic carcinoma. *Cancer* 1996, **78**:57–62.
4. Lehman GA, Uzer M: Pancreatic cancer. *Curr Pract Med* 1998, **4**:870–875.
5. van Riel JMGH, van Groeningen CJ, Pinedo HM, Giaccone G: Current chemotherapeutic possibilities in pancreaticobiliary cancer. *Ann Oncol* 1999, **10(Suppl 4)**:S157–S161.
6. Burris HA, Moore MJ, Andersen J, *et al.*: Improvements in survival and clinical benefit with gemcitabine as first-line therapy for patients with advanced pancreas cancer: a randomized trial. *J Clin Oncol* 1997, **15**:2403–2413.
7. Howden CW, Woods BL: Self-expanding metal stents for palliative treatment of malignant biliary and duodenal stenoses. *Gastrointest Endosc* 1995, **42**:104–105.

Pancreatitis, acute

Diagnosis

Symptoms

Epigastric pain: sudden onset; radiation into back (relative relief obtained by sitting forward or curling into a "fetal position"); may become increasingly severe.

Anorexia, nausea, vomiting.

Fever: less common.

Signs

Tachycardia, diaphoresis, peritoneal signs, hypotension, tachypnea: suggests more severe disease.

Ecchymosis: on flanks (Turner's sign) or periumbilically (Cullen's sign); often cited but rarely seen signs of intra-abdominal hemorrhage secondary to pancreatitis.

Peripheral fat necrosis: uncommon (more frequent in alcohol-induced pancreatitis).

Jaundice: especially in gallstone-induced pancreatitis.

Tetany: secondary to hypocalcemia.

Investigations

Amylase measurement: abnormal serum concentration (*e.g.*, >100 IU/dL); elevated lipase more specific and sensitive (both may be falsely elevated in renal failure).

Serum transaminase, alkaline phosphatase, and bilirubin measurement: elevations increase the possibility of biliary pancreatitis.

Complete blood count: to evaluate for anemia and systemic evidence of inflammation.

Serum creatinine, serum calcium: in toxic patients.

Serum lipids: in patients with unexplained pancreatitis.

Ultrasonography: to determine as soon as possible whether gallstones are causative (~80% sensitive); useful in following course of acute fluid collections (*i.e.*, pseudocysts and abscesses).

Arterial blood gases: in patients with tachypnea, shock; hypoxia indicates poor prognosis.

Contrast-enhanced CT: useful to determine extent of interstitial pancreatitis vs. necrotizing pancreatitis; done early in patients with severe presentation or in patients slow to respond to conservative therapy.

Fine-needle aspiration: to sample necrotic tissue for Gram stain and culture to ascertain presence of infected tissue.

Endoscopic retrograde cholangiopancreatography (ERCP): acutely for patients with biliary pancreatitis to remove obstructing stones from the bile duct or ampulla of patients suspected of having traumatic rupture of the pancreatic duct and traumatic pancreatitis. ERCP may aggravate acute pancreatitis and should be performed with caution to ascertain presence of gallstones of choledocholithiasis requiring endoscopic extraction and other causes in biliary tree or pancreas; in severe pancreatitis, disruption of main pancreatic duct suggests significant central necrosis; also indicated in cases of pancreatic trauma.

Complications

Anemia, hypoglycemia, hypocalcemia.

Acute fluid collections: occur early, in 30%–50% with severe disease and often in patients with mild disease; only 33%–50% of these become clinically significant pseudocysts.

Pancreatic necrosis: clinically significant in 3%–5%; up to 70% are infected necrosis; lesser degrees (<30% of the gland) often occur in clinically mild pancreatitis.

Hemorrhage: splenic artery aneurysm (an uncommon but particularly serious complication).

Multiorgan failure: acute respiratory distress syndrome, renal failure, disseminated intravascular coagulation, metabolic acidosis.

Sepsis.

Differential diagnosis

Abdominal catastrophe: any perforation of gastrointestinal tract, ruptured aneurysm, ectopic pregnancy, mesenteric infarction, ovarian cyst torsion.

Pyelonephritis, renal colic.

Peptic ulcer disease.

Cholangitis, cholecystitis.

Splenic infarction.

Ruptured esophagus (Boerhave's syndrome).

Crohn's disease.

Etiology

Alcohol in >50%.

Biliary disorders in 30%–60% of patients: gallstones, cholesterolosis, "sludge," ascariasis, sclerosing cholangitis, choledochocele, tumors.

Complication of endoscopic retrograde cholangiopancreatography.

Penetrating duodenal ulcer.

Hyperlipidemia in 1%–5%: types I (30%), IV (15%), and V (30%–40%).

Unusual causes in 1%–5%: obstructive (pancreas divisum, strictures, tumors), trauma, ischemia, infections (viruses), drugs (azathioprine, L-asparaginase, warfarin), vasculitides, transplantation, hypercalcemia, scorpion bites [2].

Epidemiology

- Gallstone-induced pancreatitis occurs more often in elderly people and women.
- Typically, 30–60 in 10^5 population are affected annually.
- The incidence is increasing.

Treatment

Diet and lifestyle

• During acute illness, patients should not ingest liquids or solids.

• Once pancreatitis has resolved, patients must eat regular meals; prolonged starvation followed by large meals must be avoided; clinical symptoms, rather than serum amylase or lipase levels, should determine when the patient may begin eating.

• Refraining from alcohol must be stressed to patients with alcohol-related pancreatitis.

Pharmacological treatment

• Supportive care involves the following:

Intravenous fluid: crystalloid and colloid (up to 12 L may be sequestered outside of the vascular compartment in the first 24–48 hours).

Pain relief with narcotics such as meperidine (50–100 mg i.m. every 4–6 hours).

Calcium supplementation as needed for patients with hypocalcemia and tetany.

Monitoring and treatment of diabetes mellitus as needed.

Pressor support: if systolic blood pressure <90 mm Hg or renal perfusion inadequate despite fluid replacement.

Antibiotics: for patients with gallstone pancreatitis.

• Glucagon, antiproteases (*e.g.*, aprotinin), somatostatin, are probably of no value in the setting of severe pancreatitis.

Nonpharmacological treatment

Nasogastric suction only for symptomatic relief of nausea and vomiting.

Oxygen administration: if oxygen saturation in arterial blood <90%; large pleural effusions should be drained.

Hemodialysis: for renal failure refractory to fluid replacement and inotropic support.

Endoscopic retrograde cholangiopancreatography and endoscopic sphincterotomy: for patients with severe pancreatitis in whom biliary tract disease (*i.e.*, biliary pancreatitis) is suspected.

Infected necrosis is a strong indication for surgery; patients who do not improve or who deteriorate over 5–10 days of conservative therapy should undergo CT scanning with needle aspiration of any regions suspicious for infection.

Drainage: for large pseudocysts (>6 cm), persisting in size, expanding, or causing symptoms; repeated percutaneous tapping increases risk of infection and abscess; internal cyst drainage via endoscopically placed stent or surgery is preferred to external drainage; abscess or infected necrosis must be treated early and aggressively preferably with surgical drainage [3,4].

Treatment aims

To provide supportive care.

To prevent further attacks.

To reduce complications and underlying disorders (*e.g.*, hyperlipidemia).

Prognosis

• Ranson's criteria of severity is predictive of mortality.

• Most patients recover after management in hospital with fluid replacement.

• Recurrent attacks are highly probable if alcohol abuse continues or if hyperlipidemia is not treated.

• Unless cholecystectomy or endoscopic sphincterotomy is performed in patients with gallstones, 10%–40% suffer recurrent attacks [2].

Follow-up and management [5]

• Further attacks can be prevented by laparoscopic cholecystectomy (for gallstones) or endoscopic sphincterotomy, stopping alcohol intake, treating hyperlipidemia and other underlying disorders.

• Follow-up is needed in patients in whom the cause has not been identified or treated or in those who have had extensive surgery for necrosis.

Key references

1. Bradley EL III: A clinically based classification system for acute pancreatitis. *Arch Surg* 1993, **128**:586–590.
2. Brugge WR: Acute and chronic pancreatitis. *Curr Pract Med* 1998, **1**:861–867.
3. Poston GJ, Williamson RCN: Surgical management of acute pancreatitis. *Br J Surg* 1990, **77**:5–12.
4. Fernandez del Castillo C, Rattner DW, Warshaw AL: Acute pancreatitis. *Lancet* 1993, **342**:475–479.
5. Steinberg WM, *et al.*: Controversies in clinical pancreatology. *Pancreas* 1996, **13**:219–225.

Pancreatitis, chronic

Diagnosis

Symptoms

• Chronic pancreatitis usually evolves over 5–20 years; symptoms, signs, and complications vary during this period [1].

Abdominal pain: in 90% of patients; often worse with eating; acute pancreatitis in 40%.

Weight loss: in 80%.

Diarrhea or steatorrhea: in 40%.

Polyphagia, polydipsia of diabetes mellitus: in 40%.

Signs

Greasy stool: in 10% on rectal examination.

Epigastric mass: in 10%.

Anemia: nonspecific anemia of chronic disease.

Jaundice: suggests biliary stricture from chronic pancreatitis.

Muscle wasting, cachexia, ecchymosis: malnourishment and evidence of malabsorption (*e.g.*, inability to absorb vitamin K) seen in patients with advanced disease.

Investigations

Serum amylase, lipase measurement: concentrations raised in acute exacerbation of pancreatitis; often normal in chronic pancreatitis.

Blood glucose measurement: at least 20% of functional parenchyma is required for euglycemia.

Abdominal radiography: pancreatic calcification has high specificity for chronic pancreatitis but limited sensitivity.

72-hour fecal fat collection: excretion of >6 g fecal fat/24 hours in patients ingesting at least 100 g of fat per day in the absence of other causes of malabsorption is highly suggestive of chronic pancreatitis.

Ultrasonography: for parenchymal changes, duct dilatation, calcification, pseudocysts, ascites; endoscopic ultrasonography is particularly good at rendering a diagnosis of chronic pancreatitis.

Contast-enhanced CT: highly sensitive for calcification; also useful to evaluate for inflammatory mass, ductal dilation, pseudocysts, ascites.

Pancreatic function tests: collection of pancreatic secretions via a nasogastric tube following stimulation by i.v. secretin or cholecystokinin; reduced lipase, bicarbonate, proteolytic enzymes confirms the presence of exocrine pancreatic insufficiency.

Endoscopic retrograde cholangiopancreatography: for changes in main duct and side branches ("minimal change pancreatitis"), stones (calcified and noncalcified) and protein plugs in duct, pseudocysts, fistulas.

Complications

Pancreatic exocrine insufficiency.

Pancreatic endocrine insufficiency.

Duodenal ulcer.

Common bile duct obstruction: secondary biliary cirrhosis (rare).

Duodenal obstruction.

Pseudocysts: pancreatic, intra-abdominal, mediastinal.

Pancreatic ascites.

Pleural effusion.

Pancreatic abscess.

Pancreatic pseudoaneurysm.

Splenic vein thrombosis: gastric fundus varices.

Narcotic dependency.

Differential diagnosis

Recurrent acute pancreatitis without chronic pancreatitis.

Idiopathic hypertrophy of head of pancreas.

Secondary pancreatic inflammation (duodenal ulceration).

Pancreatic cancer.

Celiac disease.

Bacterial overgrowth of small bowel.

Etiology

Alcohol in 60%–80% of patients.

Obstruction in 10%: ampullary stenosis, pancreas divisum, annular pancreas, stricture (trauma, tumor), irradiation, pancreatitis.

Idiopathic in 10%.

Hereditary (chronic familial pancreatitis).

Malnutrition (tropical pancreatitis).

Cystic fibrosis.

Tropical pancreatitis.

Epidemiology

• In industrialized countries, the incidence largely depends on alcohol consumption (other factors have a modifying effect): 1–10 in 100 000 population are affected annually.

• Chronic pancreatitis occurs more often in men than in women; the ratios vary from 10:1 to 2:1.

• The incidence is increasing in all countries.

Treatment

Diet and lifestyle

• Patients should eat regular meals and abstain from alcohol.

• Use of medium-chain triglycerides is occasionally helpful for patients with malnutrition and extensive fat malabsorption.

Pharmacological treatment

• When possible, therapy should be directed at the underlying cause.

For exocrine insufficiency: pancreatic enzyme therapy consisting of 28 000 IU of lipase administered with meals and titrated to control symptoms (steatorrhea, weight loss); concomitant gastric acid reduction (*e.g.*, with an H_2-receptor antagonist or proton pump inhibitor) may improve the activity of enzyme supplements [2].

For endocrine insufficiency: insulin therapy is usually required to control diabetes.

For pain

• Self-titration of pancreatic supplements containing proteases may reduce mild or moderate pain (despite the absence of overt steatorrhea) [3].

• Simple analgesics or NSAIDs can be used; however, patients often require management with narcotics.

• Celiac plexus block with alcohol can be considered, repeated if necessary.

Nonpharmacological treatment

Main pancreatic duct drainage

• Endoscopic sphincterotomy and stone extraction are suitable in only a few patients; stenting of strictures or pancreatic sphincterotomy may be helpful in select cases [4].

• Pancreaticojejunostomy or transduodenal sphincteroplasty are alternatives to endoscopic treatment; draining alone is usually insufficient in the presence of extensive parenchymal calcification, inflammation, and pain [5–8].

Surgery for pain

• Surgery can be considered in patients with intractable pain.

• For nondiabetic patients or those having an operation for the first time, treatment should be conservative and only "dominant" disease resected.

• For patients with diabetes or previous surgery, extensive surgery may be required.

• Preservation of the stomach, pylorus, duodenum, and spleen is almost always possible.

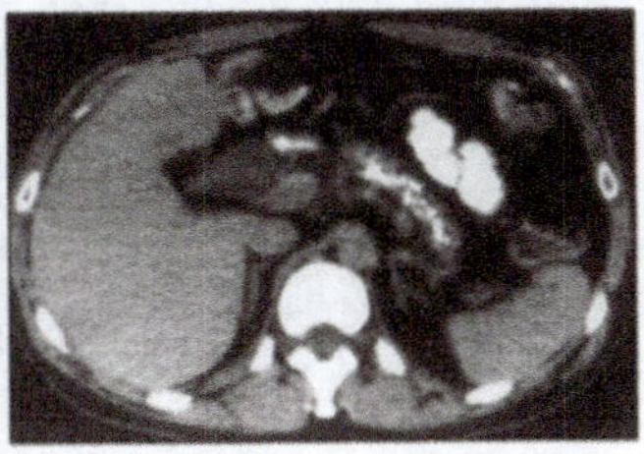

CT scan reveals numerous pancreatic stones in patient with chronic alcholic pancreatitis. Pancreas appears atrophic.

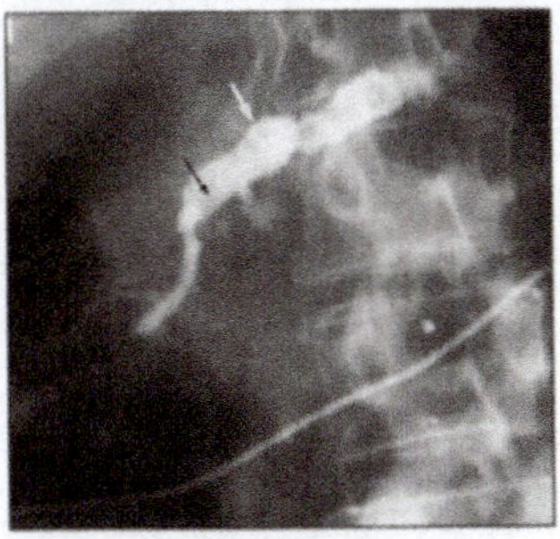

Endoscopic retrograde cholangiopancreatography reveals dilatation of main pancreatic duct (*white arrow*). There are numerous introductal calculi (*black arrow*).

Treatment aims

To eliminate the underlying cause.
To relieve pain.
To delay disease progression (duct drainage).
To treat malabsorption.

Prognosis [4]

• The disease is not always progressive.
• Pain and calcification occur after 5–10 years, and both may subsequently regress, but this is unpredictable.
• The long-term survival is often poor (~50% of patients die within 7 years) because of comorbid factors.
• Preservation of the quality of life and chronic pain management are the biggest challenges of dealing with this group of patients.

Follow-up and management

• All patients must be followed up to monitor endocrine and exocrine function and pain and to ascertain the need for operation or reoperation.

Key references

1. Steer ML, *et al.*: Chronic pancreatitis. *N Engl J Med* 1995, **332**:1482–1490.
2. Brugge WR: Acute and chronic pancreatitis. *Curr Pract Med* 1998, **1**:861–867.
3. Ihse I, Permerth J: Enzyme therapy and pancreatic pain. *Acta Chir Scand* 1990, **156**:281–283.
4. Ammann RW, *et al.*: Course of alcoholic chronic pancreatitis. *Gastroenterology* 1996, **111**:224–231.
5. Malfertheiner P, Dominquez-Munoz JE, Büchler M: Diagnosis and staging of chronic pancreatitis. In *Standards in Pancreatic Surgery*. Edited by Beger HG, *et al.* Berlin: Springer-Verlag; 1993: 297–313.
6. Nealon WH, Thompson JC: Progressive loss of pancreatic function in chronic pancreatitis is delayed by main pancreatic duct decompression. *Ann Surg* 1993, **217**:458–466.
7. Watanapa P, Williams RC: Pancreatic sphincterotomy and sphincteroplasty. *Gut* 1992, **33**:865–867.
8. Beger HG, Büchler M, Bittner R: The duodenum preserving resection of the head of the pancreas (DPRHP) in patients with chronic pancreatitis and an inflammatory mass in the head. *Acta Chir Scand* 1990, **156**:309–315.

Panic & generalized anxiety disorder

Diagnosis

Symptoms

Panic

Recurrent attacks of severe unprovoked anxiety: starting suddenly, reaching a peak within a few minutes, and lasting at least 20 minutes, with at least four of the following:

Palpitations.
Stomach churning.
Hot or cold flushes.
Shaking or trembling.
Choking or difficulty breathing.
Fear of dying.
Feelings of unreality.
Fear of losing control.
Sweating.
Chest pain or discomfort.
Feeling dizzy, unsteady, lightheaded, or faint.
Paresthesias (numbness or tingling sensations).

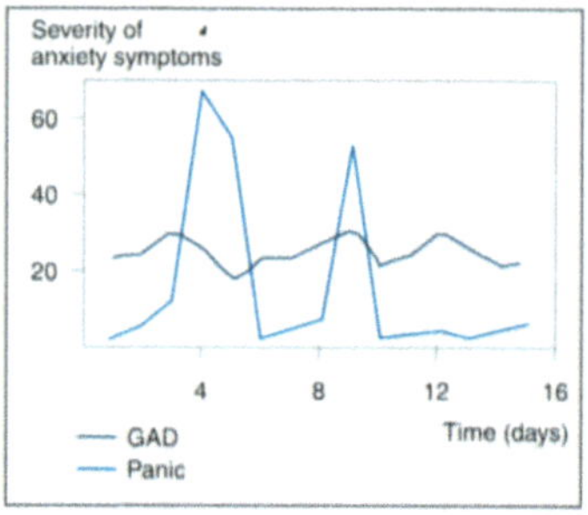

Course of pure panic disorder and pure generalized anxiety disorder (GAD).

Generalized anxiety disorder (GAD)

Relatively persistent anxiety: at least 6 months, associated with worrying and apprehension about events and other matters that do not justify excessive worry; the anxiety and worry are associated with at least three of the following symptoms:

Restlessness: feeling keyed up or on edge.
Being easily fatigued.
Difficulty concentrating or mind going blank.
Irritability.
Muscle tension.
Sleep disturbance: difficulty falling or staying asleep or restless, unsatisfying sleep.

Signs

Panic

• Physicians seldom see a panic attack in vivo because patients usually feel more secure in a medical setting. Features present on examination include the following:

Fear of having a panic attack.
Reassurance that a heart attack or other physical catastrophe is not imminent.
Wish to be physically examined.
Physiological evidence of anxiety: usually no different from generalized anxiety disorder.

Generalized anxiety disorder

Furrowed brow, hunted look, lack of confidence: evidence of long-standing anxiety.
Tachycardia: pulse 80–100 beats/min.
Sweating.
Dilated pupils.
Observed tremor.

Investigations

• Investigations should not be entered into lightly in patients with anxiety disorders because they may cause hypochondriacal concern and increased anxiety. If, however, anxiety appears for the first time in middle age or later, it may have an organic cause.

Thyroid function tests, complete blood screening, neurological assessment: may sometimes be indicated if anxiety is episodic, diurnally varied, or linked to specific somatic symptoms persistently; epilepsy and pheochromocytoma are rare but remediable causes of anxiety.

Complications

Alcohol dependence: with persistent anxiety (alcohol provides temporary relief).
Hypochondriasis: due to anxiety about bodily complaints.
Agoraphobia: due to persistent severe anxiety, particularly after panics in public places.
Social phobia: due to self-consciousness of anxiety attacks.

Differential diagnosis

Tachycardia, pulmonary emboli, organic dyspnea, thyrotoxicosis: anxiety related to physical disease.
Mixed anxiety and depressive disorder, depressive episode: anxiety due to depressive symptoms.
Posttraumatic stress: anxiety due to major unusual event (e.g., rape, major disaster).
Hypochondriasis, somatoform disease: anxiety due entirely to fear of disease or preoccupation with bodily symptoms.
Organic psychoses, schizophrenia, affective psychoses: anxiety due to psychotic symptoms, e.g., delusions or hallucinations.
Agoraphobia, social or simple phobias: anxiety due to specific stimuli, accompanied by avoidance of the stimuli.
Most GAD in the elderly is caused by depression.
Substance abuse disorders: anxiety due to alcohol or drug abuse.

Etiology

• The immediate cause of anxiety in panic and generalized anxiety disorder is unknown.
• The episodes of anxiety are unfocused or "free-floating" (generalized anxiety disorder) or spontaneous (panic).
• Both disorders are associated with life changes and events and may sometimes be a delayed reaction to the events.
• A genetic component is possible.

Epidemiology

• Panic attacks are most frequent in the 15–24-year age range and have an annual prevalence of ~2% in this group, with ~1% in the total population.
• Generalized anxiety disorder is much more common, with an annual prevalence of ~6%.
• Major depression coexists with generalized anxiety disorder and panic disorder in up to 60% of patients.

Treatment

Diet and lifestyle

• A good square meal is sometimes said to be the best tranquillizer in the world; unsurprisingly, therefore, some anxious people resolve their anxiety by overeating and getting fat. This may relieve their anxiety (good studies show that fat people are less anxious generally than thin people) but does not improve their health overall.

• Because anxious people fear trouble around every corner, they often restrict their lifestyles; this is seen to its extreme in the housebound agoraphobic.

Pharmacological treatment [1]

• The patient's view must be taken into account: some refuse drug treatment, others are equally negative about psychological treatment.
• Less effective treatments, *e.g.*, beta-blockade and relaxation training, should be avoided in patients with panic disorder.
• Combined drug and psychological treatments are acceptable and may even be more effective than individual treatments alone.
• Patients must be warned against self-medication with alcohol for anxiety and pain: it provokes worse symptoms in the longer term.
• The duration of treatment should be set in advance, whenever possible.

Standard dosage

Specific 5-HT reuptake inhibitors, e.g., paroxetine, 20-60 mg daily [2].

Benzodiazepines, e.g., clonazapam 0.5 mg twice daily; alprazolam, 0.25-6.0 mg daily.

Buspirone, 10-60 mg daily, especially useful for eldery patients [3].
Beta-blockers, e.g., propranolol, 40-120 mg daily.
Heterocyclic antidepressants, e.g., clomiprimine, 100-150 mg daily [1].

Contraindications

Benzodiazepines: caution with previous or current evidence of dependent personality or behavior or substance abuse.

Special points

Serotonin reuptake inhibitors: first-line agents, effective in most forms of anexity disorders [2].

Benzodiazepines: rapid and more effective in short term than other treatments, but tolerance and dependence make them generally unsuitable for regular treatment; may interfere with success of behavior therapy. Beta-blockers: useful if somatic symptoms of anxiety are prominent but not severe (more useful in generalized anxiety disorder).

Heterocyclic antidepressants: more effective than benzodiazepines when given for more than 4 weeks, but slow onset of antianxiety effects.

Main drug interactions

Additive effects with alcohol.

Main side effects

Sedation (not beta-blockers).

Nonpharmacological treatment

Psychological treatments [1]

Relaxation training: of some value (but less than other more intensive therapies) and can be very cheap.

Cognitive therapy: effective in both disorders, may be superior to other psychological treatments; substantially decreases relapse rates after medication taper; aimed at altering unproductive dysfunctional thinking that helps to generate and maintain anxiety; patients with panic disorders learn to decatastrophize thinking, so that attacks are avoided.

Behavior therapy: effective in treating maladaptive behaviors associated with anxiety, mainly by gradual exposure to more adaptive situations.

Combination therapies: cognitive behavior therapy, anxiety management training.

Hypnosis and alternative therapies (yoga, meditation): sometimes useful but not as effective as cognitive and behavior therapies.

Treatment aims

To alleviate symptoms.

To teach patient to recognize anxiety early.

To teach patient stress management and relaxation techniques.

Prognosis

• Prognosis is generally good except when symptoms begin early in adult life and are associated with personality disturbance.
• Markers of poor prognosis in panic disorder include coexisting depression, severe symptoms, and agorophobia.

Follow-up and management

• Drug treatment is best regarded as a temporary measure, except in patients who are persistently anxious; long-term treatment should be psychological because relapse is less likely and self-esteem is improved.

Key references

1. Nesse RM, Bamurski MA: Anxiety disorders in primary care. In: Primary Care Psychiatry. Edited by Knespe DJ, Robi MB, Schwenk TL. Philadelphia: W.B. Saunders, 1997.
2. Boyer W: Serotonin uptake inhibitors are superior to imipramine and alprazolam in alleviating panic attacks: a meta-analysis. *Int Clin Psychopharmacol* 1995, **10**:45-49.
3. Folles DG, Fuller WC: Anxiety disorders and insomnia in geriatric patients. *Pychiatric Clin North Am* 1997, **29(1)**:137–164.

Diagnosis

Symptoms

Tremor: in ~70% of patients; unilateral and usually noted in hand first; may be seen in jaw or leg. Most often unilateral at onset.

Poverty of movement, difficulty initiating movements and with repetitive movements: *e.g.*, shuffling gait, drooling, difficulty turning in bed, micrographia, softness of voice, constipation.

Rigidity: *e.g.*, poor balance, falls, muscle stiffness, pain.

Signs

Tremor: asymmetric, resting, "pill-rolling" at 3–5 Hz; usually disappears on intention; increased by anxiety; possibly postural tremor at 6–8 Hz.

Rigidity and bradykinesia: stooped, flexed posture; shuffling gait with poor swing of affected arm; cogwheel rigidity, may be enhanced by synkinesis; immobile facies, reduced blink and swallowing rates; rigidity usually noted first in axial muscles, *e.g.*, neck and shoulder.

Investigations

• No tests are available for Parkinson's disease; the diagnosis is based on clinical features alone.

• Investigation is indicated when the diagnosis is in doubt or presentation is atypical, especially in young-onset cases.

Testing of autonomic function: patients with multiple system atrophy may show abnormalities.

MRI: can show abnormal hypointensity in the putamen of patients with multiple system atrophy, can reveal strokes in some patients with parkinsonism.

Copper and ceruloplasmin measurement: in all patients with young-onset or atypical Parkinson's disease.

Huntington's genetic testing: for young presentation with family history.

Complications

Depression, anxiety.

Postural imbalance: with falls and trauma.

Cognitive and psychiatric problems: frontal lobe dysfunction, bradyphrenia, fluctuating confusional state (dementia in 25% of patients); possible overlap with other syndromes, *e.g.*, diffuse Lewy body disease, senile dementia of Lewy body type.

Complications of L-dopa: dyskinesias, motor fluctuation.

Differential diagnosis

Drug-induced parkinsonism: *e.g.*, phenothiazines, butyrophenones; usually symmetrical and reversible.

Essential tremor: bilateral; absent at rest, exacerbated by intention, or maintaining posture; improved by alcohol; possible family history; should be treated with beta-blockers or primidone when necessary.

Multiple system atrophy or progressive supranuclear palsy: symptoms and signs usually symmetrical; tremor less usual; falls frequent; additional features, *e.g.*, pyramidal or cerebellar deficits, gaze palsies, or autonomic involvement including postural hypotension, and bladder dysfunction.

Wilson's disease: 40% present with neurological features, mainly parkinsonism and hypokinetic dysarthria; liver cirrhosis or psychiatric disease also occur; Kayser–Fleischer rings visible by slit lamp in most; low serum ceruloplasmin, high urinary copper; liver biopsy shows high copper and evidence of liver cell damage; should be treated with penicillamine.

Toxin-induced parkinsonism (*e.g.*, carbon monoxide).

Mitochondrial disorders; abnormal movements, usually dystonia or chorea.

Etiology [1]

• >80% dopamine depletion occurs in the striatum at presentation; neurons are lost in the substantia nigra (dopaminergic), locus caeruleus (noradrenergic), and substantia innominata (cholinergic). Intracytoplasmic inclusions, Lewy bodies, are found in surviving neurons.

• The cause of Parkinson's disease is not known, but environmental toxins and genetic susceptibility may play a role alone or in combination.

Epidemiology

• The incidence is ~20 in 100 000, with an overall prevalence of 150 in 100 000 (500 in 100 000 for those aged >50 years).

• The male : female ratio is equal.

• Younger-onset patients tend to develop more motor fluctuations, and older-onset patients have a much higher incidence of associated dementia.

Treatment

Diet and lifestyle

• Maintaining activity is important: a multidisciplinary approach, with physical therapy, occupational therapy, speech therapy, and social work contact is helpful; patients and caregivers may need support.

• Dietary protein should be reduced during the day; a main meal at night allows more predictable absorption of L-dopa.

Pharmacological treatment [2]

At diagnosis

• Most neurologists advocate selegiline or dopamine agonists.

Standard dosage	Selegiline (Eldepryl). 5 mg twice daily.
Contraindications	Possible interaction with tricyclic antidepressants or 5-HT reuptake inhibitors.
Special points	May delay requirement for L-dopa, although mechanism of action uncertain; some symptomatic benefit.
Main drug interactions	Concurrent L-dopa dose may need to be decreased 20%–50%; should not be administered with tricyclic antidepressants.
Main side effects	Gastrointestinal upset, hypotension, confusion.

At review

• Treatment is essentially symptomatic.

• L-Dopa is prescribed when clinical features interfere with life, or postural instability is noted on examination.

• Tremor and bradykinesia respond well.

• The use of controlled-release L-dopa offers some improvement in patients with medium to advanced disease, especially in decreasing "off time"; transition to these drugs should be gradual because the bioavailability is different from that of the standard preparations; some neurologists use controlled-release preparations early to provide a more "physiological" prolonged drug exposure to dopaminergic neurons.

• Dopaminergic agonists may be used alone (early) or in combination with L-dopa.

Standard dosage	L-Dopa with a dopa decarboxylase inhibitor, initially at low dose and frequency, *e.g.*, 100 mg twice or 3 times daily, increased as necessary. Dopaminergic agonists, *e.g.*, bromocriptine or pergolide in low doses initially and built up gradually.
Contraindications	*L-Dopa:* closed angle glaucoma. *Dopaminergic agents:* hypotension, cardiac arrhythmias.
Special points	*L-Dopa:* generally, frequent small doses (up to every 2–3 hours) are better than infrequent large doses. *Dopaminergic agents:* may be used alone, but tolerance to these drugs develops quickly.
Main drug interactions	*Dopaminergic agents:* combination with L-dopa may improve control.
Main side effects	*L-Dopa:* gastrointestinal upset, postural hypotension, confusion, hallucination, dyskinesias and dystonia; neuropsychiatric side effects best treated by dose modification, but clozapine or olanzapine may be used (possible development of agranulocytosis). *Dopaminergic agents:* hypotension, hallucinations, confusion, gastrointestinal symptoms.

• Amantidine or anticholinergics may be useful adjunctive medications for tremor.

Treatment aims

To improve functional disability.

To avoid or minimize drug-related side effects.

To treat fluctuations when present.

Other treatments

• Posteroventral pallidotomy may be useful in selected patients to improve dyskinesias and motor fluctuations.

Prognosis

• Parkinson's disease progresses at variable rates.

• Patients with dementia have a significantly worse prognosis.

Follow-up and management

• The need for symptomatic treatment should be assessed.

• Correct use and titration of drugs should be monitored.

• Medical and support needs should be assessed.

Key references

1. Calne DB: Treatment of Parkinson's disease. *N Engl J Med* 1993, **329**:1021–1027.
2. Marsden CD: Parkinson's disease. *J Neurol Neurosurg Psychiatry* 1994, **57**:672–681.

Parvovirus B19 infection

Diagnosis

Symptoms

• Often no symptoms are manifest.

Mild feverish illness: in children.

Mild feverish illness with arthralgia or arthritis: in adults.

Symptoms of an aplastic crisis: in patients with hemolytic anemias or occasionally normal people; onset usually acute but self-limiting.

Symptoms of persistent severe anemia: in immunosuppressed patients.

Signs

• The illness, when accompanied by a rash, is known as erythema infectiosum, fifth disease, or slapped-cheek syndrome.

Rash: usually seen in children; appears on cheeks, giving slapped-cheek appearance; lasts 1 week; recurs for several months on exposure to sun or wind; variable but often reticular maculopapular rash may also develop on arms and legs but rarely affects palms or soles.

Lymph-node enlargement: in adults.

Arthralgia or arthritis: often involving wrists and knees in adults; can occur without rash; usually last 2–4 weeks, occasionally longer.

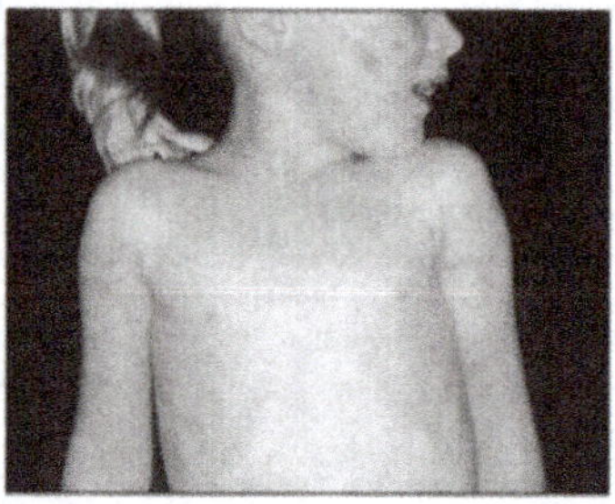

Slapped-cheek appearance of parvovirus B19 infection and reticular rash on arms. **(*See* Color Plate.)**

Investigations

Serology: IgM specific to parvovirus B19 manifest in early illness; parvovirus B19 IgG antibody develops early in illness and falls within 1–2 months.

Complications

Aplastic crisis.

Fetal anemia, hydrops fetalis, and death: especially during second trimester, although effect on pregnancy uncertain; about one-third of pregnant women with primary infection transmit it to fetus.

Differential diagnosis

Scarlet fever: parvovirus has no oral stigmata.

Measles: no Koplik's spots or marked syndrome in parvovirus infection.

Rubella, enteroviral infections, cytomegalovirus, Epstein–Barr virus, toxoplasmosis.

Etiology

• Infection is by parvovirus B19.

• Transmission is by respiratory droplets.

Epidemiology

• Infection occurs worldwide.

• Most infections are in spring or early summer.

Infectivity

• Parvovirus B19 is moderately infective.

• Immunity is apparently for life after an acute episode.

Mean incubation period

To the mild febrile illness: 6–8 days.

To the rash: 17–18 days.

Treatment

Diet and lifestyle

- People known to be infected should avoid contact with pregnant women.

Pharmacological treatment

Analgesics, *e.g.*, acetaminophen.

NSAIDs for reactive arthralgia.

Treatment aims

To relieve symptoms (if any).

Prognosis

- Prognosis is good in acquired illness.
- Mortality is 9% in recognized fetal infections.

Follow-up and management

- Follow-up is not needed.

General references

Brown KE, Young NS: Parvovirus B19 in human disease. *Am Rev Med* 1997, **48**:59–67.

Gay NJ, *et al.*: Age specific antibody prevalence to parvovirus B19: how many women are infected in pregnancy? *Comm Dis Rep* 1994, **4**:R104–R107.

Levy R, Waissman A, Blomberg G, Hagay ZJ: Infection by parvovirus B19 during pregnancy: a review. *Obstet Gynecol Surv* 1997, **52**:254–259.

Pattison JR: Human parvovirus B19. *BMJ* 1994, **308**:149–150.

Pericarditis & tamponade

Diagnosis

Symptoms

Pericarditis

Mild to severe precordial pain: on inspiration or worse on inspiration; may radiate to neck and shoulders; worse on coughing, swallowing, or sneezing; improved by leaning forward.

Dyspnea, nausea.

Tamponade

Precordial discomfort: occasionally, due to large effusions.

Cough, hoarseness, tachypnea, dysphagia: due to pressure.

Malaise, cyanosis, dyspnea, sweating, anxiety, hypotension: rapidly developing.

Signs

Pericarditis

Fever.

Pericardial, often pleuropericardial, coarse rub: best heard at left sternal edge with patient leaning forward; may come and go over minutes to hours, may decrease with development of effusion.

Initially normal venous pressure.

Tamponade

Tachycardia: nearly always present.

Low blood and pulse pressures.

Pulsus paradoxus: pulse may disappear on inspiration; may also occur in asthma.

Raised venous pressure: with prominent "y" descent and no "x" descent; may increase on inspiration.

Investigations

- For any pericardial disease, the underlying cause must always be sought.

Pericarditis

Complete blood count, ESR and urine and electrolyte measurement. TSH and T4 to exclude hypothyroidism.

Antistreptolysin O titer, antineutrophil factor, rheumatoid factor analysis. HIV test to exclude AIDS and fungal serology in immunocompromised patients or in endemic areas.

Cardiac enzyme tests: enzymes may be normal or increase, but creatinine phosphokinase MB and troponins probably not significantly increased unless accompanying myocarditis.

Paired viral antibody screening: increase in neutralizing antibodies (up to 4 times) within 3–4 weeks of onset.

Mantoux test.

ECG: changes throughout all leads; raised ST segment, PR depression, inverted T waves only in some patients, pericardial effusion (low-voltage QRS and T wave in large effusions), electrical alternans (caused by heart swinging about).

Chest radiography: normal unless pericardial fluid >250 mL; cardiac contour may be globular, with no congestion in the lungs.

Tamponade

Echocardiography: essential in any patient in whom pericardial fluid is suspected (*e.g.*, cardiomegaly on chest radiography with hypotension); right ventricular collapse characteristic of tamponade.

Complications

Relapsing or constrictive pericarditis, pericardial effusion and tamponade: complications of pericarditis.

Hypotension, renal failure: complications of tamponade.

Differential diagnosis

Pericarditis

Extension of infarct after acute myocardial infarction.

Myocardial infarction, unstable angina, ulcer dyspepsia, acute aortic dissection, spontaneous pneumothorax, pleurisy, pulmonary embolus.

Tamponade

Cardiomyopathy or constrictive pericarditis.

Etiology

Pericarditis

Viral: may be associated with pleurisy.
Autoimmune or collagen vascular diseases: SLE, scleroderma.
Rheumatic fever, rheumatoid athritis.
Myocardial infarction or cardiac surgery.
Metabolic: uremia, myxedema.
AIDS, opportunistic infections (*e.g.*, tuberculosis).

Association with neoplasia, particularly lymphoma, leukemia, carcinoma of bronchus or breast.

Tamponade

Any of the above, but particularly the following:
Carcinoma of bronchus or breast.
Uremia.
Cardiac surgery.
Viral infection (in young patients).

Epidemiology

- The incidence at postmortem examination is 2%–6%.
- The clinical incidence is <1 in 100 hospital admissions.
- More men than women are affected.
- The disorder may recur after treatment but is usually a one-off event, depending on the cause.

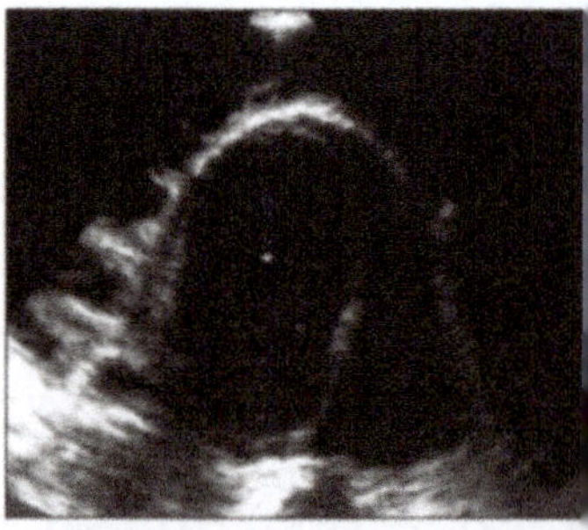

Pericardial space containing fluid (*top center*); bright pericardium (*mid center*); left ventricle (*lower center*); fibrinous strands in pericardial fluid (*lower left*).

Treatment

Diet and lifestyle

- No special dietary precautions are necessary.
- Overactivity is contraindicated until the symptoms have resolved.

Pharmacological treatment

- Drugs are used for pericarditis to decrease inflammation and treat the underlying cause.
- Aspirin usually settles both pain and fever; indomethacin is particularly useful in preventing recurrence; a short course of steroids may be needed.
- Small effusions can be followed clinically and with the aid of two-dimensional echocardiograms.

Nonpharmacological treatment

- For tamponade, pericardial aspiration may be life-saving with large effusions.
- As much fluid as possible should be drained; blood-stained effusions usually signify malignancy, but all samples should be sent for cytology and bacteriology.
- Pericardiocentesis alone frequently results in the resolution of large effusions, but recurrence is common.
- Recurrent effusions may need balloon pericardotomy or surgical drainage.
- Chemotherapy can be started if malignant disease has been confirmed.

Treatment aims

To prevent adverse hemodynamic changes of tamponade.

To diagnose and treat underlying condition.

Prognosis

- Prognosis depends on the underlying condition: it is good for viral pericarditis but poor for malignant pericardial effusion.
- Patients with viral pericarditis usually recover completely in 1–2 weeks.
- Large idiopathic chronic pericardial effusion is well-tolerated for long periods in most patients, but severe tamponade can develop unexpectedly at any time.

Follow-up and management

- Regular echocardiographic follow-up is necessary for pericardial effusions.

General references

Clifford CP, Davies GJ: Tuberculous pericarditis with rapid progression to constriction. *BMJ* 1993, **307**:1052–1054.

Sagrista-Sauleda J, *et al.*: Long-term follow-up of idiopathic pericardial effusion. *N Engl J Med* 1999, **341**:2054–2059.

Ziskind AA, *et al.*: Percutaneous balloon pericardiotomy for the treatment of cardiac tamponade and large pericardial effusions: description of technique and report of the first 50 cases. *J Am Coll Cardiol* 1993, **21**:1–5.

Diagnosis

Definition [1]

• Personality disorders are dysfunctional patterns of thinking and behavior that reflect persistent ways of relating to self and others, which deviate markedly from the norm and are invariably accompanied by impairment of social role or major subjective distress.

•The specific personality disorders that appear in adolescence can be broadly categorized into three main areas:

Flamboyant: histrionic, emotionally unstable (borderline or impulsive), dissocial.

Eccentric: paranoid/schizoid.

Fearful: anancastic, anxious/avoidant, dependent.

• Others are acquired later in life and arise as a result of organic insult, psychiatric illness, or catastrophic stress.

Symptoms and signs

Suspicion, oversensitivity, querulousness, unforgiving: paranoid.

Emotional coldness, solitude, social insensitivity: schizoid.

Impulsiveness, emotional instability, poor self-control: emotionally unstable (impulsive or borderline).

Obsessions, perfectionism, rigidity, self-doubt: anancastic.

Social sensitivity, apprehension, feelings of social inferiority: anxious, avoidant.

Reliance on others, subordination of own needs, fear of abandonment: dependent.

Callousness, irresponsibility, blaming others, aggressiveness: dissocial.

Dramatics, suggestibility, seeking center stage, shallowness: histrionic.

• Patients often place high demands on the health care system because of somatization and demand for medication. Behaviors include frequent calls, emergency visits, and prolonged office visits. Health care providers are frequently frustrated and drained, especially if the personality disorder is undiagnosed.

Investigations

History: should be corroborated with other sources if possible (with patient's permission): personality characteristics of parents, early development, adverse life events and upbringing; school/social services (history of neglect, impoverishment, or abuse); legal sources (*e.g.,* probation office); spouse, cohabitee (partners may also have personality disorders); employer.

Standardized questionnaires: usually time-consuming but highly reliable; patients are asked tightly worded questions covering specific areas of personal and social function in order to avoid biased judgement on the part of the therapist; this is particularly important in the case of disorders with antisocial characteristics.

Munich Checklist for ICD-10: a good alternative [2].

EEG: finding may be abnormal in patients with dissocial disorder.

Complications

High suicide rate.

Self-harming behavior: may lead to frequent presentations in a wide variety of health care settings, *e.g.*, emergency departments, medical wards.

Alcohol addiction and drug abuse.

Harm to others: *e.g.*, violent assault or sexual abuse of children.

Differential diagnosis

Comorbidity with mental illness (AXIS I): cross-sectional studies show that ~40% of patients also manifest AXIS I disorders when they present in clinical settings.

Schizotypal disorder: frequently overlaps with borderline and schizoid disorders.

Prodromal or residual phase of schizophrenia.

Affective disorders: hypomania may mimic dissocial disorder; depression is frequent in patients suffering from borderline disorder.

Etiology

Genetic inheritance.

Abnormal developmental biology.

Failure to negotiate critical stages of emotional development.

Childhood trauma: sexual abuse is a more frequent feature in borderline disorders.

Social theories: abnormal parenting or lack of an appropriate role model.

Epidemiology

• Because sufferers avoid society, schizoid personality disorder appears to be rare .

• The prevalence in the general population is 2%–6%; in primary care settings, 15%–34%; in psychiatric outpatients, 20%–40%; in psychiatric inpatients, 40%–60%; in forensic settings, 50%–90%.

Treatment

Diet and lifestyle

• No special precautions are necessary.

Pharmacological treatment [3]

• All drugs must be used with caution because of the dangers of overdose and abuse.

• Neuroleptics, *e.g.*, thioridazine or haloperidol in low doses, can alleviate symptoms, *e.g.*, hostility, anger, suspiciousness, and depressed mood, in borderline or dissocial conditions.

• Monoamine oxidase inhibitors may be useful in borderline conditions.

• Long-term use of benzodiazepines must be avoided because of the probability of addiction; they may cause paradoxical disinhibition.

• Mood stabilizers (lithium and carbamazepine) are most useful if there is evidence of mood swings or family history of affective disorder.

Nonpharmacological treatment

Psychotherapy

• Interpretative psychotherapies for flamboyant disorders are effective in mild to moderate conditions.

Behavior or cognitive therapy

• This is being developed but is not widely available; it is similar to therapies used in the treatment of depression and anxiety.

• Effective in decreasing symptoms in milder cases in which somatization is a prominent feature [4].

Supportive therapy

• This includes social support and is most useful for patients with severe disruptive personality disorders.

• Patients are encouraged to find practical solutions to present problems, *e.g.*, relationship difficulties, accommodation, other personal needs.

Group therapy

• Group therapy may help patients with some forms of personality disorders.

• It includes the use of therapeutic communities.

Office management

• Frequent, brief, focused visits are the mainstay. Legitimization of symptoms, brief physical examination of symptomatic areas, and specific planning for next contact should be included.

• Setting limits on between-visit and within-visit behavior (*e.g.*, phone calls, referrals, medication use) is important to limiting burden on office staff.

• Long-term objectives include increased social functions, decreased use of emergency services, decreased use of medications, and avoidance of physician and staff burnout.

Treatment aims

To alleviate subjective distress and reduce impact of dysfunctional behavior.

Prognosis

• Prognosis is usually poor in severely affected patients, but most improve with age (4th or 5th decade); improvement is more noticeable for the flamboyant group.

• The outcome is invariably worse when comorbid mental illness is present.

• Good prognostic features include intelligence and the presence of positive adaptive traits, *e.g.*, candor and introspectiveness.

Follow-up and management

• No treatment has universally proven effectiveness; the most useful approach is based on long-term supportive contact and crisis intervention when needed.

• Patients tend to arouse strong feelings in therapists; staff working in crisis situations particularly need regular support.

Danger

• Most patients with personality disorders are no more dangerous than unaffected people.

• A few people with severe disorders, especially those with paranoid or dissocial traits, can exhibit considerable aggression toward others; safety and surveillance is paramount in such circumstances.

• In community settings, the police should be involved to make the situation safe.

• Admission to secure units or forensic facilities may be needed.

Key references

1. Anonymous: *ICD-10 Classification of Mental and Behavioural Disorders. Clinical Descriptions and Diagnostic Guidelines*. Geneva: World Health Organization; 1992.
2. Bronisch T, *et al.*: The Munich diagnostic checklist for the assessment of DSM-III-R personality disorders for use in routine clinical care and research. *Eur Arch Psychiatry Clin Neurosci* 1992, **242**:77–81.
3. Stein G: Drug treatment of personality disorders. *Br J Psychiatry* 1992, **166**:67–84.
4. Speckens AM, *et al.*: Cognitive behavioural therapy for medically unexplained physical symptoms: a randomised controlled trail. *BMJ* 1995, **311**:1328–1332.

Pharyngitis

Diagnosis

Symptoms

Sore throat: with difficulty swallowing.
Concurrent coryza, laryngitis, productive cough: suggesting viral cause.
Malaise, fever, headache: common.

Signs

General

Injected mucous membranes of pharynx, tonsils, conjunctivae, and tympanic membranes.
Enlarged tonsils: sometimes with exudates.
Enlarged cervical lymph nodes.

Streptococcal infection

Grey exudates in tonsillar follicles.
Enlarged injected tonsillar and peritonsillar area.
Coated tongue with fetor.
Enlarged, tender cervical nodes.
Occasional meningismus.
Diffuse punctate erythema, flushed cheeks, circumoral pallor, reddened mucous membrane, white then red strawberry tongue: signs of scarlet fever.

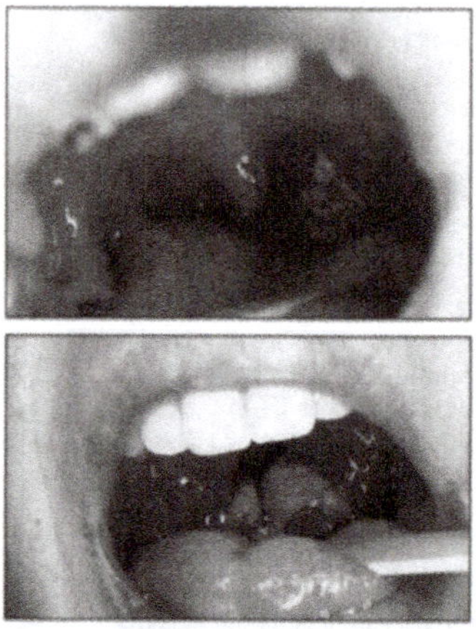

Streptococcal follicular tonsillar exudates (*top*) and confluent exudates (*bottom*) in infectious mononucleosis. (*See* Color Plates.)

Infectious mononucleosis

Prolonged fever: often for 10–14 days.
Nasal voice/"fish mouth" breathing.
Enlarged lymph nodes and splenomegaly.
Palatal petechiae and clean tongue.
Enlarged tonsils: sometimes almost meeting in middle, with confluent white exudates.
Faint maculopapular rash.

Coxsackie A virus

5–10 small aphthoid ulcers: scattered over oral cavity.
Firm vesicular lesions: along sides of fingers and on feet (usually few).
Papular lesions: especially on feet and lower legs, occasionally up to buttocks.

Diphtheria

Toxic, listless, tachycardia due to myocarditis: fever usually low-grade or nonexistent.
Adherent whitish membrane: spreading from tonsils to oropharynx or oral cavity.
Enlarged anterior cervical lymph nodes: with surrounding edema.

Investigations

Throat swab: to check for streptococcal infection and diphtheria; usually not needed for viral infections. Rapid streptococcal test.
Differential leukocyte count: elevated neutrophil leukocytosis indicates streptococcal infection; elevated, many atypical mononuclear cells indicate infectious mononucleosis.
Serology: for Epstein–Barr virus, mycoplasma.

Complications

Peritonsillar abscess, reactive phenomena (rheumatic fever, glomerulonephritis, erythema nodosum, Henoch–Schönlein purpura): with streptococcal infection.
Respiratory obstruction, hepatitis, splenic rupture: with infectious mononucleosis.
Nerve palsies, myocarditis: with diphtheria.
Erythema multiforme: with *Mycoplasma pneumoniae* infection.

Differential diagnosis

- Differential diagnosis depends on the underlying cause.

Etiology [1]

- Causes include the following:

Pharyngitis with nonspecific features
Viral infection, especially adenoviruses, enteroviruses, influenza or parainfluenza virus, Epstein–Barr virus, coronavirus.
Beta-hemolytic *Streptococcus pyogenes* group A, C, or G.
M. pneumoniae, Corynebacterium diphtheriae, Neisseria gonorrhoeae.

Pharyngitis with clinically recognizable features
Streptococcus pyogenes infection: cause of follicular tonsillitis, scarlet fever.
Epstein–Barr virus infection: cause of infectious mononucleosis.
Coxsackievirus infection: cause of hand, foot, and mouth disease (A16), herp-angina (A).
C. diphtheriae infection: cause of diphtheria.

Epidemiology

- Very common disease of adults and children.
- Adenoviral infection is the most common viral type identified in children with respiratory illnesses, which are more prevalent in crowded conditions.
- Enteroviral infection usually occurs in late summer or early autumn, with one or two types dominating (out of >70).
- Some influenza virus activity is usual each winter, with some larger outbreaks.
- Epstein–Barr virus circulates throughout childhood but is usually only manifest symptomatically in teenagers and young adults.
- Streptococcal infection occurs in late winter and early spring, especially in school children.
- Very few cases of diphtheria occur in the United States each year.

Treatment

Diet and lifestyle

• Infants should be breast-fed and subsequently provided with adequate nutrition throughout childhood.

• Respiratory secretions must be disposed of hygienically.

Pharmacological treatment [2]

• Immunization should be given as nationally recommended: *e.g.*, against diphtheria, influenza A.

• Symptomatic treatment is indicated for presumed viral infections: *e.g.*, throat lozenges, acetaminophen.

Antibiotics

• Penicillins are effective against streptococcal and diphtherial infections [3,4].

Standard dosage	Penicillin G, 1.2 MU i.m. Phenoxymethylpenicillin, 500 mg orally every 6 hours.
Contraindications	Hypersensitivity.
Special points	Erythromycin, 250 mg every 6 hours, or new macrolides are other options.
Main drug interactions	None.
Main side effects	Sensitivity reactions, diarrhea.

Antitoxin

• Antitoxin should be given immediately on clinical suspicion of diphtheria.

Standard dosage	Antitoxin 20 000–100 000 units i.v. (depending on disease severity).
Contraindications	Hypersensitivity (epinephrine should be available).
Special points	Test dose is needed before full dose because of equine origin of antitoxin.
Main drug interactions	None.
Main side effects	Sensitivity reactions, including serum sickness.

Alternative medicine

Recommended use: Purple coneflower (*Echinacea* spp.).

Common use: hyssop (*Hyssopus officinalis*); sage (*Salvia officinalis*); Lady's mantle (*Alchemilla vulgaris*); pokeroot (*Phytolacca americana*); coltsfoot (*Tussilago farfara*).

Caution: none.

Treatment aims

To provide symptomatic relief.
To reduce infectivity.
To prevent rheumatic fever (in streptococcal infections).
To neutralize circulating toxins of diphtheria promptly.

Other treatments

Drainage of peritonsillar abscess, indicated by marked inferior and posterior displacement of tonsil.
Tracheostomy for respiratory obstruction.
Tonsillectomy in children with recurrent tonsillitis that disrupts schooling.

Prognosis

• Full rapid recovery is usual.
• Occasionally, patients suffer from post-viral fatigue, especially after influenza, Epstein–Barr, or enteroviral infections.
• Mortality from diphtheria is 5%–10%; survivors usually recover completely.

Follow-up and management

• Patients who have apparently recovered from streptococcal tonsillitis may continue to have enlarged and tender cervical nodes that subsequently spread infection as cellulitis or septicemia.
• Patients with diphtheria should be followed up after 2–6 weeks for late nerve palsies and myocarditis.

Notification

• Diphtheria and scarlet fever are legally notifiable diseases in the United States.

Key references

1. McIsaac WJ, Gael V, Slaughter PM, *et al.*: Reconsidering sore throats: problems with current clinical practice. *Can Fam Physician* 1997, **43**:485–493.
2. Carroll K, Reimer L: Microbiology and laboratory diagnosis of upper respiratory infections. *Clin Infect Dis* 1996, **23**:442–448.
3. Kline JA, Runge JW: Streptococcal pharyngitis: a review of pathophysiology, diagnosis, and management. *J Emerg Med* 1994, **12**:665–680.
4. Blumer JL, Goldfarb J: Meta-analysis in the evaluation of treatment for streptococcal pharyngitis: a review. *Clin Ther* 1994, **16**:604–620.

Diagnosis

Symptoms

Palpable swelling in the soft tissue overlying the sacrococcygeal junction.

Pain.

Drainage.

Fevers, symptoms of systemic infection: unusual.

Signs

Midline localized inflammation, most commonly in the region internatal or gluteal cleft.

Possible abscess formation.

Sinus tract: directed cephalad.

Absence of perianal inflammation or other signs of a perianal fistula.

Investigations

Careful digital rectal examination and, if necessary, anoscopy: to exclude perianal inflammation or communication with the anorectum.

Complications

Chronic abscess.

Persistent or recurrent cellulitis.

Sepsis and/or osteomyelitis: rare.

Squamous cell carcinoma: rare.

Differential diagnosis

Perianal fistula/abscess.

Hidradenitis suppurativa.

Carbuncle or furuncle.

Osteomyelitis.

Etiology

Acquired process from torsion on hair growing in the gluteal cleft resulting in folliculitis and sinus formation.

- Risk factors include family predisposition, prolonged sitting, obesity.

Epidemiology

- Incidence is 26 cases per 100 000.
- It is most common in the third decade and rarely occurs preadolescence.
- Male:female ratio is 3:1.

Treatment

Diet and lifestyle

• Patients with recurrent problems benefit from shaving the hairs in the sacrococcygeal region.

Pharmacological treatment

Cellulitis should be treated with a course of antibiotics that will cover *Staphylococcus* and *Bacteroides* spp. (*e.g.*, Augmentin).

Standard dosage	Augmentin, 500 mg every 8 hours for 10 days.
Contraindications	Penicillin allergy.
Main side effects	Antibiotic-related diarrhea.

Treatment aims

To relieve pain.

To control infection.

To prevent recurrence.

Other treatments

• Patients with tender, localized nodules are best treated by surgical drainage rather than antibiotics.

• Definitive surgical management with resection of midline holes and pits that sustain abscesses is necessary in patients with recurrent disease.

• Sclerosing therapy is occasionally used to manage recurrent disease.

Prognosis

• 80% of patients are successfully treated long-term with simple drainage procedures.

Follow-up and management

• As noted earlier, removal of hair by shaving the sacrococcygeal region of the natal cleft probably reduces the recurrence of the disease.

General references

Armstrong JH, Barcia PJ: Pilonidal sinus disease: the conservative approach. *Arch Surg* 1994, **129**:914–918.

Barnett JL: Anorectal disease. In *Textbook of Gastroenterology*, edn 3. Edited by Yamada T. Philadelphia: Lippincott Williams & Wilkins; 1999:2083–2106.

Sebastian MW: Pilonidal cysts and sinuses. In *Textbook of Surgery*, edn 15. Edited by Sabiston DC, Jr. Philadelphia: WB Saunders; 1996:1330–1334.

Platelet disorders

Diagnosis

Symptoms

• Platelet disorders may be manifest by bleeding or discovered incidentally in an otherwise asymptomatic patient.

Bruising.

Bleeding: usually mucosal, *e.g.*, gingival, nasal, gastrointestinal, menorrhagic; occasionally retinal (loss of vision) or intracranial (headache); after surgical procedures.

Deafness: in some familial disorders.

Signs

Petechiae, purpura, bruises.

Retinal hemorrhages.

Thrombosis and skin microinfarcts: in thrombotic thrombocytopenic purpura.

Capillary bleeding.

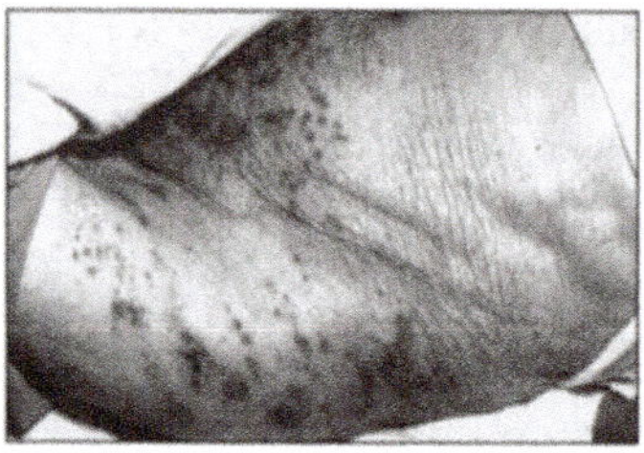

Purpura due to thrombocytopenia. (*See* Color Plate.)

Investigations

• Initial investigations are used to identify primary platelet disorder and to exclude von Willebrand's disease in patients with a strong family history and lifelong bleeding disorder.

Complete blood count: platelet count and mean platelet volume, to exclude other hematological disease and pseudothrombocytopenia due to clumping or EDTA (ethylene- diaminetetra-acetic acid)-induced aggregation.

Microscopic examination of film: for platelet morphology, to detect erythrocyte or leukocyte abnormality.

Coagulation screening: to exclude primary coagulopathy.

Biochemistry profiles: to identify renal or hepatic disease.

Platelet function tests: bleeding time, if prolonged, suggests platelet function disorder or von Willebrand's disease (drugs that affect platelet function, *e.g.*, aspirin, should be avoided for 10 days before testing); spontaneous in vitro aggregation and response to ADP (adenosine diphosphate), collagen, and ristocetin should be recorded; if abnormal, response to other agonists (*e.g.*, epinephrine, thrombin, arachidonate) should be assessed; release reaction of radiolabeled 5-HT (5-hydroxytryptamine); measurement of platelet adenine nucleotides; hereditary and some acquired platelet disorders have characteristic aggregation responses.

Bone-marrow aspiration and biopsy: in most patients with thrombocytopenia, to assess number and structure of megakaryocytes and bone-marrow function.

Platelet serology: in posttransfusion purpura and in neonates with alloimmune thrombocytopenia, to identify specific antiplatelet antigen antibodies.

Platelet-associated immunoglobulin measurement: nonspecific, often increases in immune thrombocytopenias.

Flow cytometry: to quantify platelet membrane glycoproteins, using monoclonal antibodies to detect hereditary disorders.

Complications

Iron-deficiency anemia: caused by menorrhagia or recurrent epistaxis or gastrointestinal bleeding.

Neurological impairment or death: caused by intracranial bleeding.

Differential diagnosis

Bleeding disorders

Von Willebrand's disease.
Fibrinogen disorders.

Purpura

Vasculitis: *e.g.*, Henoch-Schönlein syndrome.
Amyloid.
Senile purpura.
Scurvy.
Steroid treatment.
Collagen disorders (*e.g.*, Ehlers–Danlos syndrome).
Hereditary hemorrhagic telangiectasia (does not cause purpura but can lead to low platelet count in extreme forms).

Etiology [1,2]

Decreased production

Bone-marrow failure: leukemia, metastatic tumor, idiopathic aplasia, infiltration, abnormal production, myelodysplasia, aplastic anemia, drugs (predictable, *e.g.*, cytotoxic drugs, or idiosyncratic reactions).

Increased consumption

Immune: autoimmune (idiopathic, post-viral, HIV, associated with other autoimmune disorders), alloimmune against platelet-specific antigens, *e.g.*, HPA-1.
Drugs: *e.g.*, quinine, heparin, sulfonamides, rifampin.
Coagulopathy: disseminated intravascular coagulation, thrombotic thrombocytopenic purpura.
Hypersplenism and splenomegaly.

Hereditary

Platelet membrane glycoprotein abnormalities, e.g., Bernard-Soulier and Glanzmann's diseases.
Platelet storage pool abnormalities.
Other abnormalities, e.g., May–Hegglin anomaly.

Acquired

Platelet storage pool defects: *e.g.*, aspirin, uremia, ethanol, cirrhosis, myeloproliferative disorders.

Epidemiology

• Acquired disorders of platelet function are common and are associated with disorders such as chronic renal failure or the ingestion of aspirin.

• Chronic idiopathic thrombocytopenic purpura is relatively common (one group suggests that 0.18% of patients admitted to hospital in a 10-year period had the disease).

Treatment

Diet and lifestyle

• Patients should avoid trauma and contact sports.

Pharmacological treatment

For immune thrombocytopenia [3,4]

• In children, the onset is usually acute and often follows a viral infection; spontaneous recovery is common, and treatment is given to those with severe or life-threatening bleeding to elevate the platelet count. In adults, the onset is more insidious, and the condition almost never remits spontaneously.

Standard dosage	*Children:* immunoglobulin, 0.4 g/kg i.v.daily (in 4–6 hours) for 5 days (sometimes 1.0 g/kg daily for 2 days); or prednisone, 1 mg/kg. *Adults:* prednisone, 1 mg/kg daily initially until maximum response, then tapered off.
Contraindications	*Prednisone:* active infection, diabetes mellitus.
Main drug interactions	*See manufacturer's current prescribing information.*
Main side effects	*Immunoglobulin:* headache, hypertension, tachycardia. *Prednisone:* hypertension, diabetes mellitus, osteoporosis.

• Adults who do not respond or who relapse when steroids are reduced should be considered for splenectomy.

• Other treatments for adults in whom steroids or splenectomy fails include i.v. immunoglobulin, azathioprine, vinca alkaloids, danazol, high-dose dexamethasone, or vitamin C.

For platelet functional defects [5]

• Bleeding tendency is often mild, and specific treatment is needed for major hemorrhage or to cover surgical procedures. Antifibrinolytic agents may be helpful to control minor bleeding; antiovulatory treatment may be needed for menorrhagia.

Standard dosage	One donor platelet pack/10 kg body weight or one platelet pheresis pack should raise the platelet count. DDAVP, 0.4 μg/kg i.v. in 100 mL 0.9% saline solution in 15–20 minutes. Tranexamic acid, 0.5–1.0 g 3 times daily orally or i.v. Aminocaproic acid, 2–4 g 4 times daily orally.
Contraindications	*DDAVP:* coronary artery disease. *Tranexamic acid and aminocaproic acid:* history of thromboembolism and hematuria.
Special points	*DDAVP:* ineffective in Glanzmann's thrombasthenia.
Main drug interactions	*See manufacturer's current prescribing information.*
Main side effects	*Platelet transfusion:* allergic reactions, HLA or alloimmunization in multitransfused patients; hepatitis B (rare) or C virus transmission. *DDAVP:* nausea, tremor, vomiting, angina, myocardial infarction. *Tranexamic acid:* nausea, vomiting, diarrhea.

For bone-marrow disorders

• The risk of spontaneous hemorrhage increases when the platelet count is $<10 \times 10^9$/L. Prophylactic platelet transfusions are given to maintain the count above this level during the treatment of acute leukemia or aplastic anemia or during bone-marrow transplantation.

• In chronic thrombocytopenia due to bone-marrow failure, platelet transfusions are given for symptomatic bleeding.

For thrombotic thrombocytopenic purpura [6]

Supportive therapy of medical complications, *e.g.*, hemodialysis. Plasma exchange with fresh frozen plasma replacement (1.5 times plasma volume) for 7 days. Additional treatments include aspirin, dipyridamole, methylprednisone, and vincristine.

For alloimmune thrombocytopenia, neonatal and posttransfusion

Antigen-negative platelet transfusion, i.v. immunoglobulin, prednisone, or plasma exchange.

Treatment aims

To cure or alleviate symptoms.

Other treatments

• Splenectomy is indicated for immune thrombocytopenia in those >6 y).

• Vaccination by Pneumovax and against *H. influenzae* type b and *N. meningitidis* serogroups A and C should be given 1–2 weeks before surgery.

Lifelong antipneumococcal prophylaxis is recommended for patients who have had splenectomy.

Prognosis

• Up to 90% of children with idiopathic thrombocytopenic purpura remit spontaneously, with 50% recovering in 1 month.

• 80% of adults with idiopathic thrombocytopenic purpura remit after treatment by steroids alone or after splenectomy.

• In patients with acquired platelet function defects, prognosis related to underlying disease.

• Mortality in patients with untreated thrombotic thrombocytopenic purpura is up to 90%; 60%–80% respond to treatment.

• Alloimmune thrombocytopenias are self-limiting but potentially fatal.

Follow-up and management

• Frequency depends on the clinical severity and stability of underlying disorder.

Key references

1. George JN, Shattil SJ: The clinical importance of acquired abnormalities of platelet function. *N Engl J Med* 1991, **324**:27–38.
2. George JN, Raskob GE: Idiopathic thrombocytopenic purpura: a concise summary of the pathophysiology and diagnosis in children and adults. *Semin Hematol* 1998, **35(Suppl 1)**:5–8.
3. Tarantino MD, Goldsmith G: Treatment of acute immune thrombocytopenic purpura. *Semin Hematol* 1998, **35(Suppl 1)**:28–35.
4. Blanchette V, Freedman J, Garvey B: Management of chronic immune thrombocytopenic purpura in children and adults. *Semin Hematol* 1998, **35(Suppl 1)**:36–51.
5. Bolan CD, Alving BM: Pharmacologic agents in the management of bleeding disorders. *Transfusion* 1990, **30**:541–551.
6. Kwaan HC, Soff GA: Management of thrombotic thrombocytopenic purpura and hemolytic uremic syndrome. *Semin Hematol* 1997, **34**:159–166.

Pleural effusion

Diagnosis

Symptoms

• Patients are often asymptomatic if the effusion is small.

Breathlessness.

Chest pain: increased on deep inspiration or movement.

Positional discomfort or pain: with large effusions, causing mediastinal shift.

Symptoms of underlying disease.

Fever.

Signs

• Signs are clinically detectable only if the volume is ≥300 mL; loculated effusion may be very difficult to detect.

Decreased movement of chest wall on affected side.

Dullness to percussion.

Absent breath sounds in area of dullness.

Occasional bronchial breathing at upper margin of area of dullness.

Displaced trachea: large effusions only.

Decreased tactile tremitus.

Investigations [1,2]

Chest radiography: to assess extent of effusion and free-flowing character.

Ultrasonography: if doubt about nature of shadowing and to define loculated area for aspiration.

Aspiration: for cytology, Gram stain and Ziehl-Neelsen stain for acid-fast bacilli, culture, protein content, lactate dehydrogenase (LDH), cell count and differential, pH, glucose.

• Comparison of pleural protein content and LDH to plasma protein and LDH is essential to distinguish between transudative and exudative effusions [3].

Pleural biopsy: in experienced hands, much more reliable for diagnosis of tuberculosis and malignancy than simple aspiration.

Repeat radiography: after drainage of effusion, to visualize underlying lung.

Thoracoscopy: if doubt remains, to obtain better samples for histology.

CT: for visualizing loculated effusions and pleural and parenchymal disease.

Complications

Constrictive fibrosis of pleura and restricted lung function: caused by empyema and postpneumonic effusions.

Iatrogenic secondary infection.

Iatrogenic pneumothorax.

Unilateral pulmonary edema: after injudiciously rapid drainage (rare).

Hemorrhage: damage to intercostal vessels, especially after pleural biopsy.

Differential diagnosis

Infections: postpneumonic, tuberculosis.

Inflammation: pancreatitis, rheumatoid arthritis, SLE, polyarteritis nodosa.

Primary malignancy: mesothelioma.

Secondary malignancy: bronchogenic carcinoma, metastatic spread (especially breast, stomach, pancreas), lymphoma.

Infarction secondary to pulmonary embolism.

Etiology

Exudates

Unknown in ~20%, despite extensive investigation.

Infections: viral pleurisy, bacterial pneumonia, tuberculosis, empyema.

Secondary malignancy or secondary cancer (*e.g.*, lung, breast, stomach), leukemia or lymphoma.

Vascular: pulmonary infarction, pulmonary embolism.

Collagen disorders: rheumatoid arthritis.

Primary pleural malignancy (mesothelioma).

Uremia, chylothorax.

Transudates

Congestive heart failure, hypoalbuminemia (nephrotic syndrome and hepatic cirrhosis), constrictive pericarditis, pulmonary embolism.

Peritoneal dialysis.

Epidemiology

• Pleural effusion is frequently found with lung cancer and pneumonia.

• Tuberculosis is declining in importance but remains one of the most common causes of pleural effusion worldwide.

• Mesothelioma is rare. It is associated with asbestos exposure.

Treatment

Diet and lifestyle

• No special precautions are necessary.

Pharmacological treatment

Principles

• The principal aim is to treat any underlying cause and to treat the local problem by drainage.

• For transudates, the underlying disease must be treated.

• For infective causes (empyema, pneumonia), systemic antibiotics are indicated and intercostal drainage is essential; surgical drainage and decortication of pleura can be done if thick pleural rind develops.

• For tuberculosis, standard oral antituberculosis chemotherapy is indicated. The effusion should be aspirated to dryness. Tube drainage and surgery should be avoided if possible. *See* Tuberculosis, pulmonary *for details.*

• For malignant effusions, pleural effusion indicates inoperability; treatment is guided by symptoms. Intermittent aspiration is usually helpful. Tube drainage is the best method of preventing recurrence and achieving pleurodesis. In mesothelioma, tube drainage is best avoided if possible because of the risk of seeding tube tract [4,5].

• For noninfective nonmalignant causes, the effusion should be drained to dryness and followed with repeated chest radiographs.

• Pulmonary infarcts usually resolve without needing drainage, but formal anticoagulation with warfarin is usually appropriate (*see* Pulmonary embolism *for details*).

Chemical pleurodesis [5,6]

• Chemical pleurodesis is best done by specialists, who can consider the advantages and disadvantages in each individual case. It is usually reserved for malignant pleural effusions.

• Although many different agents ranging from antibiotics to antiseptics to antineoplastics to talc have been advocated, none is ideal.

• The agent most commonly used is talc. It may be insufflated via thoracoscopy or instilled as a slurry.

• Other approaches include the following:

Standard dosage	Doxycycline, 500 mg, or minocycline, 300 mg in 50 mL saline, after pleural fluid has been drained. A second dose may be given after 72 hours. Bleomycin, 60 U is an alternative for malignant effusions.
Contraindications	Transudate, bronchopleural fistulas, infection.
Main drug interactions	None.
Main side effects	Local pain, transient fever, hypersensitivity reaction.

Treatment aims

To achieve resolution of pleural effusion without residual fibrosis or functional deficit.

Prognosis

• Prognosis varies widely according to the underlying cause.

• If cleared by drainage, most bacterial effusions resolve, leaving some pleural scarring, which may need surgery if severe.

• Malignant effusions have poor prognosis, and treatment is mainly palliative, guided by symptoms.

Follow-up and management

• Serial chest radiographs should be taken, usually at 4–6-week intervals to assess recurrence.

• Lung function tests are needed to assess residual restrictive deficit if radiographic changes persist.

Key references

1. Collins TR, Sahn SA: Thoracentesis: complications, patient experience and diagnostic value. *Chest* 1987, **91**:817–819.
2. Bone R: The techniques of diagnostic and therapeutic thoracentesis. *J Crit Illness* 1990, **5**:371–379.
3. Light R, *et al.*: Pleural effusions: the diagnostic separation of transudates and exudates. *Ann Intern Med* 1972, **77**:507–513.
4. Keller SM: Current and future therapy for malignant pleural effusion. *Chest* 1993, **103(suppl)**:635–675.
5. Sahn S: Pleural effusion in lung cancer. *Clin Chest Med* 1993, **14**:189–200.
6. Light RW, Vargas FS: Pleural sclerosis for the treatment of pneumothorax and pleural effusion. *Lung* 1997, **175**:213–223.

Pneumocystis carinii pneumonia in AIDS

Diagnosis

Symptoms

Fever, fatigue, weight loss: for weeks before respiratory symptoms develop.

Nonproductive cough, shortness of breath: initially on exertion, then at rest with disease progression.

• The absence of respiratory symptoms does not exclude *Pneumocystis carinii* pneumonia.

Signs

Tachypnea, rales without consolidation: revealed by auscultation, but often no pulmonary abnormalities.

Investigations

• *P. carinii* pneumonia occurs in HIV-infected individuals who have a CD4 lymphocyte count $<200 \times 10^6$/L.

Complete blood count: to exclude anemia.

Plain chest radiography: may show diffuse interstitial infiltration; various other appearances, including lobar infiltrate cavity or pneumothorax, occur. Chest radiograph may be normal early in the course of the infection.

Arterial oxygen tension measurement: hypoxia commonly occurs.

Exercise oximetry: a useful noninvasive test.

Sputum analysis: obviates need for routine bronchoscopy if laboratory is experienced; sputum induced by inhaled nebulized hypertonic saline solution; samples stained by Grocott or immunofluorescent stains.

Fiberoptic bronchoscopy: reserved for patients whose induced sputum test results are not diagnostic.

Complications

Pneumothorax.

Restrictive lung disease.

Extrapulmonic *P. carinii* infection.

Acute respiratory distress syndrome.

Differential diagnosis

Bacterial pneumonia.

Pulmonary Kaposi's sarcoma.

Pulmonary tuberculosis.

Toxoplasmosis.

Pulmonary lymphoma.

Asthma.

Cytomegalovirus pneumonitis.

Lipid interstitial pneumonitis.

Histoplasmosis.

Aspergillosis.

Etiology

• The pneumonia is caused by infection by *P. carinii*.

• Acquisition may be common early in life (and controlled by the immune system) or occur shortly before the disease develops.

Epidemiology

• Most children have serological evidence of previous *P. carinii* infection by the age of 4 years; the disease was first recognized because of epidemics in orphanages after World War II.

• The disease is the most common AIDS opportunistic infection in people with HIV-induced immunosuppression, with no difference between genders or among races, although it occurs significantly less often in many developing countries.

Treatment

Diet and lifestyle

Not applicable.

Pharmacological treatment

Treatment of the disease

• The most effective agent is trimethoprim-sulfamethoxazole (TMP-SMX); in less severely ill patients, oral treatment may be used.

• Unfortunately, many patients are unable to complete a treatment course because of allergic or toxic side effects.

• Alternative treatment in bactrim-intolerant individuals with mild to moderate disease includes clindamycin and primaquine, or trimethoprim and dapsone or atovoguore. For patients with severe infection, the alternates to bactrim are pentamidine and trimetrexate.

• Corticosteroids have been shown to reduce mortality and the risk of respiratory failure in patients presenting with partial arterial oxygen pressure <70 mmHg.

Standard dosage	TMP-SMX, 15 mg/kg daily, given in 3 divided doses.
Contraindications	Hypersensitivity.
Special points	Full blood count, U&E monitoring, and liver function tests must be done.
Main drug interactions	None.
Main side effects	Nausea and vomiting (antiemetic can be given), skin rash, leukopenia, thrombocytopenia, raised liver function tests.

Prophylaxis

• Primary prophylaxis is recommended in patients with clinical evidence of immunosuppression (*e.g.*, buccal candidiasis) or other opportunistic infections or laboratory evidence (CD4 count $<200 \times 10^6$/L).

• Secondary prophylaxis should be offered to patients who have had previous episodes of *P. carinii* pneumonia.

Standard dosage	TMP-SMX, 1 tablet daily. Alternatively, dapsone, 100 mg daily, or pentamidine, 300 mg inhaled every month.
Contraindications	Allergy to sulfonamides or trimethoprim.
Special points	TMP-SMX may also reduce the incidence of subsequent toxoplasmosis and bacterial infection.
Main drug interactions	None.
Main side effects	Skin rash, nausea and vomiting, leukopenia, thrombocytopenia, raised liver function tests.

Treatment aims

To treat pneumonia.

To suppress future infection.

Prognosis

• Mortality for the first episode of *P. carinii* pneumonia is <10% but is higher for subsequent attacks.

Follow-up and management

• Complete blood count should be done after treatment because anemia is common.

• Patients should be followed up at least monthly.

General references

Masur H: Prevention and treatment of Pneumocystis pneumonia. *N Engl J Med* 1992, **327**:1853–1860.

Moe AA, Hardy WD: *Pneumocystis carinii* infection in the HIV-seropositive patient. *Infect Dis Clin North Am* 1994, **8**:331–364.

Murray JF: Pulmonary complications of HIV infection. *Am Rev Med* 1996, **47**:117–126.

Santamauro JT, Stover DE: *Pneumocystis carinii* pneumonia. *Med Clin North Am* **81**:299–318.

Pneumonia

Diagnosis

Symptoms

Common

- Onset may be abrupt or over days.

Cough: with sputum, which may be purulent, in two-thirds of patients.

Fever: possibly with rigors and diaphoresis.

Pleuritic chest pain: occasionally.

Dyspnea.

Less common

Hemoptysis, vomiting, diarrhea, myalgia.

Mental confusion: especially in patients with severe pneumonia and in elderly patients.

Signs

Fever.

Mental confusion, cyanosis, hypotension: suggesting severe illness.

Increased respiratory rate: suggesting severe illness.

Dullness on percussion.

Increased vocal fremitus.

Crackles.

Bronchial breathing: egobronchophony and whispering pectoriloquy; in one-third of patients.

Investigations [1]

To confirm diagnosis

Chest radiography: shows consolidation or infiltrates.

To assess severity

Arterial blood gas analysis: low partial oxygen pressure, raised partial carbon dioxide pressure, low pH.

Complete blood count: leukocytosis with left shift (leukocyte count <4 or $>20 \times 10^9$/L indicates high risk).

To assess cause

Blood culture: for bacteremia.

Sputum Gram stain and culture: to exclude *Legionella* and *Pneumocystis* spp. and mycobacteria.

Pleural-fluid Gram stain and culture: if fluid present.

Serology: acute and convalescent sera for antibodies to viruses, chlamydia, mycoplasma, *Coxiella* spp., and legionella.

Bronchoscopy: often needed in immunocompromised patients but rarely in others.

Complications

Empyema, lung abscess, pulmonary embolus, acute respiratory distress syndrome.

Acute renal failure, hemolysis.

Sepsis.

Death: especially in the elderly, often despite appropriate therapy.

Differential diagnosis

Pulmonary edema.

Exacerbation of chronic bronchitis.

Pulmonary embolus.

Lung cancer.

Etiology [2,3]

- Pneumococcal infection is the cause of 50%–80% of community-acquired pneumonias.
- Gram-negative organisms (*e.g.*, *Escherichia coli* and *Pseudomonas* spp.) are the cause of 50% or more of nosocomial pneumonias.
- Anaerobic bacteria (*e.g.*, bacteroides) are important in aspiration pneumonia.
- Immunocompromised patients may be infected by a huge range of microorganisms, *e.g.*, unusual bacteria and fungi, many of which would not cause infection in immunocompetent patients.

Epidemiology [3]

- Pneumonia occurs at all ages but is most frequent in very young and very old patients.
- Primary care physicians see on average 10 cases annually.
- One patient in every five seen needs hospital admission.
- Most cases occur in the winter months.
- Mycoplasma infection affects mainly teenagers and young adults.
- Legionella infection may occur in epidemics related to water systems in buildings.

Classification

Community-acquired pneumonia.

Nosocomial pneumonia.

Aspiration pneumonia: caused by inhalation of oropharyngeal secretions, during vomiting, or when consciousness is depressed.

Immunocompromised pneumonia: *e.g.*, with HIV infection, organ transplantation, cytotoxic chemotherapy.

Treatment

Diet and lifestyle

• Smoking and smoking-related diseases are a major risk factor for pneumonia; smoking education is therefore important.

Pharmacological treatment [4,5]

General guidelines

Oxygen: to maintain partial oxygen pressure in arterial blood >60 mm Hg; may cause hypercapnia in patients with chronic obstructive pulmonary disease, so arterial blood gases should be monitored.

Oral or parenteral fluids: to correct dehydration.

Nonsedative analgesia: for pleuritic chest pain.

Physical therapy: especially if large sputum volumes are difficult to expectorate.

Intensive care, including assisted ventilation: valuable for patients in whom respiratory failure worsens despite treatment.

Antibiotics [7]

• Initial treatment must be empirical; this can be modified later if indicated by microbiological results.

• Oral antibiotics are appropriate in mild infection, parenteral if infection is severe or accompanied by vomiting.

• Treatment should be for at least 7 days; severely ill patients need treatment for up to 3 weeks.

For mild community-acquired disease: azithromycin, penicillin, cephalosporin, or erythromycin.

For severe community-acquired disease: 2nd- or 3rd-generation cephalosporin (*e.g.*, cefuroxime), possibly with erythromycin.

For nosocomial infection: 2nd- or 3rd-generation cephalosporin, possibly with aminoglycoside; usually requires 2–3 weeks of therapy.

For aspiration: amoxicillin-clavulanate or clindamycin.

For immunocompromised disease: individually determined by causative pathogen.

Standard dosage	Amoxicillin, 500 mg 3 times daily. Erythromycin, 500 mg 4 times daily. Cefuroxime, 750 mg 3 times daily. Aminoglycoside guided by blood level. Clindamycin, 300 mg 3 times daily.
Contraindications	Hypersensitivity.
Main drug interactions	Warfarin.
Main side effects	Diarrhea.

Prophylaxis

Annual influenza vaccination: for patients >65 years of age or those with chronic heart or lung disease, renal failure, or diabetes mellitus and for immunosuppressed patients.

Pneumococcal vaccination: for patients who are >65 years of age; asplenic; or have sickle cell disease, chronic renal failure, or chronic lung, heart, or liver disease; and those with diabetes mellitus or who are immunocompromised.

Criteria for hospitalization: age >65 years, co-existing illnesses (*e.g.*, diabetes, chronic obstructive pulmonary disease), tachypnea, tachycardia, hypotension, signs of sepsis, leukopenia, or severe leukocytosis.

Treatment aims

To improve oxygenation.

To achieve rapid resolution of pneumonia and return to normal activities.

To prevent death or sepsis.

To relieve symptoms.

Prognosis [6]

• Pyrexia usually settles within 48 hours of starting treatment.

• Lethargy after pneumonia often lasts weeks or months.

• Radiographic shadowing is slow to clear and lags behind clinical recovery.

• Death is unusual in patients managed at home.

• 5%–10% of patients admitted to hospital die.

• Up to 50% reaching intensive care die.

• The mortality in nosocomial pneumonia is up to 30% and may be higher in immunocompromised patients.

Follow-up and management

• Patients should be seen 6 weeks after presentation, and chest radiography repeated to confirm recovery and exclude underlying lung disease, especially lung cancer.

Key references

1. Fine M, Smith D, Singer D: Hospitalization decision in patients with community-acquired pneumonia: a prospective study. *Am J Med* 1990, **89**:713–721.
2. Fang G, *et al.*: New and emerging etiologies for community-acquired pneumonia with implications for therapy. A prospective multicenter study of 359 cases. *Medicine* 1990, **69**:307–316.
3. Bartlett JG, Mundy LM: Community-acquired pneumonia. *N Engl J Med* 1995, **333**:1618–1624.
4. Bartlett JG, Breiman RF, Mandell LA, File TM Jr: Community-acquired pneumonia in adults: guidelines for management. Guidelines from the Infectious Disease Society of America. *Clin Infect Dis* 1998, **26**:811–838.
5. Niederman MS, *et al.*: American Thoracic Society guidelines for the initial management of adults with community-acquired pneumonia: diagnosis, assessment of severity, and initial antimicrobial therapy. *Am Rev Respir Dis* 1993, **148**:1418–1426.
6. Fine MJ, Smith MA, Carson CA, *et. al.*: Prognosis and outcome of patients with community-acquired pneumonia: a meta-analysis. *JAMA* 1996, **275**:134–141.
7. The choice of antibacterial drugs. *Med Lett Drugs Ther* 1999, **41(1064)**:95–104.

Polycystic ovarian syndrome

Diagnosis

Symptoms

Oligomenorrhea or amenorrhea with sometimes heavy menses: endometrium remains estrogenized, in contrast with other causes or anovulation.

Infertility: due to anovulation.

Mild androgenism: hirsutism, acne, seborrhea [1].

Severe virilization (rare): alopecia, voice change, clitoromegaly.

Signs

• The signs associated with polycystic ovarian syndrome are extremely variable; in most women, the endocrine disturbance is subtle and the disorder has no outward signs.

Obesity.

Central adiposity.

Mild hypertension.

Hirsutism: documented by photography or Ferriman–Gallway score [1].

Acanthosis nigricans: feature of severe insulin resistance.

• Abdominal and pelvic examinations are rarely helpful but should be done to exclude ovarian masses.

Investigations [2,3]

• The aims are to make a positive diagnosis, to exclude other causes of anovulation, infertility, recurrent miscarriage and virilization as appropriate, and to screen for insulin resistance or frank diabetes mellitus (type 2).

• Diagnosis of polycystic ovarian syndrome should incorporate both an endocrine and a morphological assessment.

For the disorder

Chronic anovulation, hyperandrogenism: diagnostic criteria.

• The presence or absence of ovarian cysts is an unreliable finding, and not a diagnostic criterion.

To rule out other causes of amenorrhea

Pelvic examination.

Ultrasonography: to examine endometrium, possibly with endometrial biopsy (menstrual disorder); to diagnose ovarian tumors (virilization).

Serum testosterone measurement: tumor more likely if concentrations are markedly elevated.

For cardiovascular risk factors

Blood pressure measurement.

Evidence of insulin resistance or frank diabetes.

Serum lipid measurements.

Complications

Endometrial cancer: despite anovulation, ovaries continue to secrete estradiol.

Diabetes mellitus, myocardial infarction, stroke: related to insulin resistance [4].

Recurrent miscarriages: probably due to elevated androgen levels.

Differential diagnosis

Classic polycystic ovarian syndrome.

Hypothyroidism.

Cushing's syndrome.

Acromegaly.

Androgen-secreting tumor.

Estrogenized amenorrhea.

Granulosa cell tumor.

Etiology [3]

• Excess androgen production is of unclear etiology, often combined with insulin resistance.

Epidemiology [3]

• 10%–20% of apparently normal women are found to have polycystic ovaries on ultrasonography.

• 1% of young women (aged 15–40 years) have clinically evident disease.

• Family studies show the prevalence of polycystic ovaries to be high among asymptomatic close relatives (80%).

• The disease is a factor in ~10% of couples with infertility.

Treatment

Diet and lifestyle

• In view of the increased risk of cardiovascular disease, advice should be given about diet, smoking, lipid management, and exercise.

• A calorie-restricted diet may help by decreasing insulin resistance.

• Women with oligo- or amenorrhea not wishing to conceive should be warned of the small risk of conception.

Pharmacological treatment [3,5]

• Pregnancy must be ruled out before treatment begins.

• Polycystic ovarian syndrome is a diagnosis of exclusion, and other causes of amenorrhea must be investigated and ruled out.

For menstrual disorder

Combined oral contraceptive to improve regularity or reduce flow.

Cyclical progesterone or combined oral contraceptive to prevent endometrial neoplasia in women with oligo- or amenorrhea.

For anovulatory infertility

• Treatment should be carried out in conjunction with an appropriate specialist.

Antiestrogen treatment (clomiphene): acts through the hypothalamus.

Exogenous gonadotropin treatment: involves direct ovarian stimulation with human menopausal gonadotropin (hMG) or human follicle-stimulating hormone (hFSH), with human chorionic gonadotropin (hCG) to trigger ovulation.

Typical dosages	*Antiestrogen:* clomiphene, 100 mg orally daily on days 2–6 of cycle for up to 3 cycles. *Exogenous gonadotropin:* hMG or hFSH, 75 U daily.
Contraindications	Pregnancy, hormone-dependent tumors, undiagnosed abnormal menstruation.
Special points	*Antiestrogen:* near-normal conception rates expected; low risk of high-order multiple pregnancy (8% twin rate) and ovarian hyperstimulation; minimal monitoring needed (midluteal serum progesterone measurement). *Gonadotropin:* risk of multiple pregnancy and ovarian hyperstimulation; detailed monitoring mandatory (serial follicle scanning and estradiol measurement).
Main drug interactions	None.
Main side effects	*Antiestrogen:* hot flushes, mild abdominal discomfort, visual disturbance (rare). *Gonadotropin:* nausea, abdominal discomfort, allergy.

For virilization

Combined oral contraceptive: usual precautions for oral contraceptive use.

Flutamide or spironolactone: both are antiandrogens and may feminize a developing male fetus; therefore, contraception is of critical importance.

Special considerations

• Insulin-sparing agents such as metformin and thiozalidmediones (rosiglitazone and piaglitazone) are being evalutated as treatments for polycystic ovarian syndrome.

Treatment aims

To prevent long-term health risks, particularly those related to diabetes.

To alleviate symptoms.

To restore fertility.

Other treatments

Shaving, bleaching, electrolysis: for hirsutism.

Laparoscopic ovarian surgery: electrodiathermy or laser drilling; 80% ovulation rate; near-normal conception rate; normal twin rate and low miscarriage rate; effect lasts ~9 months on average.

Prognosis

• Acne and seborrhea respond within a few weeks, but the duration of the hair cycle means that improvement in hair growth may take many months.

• Symptoms generally return quickly after withdrawal of treatment.

Follow-up and management

• Follow up varies according to the disorder.

Key references

1. Fox R, *et al.*: Oestrogen and androgen states in oligo-amenorrhoeic women with polycystic ovaries. *Br J Obstet Gynaecol* 1991, **98**:294–299.
2. Fox R, *et al.*: Polycystic ovarian disease: diagnostic methods. *Contemp Rev Obstet Gynaecol* 1992, **4**:84–89.
3. Frank S: Polycystic ovary syndrome. *N Engl J Med* 1995, **333**:853–861.
4. Conway GS, *et al.*: Risk factors for coronary artery disease in lean and obese women with polycystic ovary syndrome. *Clin Endocrinol* 1992, **37**:119–125.
5. Jacobs HS: Polycystic ovary syndrome: aetiology and management. *Curr Opin Obstet Gynecol* 1995, **7**:203–208.

Diagnosis

Symptoms

Polymyalgia rheumatica

Pain and stiffness: bilateral and symmetrical, affecting neck, shoulder, and pelvic girdles; stiffness usually predominant, particularly severe after rest, and may prevent patient getting out of bed [1].

Malaise.

Depression.

Giant-cell arteritis

Headache: in two-thirds or more of patients; severe pain, usually localized in the temple but may be occipital or be less defined and precipitated by brushing the hair [2,3].

Pain on chewing: due to claudication of muscles of mastication, in up to two-thirds of patients.

Visual disturbances: in 25%; visual loss evident in <10%.

Malaise.

Depression.

Scalp tenderness.

Signs

Polymyalgia rheumatica

Unimpaired muscle strength: although pain makes interpretation of muscle testing difficult.

Tenderness of involved structures: with restriction of shoulder movement, if diagnosis delayed [1].

Peripheral synovitis: uncommon and transient.

Giant-cell arteritis

Scalp tenderness: particularly around temporal and occipital arteries; may disturb sleep [2].

Thickened, tender, and nodular arteries: with absent or reduced pulsation.

Partial or complete visual loss: due to anterior ischemic optic neuropathy [2,3].

Investigations

Baseline clinical investigations

• These are used to make the diagnosis and exclude other diagnoses.

ESR measurement: rate usually greatly raised, but can be normal [4].

Acute-phase protein (*e.g.*, CRP) measurement: concentration usually raised.

Complete blood count.

Biochemical profile.

Rheumatoid factor test.

Serum protein electrophoresis.

Thyroid function test.

Chest radiography.

Specific investigations

Temporal artery biopsy: for suspected giant-cell arteritis, not for polymyalgia rheumatica; findings can be focal, may be normal [2].

Segmental: skip areas.

Complications

Visual loss: in up to 10% of patients, permanent blindness in giant-cell arteritis [5]; usually not reversible.

Differential diagnosis

Neoplastic disease.

Joint disease: osteoarthritis (particularly of cervical spine), rheumatoid arthritis, connective tissue disease.

Multiple myeloma.

Leukemia.

Lymphoma.

Muscle disease: polymyositis, myopathy.

Infections: e.g., bacterial endocarditis.

Bone disease: particularly osteomyelitis.

Hypothyroidism.

Parkinsonism.

Depression.

Etiology

• A distinct prodromal event is often noted, resembling influenza, although viral studies are negative.

• HLA-DR4 is increased in both polymyalgia rheumatica and giant-cell arteritis.

• Lymphocytes in arteritic lesions express the T-cell phenotype, and the $CD4^+$ subset predominates.

Epidemiology

• The peak age is 60–75 years.

• The female:male ratio is 3:1.

• The annual incidence of biopsy-positive disease is 6.7 in 100 000 people (16.8 in 100 000 >55 years of age).

• The disease occurs predominantly in northern Europe and northern United States.

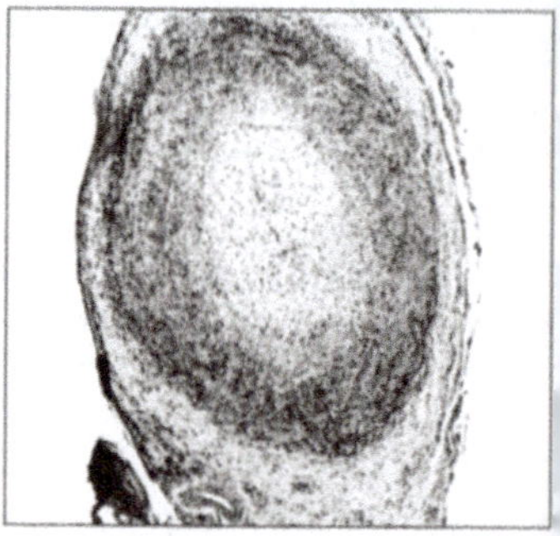

Occlusion of lumen due to intimal proliferation and inflammation of the media.

Treatment

Diet and lifestyle

• No special precautions are necessary.

Pharmacological treatment

• Patients with giant-cell arteritis should be referred as an emergency to a specialist to arrange a biopsy and to initiate treatment.

• Immediate treatment by a systemic corticosteroid has long been recognized as mandatory in patients with giant-cell arteritis in order to prevent serious vascular complications, particularly blindness.

• Corticosteroids are usually also needed for patients with polymyalgia rheumatica.

• Many patients remain on treatment for years.

• Methotrexate may be helpful in select patients as a steroid-sparing agent.

For polymyalgia rheumatica

Standard dosage	Prednisolone, 10–20 mg initially for 1 month, reduced by 2.5 mg every 2 weeks to 10 mg daily, then 1 mg daily every 2–4 weeks; maintenance dose 5–7 mg daily for 6–12 months; final reduction, 1 mg every 4 weeks [6].
Contraindications	Systemic infections; caution in pregnancy, hypertension, diabetes mellitus, osteoporosis, glaucoma, epilepsy, peptic ulceration.
Special points	In patients whose prednisolone dosage cannot be reduced because of recurring symptoms or who develop serious steroid-related side effects, azathioprine has been shown to have a modest steroid-sparing effect, and methotrexate may be more effective [7].
Main drug interactions	Rifampin and phenytoin reduce corticosteroid concentrations; anticoagulant dosage may need adjustment; reduced effect of NSAIDs.
Main side effects	Weight gain, edema, increased intraocular pressure, cataracts, glaucoma, gastrointestinal disturbances, peptic ulceration, diabetes, osteoporosis, skin atrophy [8].

For giant-cell arteritis without visual symptoms

Prednisolone, 40–60 mg daily initially for 8 weeks, reduced by 5 mg every 2 weeks to 10 mg daily; then as for polymyalgia rheumatica [9,10].

For giant-cell arteritis with possible or definite ocular involvement

Prednisolone, 60–80 mg daily initially for 8 weeks, reduced to 20 mg daily over next 4 weeks; then as for uncomplicated giant-cell arteritis [9,10].

Treatment aims

To relieve pain and symptoms.

To reduce the incidence of complications.

Prognosis

• Untreated, patients have prolonged ill health, and up to 20% of those with giant-cell arteritis go blind or develop vascular complications.

• Treated, between one-third and one-half of patients can discontinue treatment after 2 years.

Follow-up and management

• Treatment is monitored clinically and by acute-phase response (ESR, CRP).

• Long-term low-dose maintenance prednisolone ≤3 mg, is sometimes needed.

Key references

1. Lestico MR, *et al.*: Polymyalgia rheumatica. *Clin Pharmacol* 1993, **12**:571–580.
2. Chmelewski WL, *et al.*: Presenting features and outcomes in patients undergoing temporal artery biopsy: a review of 98 patients. *Arch Intern Med* 1992, **152**:1690–1695.
3. Reech KA, *et al.*: Neurologic manifestations of giant cell arteritis. *Am J Med* 1990, **89**:67–72.
4. Kyle V, Cawston TE, Hazleman BL: Erythrocyte sedimentation rate and c reactive protein in the assessment of polymyalgia rheumatica/giant cell arteritis on presentation and during follow-up. *Ann Rheum Dis* 1989, **48**:667–671.
5. Wilke WS, Hoffman GS: Treatment of corticosteroid resistant giant cell arteritis. *Rheum Dis Clin North Am* 1995, **21**:59–71.
6. Kyle V, Hazleman BL: Treatment of polymyalgia rheumatica and giant cell arteritis. I. Steroid regimens in the first two months. *Ann Rheum Dis* 1989, **48**:658–661.
7. Krall PL, Mazanec DJ, Wilke WS: Methotrexate for corticosteroid-resistant polymyalgia rheumatica and giant-cell arteritis. *Cleve Clin J Med* 1989, **56**:253–277.
8. Kyle V, Hazleman BL: Treatment of polymyalgia rheumatica and giant cell arteritis. II. Relation between steroid dose and steroid associated side effects. *Ann Rheum Dis* 1989, **48**:662–666.
9. Behn AR, Perera T, Myles AB: Polymyalgia rheumatica and corticosteroids: how much for how long? *Ann Rheum Dis* 1983, **42**:374–378.
10. Hunder GG: Giant cell arteritis and polymyalgia rheumatica. *Med Clin North Am* 1997, **81**:195–219.

Postpartum depression

Diagnosis

Definition

- Postpartum depression is defined as a new episode of depression in a woman who has been well for at least the previous 6 months, with onset in the first 90 days postpartum.
- The illness may be manifest later in the puerperium.

Symptoms and signs

Postpartum "blues" [1]

- Develops within first 2 weeks after delivery; peak symptoms occur between 3rd and 7th day after delivery.

Insomnia, anxiety, tearfulness, headaches, irritability, appetite changes, feeling overwhelmed and oversensitive.

- Patients do not meet criteria for major depressive disorder (*see* Depression).

Postpartum depression

- It can occur up to 6 months after delivery; severe cases present early (within the first 6 weeks).
- Patients meet criteria for major depressive disorder (*see* Depression), characterized by depressed mood and/or loss of interest in activities; disrupted sleep and early-morning wakening; psychomotor retardation; or overvalued ideas or delusion of unworthiness, incompetence, and guilt; suicidal thoughts.
- Frequent intrusive, obsessional thoughts of failure as a mother or harm coming to the child are common manifestations.

Postpartum psychosis (bipolar or manic-depressive psychosis)

- Onset is abrupt and occurs between days 3 and 16 in most women. Within a week, a diagnosis of acute severe affective psychosis becomes clear.

Perplexity, agitation, confusion (first few days) followed by hallucinations, delusions, emotional and behavioral disturbances: one-third of patients manifest manic symptoms (overactivity, elation, pressure of speech, flight of ideas), two-thirds manifest depressive symptoms (*see* above).

Investigations

- No special clinical investigation is needed beyond the normal physical postpartum investigations, including history, physical examination, and hemoglobin and thyroid-stimulating hormone levels.

Complications

Delayed detection and treatment of severe depression, physical morbidity.

Suicide and infanticide: rare but tragic and often avoidable.

Failure to establish relationship with child.

Removal of child by family or social services.

Lasting problems in child's social, emotional, and cognitive development and physical health.

Marital difficulties.

Differential diagnosis

Transient hypothyroidism or thyrotoxicosis, profound anemia (fatigue), pituitary or adrenal disorders.

Acute confusional state (delirium, organic brain syndrome): rare, caused by infection, eclampsia, or other neurological disorder.

Distress: caused by social, marital, or relationship problems.

Etiology [2]

- Biological and psychological factors are important.
- No evidence suggests that the hormonal profile of mentally ill mothers differs from that of normal women; the postpartum drop to low progesterone concentrations is probably responsible for the "blues."
- Manic-depressive illness in a first-degree relative indicates a 1 in 3 risk for postpartum psychosis.
- Previous postpartum depression indicates a 1 in 3 risk after subsequent deliveries; previous nonpostpartum depression indicates a 1 in 5 risk or higher.
- Infertility, assisted reproduction, previous obstetric loss, or traumatic delivery may contribute to severe depressive illness.
- Marital conflict, social adversity, lack of confidante, single status, low socio-economic status all increase the risk of a mild depressive episode.

Epidemiology

- 85% of new mothers experience a depressed mood after birth.
- 5%–20% of women who deliver develop postpartum depression.
- Two in 1000 women who deliver are admitted to a psychiatric hospital suffering from a postpartum psychosis.

Treatment [3]

Diet and lifestyle [1]

• Counseling expectant mothers and fathers during the prenatal period about the symptoms and prevalence of postpartum depression will better prepare them for their upcoming roles and occupational changes.

• Expectant mothers should be taught to avoid self-blame if they are unable to meet their expanded responsibilities.

• Stress reduction and family therapy may also help women cope with the emotional and physical demands of their families.

Pharmacological treatment

• Women suffering from severe depression, with active suicidal or infanticidal ideation, and with postpartum psychosis should be treated in an inpatient psychiatric unit.

• Most postpartum depressive illnesses can be managed at home if the patient is not suicidal or infanticidal.

Postpartum "blues"

• Brief in-office counseling and supportive therapy are usually sufficient. Women with complicated social situations (*e.g.*, marital relational problems, threats of domestic violence) will benefit from more intense counseling services from a trained therapist.

Postpartum depression

• Most women (~60%) respond satisfactorily to antidepressants, such as selective serotonin reuptake inhibitors (SSRIs) or tricyclic antidepressants (TCAs). Both classes of antidepressants are excreted in breast milk, although concentrations are small for SSRIs. Long-term effects on neonates are unknown. Breast-feeding should either be discontinued (especially TCAs) or timed to avoid peak concentrations (SSRIs).

• Excessive sedation should be avoided because of childcare responsibilities.

• Women should always be referred to a psychiatrist if they are severely distressed, in a state of hopeless despair, or suicidal. *See* Depression *for details.*

Postpartum psychosis

• The immediate priority is to sedate the patient with neuroleptics to a level that makes her safe, allows adequate nutrition, and reduces her agitation, confusion, and fear.

• Treatment often requires both antipsychotic and antidepressant medication.

Standard dosage	Haloperidol, 5–20 mg daily orally for acute psychosis; alternatively risperidone, 1–3 mg twice daily.
Contraindications	*Neuroleptics:* hypersensitivity; caution in cardiovascular disease, hepatic impairment, epilepsy.
Special points	If no response occurs within 7 days, electroconvulsive therapy or lithium carbonate can be tried. Postpartum women are very sensitive to the extrapyramidal side effects of neuroleptic agents; close monitoring is needed. SSRIs and TCAs take effect in 10–14 days. No psychotropic drug is of proven safety in breast-feeding.
Main drug interactions	*Neuroleptics:* antagonize anticonvulsants.
Main side effects	*Neuroleptics:* sedation, extrapyramidal effects, acute dystonias, akasthesia, parkinsonism.

Treatment aims

To provide early detection and prompt treatment in the setting most appropriate for safe recovery.

To give priority to the needs of the baby.

To avoid unnecessary separation of mother and baby.

To provide social and psychological support.

Psychosocial treatment

Adjunctive psychotherapy and specific counseling for all patients.

• Nondirective or cognitive therapy (6 sessions at weekly intervals) is effective for mild depressive illness.

• Practical social support and addressing of concurrent problems are essential.

• Psychosocial treatment is as effective as antidepressants for mild depressive illness.

Prognosis

• With early intervention and effective treatment the prognosis is excellent; improvement begins within 2 weeks and recovery within 6–8 weeks.

• Without treatment the illness may be prolonged, although 60% of patients recover spontaneously within 6 months.

Follow-up and management

• Treatment should continue for at least 6 months after the patient has recovered, longer in the case of a relapse.

• Patients with previous manic-depressive episodes should take lithium or valproic acid.

• For serious mental illness, the risk follows every childbirth: 1 in 3–5 risk of recurrent postpartum depression.

Key references

1. Susman JL: Postpartum depressive disorders. *J Fam Pract* 1996, **43(suppl)**:S17–S24.
2. O'Hara MW: Social support, life events and depression during pregnancy and the peurperium. *Arch Gen Psych* 1986, **43**:569–573.
3. Cooper PJ, *et al.*: Fortnightly review: postnatal depression. *BMJ* 1998, **316**:1884–1886.

Postpoliomyelitis syndrome

Diagnosis

Symptoms

In patients with known prior poliomyelitis infection:

Neuromuscular symptoms such as pain, cramps, myalgia, arthralgia (post-polio syndrome).

Weakness, slowly progressive (54% to 87% previously affected muscles; 33% to 77% previously unaffected), muscle atrophy, fatigue (PPMA).

Lower extremities affected more frequently than upper.

Dysarthria, dyspnea in 42%.

Symptoms begin 20–40 years after initial polio infection.

Signs

In patients with known prior poliomyelitis infection:

Weakness, atrophy, fasciculations.

Hyperreflexia, extensor plantar responses.

Spasticity (rare).

Sensation should be unaffected.

Investigations

Electromyography: confirm denervation in affected, unaffected muscles, find evidence (giant motor units) of prior polio, and exclude other neuromuscular disorders.

Erythrocyte sedimentation rate, thyroid function tests, creatine kinase.

Radiographs as indicated for arthralgias.

Pulmonary function tests, swallowing studies as indicated by symptoms.

The following do not add to specificity of diagnosis, may be needed to exclude other considered diagnoses:

Muscle biopsy confirms prior denervation; spinal fluid examination reveals normal routine studies.

Viral assays.

Complications

Sleep apnea (central and obstructive), joint derangements (in 60%, due to lack of support by weakened muscles), falls, aspiration, choking.

Differential diagnosis

Confirm history of polio. Diagnosis of exclusion.

Neuromuscular disorders producing similar symptoms: polyneuropathy, myopathy, myasthenia gravis, spinal cord disease, spinal stenosis, polyradiculopathy, nerve entrapments (*e.g.*, carpal tunnel syndrome).

Musculoskeletal disorders producing similar symptoms: arthritis, tendonitis, polymyalgia rheumatica, fibromyalgia.

Central nervous system disorders producing similar symptoms: multiple sclerosis.

Other disorders producing fatigue and weakness: hypothyroidism

Differentiate from ALS by slow rate of progression.

Epidemiology

First recognized in 1875. Estimated > 600,000 in United States with history of paralytic poliomyelitis and thus at risk.

Develops in 22% to 68% of exposed patients.

Last US "wild" case was 1979; last case in Americas in Peru, 1991.

Eight vaccine-related cases of polio per year.

Number of potential patients decreasing yearly.

No increased risk of motor neuron disease after polio.

Treatment

Diet and lifestyle

Avoid obesity.
Altered food consistency may be required if progressive dysphagia present.

Pharmacological treatment

Anecdotal and open label reports have suggested amantadine and pyridostmine to treat fatigue and weakness, respectively. No significant improvement in controlled trials. Creatine has been shown effective in slightly improving neuromuscular weakness and fatigue.

High-dose steroids and insulin-like growth factor (IGF-1) are ineffective.

Nonsteroidal antiinflammatory agents for arthralgia.

Nonpharmacological treatment

Nonfatiguing exercise, reconditioning, stretching.

Bracing of weak limbs (*e.g.*, ankle foot orthosis for foot drop), assistive devices as needed. Percutaneous feeding tubes for severe dysphagia (rarely required).

Treatment aims

Maintain function and fitness; overcome weakness with bracing, assistive devices. Energy-saving principles to avoid fatigue.

Prognosis

Weakness progresses only slowly if at all; summed MRC decreases 1%/year.

Follow-up and management

Follow-up to exclude more rapid decline or other finding suggesting alternative diagnosis.
Physical therapy to maintain joint range of motion.
Continued evaluation for assistive devices as weakness progresses.
Monitor changes in ventilatory function in those with dyspnea.

General references

Aurlien D, *et al.*: The postpolio syndrome-a critical comment to the diagnosis. *Acta Neurol Scand* 1999, **100**:76–80.

Kid D, *et al.*: Late functional deterioration following paralytic poliomyelitis. *Q J M* 1997, **90**:189–196.

Spector SA, *et al.*: Strength gains without muscle injury after strength training in patients with postpolio muscular atrophy. *Muscle Nerve* 1996, 19:1282–1290.

Thorsteinsson G: Management of postpolio syndrome. *Mayo Clin Proc* 1997, **72**:627–638.

Trojan DA, *et al.*: A multicenter, randomized, double-blinded trial of pyridostigmine in postpolio syndrome. *Neurology* 1999, **53**:1225–1233.

The post-polio syndrome: advances in the pathogenesis and treatment. Conference proceedings. Bethesda, Maryland, April 27–30, 1994. *Ann NY Acad Sci* 1995, **753**:1–412.

Pressure ulcers

Diagnosis

Symptoms and signs

• Pressure ulcers should be assessed for location; stage (*see* table); size; presence of sinus tracts, undermining, tunneling, exudate, necrotic tissue, and granulation tissue or epithelialization.

• Characteristics should be thoroughly documented.

• Pain associated with pressure ulcers should be assessed and treated with analgesics while the ulcer is healing.

Pressure ulcer staging

Stage I	Nonblanchable erythema of intact skin
Stage II	Partial-thickness skin loss involving epidermis and/or dermis; the ulcer is superficial and appears as an abrasion, blister, or shallow crater
Stage III	Full-thickness skin loss involving damage or necrosis of subcutaneous tissue superficial to fascia; appears as deep crater with or without undermining of adjacent tissue
Stage IV	Full-thickness skin loss with extensive destruction, tissue necrosis, or damage to muscle, bone, tendon, or joint capsule; undermining and sinus tracts may be present

Risk factors

Bed- and chair-bound status: especially with impaired ability to reposition.

Incontinence: fecal incontinence presents greater risk than urinary incontinence.

Poor nutritional status: albumin <3.5 mg/dL, total lymphocyte count <1800, patient not eating, weight <80% of ideal body weight. Vitamin deficiencies are common among nursing home residents and may contribute to ulcer formation and persistence.

Chronically moist or dry skin.

Friction and shear forces: pressure lateral to surface of the skin, as when repositioning patients by sliding or when patients sit up in bed without foot support.

• Risk assessment should be carried out periodically among patients with one or more risk factors. Serial use of assessment scales such as the Norton Scale (*see* table) help to measure patients' degree of risk and identify changes in risk status over time.

Norton scale*

Physical condition	Mental condition	Activity	Mobility	Incontinent
Good = 4	Alert = 4	Ambulant = 4	Full = 4	Not = 4
Fair = 3	Apathetic = 3	Walk with help = 3	Slightly limited = 3	Occasional = 3
Poor = 2	Confused = 2	Chair-bound = 2	Very limited = 2	Usually (urine) = 2
Very bad = 1	Stupor = 1	Bed-bound = 1	Immobile = 1	Doubly = 1

*Scores are the total of individual scales (range, 5–20).

Investigations

Swab cultures: reflect surface colonization and have no diagnostic value.

Needle aspiration or tissue biopsy: should be used when necessary to obtain cultures.

Plain radiograph of underlying bone and nuclear medicine bone scan: for nonhealing pressure ulcers under appropriate treatment, may help diagnose underlying osteomyelitis.

Complications

Osteomyelitis, bacteremia, advancing cellulitis: most common.

Endocarditis, heterotopic bone formation, maggot infestation, meningitis, perineal-urethral fistula, squamous cell carcinoma in the ulcer, sinus tract, or abscess formation: less common.

Differential diagnosis

• Commonly overlooked causes of non-healing ulcers include underestimate of ulcer stage, underlying osteomyelitis, and other complications such as squamous cell carcinoma (see Complications).

• Pyoderma gangrenosum (rapidly expanding ulcer; may be associated with inflammatory bowel disease or other causes, or may be idiopathic).

• Ecthyma gangrenosum (neutropenic patients; usually due to *Pseudomonas* infection).

Etiology

• Pressure ulcers occur as a result of inadequate blood flow to capillaries in soft-tissue beds, in part due to mechanical pressure over the involved area.

• Tissue-threatening compromise of microvessel blood flow is a function of both pressure and time, and can occur as a result of high pressures for brief periods (*e.g.*, sitting on ischial tuberosities), low pressure for prolonged periods (*e.g.*, heel pressure in bedbound patients), or both (*e.g.*, trochanteric pressure in bed-bound patient).

Epidemiology

• Pressure ulcers occur in 10% of hospitalized patients; 20%–25% of nursing home residents; 60% of hospitalized quadreplegic patients; 66% of elderly patients admitted to hospitals for femoral fracture.

• 25% of nonhealing pressure ulcers are associated with underlying osteomyelitis.

• Total annual national cost of pressure ulcer treatment is estimated at $1.3 billion.

Treatment

Diet and lifestyle

Prevention

• Minimize risk factors through skin care, ensuring adequate dietary intake, maximizing mobility.

• Skin massage over bony prominences may lead to deep tissue trauma and thus should not be used.

• Reposition patients at risk at least every 2 hours, using a written schedule. Because of higher pressure loads, seated patients must be repositioned every hour, by returning to bed if necessary. Seated patients who are able should be taught to reposition themselves every 15 minutes.

• Pillows or foam wedges should be used to keep bony prominences (knees, ankles) from direct contact with one another.

• Patients who are completely immobile should have a care plan that includes the use of devices that totally relieve pressure on the heels (*e.g.*, by raising them off the bed).

• Static support surfaces (foam rubber, "egg-crate" cushions) are helpful in patients who can be periodically repositioned (or reposition themselves). Doughnut cushions should be avoided.

Debridement

• Devitalized tissue should be removed. Sharp debridement is necessary with advancing cellulitis or sepsis. Debridement by a surgeon is indicated for large ulcers or if the primary physician is inexperienced. Mechanical (*e.g.*, wet-to-dry dressings, hydrotherapy, wound irrigation, and dextranomers) or enzymatic (*e.g.*, collagenase) debridement is effective for small wounds.

Wound cleansing

• Normal saline should be used to cleanse most wounds, initially at each dressing change. Antiseptic agents and skin cleansers are cytotoxic to normal tissues and should generally be avoided. Wound should be irrigated under mild pressure (*e.g.*, syringe with 19-gauge needle), adequate to remove bacteria and debris. Whirlpool treatment may be necessary for thick exudate, slough, or necrotic tissue.

Wound dressing

• After debridement and wound cleansing, moist dressings (*e.g.*, continuously moist saline gauze, hydrocolloid dressing such as Duoderm) are preferable to dry dressings.

• Dynamic support surfaces (air-fluidized, low-air loss, and alternating air support devices) are expensive but should be considered in patients with stage III or IV pressure ulcers on multiple turning surfaces.

Pharmacological treatment

• Stage II, III, and IV pressure ulcers are uniformly colonized with bacteria. Colonization per se need not (and should not) be treated with antimicrobial agents. Minimizing bacterial colonization enhances healing, however, and is best achieved through wound debridement and cleansing (*see* Wound dressing).

• Wound infection (purulence, foul odor) is initially managed by increasing the frequency of wound cleansing.

• For infected ulcers that produce exudate after 2–4 weeks of aggressive wound cleansing, or appear clean but nonhealing, a 2-week trial of a topical antibiotic is appropriate. The antibiotic should be effective against gram-negative, gram-positive, and anaerobic organisms (*e.g.*, silver sulfadiazine, triple antibiotic). If resistant staphylococcal organisms are prevalent in the nursing home, mupirocin ointment should be used and susceptibility demonstrated.

• Choice of topical antimicrobial agents can be guided by culture of material obtained through needle aspiration or biopsy of ulcer tissue. Swab cultures are not helpful in guiding therapy, because all open pressure ulcers are colonized with bacteria.

• Appropriate systemic antibiotic therapy should be given for patients with bacteremia, sepsis, advancing cellulitis, or osteomyelitis. Systemic antibiotics are not required for pressure ulcers with clinical signs only of local infection.

Treatment aims

To achieve complete healing.

To provide patient comfort (in terminal illness).

Other treatments

• Electrical stimulation therapy, using proper equipment and trained personnel, may be helpful for stage III and IV and recalcitrant stage II ulcers.

• Hyperbaric oxygen, infrared, ultraviolet, and low-energy laser irradiation, and ultrasound therapy have not been demonstrated to be of benefit.

• Various topical treatments (sugar, vitamins, hormones), growth factors, and skin equivalents have not been demonstrated to be of benefit.

• Operative repair (*e.g.*, skin grafts, skin flaps, musculocutaneous flaps) should be considered for clean stage III or stage IV pressure ulcers not responding to optimal care.

• Vitamin C and zinc nutritional supplements may aid healing in the presence of deficiencies.

• Research on exogenous growth factors to accelerate the healing process is being done.

Prognosis

• A clean pressure ulcer should show evidence of some healing within 2–4 weeks. If no progress can be demonstrated, re-evaluate the adequacy of the overall treatment plan as well as adherence to the plan, including risk factor modification.

Follow-up and management

Monitor at least weekly, with documentation of pressure ulcer characteristics and revision of management plan as appropriate.

General references

Pressure Ulcers in Adults: Prediction and Prevention. Rockville: Agency for Health Care Policy and Research, Public Health Service, U.S. Department of Health and Human Services; 1992 [AHCPR Publication 92-0047.] (Available at U.S. National Library of Medicine's Health Services/Technology Assessment Text (HSTAT) web page: http://text.nlm.nih.gov/).

Pressure Ulcers in Adults: Treatment. Rockville: Agency for Health Care Policy and Research, Public Health Service, U.S. Department of Health and Human Services; 1994. [AHCPR Publication 94-0075.]

Prostate cancer

Diagnosis

Symptoms

• Many prostate cancers are asymptomatic at the time of diagnosis; initiated by an elevation in a serum prostate-specific antigen (PSA) screening study.

Urinary hesitancy, frequency, urgency, incontinence.

Decreased urinary stream.

Nocturia.

Signs

Presence of induration, enlargement, or a discrete mass within the prostate on digital rectal examination.

Bone pain (metastatic disease).

Investigations

For screening [1,2]

• Serum PSA is frequently used as a screening assay. However, there is no universally acceptable role for screening because of the inability to identify patients who will develop clinically significant disease and to balance these patients with those who will undergo unnecessary therapeutic interventions for clinically insignificant neoplasms.

For diagnosis

• The need to pursue a diagnosis of prostate cancer depends on symptoms, findings on physical examination, and identification of an elevated serum PSA level.

Digital rectal examination: only 25%–50% of men with an abnormal examination will have prostate cancer.

Transrectal ultrasonography.

Transrectal ultrasonography–guided transrectal needle biopsy.

PSA determination.

Prostatic acid phosphatase: less valuable since PSA was discovered.

Bone scanning: when metastatic disease to bone is suggested.

Computed tomography and magnetic resonance imaging: not useful for diagnosis but may be helpful in specific circumstances.

Staging: Tumor staging systems, such as the TNM and American Urologic Association (AUA) staging systems, define the extent of disease within and beyond the prostate gland.

AUA Staging System

Stage A	Tumor found incidentally at transurethral retrograde prostatectomy.
Stage B	Tumor(s) confined to the prostate gland.
Stage C	Tumors that have extended through the glands' capsule.
Stage D	Tumors that have spread to regional lymph nodes or to distant sites.

Complications

Pain, metastases to bone, urinary tract infection, spinal cord compression, benign prostatic hypertrophy.

Differential diagnosis

Benign prostatic hypertrophy.

Transitional cell carcinoma.

Small cell tumors.

Carcinosarcoma.

Lymphoma.

Germ cell tumors.

Mesenchymal neoplasms.

Etiology

Inactivation of several tumor suppressor genes (*e.g., p53, RB*) and overexpression of oncogenes (*e.g., H-ras, bcl-2*) have been implicated in prostate carcinogenesis.

Epidemiology

The incidence of a diagnosis of prostate cancer is increasing.

Median age at diagnosis in the United States is 66 years.

Prostate cancer is responsible for 36% of newly diagnosed cancers and is the second leading cause of cancer deaths in men.

Increasing risk with age: although it is estimated that 70% of men older than 80 years of age have some histologic evidence of prostate cancer, many of these cancers never become clinically evident or significant.

Histologic grading

Determines the biologic potential of the tumor.

Gleason grading system is the one most commonly used. A score of 1–5 is assigned for the primary and secondary growth patterns of a tumor; a score of 1 represents the most differentiated, with discrete gland formation; a score of 5 represents very undifferentiated tumors, with nearly complete loss of glandular structures. The two scores are added together to give a total of 2–10. The higher the score, the more likely the presence of extracapsular spread, lymph node involvement, and eventual metastases.

Treatment [3–5]

Diet and lifestyle

• Patients should be encouraged to live as normal a life as possible.

• Counseling for patients and their sexual partner may be needed for changes in sexual function associated with therapy.

General principles

• Type of treatment depends on disease stage, age of the patient, and biologic behavior of the tumor.

• Treatment should be given under specialist supervision.

Surgical treatment

• Surgery is mainstay of therapy for organ-confined disease and for relieving symptoms related to prostate gland involvement.

• Many surgical approaches are available. The approach chosen depends on the indication for surgery.

• Pelvic lymph node resections are typically performed during open prostatectomies to assess for involvement by tumor.

Radiation therapy

• A viable alternative to surgery for cure of localized prostate cancer.

• Can be delivered via external-beam or brachytherapy approaches.

Hormonal therapy

• Hormonal therapies primarily used for locoregional and metastatic disease.

• Estrogen (*e.g.*, diethylstilbestrol, fosfestrol), progestational agents (*e.g.*, medroxyprogesterone, megestrol, cyproterone acetate), gonadotropin-releasing hormone analogues (*e.g.*, leuprolide, goserelin), adrenal enzyme synthesis inhibitors (*e.g.*, ketoconazole, aminoglutethimide), and antiandrogens (*e.g.*, cyproterone acetate, megestrol, medroxyprogesterone, flutamide) are used in specific clinical settings.

• Orchiectomy can be considered an alternative form of hormonal therapy.

Chemotherapy

• Primarily reserved for palliation of symptoms in patients with advanced disease.

• Clinical trials are in progress to evaluate and compare old and new agents for effectiveness.

Complications of therapy

Surgery: urinary incontinence, impaired sexual potency.

Radiation therapy: diarrhea, rectal discomfort, rectal bleeding, rectal fistula, rectal perforation, frequency of urination, hematuria, dysuria.

Hormonal therapy: cardiovascular disease, transient exacerbation of prostate cancer symptoms ("flare") with gonadotropin-releasing hormone analogues, somnolence, fatigue, rashes, hypothyroidism, hepatotoxicity, gynecomastia, hot flashes, diarrhea.

Chemotherapy: depends on drug(s) used.

Treatment aims

To provide a cure, when possible.

To alleviate symptoms.

To provide effective palliation when cure is impossible.

Prognosis

Prognosis depends on age at diagnosis, state of disease, and biologic behavior of cancer.

If prostate cancer is organ-confined at the time of diagnosis, it may not have a significant impact on the survival until 10–15 years later.

Follow-up and management

Routine monitoring of PSA level and patient's symptoms is necessary.

Additional interventions with medications or mechanical devices to enhance sexual potency that has been lost because of therapy should be made available when possible.

Key references

1. Brawer MK: Prostate-specific antigen: current status. *CA Cancer J Clin* 1999, **49**:264–281.
2. Hahnfeld LE, Moon TD: Prostate cancer. *Med Clin North Am* 1999, **83**:1231–1245.
3. Garnick MB, Fair WR: Prostate cancer: emerging concepts (part 1). *Ann Intern Med* 1996, **125**:118–125.
4. Garnick MB, Fair WR: Prostate cancer: emerging concepts (part 2). *Ann Intern Med* 1996, **125**:205–212.
5. Henry RY, O'Mahony D: Treatment of prostate cancer. *J Clin Pharm Ther* 1999, **24**:93–102.

General reference

Osterling J, Fuks Z, Lee CT, Scher HI: Cancer of the prostate. In *Cancer: Principles and Practice of Oncology*, edn 5. Edited by De Vita VT Jr, Hellman S, Rosenberg SA. Philadelphia: Lippincott-Raven; 1997: 1322–1386.

Diagnosis

Symptoms

Symptoms of venous or arterial thrombosis.

Signs

• Patients to investigate include those with the following:

Venous thromboembolism before the age of 40–45 years.

Recurrent venous thrombosis or thrombophlebitis.

Thrombosis in an unusual site: *e.g.*, mesenteric vein, cerebral vein.

Unexplained neonatal thrombosis.

Skin necrosis.

Arterial thrombosis before the age of 30 years.

Relatives with a specific defect.

Unexplained prolonged coagulation screening tests.

Recurrent fetal loss, idiopathic thrombocytopenic purpura, SLE.

Investigations

• Functional and immunological assays are needed for a precise diagnosis.

• Screening tests and functional assays should be performed on fresh citrated blood samples collected with minimal venous stasis on all patients being investigated for a prothrombotic state.

Complete blood count and film.

Measurement of prothrombin, activated partial thromboplastin, and thrombin time; fibrinogen.

Assays for antithrombin III, protein C, protein S, activated protein C resistance (factor V Leiden), plasminogen, heparin cofactor II, anticardiolipin antibodies, lupus anticoagulant, factor XII, dysfibrinogenemia, homocystinuria, and prothrombin 20210.

Fibrinolytic tests: before and after stimulation (*i.e.*, venous occlusion or DDAVP).

Fibrin plate, tissue-type plasminogen activator, and PA1-1 assays.

Platelet activation markers analysis: *i.e.*, GMP-140 expression, plasma β-thromboglobulin.

Complications

Arterial and venous thrombosis and embolism.

Differential diagnosis

Hyperviscosity.

Etiology

Common acquired causes of thrombosis

Diabetes mellitus, hyperlipidemia, malignancy, myeloproliferative disorders, chronic liver disease, SLE, paraproteinemias, nephrotic syndrome, antiphospholipid syndrome.

• These disorders cause predisposition to thrombosis in a multifactorial way; specific homeostatic assays are generally unhelpful in the investigation and management of individual patients.

Inherited defects with increased tendency to thrombosis

Antithrombin III, protein C, protein S, factor V Leiden, plasminogen, heparin cofactor II, factor XII, dysfibrinogenemia, homocystinuria, prothrombin 20210.

• Most of these disorders represent autosomal-dominant traits with variable penetrance.

• Deficiency in the heterozygous state predisposes to thrombosis either spontaneously or in association with other high-risk factors.

Pathophysiology

• The balance of the hemostatic mechanism can be shifted in favor of thrombosis in the following circumstances:

Increased coagulation system activity.

Increased platelet activity.

Decreased fibrinolytic activity.

Damaged vascular endothelial activity.

Epidemiology

• Epidemiological studies have shown an increased incidence of thrombotic events associated with raised concentrations, particularly of fibrinogen, factor VII, and factor VIII:C, with a frequency of 1 in 2000–5000.

High-risk factors for thrombosis

Surgical and nonsurgical trauma.

Age.

Immobilization.

Heart failure.

Prior venous thrombosis and varicose veins.

Paralysis of lower limbs.

Obesity.

Estrogen treatment.

Pregnancy and puerperium.

Smoking.

Raised blood viscosity.

Treatment

Diet and lifestyle

- No special precautions are necessary.

Pharmacological treatment [2]

Prophylaxis for venous thromboembolism [3]

- The degree of risk must be assessed depending on the predisposing factors.

Low risk: early ambulation, graduated compression stocking.
Moderate risk: standard unfractionated heparin, 5000 U s.c. every 8–12 hours.
High risk: low molecular weight heparin, s.c. every 12–24 hours, dose depending on type of heparin.

- The degree of risk for surgical prophylaxis may be defined as follows:

Low risk: <40 years, minor surgery lasting <1 hour.
Moderate risk: >40 years, abdominal or thoracic surgery lasting >1 hour.
High risk: >40 years, knee and hip orthopedic surgery, obesity, and malignancy.

Heparin

Standard dosage [4]	Unfractionated heparin, 5000 U i.v. bolus, followed by 1000–2000 U/h i.v.; or 80 U/kg i.v. bolus, followed by 18 U/kg/h i.v., for 5–7 days. Low molecular weight heparin s.c. once to twice daily [5].
Contraindications	Rare hypersensitivity, risk of bleeding complications.
Special points	Activated partial thromboplastin time must be monitored 6 hours after start of treatment for unfractionated heparin, then at least every 24 hours, with dose adjustment to maintain ratio at 1.5–2.5 times control.
Main drug interactions	Drugs that interfere with platelet aggregation or coagulation.
Main side effects	Bleeding, thrombocytopenia, rebound thrombosis, osteoporosis (if treatment lasts >3 months), rare alopecia, skin rash.

- Heparinization can be reversed by administering protamine sulfate, 1 mg, which neutralizes ~100 U heparin; maximum dose, 40 mg i.v. in 10 minutes.

Warfarin [6]

Standard dosage	Warfarin, 5 mg orally on days 1, 2, and 3; then adjusted daily according to prothrombin time.
Contraindications	Pregnancy.
Special points	Prothrombin time must be monitored, with results expressed as INR with therapeutic range of 2.0–4.5.
Main drug interactions	Many medications potentiate or antagonize effect; for any new medication, prothrombin time should be checked.
Main side effects	Bleeding, skin necrosis after first few days of treatment in the case of protein C or S deficiency.

- Anticoagulant effects can be reversed by an infusion of fresh frozen plasma or factor II, IX, and X concentrate if bleed is life-threatening; vitamin K_1, 1–2 mg i.v., takes 6–24 hours to reverse warfarin effect.

Antiplatelet agents

- These are indicated for prophylaxis and prevention of further arterial thrombotic events when platelet activation has been shown to be a primary pathological factor, particularly myocardial ischemia and cerebrovascular thrombotic strokes, including transient ischemic attack, for secondary thrombocytosis (>800 × 10^9/L), and for essential thrombocythemia.

Aspirin, 75 mg orally daily or 300 mg twice weekly, or dipyridamole, up to 100 mg orally 3 times daily (dipyridamole may cause severe headaches).

Treatment aims

To prevent thrombosis.

Prognosis

- Prognosis depends on the underlying cause and the degree of risk of arterial or venous thrombosis or embolism.

Follow-up and management

- Lifelong expert management is needed.

Therapeutic ranges for oral anticoagulation

INR 2.0–2.5: prophylaxis of deep-vein thrombosis.

INR 2.0–3.0: treatment of deep-vein thrombosis, pulmonary embolism, systemic embolism, prevention of venous thromboembolism in myocardial infarction, mitral stenosis with embolism, transient ischemic attacks, atrial fibrillation.

INR 3.0–4.5: recurrent deep-vein thrombosis and pulmonary embolism, arterial disease including myocardial infarction, mechanical prosthetic heart valves (tissue prosthetic values can be controlled at 2.0–3.0).

Key references

1. Sacher RA: Thrombophilia: a genetic predisposition to thrombosis. *Trans Am Clin Climatol Assoc* 1999, **110**:51–61.
2. Hirsch J, Weitz JI: New antithrombotic agents. *Lancet* 1999, **353**:1431–1436.
3. Lowe GDO: Risk of and prophylaxis for venous thromboembolism in hospital patients. *BMJ* 1992, **305**:567–574.
4. Raschke RA, Reilly BM, Guidry JR, *et al.*: The weight-based heparin dosing nomogram compared with a "standard care" nomogram. *Ann Intern Med* 1993, **119**:874–881.
5. The Columbus Investigators: Low molecular weight heparin in the treatment of patients with venous thromboembolism. *N Engl J Med* 1997, **337**:657–662.
6. Poller L: Oral anticoagulation. *J Clin Pathol* 1990, **43**:177–183.

General reference

Thomas DP, Roberts HR: Hypercoagulability in venous and arterial thrombosis. *Ann Intern Med* 1997, **126**:638–644.

Diagnosis

Symptoms

Uncomfortable sensation provoking the desire to scratch.

Signs

Erythema.
Excoriations.
Lichenification.

Cutaneous disorders associated with pruritus

Inflammatory: atopic dermatitis, lichen simplex chronicus, urticaria, contact dermatitis, lichen planus, drug reaction, seborrheic dermatitis, pityriasis rosea.

Infectious: scabies, pediculosis (lice), pinworms, insect bites/stings, candidiasis, superficial fungal infection, cutaneous bacterial infection, folliculitis, condyloma acuminata.

Immune-mediated: bullous pemphigoid, pemphigus, dermatitis herpetiformis.

Environmental: xerosis, polymorphous light eruption.

Miscellaneous: essential pruritus.

Internal disorders associated with pruritus

Uremia: chronic renal failure (more commonly associated with hemodialysis than peritoneal dialysis).

Liver disease: obstructive biliary disease (primary sclerosing cholangitis, primary biliary cirrhosis, choledocholithiasis, carcinoma, hepatitis C, or drug-induced cholestasis).

Malignancy: Hodgkin's lymphoma (pruritus may precede diagnosis by as much as 5 years); non-Hodgkin's lymphoma; leukemia; mycosis fungoides; multiple myeloma; breast, lung, pancreatic, or gastric carcinoma.

Hematologic: polycythemia rubra vera (pruritus triggered by a sudden drop in temperature), paraproteinemia, rarely in iron deficiency anemia.

Endocrine: hypothyroidism or hyperthyroidism, diabetes mellitus, mastocytosis, carcinoid syndrome.

Neurologic: multiple sclerosis, notalgia paresthetica, cerebral lesions.

Infectious:HIV, viral exanthems (*e.g.*, herpes, varicella), parasitosis.

Psychiatric: depression, neurotic excoriations, severe stress.

Drug-induced: aspirin, morphine, codeine, scopolamine, phenothiazines, anabolic steroids, oral contraceptives, erythromycin estolate, quinidine.

Investigations

• The patient should be questioned and examined for skin lesions to determine the direction of investigation (*i.e.*, cutaneous vs systemic). A careful history regarding the nature of the itch, any new medications, exposures (fiberglass, mites), foreign travel, and the relationship of the pruritus to activities such as bathing should be elicited.

• For suspected systemic sources: complete blood count and differential, liver function tests (including alkaline phosphatase for obstructive disease), renal function testing, thyroid function tests, glucose, and chest radiography.

• Skin scraping: may see mites, ova, or fecal pellets in scabies; hyphae in fungal infection.

• Skin biopsy: useful for some inflammatory cutaneous conditions.

• Patch testing: may be helpful in pruritus caused by contact dermatitis.

• Pediculosis pubis: more than one third of patients have a concurrent sexually transmitted disease and should be tested for such disease.

Complications

Lichenification: from chronic scratching or rubbing.
Secondary infection: of excoriated areas.
Psychological distress: in recalcitrant cases.

Differential diagnosis

Not applicable.

Etiology

• The sensation of pruritus originates from stimulation of nerve endings in the dermoepidermal junction. Free nerve endings connect to unmyelinated C-fibers that carry the impulse to the central nervous systems. Pain and itch share the same neural pathway (spinothalamic tract) but are thought to be distinct sensations.

• An opiate-sensitive scratch center appears to exist at the floor of the fourth ventricle.

• Histamine is the primary chemical mediator, and its release from mast cells can stimulate C-fibers. Other factors (substance P, interleukin-2) may be involved.

• Prostaglandins affect the perception of itch by lowering the threshold of C-fiber response. Serotonin acts on peripheral serotoninergic receptors and opioids can act centrally to induce itch.

• Systemic causes of pruritus are poorly understood. The pruritus of liver disease may relate to the build-up of bile salts in the serum and tissues. Opiate and serotonergic mediators probably play a role. The pruritus of chronic renal failure may involve metabolic derangements due to dialysis or the natural history of renal failure itself. Neurologic disorders can interfere with pathways that modulate pruritus.

Epidemiology

Dry skin is the most common cause of pruritus without primary cutaneous disease.
Systemic disease may be detected in 10%–50% of patients with generalized pruritus; uremia is the most prevalent culprit, with 60%–80% of dialysis recipients experiencing itch.

Treatment

Diet and lifestyle

• Encourage brief lukewarm baths or showers with limited use of mild soaps, followed by liberal use of emollient creams or ointments (more moisturizing than lotions).

• Avoid irritants, *e.g.*, dry ambient environment; contact with wool, fiberglass, fragrances (in detergents and fabric softener); scratching.

• Trimming the fingernails may be of some help.

Pharmacological treatment

• Treatment should be aimed at treating the underlying disease and relieving the itching.

Topical symptomatic relief

Camphor or menthol: 0.25% lotion as needed.

Doxepin: 5% cream up to four times daily; can cause sedation.

Pramoxine hydrochloride: 1% cream up to four times daily; prescription form formulated with 1%–2% hydrocortisone cream.

Low- to mid-potency topical steroids: may be helpful for controlling dermatitis; can cause skin atrophy, hypothalamic pituitary axis suppression, and other sequelae of oral steroid use because of systemic absorption when used for prolonged duration and/or on extensive areas of skin.

Systemic symptomatic relief

Antihistamines (diphenhydramine, hydroxyzine, doxepin): can cause drowsiness, anticholinergic effects.

Nonsedating antihistamines (cetirizine, loratadine, fexofenadine): sometimes helpful.

Corticosteroids (prednisone, dexamethasone): temporary control of an acute flare or recalcitrant disease.

Treatment aims

Treating the underlying disease.

Relieving symptoms.

Other treatments

Uremia: phototherapy, oral activated charcoal, renal transplantation.

Liver disease: cholestyramine, phototherapy, naloxone (parenteral opioid antagonist), ondansetron (5-HT3 antagonist).

Scabies: 5% permethrin cream in infants or adults; 1% lindane cream or lotion in adults; ivermectin, 200 µg/kg single oral dose for resistant cases.

Idiopathic pruritus: capsaicin (substance P antagonist) may be of some help in chronic pruritus; cold stimuli; vibration and transcutaneous electrical nerve stimulation (TENS) are effective short-term therapy; parenteral propofol (subhypnotic doses) inhibits spinal afferents; acupuncture; psychotherapy.

Prognosis

Generally good with treatment of underlying cause.

Follow-up and management

Follow-up should be geared toward treatment of underlying disease states.

General references

Denman ST: A review of pruritus. *J Am Acad Dermatol* 1986, 14:375–392.

Gilchrest B: Pruritus: pathogenesis, therapy, and significance in systemic disease states. *Arch Intern Med* 1982, **142**:101–105.

Greaves MW, Wall PD: Pathophysiology of itching. *Lancet* 1996, 348:938–940.

Kam PCA, Tan KH: Pruritus—itching for a cause and relief? *Anaesthesia* 1996, **51**:1133–1138.

Millikan LE: Treating pruritus: what's new in safe relief of symptoms. *Postgrad Med* 1996, **99**:173–184.

Yosipovitch G, David M: The diagnostic and therapeutic approach to idiopathic generalized pruritus. *Int J Dermatol* 1999, **38**:881–887.

Psoriasis

Diagnosis

Symptoms

Pruritus: in 20% of patients.

Unpleasant odor: in severe extensive cases.

Joint pain, tenderness, and morning stiffness: in cases with psoriatic arthritis.

Chills: secondary to loss of body heat in patients with generalized psoriasis.

Signs

Scalp

Scaling.

Skin

Psoriatic plaques: classic lesion is a red plaque with sharply demarcated borders and a thick, silver scale; most common on elbows, knees, extensor surfaces, and areas of trauma; some patients have pustules (pustular psoriasis); the face is usually spared.

Auspitz sign: removal of scale causes pinpoint bleeding.

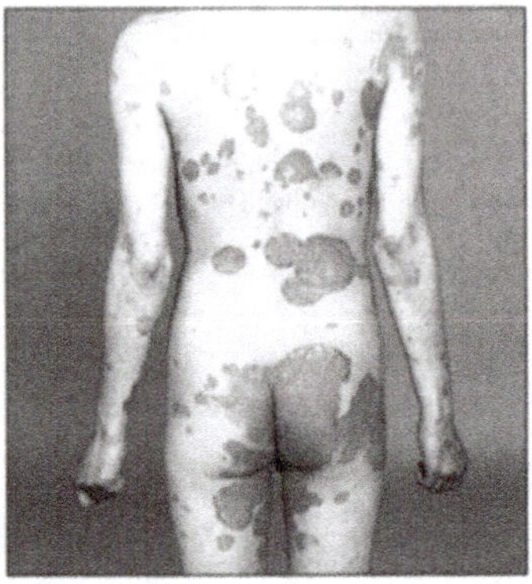

Chronic plaque psoriasis. (*See* Color Plate.)

Oral mucosa

Glossitis or geographic tongue: in 10% of patients.

Nails

• 50% of patients have nail involvement.

Pitting.

Subungual keratotic debris.

Onycholysis.

Discoloration: yellow-brown ("oil spots").

Musculoskeletal system

Asymmetrical oligoarticular arthritis: most common. (*See* psoriatic arthritis for more details.)

Investigations

HIV test: if there is a history of sudden onset of severe psoriasis with no family history and no previous personal history.

Antistreptolysin O (ASO) titer: if guttate flare from recent streptococcal infection is suspected.

Complications

Exfoliative erythroderma.

Generalized pustular psoriasis: sheets of sterile pustules and erythema; with associated fever, leukocytosis, arthralgias, skin tenderness, and malaise.

Psoriatic arthropathy.

Ankylosing spondylitis.

Differential diagnosis

Lichen planus.

Tinea corporis.

Seborrheic dermatitis.

Reiter's disease.

Pityriasis rosea.

Secondary syphilis.

Subacute cutaneous lupus erythematosus.

Premycosis fungoides (parapsoriasis).

Drug reaction.

Atopic eczema: especially patients with advanced lichenification.

Etiology

• Psoriasis is a multifactorial disease with a definite genetic predisposition.

Positive family history in 30% of cases.

• Histocompatibility antigen HLA-Cw6 is strongly associated (relative risk of 24).

• The presence of HLA-B17 or B27 is associated with more severe disease or associated arthritis.

• Although immunological abnormalities of humoral and cell-mediated immunity have been described, no specific circulatory immune abnormalities have been identified.

• Epidermal transit time is rapidly increased (6–9-fold).

• Studies have suggested that altered cellular metabolism of vitamin A may play a role.

Precipitating factors

Streptococcal infections.

Trauma: Koebner's phenomenon.

Drugs: beta-blockers, antimalarials, lithium, NSAIDs, oral corticosteroid withdrawal.

Stress.

Sunlight: a small subset of patients actually worsen with sun exposure (especially sunburn).

Alcoholism: may be related to decreased compliance in alcoholic patients.

Epidemiology

• Incidence is 1%–3% of world population [3].

• It affects 2–8 million people in the United States.

• Peak onset is in the second decade of life, but it may appear at any age.

Treatment

Diet and lifestyle

- Avoid physical trauma to the skin.

Pharmacological treatment

- Generalized pustular psoriasis or exfoliative erythroderma should be referred to a specialist immediately.

Topical treatment

Coal tar: safe and effective in plaque psoriasis; messy to apply (limiting compliance).
Steroids: effective and cosmetically acceptable; long-term use needs close supervision.
Vitamin D_3 analogues: calcipotriene appears safe and effective in limited areas of mild to moderate psoriasis; may be irritating on the face.
Phototherapy: ultraviolet B useful for chronic plaque and guttate psoriasis, alone or with other treatments such as topical applications.
Tazarotene (a recently developed receptor-selective retinoid): efficacious in mild to moderate plaque psoriasis. Once-daily application of a 0.1% or 0.05% gel.
Tazarotene: applied once daily in conjunction with a potent topical steroid; often leads to local irritation; contraindicated during pregnancy.
Anthralin: 0.1% to 1% cream, applied once daily; not recommended for use on face or acutely inflamed lesions; may be irritating and can cause skin and hair discoloration.

Systemic therapy

- Treatment should be given under supervision of a specialist.
- Long-term photochemotherapy is complicated by increased risk of cutaneous squamous cell carcinoma.

Standard dosage	Determined by specialist with systemic therapy experience.
Contraindications	*Acitretin:* childbearing potential, pre-existing hepatic disease, hypertriglyceridemia. *Methotrexate:* history of hypersensitivity to drug, hepatic disease, alcohol abuse, pregnancy. *Cyclosporine:* hypertension, renal insufficiency, underlying systemic infection.
Special points	*Acitretin:* effective in acral or generalized pustular psoriasis; teratogenic potential is present for up to 3 years after drug cessation. *Methotrexate:* oral or i.m.; used in widespread plaques, acute generalized pustular psoriasis, erythrodermic psoriatic arthropathy; should first be given with test dose; monitor CBC, liver function tests, periodic liver biopsy, depending on total dosage ingested. *Cyclosporine:* best for short-term treatment of erythrodermic or pustular psoriasis; side effects limit long-term use; may be used for severe refractory psoriasis, psoriatic arthropathy; monitor blood pressure, serum creatinine levels, creatinine clearance.
Main drug interactions	*Methotrexate:* trimethoprim-sulfamethoxazole, alcohol, NSAIDs, probenecid, retinoids. *Cyclosporine:* use caution with medications that affect renal function and drugs that inhibit the cytochrome P-450 system.
Main side effects	*Acitretin:* drying of skin and mucosa, elevated liver enzyme and triglyceride levels, myalgias, teratogenicity. *Methotrexate:* gastrointestinal, bone marrow suppression, immunosuppression, dose-dependent risk for hepatic fibrosis/cirrhosis, teratogenic effects, abortifacient. *Cyclosporine:* dose-dependent hypertension and nephrotoxicity, electrolyte imbalances, immunosuppression.

Alternative medicine

Recommended: none.
Common use: angelica (*Angelica archangelica*); cleavers (*Gallium aparine*); Yellow dock (*Rumex crispus*); figwort (*Scrophularia nodosa*); gotu kola (*Centella asiatica* or Hydrocotyle).
Caution: none.

Treatment aims

To control and prevent severe disease.

Prognosis

- Psoriasis is usually a chronic disease characterized by flares and remissions.

Follow-up and management

Individualized for each patient.

General references

Farber EM, Nall ML: The natural history of psoriasis in 5600 patients. *Dermatologica* 1974, **148**:1–18.

Greaves MW, Weinstein GD: Treatment of psoriasis. *N Engl J Med* 1995, **332**:581–588.

Highton A, Quell J: Calcipotreine ointment 0.005% for psoriasis: a safety and efficacy study. Calcipotreine study group. *J Am Acad Dermatol* 1995, **32**:67–72.

Koo J: Systemic sequential therapy of psoriasis: a new paradigm for improved therapeutic results. *J Am Acad Dermatol* 1999, **41(3 Pt 2)**:S25–S28.

Nickoloff BJ: The immunologic and genetic basis of psoriasis. *Arch Dermatol* 1999, **135**:1104–1110.

Saurat JH: Retinoids and psoriasis: novel issues in retinoid pharmacology and implications for psoriasis treatment. *J Am Acad Dermatol* 1999, **41(3 Pt 2)**:S2–S26.

Weinstein GD: Safety, efficacy and duration of therapeutic effect of tazarotene used in the treatment of plaque psoriasis. *Br J Dermatol* 1996, **135(suppl 49)**:32–36.

Zelickson BD, Muller SA: Generalized pustular psoriasis: a review of 63 cases. *Arch Dermatol* 1991, **127**:1339–1345.

Pubertal abnormalities

Diagnosis

Symptoms

Precocious puberty

Pubertal development <8 years in girls, <9 years in boys.

Rapid growth.

Menstruation in girls.

Advanced skeletal maturation.

Behavioral disturbance.

Delayed puberty

Lack of pubertal development >14 years in girls, >15 years in boys.

Lack of pubertal growth spurt.

Small external genitalia in boys.

Possible anosmia.

Social difficulties.

Signs

Precocious puberty

Secondary isosexual sexual development.

Tall stature.

Short stature.

Cutaneous pigmentation: McCune-Albright syndrome.

Acne, clitoromegaly: indicating virilization in girls.

Delayed puberty

Lack of secondary sexual development.

Gynecomastia in boys.

Family history of delayed puberty.

Signs of Turner's syndrome in girls.

Chronic pediatric illness: *e.g.*, Crohn's disease, thalassemia.

Investigations [1,2]

Precocious puberty

Usually divided into gonadotropin-dependent (hypothalamic or pituitary) or gonadotropin-independent (*see* Etiology).

Hormone measurement: for gonadotropin and sex steroid concentrations.

MRI or CT of hypothalamic–pituitary region: to exclude structural lesion.

Ovarian ultrasonography: to assess ovarian development.

Adrenal CT: for precocious puberty secondary to adrenal tumors.

Delayed puberty

Hormone measurement: for gonadotropin and sex steroid concentrations.

Complete blood count, electrolytes analysis, liver function tests: to exclude chronic disease.

Karyotyping: in girls.

MRI or CT of hypothalamic–pituitary region: to exclude structural lesion.

Ovarian ultrasonography: to assess ovarian development.

Test of smell: to exclude Kallmann's syndrome.

Clomiphene test: in older patients, to exclude gonadotropin-releasing hormone deficiency.

Complications

Precocious puberty

Progression of pubertal development.

Early menstruation.

Premature completion of skeletal maturation.

Adult short stature.

Delayed puberty

No secondary sexual development.

Absence of pubertal growth spurt.

Emotional, physical immaturity.

Infertility.

Differential diagnosis

Not applicable.

Etiology [1,2]

True precocious puberty (gonadotropin-dependent)

Idiopathic (principally girls).

Structural lesions of hypothalamic region (tumors).

Postcranial irradiation.

Hydrocephalus.

Hypothyroidism.

Pseudoprecocious puberty (gonadotropin-independent)

McCune–Albright syndrome.

Familial male precocious puberty.

Adrenal tumors.

Congenital adrenal hyperplasia.

Gonadal tumors.

Human chorionic gonadotropin–secreting tumors.

Exogenous sex steroids.

Delayed puberty

Constitutional.

Chronic pediatric illness.

Malnutrition.

Hypopituitarism (idiopathic, tumors).

Isolated gonadotropin-releasing hormone deficiency and anosmia (Kallmann's syndrome).

Hyperprolactinemia.

Intensive exercise.

Turner's or Klinefelter's syndromes.

Radiotherapy, surgery, chemotherapy, autoimmunity.

Epidemiology

- No reliable estimates are available.

Treatment

Diet and lifestyle

- No special precautions are necessary.

Pharmacological treatment [1,2]

Should be carried out in conjunction with an appropriate specialist.

For central precocious puberty

- Primary CNS lesions, *e.g.*, tumors, must be treated.

Gonadotropin-releasing hormone analogue fixed dose s.c. injection monthly or cyproterone acetate, 50–100 mg daily; treatment continued until appropriate age for puberty to progress.

- Long-term cyproterone treatment may induce adrenal insufficiency.

For gonadotropin-independent precocious puberty

Treatment of underlying disease (*e.g.*, congenital adrenal hyperplasia).

Androgen antagonists (spironolactone).

Inhibitors of steroid synthesis (ketoconazole).

For delayed puberty

- The primary cause must be treated, *e.g.*, chronic illness, pituitary tumor, hyperprolactinemia.

For boys: testosterone, from 50 mg every 2 weeks to 300 mg every 3 weeks i.m. depending on age.

For girls: ethinyl estradiol, 2–10 μg daily, increasing to 30 μg daily with norethindrone or medroxyprogesterone acetate, 5 mg daily on days 1–14 of each calendar month.

Treatment aims

To replace hormones.

Prognosis

- Prognosis is good unless the disorder is caused by a tumor.

Follow-up and management

- Patients should be checked every 3–6 months to ensure that treatment is effective.

Key references

1. Bridges NA, Brook CDG: Premature sexual development. In *Clinical Endocrinology*. Edited by Grossman A. Oxford: Blackwell Scientific Publications; 1992:837–846.
2. Stanhope R, Albanese A, Shalet S: Delayed puberty. *BMJ* 1992, **305**:790.

Pulmonary complications of immunosuppression

Diagnosis

Symptoms

• Symptoms may be minimal.

Dyspnea, cough, sputum production, hemoptysis, chest pain, weight loss, fever.

• Hemoptysis with chest pain suggests Kaposi's sarcoma in those with AIDS but pneumonia in those with other forms of immunosuppression.

Signs

Tachypnea.

Cyanosis: indicating respiratory failure.

Consolidation: suggesting bacterial infection.

Collapse: suggesting infection or neoplasia.

Pleural effusion: suggesting mycobacterial infection or neoplasia.

Investigations

• The choice of investigation depends on the physical signs and symptoms and the degree of immunosuppression.

To assess degree of immunosuppression

Complete blood count, differential leukocyte count: in patients with acquired immunosuppression, *e.g.*, to assess neutropenia, after organ transplantation.

Immunoglobulin measurement, CD4 count: in patients with acquired immunosuppression; normal CD4 count in early stages of HIV infection, bacterial infection common; low CD4 count in late stages of HIV infection, opportunistic infection or neoplasia more likely.

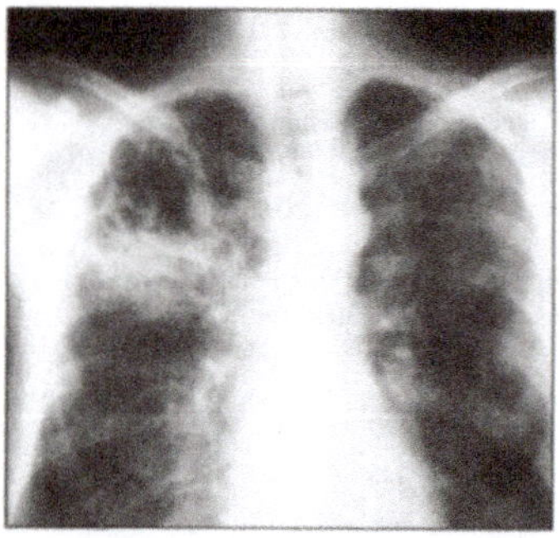

Chest radiograph showing cavitating aspergilloma.

To assess pulmonary complications of immunosuppression

Chest radiography: to identify focal or generalized abnormality.

CT: to assess pulmonary abnormalities in more detail (*e.g.*, intrathoracic lymph nodes).

Oximetry or arterial blood gas measurement: at rest or exercise, essential for early detection of respiratory failure.

Sputum for special stains and cytology: in patients with nonproductive coughs, sputum may be induced by inhalation of 3% nebulized saline solution.

Bronchoscopy, bronchoalveolar lavage, transbronchial biopsy, open lung biopsy: for tissue diagnosis.

Mediastinoscopy: if mediastinal lymph-node disease has been identified.

Complications

Respiratory failure.

Disseminated infection.

Disseminated secondary malignancy.

Differential diagnosis

• The diagnosis depends on the course, stage, and degree of immunosuppression, in addition to local pathogenic load, which may differ in community, hospital, or geographical location.

P. carinii pneumonia (*see Pneumocystis carinii* pneumonia in AIDS *for details*).

Bacterial infection (including mycobacteria).

Viral infection (*e.g.*, cytomegalovirus).

Fungal infection (*e.g.*, aspergillus, candida).

Parasitic infection (*e.g.*, *Strongyloides*).

Kaposi's sarcoma.

Secondary B cell lymphoma.

Secondary carcinoma.

Lymphocytic interstitial pneumonitis.

Graft-versus-host disease or rejection episodes in transplant recipients.

Etiology

Congenital causes

Genetically determined absence or reduction in immune response, *e.g.*, X-linked infantile hypogammaglobulinemia (Bruton type).

Acquired causes

HIV infection.

Organ transplantation.

Drug treatment, *e.g.*, steroids, azathioprine, cyclosporine (used in rheumatoid arthritis, asthma, ulcerative colitis).

Causes of relative immunosuppression

Diabetes.

Old age.

Epidemiology

• 1 in 100 000 people suffers from congenital immunosuppression.

• The incidence of acquired immunosuppression is increasing with the use of immunosuppressive drugs, organ transplantation, and HIV infection.

Treatment

Diet and lifestyle

• Excessive alcohol consumption should be avoided.

• Cigarette smoking should be stopped because of the increased incidence of pulmonary complications in immunosuppressed patients who smoke.

Pharmacological treatment

• Treatment depends on diagnosis, which should be as accurate as possible.

• In deteriorating patients, treatment must be started empirically, depending on the most probable cause or agent; this is determined by the combination of symptoms, signs, degree of immunocompromise, stage of immunocompromise, and local pathogenic load.

Antibiotics

• If a specific organism is not detected and the patient is deteriorating, antibiotics may be used when there is purulence on the Gram stain.

Antituberculous drugs

• Four-drug treatment (ethambutol, rifampin, pyrazinamide, isoniazid) is recommended until sensitivity is available.

Antiviral agents

• Treatment should be initiated only if diagnosis is established.

For cytomegalovirus disease: Ganciclovir, 6 mg/kg twice daily initially, then maintenance dose depending on response.

Foscarnet, 90 mg/kg continuous infusion over 90 minutes twice daily depending on renal function.

• Renal function and leukocyte count must be monitored.

Antifungal agents

• Treatment should be initiated only if diagnosis is established.

Amphotericin B, 0.5 mg/kg daily i.v., increasing to 1 mg/kg daily, depending on renal function.

Itraconazole, 200 mg daily.

Antiparasitic agents

Trimethoprim, 15 mg/kg, may be used for *Pneumocystis* spp. infection.

Chemotherapy

• Chemotherapy may be used in certain patients with Kaposi's sarcoma or secondary B cell lymphoma or carcinoma.

• The choice of treatment is determined locally, and the use of chemotherapy combined with radiation therapy for symptomatic treatment must be considered.

Treatment aims

To eradicate infection and to prevent recurrence.

To relieve symptoms of secondary neoplasia or Kaposi's sarcoma.

Other treatments

Controlled oxygen therapy.

Continuous positive airways pressure.

Mechanical ventilation: needs careful consideration, ideally with the patient or a relative, before initiation.

Prognosis

• Prognosis depends on the cause of immunosuppression and the form of pulmonary complication.

• Mortality is 10%–20% in transiently neutropenic patients with bacterial infection.

• If the immunosuppression is reversible, recurrence is unlikely after the patient has recovered from an acute event.

Follow-up and management

• In continuing immunosuppression, follow-up and management depend on the specific diagnosis: for example, HIV-infected patients may need prolonged prophylactic treatment against recurrence of *P. carinii* infection.

General references

Dichter JR, Levine SJ, Shelhamer JH: Approach to the immunocompromised host with pulmonary symptoms. *Hematol Oncol Clin North Am* 1993, **7**:887–912.

Lartholory O, Dupont B: Antifungal prophylaxis during neutropenia and immunodeficiency. *Clin Microbiol Rev* 1997, **10**:477–504.

Verra F, *et al.*: Bronchoalveolar lavage in immunocompromised patients: clinical and functional consequences. *Chest* 1992, **101**:1215–1220.

Wade JC: Treatment of fungal and other opportunistic infections in immunocompromised patients. *Leukemia* 1997, **11(suppl 4)**:S538–S539.

Pulmonary embolism

Diagnosis

Symptoms

Pleuritic chest pain, dyspnea, hemoptysis: indicate acute minor pulmonary embolism.

Acute-onset dyspnea, syncope, central chest pain: indicate acute massive pulmonary embolism.

Gradual-onset dyspnea, pleuritic chest pain, decreasing exercise tolerance: indicate subacute massive pulmonary embolism.

Increasing dyspnea, effort syncope: indicate chronic pulmonary embolism.

Signs

• Pulmonary embolism manifests in several ways, depending on extent of pulmonary vascular obstruction, time during which obstruction accumulates, presence/absence of preexisting heart or lung disease.

Shortness of breath, pleural rub, signs of pleural effusion: indicate pulmonary infarction.

Tachypnea or hyperventilation, reduced cardiac output, right heart failure: indicating massive pulmonary embolism.

Evidence of right ventricular dysfunction: bulging neck veins with V waves, left parasternal lift, accentuated pulmonic component of S2, systolic murmur at the left lower sternal border that increases in intensity during inspiration; may be obscured by obesity or barrel-shaped chest. Bulging neck veins may be replaced by profound hypoxemia when right-to-left shunting occurs through a patent foramen ovale.

Pulmonary hypertension: indicating chronic pulmonary embolism.

Investigations

• The diagnosis of pulmonary embolism needs a high index of clinical suspicion, combined with the results of investigations that may confirm or refute these suspicions.

• Combining noninvasive diagnostic tests may be useful. A normal D-dimer ELISA and venous ultrasonography can help rule out pulmonary embolism; echocardiography showing right ventricular hypokinesis combined with positive findings on ultrasonography of legs is virtually pathognomonic of pulmonary embolism.

D-dimer ELISA and venous Doppler ultrasonography: useful when clinical likelihood is low. D-dimer ELISA lacks specificity but is best suited for the emergency department or physician's office when the patient does not have associated systemic illnesses. The assay usually requires 3–4 hours to perform.

Pulmonary angiography: allows definitive diagnosis; invasive; needs specialized facilities.

Chest radiography: focal oligemia (Westermark's sign), a peripheral wedge-shaped density over diaphragm (Hampton's hump), enlarged right descending pulmonary artery (Palla's sign).

ECG: T-wave inversion in anterior leads, especially V1–V4. Probably reciprocal changes reflecting inferoposterior ischemia due to compression of the right coronary artery by the right ventricle as a result of pressure overload. Sinus tachycardia usual. New-onset right bundle-branch block or atrial fibrillation uncommon. The classic S1, Q3, T3 pattern nonspecific and unusual.

Perfusion scanning: Normal results are associated with recurrent pulmonary embolism, even if anticoagulants are withheld. Whereas normal results or results indicating a high probability of disease are extremely helpful, nondiagnostic results are difficult to interpret. Only rarely does ventilation scanning clarify the interpretation of perfusion lung scans.

Spiral CT of chest with contrast: best suited for pulmonary embolism in the proximal pulmonary vascular tree. However, if there is strong suspicion, contrast pulmonary angiography that focuses on distal pulmonary vasculature should be performed.

Gadolinium-enhanced magnetic resonance pulmonary angiography: reveals anatomical features and assesses right ventricular function.

Echocardiography: About 40% of patients with pulmonary embolism have right ventricular abnormalities. Useful to identify aortic dissection or pericardial tamponade, which may mimic pulmonary embolism. McConnell sign of pulmonary embolism is pattern of regional right ventricular dysfunction in which apical wall motion remains normal despite hypokinesis of the free walls.

Complications

Death, pulmonary infarction, infection, cavitation, or hypertension.

Differential diagnosis

• Pulmonary embolism has a wide differential diagnosis and hence its reputation as "The Great Masquerader."

Acute massive pulmonary embolism.

Septicemia; myocardial infarction; hypovolemia; pericardial tamponade; dissection of aorta.

Subacute massive pulmonary embolism.

Pulmonary edema; pneumonia; hyperventilation; exacerbation of chronic obstructive pulmonary embolism; asthma; bronchitis; lung cancer; rib fracture; pneumothorax; costochondritis; musculoskeletal chest pain.

Chronic pulmonary embolism.

Primary pulmonary hypertension.

Chronic pulmonary embolism

Primary pulmonary hypertension.

Etiology

• >90% of pulmonary emboli originate as deep venous thrombosis of the lower extremities.

• Common causes include the following:

Surgery within past 1 month.

Medical illness (*e.g.*, myocardial infarction or stroke).

Immobility, cancer, obesity, or oral contraception.

Pregnancy or estrogen therapy.

Indwelling central venous lines.

Hypercoagulable states, which may be acquired (*e.g.*, lupus anticoagulant, anti-cardiolipin antibodies) or inherited (*e.g.*, antithrombin III deficiency, protein C deficiency).

Epidemiology

• At necropsy, pulmonary embolism has been found in 9%–26% of all patients; it was suspected before death in only ~16%.

• In the International Cooperative Pulmonary Embolism Registry of 2454 patients, the 3 months mortality rate was 17.5%.

• Deaths are more common in women and increase with age.

• In Medicare recipients who are 65 years of age or older men had higher fatality rates and blacks had higher fatality rates than whites.

Treatment

Diet and lifestyle

• Patients should avoid periods of sustained immobility, *e.g.*, during longhaul flights.

Pharmacological treatment

Unfractionated heparin:

• Heparin is the cornerstone of management. It accelerates the action of antithrombin III, thereby preventing an additional thrombus from forming and permitting endogenous fibrinolysis to lyse some of the clot.
• Initial therapy with oral anticoagulant and no heparin may paradoxically intensify hypercoagulability and increase the frequency of recurrent venous thromboembolism.
• If no contraindications, patients with moderate or high clinical likelihood should receive a bolus dose of unfractionated heparin (~5000–10 000 U), followed by continuous infusion initiated at dosage of 18 U/kg body weight/hour, not exceeding 1600 U/h. Usually rapidly results in a therapeutic partial thromboplastin time of 60–80 seconds. Use of a heparin nomogram facilitates proper dosing.
• Heparin-induced thrombocytopenia causes venous thrombosis more often than arterial thrombosis. Although rapid loading of warfarin used to be recommended, it may precipitate venous gangrene of the limbs. Alternatives include a heparinoid or a direct thrombin inhibitor.

Low-molecular-weight heparin:

• As effective as unfractionated heparin to treat hemodynamically stable pulmonary embolism.

Warfarin:

• Can be safely started once therapeutic partial thromboplastin time or heparin level is achieved.
• Loading dose of warfarin does not shorten the 5-day period needed to achieve anticoagulation, and an initial dose of 5 mg is often sufficient. True anticoagulation requires depletion of factor II, which takes about 5 days; at least 5 days of heparin therapy is recommended.
• The target international normalized ratio (INR) initially should be 3.0 because concomitant administration of unfractionated heparin usually prolongs heparin by an additional 0.5, thus yielding an effective INR due to warfarin alone of 2.5.
• After hospital discharge, the risk of bleeding complications and thromboembolic events can be minimized by intensive clinical monitoring. Home monitoring devices for prothrombin time have been recently approved by the FDA.
• Optimal duration of therapy is not known. Lifelong therapy is recommended in patients with recurrent pulmonary embolism. Several years of therapy is recommended for patients with deficiency of antithrombin III, protein C, or protein S. It is unclear whether patients with factor V Leiden mutation and pulmonary embolism should receive prolonged courses of anticoagulation.

Thrombolysis with anticoagulation:

• Can be life-saving in massive pulmonary thromboembolism with hemodynamic collapse.
• There appears to be 14-day window for its effective administration.
• Patients treated with anticoagulation do better than those treated with thrombolysis alone.
• Potential benefit must be weighed against risk of major hemorrhage.

Nonpharmacological treatment

Inferior vena caval filter:

• Useful when anticoagulation is contraindicated.
• Not useful in proximal deep venous thrombosis with free-floating thrombi.
• In rare cases, massive edema of legs may develop.
• Vena caval filter with anticoagulation did not reduce mortality rate compared to anticoagulation alone.

Transvenous catheter embolectomy:

• Warranted when thrombolysis is contraindicated or unsuccessful.
• High-velocity jets of saline draw the thrombus toward the catheter and pulverize the clot.
• During treatment, dobutamine or norepinephrine may be required to maintain the mean arterial pressure and ensure adequate perfusion of the right coronary artery.

Open surgical embolectomy:

• Patients with chronic cor pulmonale due to chronic thrombi may be candidates.
• Patients undergo cardiopulmonary bypass and hypothermia before incisions are made into the pulmonary arteries to remove organized thrombi.
• Pulmonary hypertension may improve, resulting in better quality of life.
• Mortality rate in selected patients in experienced centers is 5%–10%.
• Major causes of death include inability to remove sufficient thrombi at surgery, severe reperfusion-associated lung injury.

Treatment aims

To reduce morbidity of acute episode.
To prevent recurrence of pulmonary embolism or chronic pulmonary hypertension.

Prophylactic treatment

• Most deaths from pulmonary emboli are sudden or occur in patients in whom diagnosis was not suspected; significant reduction in mortality is achieved only by adequate prevention.
Physical measures: early mobilization, pneumatic calf compression, and graduated compression stockings.
Drugs: unfractionated heparin, 5000 U s.c. every 8–12 hours; low-molecular-weight heparin, 3500–5000 U once daily, depending on the type used, or low-dose warfarin.
• Percutaneous or surgical placement of inferior vena cava filter may prevent subsequent embolism in patients with recurrent pulmonary embolism despite effective anticoagulation.

Prognosis

• One-third of acute or subacute pulmonary emboli result in sudden death or are undiagnosed during life.
• Patients with untreated clinically apparent pulmonary emboli have a 30% mortality from recurrent emboli; this is reduced to 8% with effective treatment.
• Survivors of the acute or subacute episode usually have no clinical sequelae.
• Chronic pulmonary embolism carries a grave prognosis and pharmacological treatment is generally ineffective; elective thromboendarterectomy may produce long-term improvement in some patients.
• Patients who have had pulmonary emboli are at increased risk of further thromboembolic episodes when exposed to situations in which thrombosis might occur.

Follow-up and management

• Oral anticoagulant treatment and monitoring are continued for at least 3–6 months but may be continued indefinitely if underlying risk factors cannot be controlled.

General references

Carson JL, Kelley MA, Duff A, *et al.*: The clinical course of pulmonary embolism. *N Engl J Med* 1992, **326**:1240–1245.

Goldhaber SZ: Pulmonary embolism. *N Engl J Med* 1998, **339**:93–104.

Pulmonary hypertension

Diagnosis

Symptoms

• **Dyspnea:** predominant symptom with primary pulmonary hypertension. The disease often has an insidious onset in an otherwise healthy person. The disease is typically diagnosed late in its course. Dyspnea on exertion is often the earliest presenting complaint.

Easy fatiguability, exertional chest pain, syncope, near syncope, cough, hemoptysis, hoarseness (due to compression of the left recurrent laryngeal nerve by a dilated pulmonary artery).

Angina: can occur from right ventricular ischemia.

Congenital heart disease, pulmonary embolism, pulmonary fibrosis, polycythemia vera, chronic obstructive pulmonary disease (COPD): with secondary pulmonary hypertension, symptoms of the underlying disease often predominate.

Signs

• Patients with mild and moderate disease may have no signs or may develop dyspnea with minimal exertion.

Increased P2 (pulmonic component to the second heart sound): physical examination may disclose this as the disease becomes moderate.

Diastolic murmur of pulmonic regurgitation: seen in severe disease.

Evidence of right ventricular dilatation with a peristernal heave, signs of right ventricular failure (increased jugular venous distention, hepatomegaly, ascites, and pedal edema): often present with severe disease.

Right ventricular S3: may be heard.

Reduced carotid pulse.

Investigations

Chest radiography: shows enlarged central pulmonary artery and clear lung fields in primary pulmonary hypertension.

Pulmonary function tests: often normal other than a reduced diffusing capacity for carbon monoxide; may show a mild restrictive pattern.

Arterial blood gases: show hypoxemia and hypocapnea in moderate and severe disease.

ECG: shows right ventricular hypertrophy often with acute right ventricular strain (S wave in lead I and Q wave and inverted T wave in lead III).

Echocardiography: may demonstrate enlargement of pulmonary arteries with right atrial dilatation. Enlargement of the right ventricle and parodoxical septal motion are often seen. Doppler echocardiography can estimate, often quite accurately, the level of pulmonary artery systolic and mean pressures.

Nuclear ventilation–perfusion scanning: helpful to rule out chronic pulmonary embolism as a secondary cause of pulmonary hypertension.

CT: can visualize the left and right ventricular size as well as the major pulmonary arteries. CT of the lungs is useful in ruling out underlying pulmonary causes of secondary pulmonary hypertension.

Cardiac catheterization: provides precise measurement of pulmonary arterial, capillary, and venous pressures. The severity of right ventricular failure can be quantified with cardiac output measurements and wall motion can be examined. Cardiac catheterization also can identify patients with congenital or acquired intracardiac shunts.

Pulmonary angiography: best method for identifying pulmonary embolism as a secondary reason for the development of pulmonary hypertension.

Complications

Severe right heart failure with cor pulmonale: occurs in severe disease.

Progressive right ventricular failure: leads to disability and death.

Sudden death: occurs more frequently in patients with primary pulmonary hypertension.

Differential diagnosis

Mitral stenosis.

Recurrent pulmonary emboli.

Congenital cardiac defects.

Sickle cell anemia.

Collagen vascular diseases.

• Most of these, when severe, can cause secondary pulmonary hypertension.

• Differentiating primary pulmonary hypertension from secondary pulmonary hypertension is necessary. Primary pulmonary hypertension classically presents as dyspnea that is not explained by other causes (intrinsic pulmonary disease, intrinsic cardiac disease, or severe anemia).

• Deconditioning with dyspnea can sometimes mimic early primary pulmonary hypertension.

Etiology and epidemiology

• Etiology of primary pulmonary hypertension is usually idiopathic. Women outnumber men in a ratio of ~4:1.

• Postulated causes for pulmonary hypertension include autoimmune disorders due to the high frequency of antinuclear antibodies seen in some cases of pulmonary hypertension.

• Appetite suppression medication has been implicated as a possible mechanism. One of these agents was used in Europe in the late 1960s and was linked to an increase in unexplained hypertension.

• 7% of cases of pulmonary hypertension are familial, with an autosomal dominant method of transmission with variable expression.

• Secondary pulmonary hypertension is due to the underlying disease. Major causes of secondary pulmonary hypertension include massive acute pulmonary embolism or chronic recurrent embolization, COPD, living at high altitude with hypoxia, congenital heart disease, severe pulmonary vascular or parenchymal disease (including interstitial lung diseases, parasitic lung diseases, collagen vascular diseases, granulomatous lung diseases, and i.v. drug use), severe left ventricular failure, sickle cell anemia, chronic liver disease, and mitral stenosis.

Treatment

Diet and lifestyle

• Because of the link to appetite suppressant drugs, which are amphetamine-like in nature, caution is appropriate in the use of these agents for managing obesity. It is likely that there is some unknown susceptibility factor for this association. It should be stressed that this association is suspected but not proven.

Pharmacological treatment

• Pharmacological treatment for secondary pulmonary hypertension should be directed at the underlying cause.

• No satisfactory treatment exists for primary pulmonary hypertension. Logically, treatment that would decrease the pulmonary artery pressure or reduce pulmonary vascular resistance directly would be of benefit. However, most agents that achieve this also decrease cardiac output and systemic blood pressure. If pulmonary artery pressures are reduced in proportion to the decrease in cardiac output, there is little net benefit.

• General therapeutic measures include supplementing oxygen as needed to increase the arterial oxygen saturation above 85%. This permits adequate tissue oxygenation, thereby preserving functional ability and patient activity. Oxygen usually ameliorates patient dyspnea. Because hypoxia is a potent pulmonary vasoconstrictor, oxygen therapy often can result in some decrease in pulmonary artery pressures.

• Vasodilating agents have not uniformally been successful. Calcium channel blockers in high doses, *e.g.*, diltiazam, 120 mg 3 times daily, may be helpful. Unfortunately, only a minority of patients with primary pulmonary hypertension exhibit pulmonary vasoconstriction and benefit from medications that dilate pulmonary vessels. Most recently, epoprostenol has been tried and has been successful in some patients. Studies suggest that epoprostenol may decrease pulmonary pressures and increase exercise capacity. Vasodilator treatment for primary pulmonary hypertension should be started with a pulmonary artery catheter in place. Initial pharmacological evaluation can then proceed under direct monitoring of systemic and pulmonary arterial pressures, and cardiac output. The treatment of primary pulmonary hypertension remains unsatisfactory. Virtually every class of vasodilator drug has been investigated for treatment of primary pulmonary hypertension.

• Diuretic therapy may relieve dyspnea and peripheral edema but must be used cautiously so as to not markedly decrease cardiac output.

• Oral anticoagulant therapy has been advocated by some, suggesting that in situ thrombosis may occur. Some have suggested that anticoagulants increase survival; however, they do not reverse the disease.

• Heart/lung transplantation should be considered in patients with primary pulmonary hypertension. Patients who have <1 year predicted survival because of their disease are the best candidates. Recurrence of the disease has not been reported in transplantation patients.

• Inhaled nitric oxide is being studied for long-term use. It has shown promise in acute short-term management.

Treatment aims

To reduce pulmonary artery pressure and minimize hypoxemia.

Prognosis

• Prognosis for primary pulmonary hypertension is poor. Mean survival of 2–3 years from time of diagnosis is the rule. Only rare patients survive >10 years. Sudden death is not uncommon.

Follow-up and management

• Routine monitoring of arterial oxygen levels is necessary.

• Patients should be monitored for disease progression.

General references

Abenhaim L, Moride Y, Brenot F, *et al.*: Appetite-suppressant drugs and the risk of primary pulmonary hypertension: International Primary Pulmonary Hypertension Study Group. *N Engl J Med* 1996, **335**:609–616.

D'Alonzo GE, Barst RJ, Ayres SM, *et al.*: Survival in patients with primary pulmonary hypertension: results from a National Prospective Registry. *Ann Intern Med* 1991, **115**:343.

Rubin LJ: Primary pulmonary hypertension. *N Engl J Med* 1997, **336**:111–117.

Diagnosis

Symptoms

Symptoms of hypertension.

Symptoms of associated coronary, cerebral, and peripheral vascular disease: in atherosclerotic disease.

Acute dyspnea: in "flash" pulmonary edema.

Signs

Hypertension: typically severe, requiring >2–3 antihypertensive medications.

Epigastric or renal angle bruits.

Femoral bruits and absent leg pulses: in atherosclerotic disease.

Investigations

Plasma creatinine measurement.

24-hour urinary protein excretion measurement: non-nephrotic range or occasionally nephrotic range proteinuria can be seen with renal artery stenosis.

Plasma renin activity: elevated levels (>10) in patients in normal sodium balance is indicative of renal artery stenosis.

Renal ultrasonography: to measure kidney size (kidneys <8 cm long seldom worth revascularization); renal size asymmetry consistent with renal artery stenosis.

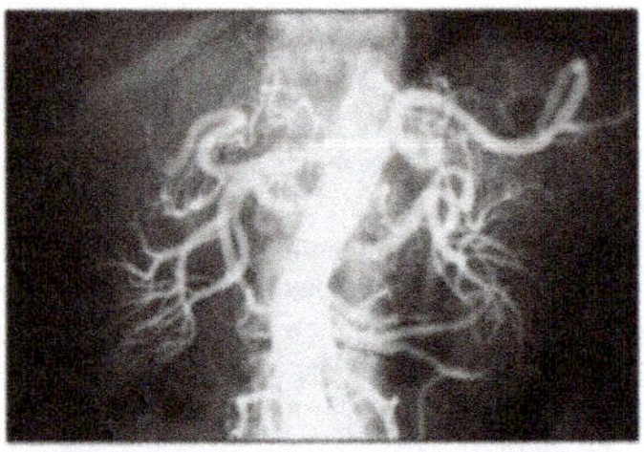

Widespread atherosclerotic disease in presence of renovascular disease, shown on angiography.

Nuclear medicine scanning: paired pre- and postcaptopril scans may increase sensitivity and specificity.

Renal angiography: use limited in patients with chronic renal insufficiency and severe aortosclerosis.

• Other examinations are those for atherosclerotic disease elsewhere.

Magnetic resonance angiography: no nephrotoxic contrast; expensive.

Spiral or helical CT scan: may well replace angiography and magnetic resonance angiography.

Complications

Malignant hypertension.

Chronic renal insufficiency.

End-stage renal disease: some patients may not need chronic dialysis if renal artery stenosis is diagnosed and treated.

Differential diagnosis

Other causes of hypertension.

Other causes of renal failure.

Left ventricular dysfunction.

Etiology

Fibromuscular disease: medial muscular hyperplasia.

Atherosclerotic disease: as for atherosclerosis elsewhere.

Large-vessel vasculitis, e.g., Takayasu's arteritis.

Epidemiology

• Fibromuscular disease is rare (more common in younger female patients).

• Atherosclerotic disease occurs in 30% of patients with abnormal coronary angiograms and 42% with abnormal peripheral angiograms.

Treatment

Diet and lifestyle

• Patients should take measures to alleviate risk factors for atherosclerotic disease, *e.g.*, stopping smoking, losing weight, and reducing lipids.

Pharmacological treatment

• Hypertension is treated by the usual agents (*see* Hypertension *for details*), except in the following cases:

Fibromuscular dysplasia or bilateral renal artery stenosis: angiotensin-converting enzyme (ACE) inhibitors should be avoided because they may reduce renal function in kidneys with renal artery stenosis.

Atherosclerotic disease: beta-blockers should be avoided because most patients have peripheral vascular disease; ACE inhibitors may reduce renal function.

Angiographic treatment

• Newer experience with angioplasty and stenting is promising, especially for complicated medical cases.

• Risk of procedure-related atheroembolism is substantial in atherosclerotic individuals.

Note: the use of stenting even allows angioplasty management of ostial lesions.

Surgical treatment

Remains the gold standard for cases that appear amenable to reconstruction and have well-defined humoral hypertension and/or renal vascular-related renal failure.

Treatment aims

To control hypertension.

To preserve renal function.

To prevent "flash" pulmonary edema.

Prognosis

• The 5-year survival rate is 92% for fibromuscular disease and 67% for atherosclerotic disease; age is a major factor.

• Renal artery stenosis may recur, especially after angioplasty.

Follow-up and management

• Blood pressure and plasma creatinine measurement and imaging studies should be repeated, with re-angiography, if restenosis is possible.

General references

Dean RH, Benjamin ME, Hansen KJ: Surgical management of renovascular hypertension. *Curr Probl Surg* 1997, **34**:209–308.

Greco BA, Breyer JA: The natural history of renal artery stenosis: who should be evaluated for suspected ischemic nephropathy? *Semin Nephrol* 1996, **16**:2–11.

Kothari SS: ACE inhibitors and unilateral renal artery stenosis: what price? *Int J Cardiol* 1996, **53**:199–201.

Novick AC: Options for therapy of ischemic nephropathy: role of angioplasty and surgery. *Semin Nephrol* 1996, **16**:53–60.

Rubin GD: Spiral (helical) CT of the renal vasculature. *Semin Ultrasound CT MR* 1996, **17**:374–397.

Salvetti A, *et al.*: Renal artery stenosis in the nineties: screening dilemmas. *Contrib Nephrol* 1996, **119**:45–53.

Renal failure, acute

Diagnosis

Symptoms

• The clinical features are usually dominated by those of the primary condition.

Nausea, vomiting, dysgeusia, pruritus, malaise, lethargy, myoclonus: features of uremia develop if diagnosis unduly delayed.

Seizures and coma: in severe cases.

Signs

Oliguria.
Edema.
Pericardial rub.
Asterixes.
Myoclonus
Jugular venous distension.
Gallop rhythm.
Cognitive impairment.

Investigations

• Priorities are the detection and documentation of possibly life-threatening complications, exclusion of prerenal and postrenal factors, diagnosis of intrinsic renal disease, distinction of acute from chronic renal failure, and monitoring of response to treatment.

Blood electrolytes/chemistries: assess for hyperkalemia, acidosis, hyponatremia, hyperphosphatemia, hypo/hypercalcemia, degree of chemical uremia.

Complete blood count: with differential for eosinophilia, suggesting acute interstitial nephritis or atheroembolic disease.

Central venous pressure monitoring and pulmonary capillary wedge pressure measurement: using Swan–Ganz catheter, if in any doubt about prerenal factors.

Chest radiography: assess for hypervolemia.

Echocardiography: to exclude prerenal factors or pericardial changes, hyperkalemia.

Ultrasonography: to exclude postrenal factors.

Urine sodium creatinine and osmolality: can identify prerenal acute renal failure.

Urinalysis: proteinuria, cells, casts, other features of intrinsic renal disease. Quantify protein loss by 24 h urine collection or spot urine protein creatinine ratio.

Urine: for eosinophils.

Serology: for glomerulonephritis and vasculitis.

Creatine kinase, haptoglobin, lactate dehydrogenase measurement: for rhabdomyolysis and hemolysis.

Blood film: for schistocytes and platelet count, to detect microangiopathic hemolytic anemia.

Blood cultures: for sepsis.

Coagulation tests, fibrinogen and fibrin degradation products analysis: for disseminated intravascular coagulation.

Renal biopsy: possibly indicated in patients with acute renal failure when intrinsic renal disease is suspected and may require specific therapy.

Ultrasonography, alkaline phosphatase measurement, bone radiography: for kidney size, evidence of metabolic bone disease, and anemia, respectively, to distinguish acute from chronic renal failure.

Immunoglobulin and protein electrophoresis: for myeloma in elderly patients.

Complications

Sepsis, acute respiratory distress syndrome (noncardiogenic pulmonary edema): usually seen in patients with multiple organ failure.

Gastrointestinal hemorrhage: caused by gastric stress ulceration.

Bleeding: uremic platelet–endothelial dysfunction and sepsis lead to bleeding diathesis.

Opportunistic infections, poor wound healing, muscle wasting: due to hypercatabolic state associated with uremia and infection.

Hypertension: often related to fluid overload, sometimes to primary renal disease.

Hypotension: often related to sepsis, occasionally to occult myocardial ischemia.

Hyperkalemia: especially in presence of acidosis and tissue breakdown.

Differential diagnosis

Prerenal: inadequate perfusion of otherwise normal kidneys.

Intrinsic renal disease: *e.g.*, acute or rapidly progressive glomerulonephritis.

Postrenal: blockage to flow of urine from otherwise normal kidneys.

Etiology

• Etiology is often complex, with more than one mechanism at play. Causes include the following:

Prerenal

Shock.

Hepatorenal syndrome.

Angiotensin-converting enzyme inhibitors.

Nonsteroidal antiinflammatory drugs.

Cyclooxygenase-2 inhibitors drugs.

Vascular: renal-artery embolus or thrombosis, dissection of aorta.

Renal

Acute tubular necrosis (the most common hospital-acquired renal failure): ischemia, toxins.

Acute glomerulonephritis.

Acute interstitial nephritis.

Atheroemboli.

Infection: bilateral pyelonephritis.

Thrombotic microangiopathies: *e.g.*, hemolytic uremic syndrome, thrombotic thrombocytopenic purpura, related conditions.

Pigment nephropathy: rhabdomyolysis, intravascular hemolysis.

Multiple myeloma: light-chain nephropathy.

Acute bilateral renal vein thrombosis.

Postrenal

Intraureteral obstruction: papillary necrosis, stones, tumors, blood clots.

Extraureteral: prostatism, extrinsic tumors, neurogenic bladder, urethral structures, retroperitoneal fibrosis, endometriosis.

Epidemiology

• ~50 people in 1 million annually develop acute renal failure needing dialysis.

• Most acute renal failure develops in the context of other acute illnesses.

Treatment

Diet and lifestyle

• Acute renal failure is a medical emergency, usually occurring in hospital; diet is modified to supply sufficient energy while minimizing accumulation of toxins (protein 40–60 g, sodium 40–60 mEq, potassium 40–60 mEq daily).

• In the maintenance support of acute renal failure, more rigorous protein (>1.0 g/kg/day) and calorie (>25 kcal/kg/day) nutrition is recommended, with appropriate control for fluid balance.

• Acute renal failure generally occurs in the setting of other acute illnesses.

Pharmacological treatment

For acute tubular necrosis

Diuretics only after restoration of euvolemia and maximization of cardiac output: escalating doses of a loop diuretic (bumetanide, 2–5 mg i.v. every 4–6 hours depending on urine flow rate) may restore urine flow; contraindicated in presence of obstruction, before hypovolemia is corrected.

For focal necrotizing and crescentic glomerulonephritis

Steroids, cyclophosphamide, and possibly plasma exchange only after biopsy confirmation if possible.

For acute interstitial nephritis

Withdrawal of offending drugs, possibly corticosteroid therapy.

For infection

High-dose prolonged course of appropriate antibiotic (at least 4–6 weeks).

For hemolytic uremic syndrome and thrombotic thrombocytopenic purpura

Plasma exchange with fresh frozen plasma (*see* Hemolytic uremic syndrome *for details*).

For pigment nephropathy, myeloma kidney

Forced alkaline diuresis: 0.9% saline, 500 mL alternating with 1.26% sodium bicarbonate solution, 500 mL every 4 hours with goal urine pH >8; bumetanide, 1–5 mg i.v. 8-hourly to maintain urine flow rate ≥100 mL/h; contraindicated in oliguria unresponsive to volume repletion and diuretics.

Nonpharmacological treatment

Optimization of vascular and extracellular fluid volume.

Maximization of perfusion of vital organs and exclusion of urinary obstruction.

Control of acidosis and hyperkalemia.

Enteral feeding, total parenteral nutrition if necessary; fluid balance must be controlled before feeding.

H2 blockers to prevent gastric stress ulceration.

Renal replacement therapy (dialysis or hemofiltration)

Indicated emergently for any combination of volume overload and congestive heart failure, hyperkalemia, severe acidosis, or symptomatic uremia in an oliguric patient.

Indicated semi-electively to support acute multisystem organ failure, nutritional administration, and fluid requirements in patients with moderate or severe renal failure who cannot be managed with diuretic therapy alone.

Uremic bleeding: consider i.v. vasopressin (0.3–0.6 mg/kg) × 1 dose, then conjugated estrogens (0.6 mg/kg/day) × 5 days.

Treatment aims

To prevent development of acute tubular necrosis.

To relieve obstruction and prevent progressive renal damage.

To identify primary treatable renal disease.

To replace renal function.

Prognosis

• In acute tubular necrosis, the prognosis for survival depends roughly on the number of additional organs that are failing.

• Many patients with acute tubular necrosis have near-complete recovery of renal function and do not develop chronic renal disease.

• Some patients make only a partial recovery. These patients may recover renal function for some months or years before developing hypertension and progressive chronic renal failure.

Follow-up and management

• Long-term follow-up is recommended in patients with persistent hypertension, impaired renal function, hematuria, or proteinuria.

General references

Alkhunaizi AM, Schrier RW: Management of acute renal failure: new perspectives. *Am J Kidney Dis* 1996, **28**:315–328.

Bellomo R, Ronco C: Acute renal failure in the intensive care unit: adequacy of dialysis and the case for continuous therapies. *Nephrol Dial Transplant* 1996, **11**:424–428.

Marik PE, Iglesias J: Low-dose dopamine does not prevent acute renal failure in patients with septic shock and oliguria. NORASEPT II Study Investigators. *Am J Med* 1999, 107:387–390.

Star RA: Treatment of acute renal failure. *Kidney Int* 1998, 54:1817–1831.

Thadhani R, Pascual M, Bonventre JV: Acute renal failure. *N Engl J Med* 1996, **334**:1448–1460.

Renal failure, chronic

Diagnosis

Definition

• Irreversible renal impairment is most often recognized by persistently high urea (blood urea nitrogen [BUN]) and creatinine concentrations; it often progresses to end-stage renal failure.

Mild: glomerular filtration rate (GFR) 20–50 mL/min; creatinine 1.5–3.0 mg/dL.

Moderate: GFR 10–20 mL/min; creatinine 3.0–7.0 mg/dL.

Severe: GFR <10 mL/min; creatinine >7.0 mg/dL.

Symptoms

Constitutional symptoms, fatigue, reduced stamina, dyspnea on exertion.

Pruritus, malaise, anorexia, sleep disorders.

Drowsiness, twitching, blunting of intellect, diarrhea: late seizures and coma.

Symptoms of underlying disease.

Signs

Anemia.

Hypertension.

Pallor and pigmentation.

Pruritus, scratch marks, bruising.

Red eyes: high calcium–phosphate product, uremia.

Edema.

Peripheral neuropathy: sensory common, motor only in severe uremia.

Proximal myopathy: severe metabolic bone disease, nutritional deficiency.

Kussmaul's respiration: when acidosis is severe.

Pericarditis: causing tamponade when renal failure severe.

Investigations

Serum electrolytes, urea (BUN), creatinine, creatinine clearance, 24-hour urinary protein, calcium and phosphate measurement.

Plain radiography of abdomen: to detect calculi and nephrocalcinosis.

Ultrasonography of kidneys: to measure size and exclude obstruction.

Kidney biopsy: for changes specific to underlying disease; contraindicated for small kidneys or very late chronic disease.

Immunoglobulin electrophoresis, Bence–Jones protein measurement: to diagnose multiple myeloma in elderly patients.

Renal artery imaging: consider spiral CT or magnetic resonance angiography if renal artery stenosis suspected.

Complications

Anemia.

Renal osteodystrophy.

Hypertension.

Bleeding (platelet dysfunction).

Peripheral neuropathy.

Pericarditis.

Acute or chronic renal failure: aggravated by hypovolemia, hypertension, infection, toxic agents, overzealous control of blood pressure.

Accelerated atherosclerosis: increased risk of stroke, heart attack, and peripheral vascular disease.

Differential diagnosis

Acute renal failure: short history, examination shows features of underlying disease, normal hemoglobin, no evidence of renal osteodystrophy, normal or enlarged kidneys.

Etiology

• The cause varies depending on the patient's age; the following may have a role:

Chronic glomerulonephritis in 20%–30% of patients.
Diabetes mellitus in 20%–30%.
Hypertension in 20%–30%.
Chronic interstitial disease in 10%–20%.
Polycystic kidney disease in 10%.
Renovascular disease in ~10%.
Drugs in 2.5%.
Hypertension in 20%–30%.
Hereditary nephritis in affected families.
In elderly patients: multiple myeloma, atherosclerotic renal artery stenosis, obstruction, and amyloid.
In children: congenital absence or dysplasia, obstruction: posterior urethral valves, juvenile nephronophthisis (cystic disease).
Family or previous history of renal disease (e.g., childhood urinary tract infection).

Epidemiology

• The annual incidence of chronic renal failure progressively to end-stage renal disease is 100–500/million depending on race and location.

Progression

• Although chronic renal failure often progresses to end-stage renal failure, function may not deteriorate quickly and, in some patients, remains stable, although significantly impaired, for several years.

• Measurement of serum creatinine is the most useful clinical test in assessing progression (serum creatinine is related to muscle mass and renal function).

• Serum creatinine rises exponentially with deteriorating renal function.

• A mild increase in serum creatinine may signal serious early loss of function.

• Plotting reciprocal serum creatinine values against time is a useful indicator of progression of renal failure.

Treatment

Diet and lifestyle

• Patients should eat a high-energy diet, with potassium restriction and protein intake restricted to 0.5–0.75 g/kg body weight daily; in later stages of chronic renal failure, decreased protein intake can help to control symptoms of nausea, vomiting, and anorexia.

• Phosphate intake should be restricted, and absorption reduced by phosphate binders (calcium carbonate in preference to aluminium hydroxide).

• Vitamin D supplementation is sometimes needed, using newer synthetic preparations.

Pharmacological treatment

• Specific treatment is directed at the underlying cause.

• Nephrotoxic drugs and NSAIDs must be avoided, and doses of other drugs must be adjusted for the degree of renal failure.

• Angiotensin-converting enzyme (ACE) inhibitors may help to control blood pressure, particularly in diabetic patients; diastolic pressure should be <90 mm Hg. Care is needed with these agents when renal artery stenosis is suspected or when serum creatinine is chronically elevated to levels >3.0 mg/dL.

• Erythropoietin can be used to treat anemia and improve well-being.

• Progression to end-stage chronic renal failure can be slowed by some or all of the following:

Aggressive control of systemic hypertension (120–130/70–80 mm Hg).

Reduction of glomerular blood pressure, using ACE inhibitors or calcium channel blockers.

Low-protein diets (in some patients).

Addressing the risk factors for accelerated atherosclerosis.

Nonpharmacological treatment

• Hemodialysis or peritoneal dialysis can be used to treat uremia, the prognosis depending on age, underlying renal diagnosis, and adequacy of the treatment regimen.

• Transplantation provides best long-term prognosis and quality of life, and all efforts should be made at the earliest reasonable time to evaluate patients with progressive chronic renal failure for transplant.

Treatment aims

To delay progression to end-stage renal failure.

To prevent renal bone disease.

To control hypertension.

To prevent acute or chronic renal failure (*e.g.*, by avoiding urinary tract infection, correcting obstruction).

Prognosis

• Timely dialysis or transplantation prolongs life.

• Comorbidity of multisystem diseases may limit survival.

Follow-up and management

• After chronic renal failure has been diagnosed, progress must be monitored at regular intervals; important parameters include the following:

Weight (for nutrition and fluid status).

Blood pressure (control may retard progression).

Urea/BUN (may alter with increased catabolism or protein intake).

Creatinine.

Hemoglobin.

Serum calcium (iatrogenic hypercalcemia must be avoided: calcium is nephrotoxic).

Serum phosphate.

Serum alkaline phosphatase.

Albumin (particularly helpful in assessing nutrition).

General references

Bushinsky DA: Bone disease in moderate renal failure: cause, nature and prevention. *Annu Rev Med* 1997, **48**:167–176.

Dunn CJ, Markham A: Epoetin beta: a review of its pharmacological properties and clinical use in the management of anaemia associated with chronic renal failure. *Drugs* 1996, **51**:299–318.

Holm EA, Solling K: Dietary protein restriction and the progression of chronic renal insufficiency: a review of the literature. *J Intern Med* 1996, **239**:99–104.

Hood VL, Gennari FJ: End-stage renal disease: measures to prevent it or slow its progression. *Postgrad Med* 1996, **100**:163–166, 171–176.

Lundin AP, Port FK: Adequacy of treatment for end-stage renal disease in the United States. *Adv Intern Med* 1996, **41**:323–363.

Steinman TI: Kidney protection: how to prevent or delay chronic renal failure. *Geriatrics* 1996, **51**:28–35.

Renal stones

Diagnosis

Symptoms

• Previous renal stone disease and/or hematuria is common.

• Severe, intermittent, colicky abdominal pain, typically flank with possible radiation to groin, with no position of comfort.

Nausea, vomiting, diaphoresis, frequency, dysuria.
Chills and fever: if complicated by obstruction and infection.

Signs

Extreme restlessness, diaphoresis.
Hematuria: typically microscopic, may be gross.
Frequency of urination, tachycardia.
Flank tenderness on affected side, possible mild abdominal tenderness with deep palpation without peritoneal signs.
Fever: if associated with urinary tract infection.

Investigations

Acute evaluation

Plain radiography of abdomen: is generally useful in rapidly demonstrating the presence and size of calcium-containing stones (radiopaque), but does not yield functional data.

Intravenous pyelography (IVP): excellent in assessing all aspects of stone imaging and is readily available; however, is limited by need for i.v. contrast dye exposure.

Renal ultrasonography: also yields comprehensive stone imaging data; however, it will not detect midureteral stones and is somewhat operator dependent.

Spiral or helical CT without contrast: the best imaging option and yields comprehensive data on all stone types and locations.

Collection and straining all urine: to capture and save stone when it passes.

Serum chemistries: electrolytes, creatinine, complete blood count, urine culture.

• Must quickly rule out urinary tract infection proximal to an obstructing stone, *i.e.*, obstructive pyelonephritis. This could be potentially life-threatening because of urosepsis, and will cause significant kidney damage if it persists.

Basic evaluation

• This evaluation should be considered in patients with uncomplicated, first-time renal stones.

Detailed history: to assess medical, lifestyle, dietary risk factors for renal stone disease.

Submit stone for radiographical diffraction crystallography evaluation, screen urine for cystine using nitroprusside test.

Screening blood tests: electrolytes, calcium, phosphorus, uric acid, creatinine. Children with first-time stones should be referred to a urologist.

Complete evaluation

• This evaluation should be done in patients with recurrent stone disease or who are in unusual demographic risk groups (*e.g.*, black females, children). It includes all the features of the basic evaluation in addition to the following:

Collect 24-hour urine on at least two occasions for the following values (includes optimal values):

Volume: >2 L	**Citrate:** >320 mg
Calcium: <300 mg in men, <250 mg in women	**Sodium:** <200 mEq
Oxalate: <40 mg	**Phosphorus:** <1100 mg
Uric acid: <800 mg in men, <750 mg in women	**pH:** >5.5 and <7.0

• Consider IVP, if not already done, to rule out medullary sponge kidney.

Complications

Chronic renal failure, pyelonephritis, perinephritic abscess, urosepsis.

Acute renal failure: if obstruction of single functioning kidney or if bilateral obstruction.

Recurrent stone formation, ureteral scarring.

Differential diagnosis

Pyelonephritis.
Salpingitis.
Appendicitis.
Diverticulitis.
Ectopic pregnancy.
Ovarian torsion.

• Always consider a full differential of abdominal pain.

Etiology

• There are four main types of renal stones as defined by the predominant component of the stone; their prevalence and typical causes follow:

Calcium stones: prevalence, ~80%; typical causes include hypercalcuria, hypocitruria, hyperuricosuria, hyperoxaluria, low urine volume, idiopathic.

Uric acid stones: prevalence, ~10%; typical causes include hyperuricosuria, hyperuricemia, low urine pH, low urine volume.

Cystine stones: prevalence, ~1%; typical causes, hereditary defect of tubular amino acid transport.

Struvite stones: prevalence, ~10%; typical causes, urinary tract infection with urease-positive organisms ("staghorn calculus").

• Drugs associated with renal stone formation: triamterene sulfonanlides, indinavir, carbonic anhydrase inhibitors.

Epidemiology

• Typical estimates of the prevalence of renal stone disease are as high as 3%–5%.

• Renal stone disease is 2–3 times more prevalent in males than in females.

• Renal stone is reported 3–4 times more frequently in whites than in blacks.

• The typical patient with renal stones is a white man between 20 and 50 years of age.

Treatment

Diet and lifestyle

Increased fluid intake: approximately 3 L water intake per day, including 8–12 oz at bedtime.

• Avoid dehydration and natural diuretics such as coffee or tea.

• Avoid high-salt and/or high-protein diet; both may increase calcium and uric acid excretion and decrease citrate excretion.

• Maintain moderate calcium intake to bind oxalate in gut and prevent osteoporosis.

• Dietary recommendations may vary depending on stone work-up; general guidelines include the following:

Start a low-oxalate diet if hyperoxaluria.

Consider decreased purine diet for hyperuricosuria.

Cystine stone disease requires very aggressive water intake because it is necessary to achieve a urine output of 3–3.5 L/day; urine flow should be as high at night as during day; maintain cystine concentration below 250 mg/L in the urine.

Pharmacological treatment

Short-term management

Prophylactic antibiotic: if more than 5 leukocytes/high-power field.

Narcotic pain medication.

Admit and initiate i.v. antibiotics: if obstructive pyelonephritis is possible.

Long-term management

• The following measures are dependent on data obtained from stone analysis and 24-hour urine studies.

Calcium stones:

Idiopathic hypercalciuria: hydrochlorothaizide, 25 mg daily; potassium citrate: 25–30 mEq twice daily.

Hyperuricosuria: allopurinol, 100 mg twice daily.

Hyperoxaluria: calcium carbonate, 1 g 3 times daily after meals.

Hypocitraturia: potassium citrate or potassium-magnesium citrate, 25–30 mEq twice daily; sodium citrate if potassium citrate not tolerated.

Uric acid stones: sodium bicarbonate, 650 mg 4 times daily (to achieve urine pH >7.0); allopurinol, 100 mg twice daily.

Struvite stones: consider long-term antibiotic suppression (trimethoprim-sulfamethoxazole).

Cystine stones: sodium bicarbonate, 650 mg 4 times daily; aggressive water intake (*see* Diet and lifestyle). Penicillamine, to bind cystine, is often necessary (needs careful monitoring for side effects).

Nonpharmacological treatment

Expectant management with hydration, 2.5–3 L/day (drinking at time of all voidings).

Treatment depends on stone size:

< 4 mm: will pass spontaneously in 90%–95% (80% within 4 weeks).

4–10 mm: decreased likelihood of passing; consider urologic consult.

≥ 10 mm: urologic intervention.

With obstructing or large stones (≥ 0.5 cm) that are not passing:

Extract cystoscopically if located in the lower ureter.

If the stone is located in the upper ureter or renal pelvis, consider extracorporeal shock-wave lithotripsy (ESWL*), percutaneous nephrolithotomy, endourologic procedures, or open surgery.

Most patients will not require admission if stone is < 5 mm.

*ESWL is contradicted in obstruction, pregnancy, and aortic or renal artery aneurysm.

Treatment aims

To preserve native renal function.

To reduce or eliminate episodes of recurrent stone formation.

Prognosis

• Recurrent stone disease may result in chronic renal insufficiency, however, end-stage kidney disease is uncommon.

• Recurrent struvite stone is associated with the highest rate of progressive renal deterioration (28% over 7-year period).

• ESWL has made a revolutionary improvement in morbidity due to stone disease.

Follow-up and management

• During acute period of stone passage, follow on an every-day to every-week interval in order to monitor progress of stone movement.

• If stone is in a fixed position for 4 weeks, surgical intervention will likely be required.

• Formal evaluation of renal stone disease is typically initiated 1 month after stone passage.

• After stone passage, plan a 2-year period of therapy with regular checks.

General references

Begun FP, Foley WD, Peterson A, White B: Urolithiasis: patient evaluation, laboratory and imaging studies. *Urol Clin North Am* 1997, **24**:97–116.

Bushinsky DA: Nephrolithiasis: *J Am Soc Nephrol* 1998, 9:208–924.

Goldfarb DS, Coe FL: Prevention of recurrent nephrolithiasis. *Am Fam Physician*, 1999,60:2269–2276.

Hesse A, Tiselius H-G, Janen A: *Urinary Stones: Diagnosis, Treatment, and Prevention of Recurrance*. Basel, New York: Karger; 1997.

Pak CY: Southwestern Internal Medicine Conference: Medical management of nephrolithiasis: a new, simplified approach for general practice. *Am J Med Sci* 1997, **313**:215–219.

Rivers K, Shetty S, Menon M: When and how to evaluate a patient with nephrolithiasis. *Urol Clin North Am* 2000, 27:203–213.

Diagnosis

Definition

• Renal tubular acidosis (RTA) is a disorder of renal hydrogen secretion or bicarbonate reabsorption.

• The following types of RTA have been defined:

Distal (type 1): defect in distal hydrogen secretion, probably related to defect in hydrogen ATPase.

Proximal (type 2): decreased proximal bicarbonate reabsorption, probably a defect in brush border sodium-hydrogen exchanger.

Hyporeninemic hypoaldosteronism (type 4): decreased distal acidification due to lack of aldoseterone and decreased distal sodium reabsorption (most commonly associated with diabetes mellitus).

Symptoms

• Renal tubular acidosis has no specific symptoms.

Weakness, musculoskeletal pains, low back pain: in distal RTA.

Failure to thrive: in children with proximal RTA; often associated with Fanconi's syndrome or other chronic renal disease and symptoms, including bone pain from osteomalacia.

Symptoms of diabetes mellitus: in hyporeninemic hypoaldosteronism (frequent association).

Symptoms of renal stone disease: in distal RTA.

Signs

• These are rare.

Weakness leading to paralysis: in proximal and distal RTA (due to hypokalemia).

Signs of diabetes mellitus: in hyporeninemic hypodosteronism.

Investigations

• The diagnosis of renal tubular acidosis is indicated by a hyperchloremic metabolic acidosis defined from blood-gas analysis with a normal plasma anion gap, defined by $(Na^+ + K^+) - (Cl^- + HCO_3^-)$; this differentiates it from an increased anion gap acidosis such as in lactic acidosis.

Plasma potassium analysis: to detect hypokalemia in patients with distal or proximal RTA.

Urine electrolytes to evaluate urine anion gap [Na + K - Cl]. Negative anion gap suggests extrarenal versus proximal RTA etiology. Positive anion gap requires further evaluation for distal RTA versus aldosterone deficit.

Short ammonium chloride loading test: if urine pH >6.0 to diagnose type 1 disease.

Sodium bicarbonate loading test: if urine pH <6.0 to diagnose type 2 disease.

Plain abdominal radiography: in distal RTA, to look for nephrocalcinosis.

Complications

• These may be renal related, as in type 1 disease, or may be due to general complications of the underlying disease, as in type 4 disease.

Nephrocalcinosis and nephrolithiasis: distal RTA.

Diabetes mellitus leading to renal failure from diabetic nephropathy: most common condition associated with hyporeninemic hypoaldosteronism.

Hypokalemia: distal and proximal RTA; may be severe, resulting in paralysis.

Hyperkalemia: hyporeninemic hypoaldosteronism.

Childhood growth retardation: type 1 and type 2 disease.

Osteitis fibrosa: children.

Osteopenia: adults.

Differential diagnosis

Distal RTA with nephrocalcinosis

Medullary sponge kidney, idiopathic hypercalciuria, hyperparathyroidism.

• Laxative abuse or chronic diarrhea can lead to a hyperchloremic acidosis with an abnormal short ammonium chloride loading test; this can be differentiated by the urinary anion gap, which is negative in patients with diarrhea but positive in patients with distal RTA.

Etiology

Causes of distal RTA

Idiopathic, Sjögren's syndrome, SLE, primary biliary cirrhosis, amphotericin, lithium, multiple myeloma, obstructive uropathy inherited defects in distal nephron anion and proton transporters.

Causes of proximal RTA

Idiopathic, cystinosis, Fanconi's syndrome, Wilson's disease, primary hyperparathyroidism, acetazolamide, consider multiple myelomas in adults.

Causes of hyporeninemic hypoaldosteroism

Diabetes mellitus (most important in clinical practice), urinary obstruction, sickle cell disease, interstitial nephritis; mimicked by potassium-sparing diuretics.

Epidemiology

• Distal and proximal RTAs are typically diagnosed in childhood.

• Distal RTA also occurs in adults.

• Distal and proximal RTAs are rare; hyporeninemic hypoaldosteroism occurs relatively frequently.

Causes of normal anion gap acidosis

Failure of renal acidification due to renal tubular acidosis or acetazolamide.

Gastrointestinal loss of bicarbonate due to diarrhea, purgative abuse, pancreatic fistula, ureteric diversion (*e.g.*, ureterosigmoidostomy).

Ingestion of acid (*e.g.*, hydrochloric).

Parenteral nutrition.

Treatment

Diet and lifestyle

• No special precautions are necessary.

Pharmacological treatment

For distal and proximal RTA

• Patients should be given oral sodium bicarbonate up to 1–2 mEq/kg (distal) or 3–5 mEq/kg (proximal) daily, titrated to improve acidosis.

• Potassium and, in type 2 disease, vitamin D supplements may also be needed.

• Acidosis is not completely corrected by oral supplements.

For hyporeninemic hypoaldosteronism

• Fludrocortisone or diuretics (loop or thiazide) with sodium bicarbonate if acidemia is substantial ($HCo_3 < 18$). Often, no treatment is needed.

• Potassium-sparing diuretics, NSAIDs, angiotensin-converting enzyme inhibitors, angiotensin receptor blockers which worsen hyperkalemia, must be avoided.

Standard dosage Fludrocortisone, 100–400 µg daily.
Bumetanide, 1–5 mg, and sodium bicarbonate up to 4 g daily.

Contraindications *Fludrocortisone*: volume overload.
Bumetanide: volume depletion.
Sodium bicarbonate: volume overload.

Main drug interactions None.

Main side effects Fluid overload if inadequate diuretic given with sodium bicarbonate.

Treatment aims

To prevent nephrocalcinosis and nephrolithiasis in type 1 disease.

To treat bone disease with vitamin D if deficiency present in type 2 disease.

To avoid life-threatening hyperkalemia caused by concomitant medication in type 4 disease.

To correct significant acidemia.

Prognosis

• Distal RTA can progress to renal failure (not usual).

• The prognosis for RTA in general depends on the associated conditions.

Follow-up and management

• Acidosis and, in distal RTA, nephrocalcinosis and nephrolithiasis must be monitored.

General references

Dell KM, Guay-Woodford LM: Inherited tubular transport disorders. *Sem Nephrol* 1999, **19**:364–373.

DuBose TD Jr.: Hyperkalemic hyperchloremic metabolic acidosis: pathophysiologic insights. *Kidney Int* 1997, **51**:591–602.

Gregory MJ, Schwartz GJ: Diagnosis and treatment of renal tubular disorders. *Sem Nephrol* 1999, **18**:317–329.

Kamel KS, *et al.*: A new classification for renal defects in net acid excretion. *Am J Kidney Dis* 1997, **29**:136–146.

Kim GH, Hans JS, Kim YS, *et al.*:Evaluation of urine acidification by urine anion gap and urine osmolal gap in chronic metabolic acidosis. *Am J Kidney Dis* 1996, **27**:42–47.

Laski ME, Kurtzman NA: Acid-base disorders in medicine. *Dis Mon* 1996, **42**:51–125.

Petersen-Smith AM: Renal tubular acidosis: when kids won't grow. *J Pediatr Health Care* 1995, **9**:131–133.

Smulders YM, *et al.*: Renal tubular acidosis: pathophysiology and diagnosis. *Arch Intern Med* 1996, **156**:1629–1636.

Restrictive cardiomyopathy & constrictive pericarditis

Diagnosis

Symptoms

Because restrictive cardiomyopathy affects either or both ventricles, it may cause symptoms and signs of right or left ventricular failure.

Dyspnea, fatigue, ankle or abdominal swelling.

Signs

Restrictive cardiomyopathy

Jugular venous pulse

Raised jugular venous pressure; inspiratory increase in jugular venous pressure; Kussmaul's sign.

Heart

Palpable apex beat; mild or moderate cardiomegaly; third or fourth heart sounds; peripheral edema; ascites.

Constrictive pericarditis

Jugular venous pulse

Raised jugular venous pressure, with rapid diastolic "y" descent; Kussmaul's sign.

Heart

Diffuse or impalpable apex beat; intercostal indrawing of apex in systole: Broadbent's sign; early diastolic pericardial "knock;" widened splitting of second heart sound.

Investigations

• The two conditions overlap considerably, and separating them on clinical findings and investigations may be impossible; thoracotomy may be needed to exclude or confirm the diagnosis.

Chest radiography: *restrictive cardiomyopathy*, shows mild or moderate cardiomegaly; *constrictive pericarditis*, shows normal heart size and pericardial calcification.

ECG: *restrictive cardiomyopathy*, shows low-voltage complexes; shows T-wave changes, bundle branch block, or atrial arrhythmias; *constrictive pericarditis* shows low-voltage complexes; shows nonspecific T-wave flattening and atrial fibrillation.

Echocardiography: *restrictive cardiomyopathy*, shows myocardial thickening and characteristic "ground glass" appearance (in amyloid heart disease); idiopathic restrictive cardiomyopathy, demonstrates biatrial enlargement, nondilated ventricles, normal ventricular thickness, and preserved systolic function (usually); *constrictive pericarditis*, shows normal myocardial thickness and may reveal thickened pericardium; *both*, show normal ventricular dimensions with enlarged atria and good systolic and poor diastolic dysfunction.

Doppler echocardiography: *restrictive cardiomyopathy*, decreased right ventricular and left ventricular velocities with inspiration, inspiratory augmentation of hepatic-vein diastolic flow reversal, mitral and tricuspid regurgitation common; *constrictive pericarditis*, increased right ventricular systolic and decreased left ventricular systolic velocity with inspiration, expiratory augmentation of hepatic-vein diastolic flow reversal.

CT or MRI: *restrictive cardiomyopathy*, shows myocardial thickening and normal pericardium; *constrictive pericarditis*, shows normal myocardial thickness and pericardial thickening and calcification.

Cardiac catheterization: *restrictive cardiomyopathy*, shows left ventricular filling pressure exceeding right ventricular filling pressure and pulmonary artery systolic pressure often > 45 mm Hg with myocardial biopsy diagnostic; *constrictive pericarditis*, shows identical left and right ventricular filling pressures and pulmonary artery systolic pressure usually < 45 mm Hg, with normal myocardial biopsy; *both*, show rapid "y" descent in atrial pressure and early dip in diastolic pressure, with pressure rise to plateau in mid-diastole or late diastole.

Complications

Systemic hypotension.

Atrial and ventricular arrhythmias.

Progressive heart failure: in constrictive pericarditis, the heart itself is not failing, but the resulting clinical features are similar to those of restrictive cardiomyopathy.

Hepatic failure: resulting from chronic hepatic venous congestion.

Nephrotic syndrome.

Conduction abnormalities: in restrictive cardiomyopathy.

Differential diagnosis

Biventricular heart failure: myocardial infarction, myocardial ischemia, dilated cardiomyopathy.

Myocardial thickening: hypertension, aortic stenosis, hypertrophic cardiomyopathy.

Cardiac tamponade.

Nephrotic syndrome.

Etiology

Restrictive cardiomyopathy

Infiltrative

Amyloidosis.

Sarcoidosis.

Storage diseases.

Glycogen storage disorders.

Hemochromatosis.

Fabry's disease.

Noninfiltrative

Collagen vascular disorders, e.g., scleroderma.

Pseudoxanthoma elasticum.

Diabetic cardiomyopathy.

Endomyocardial fibrosis.

Endomyocardial fibrosis.

Eosinophilia.

Neoplastic infiltration.

Myocardial fibrosis of any origin.

Carcinoid heart disease.

Anthracycline toxicity.

Drugs causing fibrous endocarditis (methysergide, serotonin, busulfan, ergotamine, mercurial agents).

Idiopathic: occurs in the absence of any identifiable cause.

Constrictive pericarditis

• Most causes are unknown.

Tuberculosis (<15% of patients).

Chronic renal failure.

Connective tissue disorder.

Neoplastic infiltration.

Irradiation (often years earlier).

Postpurulent pericarditis.

Hemopericardium after surgery (rare).

Epidemiology

• Both conditions are rare.

• All age groups are affected.

• Glycogen storage disorders are incompatible with progression to adult life.

Treatment

Diet and lifestyle

- Patients' daily activities are restricted by fatigue, breathlessness, and fluid retention.

Pharmacological treatment

Restrictive cardiomyopathy

Amyloid: digitalis and calcium-channel blockers should be avoided. In amyloidosis due to plasma cell dyscrasia, chemotherapy with bone-marrow transplantation has been used with some success.

Hemochromatosis iron chelating agents, *e.g.*, desferrioxamine.

- Corticosteroids and cytotoxic drugs are effective only during the acute myocardial phase of eosinophilia.

Constrictive pericarditis

- Surgery is the only satisfactory treatment.
- Patients with tuberculous pericarditis should be pretreated with antituberculous therapy; if the diagnosis is confirmed after pericardial resection, full antituberculous therapy should be continued for 6–12 months after resection.

Nonpharmacological treatment

Restrictive cardiomyopathy

Permanent pacing for conduction abnormalities in amyloid.

Bimonthly phlebotomy often for 2–3 years to reduce iron storage in hemachromatosis.

Endocardial resection after fibrosis is established in eosinophilia.

Transplantation occasionally. When transplantation has been performed to treat cardiac amyloidosis or sarcoidosis, recurrence in the explanted heart can occur and therefore transplantation is not usually considered as a viable option.

Constrictive pericarditis

Complete surgical resection of the pericardium (myocardial inflammation or fibrosis may delay symptomatic response).

Treatment aims

To relieve symptoms.

To remove underlying causes.

Prognosis

- Prognosis is good after resection for constrictive pericarditis.
- Restrictive cardiomyopathy has poor prognosis, particularly due to amyloidosis or malignancy. In idiopathic restrictive cardiopathy, the prognosis is poor in men >70 years old with higher NYHA class and a left atrial dimension >60 mm.

Follow-up and management

- Management is purely palliative.

General references

Ammash NM, *et al.*: Clinical profile and outcome of idiopathic restrictive cardiomyopathy. *Circulation* 2000, **101**:2490–2496.

Falk RH, Skinner M: The systemic amyloidoses: an overview. *Adv Intern Med* 2000, **45**:107–137.

Kushwaha SS, Fallon JT, Fuster V: Restrictive cardiomyopathy. *N Engl J Med* 1997, **336**:267.

Rheumatic fever, acute

Diagnosis

Symptoms

• Acute rheumatic fever is a multisystem disorder occurring 1–5 weeks after group A streptococcal infection.

• Its manifestation is variable, involving any of the following:

Joint pain (migratory polyarthropathy): ranging from simple pain to disabling arthritis; classically involves large joints in succession, with "overlapping" involvement.

Breathlessness and chest pain (pancarditis): cardiac failure with occasional clinical pericardial involvement.

Rapid purposeless involuntary movements (Sydenham's chorea): including slurred speech, jerky movements, facial tics and grimacing, emotional lability; manifest only during wakefulness; may occur as late isolated feature of disease.

Subcutaneous nodules: painless firm lesions (up to 2 cm diameter) over bony prominences and tendons; tend to appear late and last 1–2 weeks.

Erythema marginatum: red rash extending circumferentially on trunk and proximal limbs; changes rapidly over minutes.

Signs

Joint involvement: joints may be exquisitely tender, red, swollen; refusal to bear weight (especially in children).

Signs of cardiac failure, tachycardia, cardiomegaly, pericardial rub, mitral regurgitation, Carey–Coombs aortic regurgitation, first-, second-, or third-degree atrioventricular block.

Chorea: "bag of worms" tongue of chorea (fasciculation on protrusion), "Milkmaid's grip" (squeezing and relaxing motion on gripping the hand), pendular knee jerks.

Skin rash and nodules.

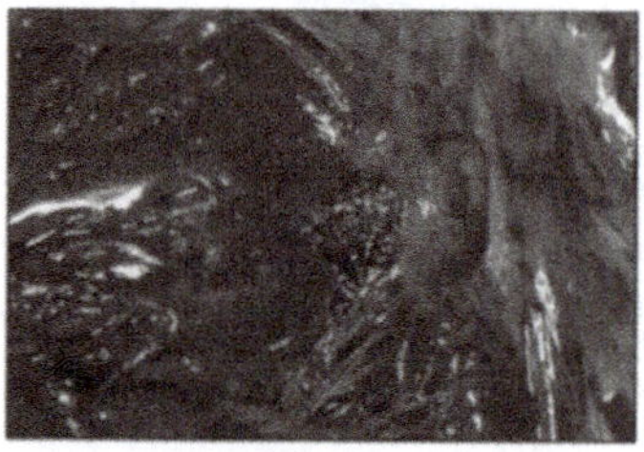

Vegetation on mitral valve, the major reason for continued prophylaxis after rheumatic heart disease. (See Color Plate.)

Investigations

• No single test is diagnostic; the diagnosis is simplified by application of the Duckett-Jones criteria.

• The most important laboratory contribution is evidence of antecedent streptococcal infection.

• No significant laboratory abnormality may be seen in pure chorea.

Throat swab: usually negative, but positive result indicates increased disease activity.

Antistreptolysin O, anti-DNAse B, antihyaluronidase titers: if all three done, 95% chance of positive result.

Complete blood count: leukocytosis common; moderate normochromic, normocytic anemia often seen.

ESR, CRP measurement: usually raised.

Liver function tests: aspartate transaminase possibly raised.

Urinalysis: sediment positive for leukocytes and erythrocytes (not pathognomonic of glomerulonephritis).

ECG: shows tachycardia and first-, second-, or, rarely, third-degree heart block.

Echocardiography: shows myocardial thickening and dysfunction, pericardial effusion, and valvular dysfunction.

Complications

Recurrent episodes: with continuing evidence of inflammatory activity.

Rheumatic heart disease: major long-term sequela.

Differential diagnosis

Other causes of polyarthropathy, fever, and cardiac involvement.

Viral arthritides, *e.g.*, rubella, hepatitis B.

Septic arthritis *e.g.*, *Neisseria* spp. infection.

Infective endocarditis.

Acute rheumatoid arthritis.

Stills' disease.

Serum sickness, *e.g.*, after penicillin.

Systemic lupus erythematosus.

Prepurpuric phase Henoch–Schönlein purpura.

Lyme disease.

Etiology

• Acute rheumatic fever is an exudative, proliferative inflammation of connective tissues, especially heart, joints, and subcutaneous tissues.

• It occurs only after group A streptococcal infection of the upper respiratory tract.

• Particular serotypes, *e.g.*, types 5 and 18, are often implicated, whereas others, *e.g.*, type 12, are not.

Epidemiology

• The incidence of acute rheumatic fever mirrors that of acute streptococcal pharyngitis in a population.

• The peak incidence is at 5–15 years; it is rare in children aged <4 years but well described in adults.

• The overall male:female ratio is equal; women, however, are more likely to develop Sydenham's chorea and mitral stenosis.

Duckett-Jones criteria for diagnosing acute rheumatic fever

Modified by the American Heart Association.

• Acute rheumatic fever is indicated by two major or one major and two minor criteria if supported by evidence of preceding streptococcal infection.

Major manifestations

Carditis.

Polyarthritis.

Chorea.

Erythema marginatum.

Subcutaneous nodules.

Minor manifestations

Previous rheumatic fever or rheumatic heart disease.

Arthralgia.

Fever.

Raised ESR and CRP concentration, leukocytosis, prolonged PR interval.

Treatment

Diet and lifestyle

• Strict bed or chair rest is advised with mobilization according to clinical status.

Pharmacological treatment

Antibiotics

• Antibiotics do not modify an acute attack or influence the development of carditis.

• They are used to eradicate streptococci from the pharynx and tonsils to prevent recurrence and further valve damage, as prophylaxis for all rheumatic carditis patients, or to cover dental extractions and other surgical interventions (long-term penicillin G benzathine, i.m. 4-weekly).

Standard dosage	Penicillin V, 500 mg 4 times daily for 10 days (adults; *see manufacurer's current prescribing information for children*). Erythromycin, 250 mg 4 times daily for 10 days (adults; *see manufacurer's current prescribing information for children*).
Contraindications	Hypersensitivity.
Special points	Shorter courses may not eradicate streptococci from pharynx.
Main drug interactions	Oral anticoagulants, theophylline preparations (erythromycin).
Main side effects	Hypersensitivity and rash (penicillin), gastrointestinal intolerance.

Anti-inflammatory agents

• These do not cure or prevent subsequent development of rheumatic disease.

• Early indiscriminate use may obscure diagnosis in mild cases.

Standard dosage	Aspirin, 80–100 mg/kg daily (children), 6–8 g daily (adults); reduced after 2 weeks and continued for 6–8 weeks. *For more severe carditis or patients intolerant of high-dose salicylates:* prednisolone, 40–60 mg daily for 2 weeks, reduced over next 3–4 weeks, followed by aspirin.
Contraindications	*Aspirin:* breast-feeding, gastrointestinal ulceration, hemophilia. *Prednisolone:* current acute gastrointestinal blood loss.
Special points	*Aspirin:* one of the few indications for aspirin treatment in childhood. *Prednisolone:* possible adrenal suppression on sudden withdrawal.
Main drug interactions	*Aspirin:* anticoagulants. *Prednisolone:* danger of gastrointestinal hemorrhage if combined with NSAIDs.
Main side effects	*Aspirin:* hypersensitivity, gastrointestinal bleeding. *Prednisolone:* glucose intolerance, Cushing's syndrome, growth retardation.

Other options

Diuretics, possibly with angiotensin-converting enzyme inhibitors.

Digoxin.

Anticoagulants.

• Use is determined by the degree of carditis or cardiac failure and the stage of illness.

Treatment aims

To eradicate current streptococcal infection and prevent reinfection.

To prevent further episodes of acute disease.

To relieve acute arthritic symptoms.

To prevent infective endocarditis on valves already damaged by carditis.

Prognosis

• Untreated acute rheumatic fever usually lasts up to 3 months.

• Severe carditis extends acute illness to 6 months.

• Most patients with valvular disease develop cardiological complications needing intervention by middle age.

• 6% of patients free of carditis during an acute attack have rheumatic heart disease at 10 years.

• 30% of patients with mild carditis and no pre-existing disease have murmurs at 10 years.

• 40% of patients with apical or basal murmurs in an acute attack have residual disease at 10 years.

• 70% of patients with cardiac failure or pericarditis in an acute attack have residual disease at 10 years.

• Exceptions are patients with "pure" chorea, who frequently develop rheumatic heart disease despite absence of signs of carditis at outset.

Follow-up and management

• Patients must be kept under strict supervision until signs of acute inflammation have subsided.

• Penicillin or alternative prophylaxis is needed at least until the age of 18 years (some clinicians advocate life-long prophylaxis).

• Adequate prophylaxis is needed for minor surgical interventions, *e.g.*, dental treatment.

General references

Homer C, *et al.*: Clinical aspects of acute rheumatic fever. *J Rheumatol* 1991, **18(suppl 29)**:2–12.

Simmons NA: Recommendations for endocarditis prophylaxis. *J Antimicrob Chemother* 1993, **31**:437–438.

Veasy LG, Hill HR: Immunologic and clinical correlations in rheumatic fever and rheumatic heart disease. *Pediatr Infect Dis J* 1997, **16**:400–407.

Rhinosinusitis

Diagnosis

Symptoms

Acute rhinosinusitis

Headache or facial pain: involving the maxillary, frontal, and ethmoid sinuses (pain directly over sinuses) or sphenoid sinuses (the great masquerader): pain may be retro-orbital, temporal, vertex, or occipital with sphenoid sinusitis.
Purulent nasal discharge.
Maxillary toothache.
Poor response to decongestants.
Fever, malaise, cough, wheezing, postnasal drip, edema or erythema over sinuses.

Chronic sinusitis

Headache or facial pain: typically less severe than acute sinusitis, unless the infection involves frontal or sphenoid sinuses.
Purulent rhinorrhea: anteriorly and/or posteriorly (note: isolated sphenoid sinusitis may present as only posterior rhinorrhea).
Nasal congestion.
Low-grade fever, malaise, halitosis, cough, wheezing edema, erythema over sinuses: less severe.

Signs

Purulent nasal secretions.
Nasal congestion and mucosal erythema.
Sinus tenderness on percussion or palpation: often nonspecific.
Abnormal translumination compared with contralateral side.
Facial edema or erythema.

Investigations

• Typically, diagnosis is made on clinical basis.

Indications for CT scan

To define extent of disease after "maximum medical treatment": in patients with chronic sinusitis who have been treated with 4 weeks of broad-spectrum antibiotics and topical steroid therapy.
Full CT scan: indicated in cases of suspected fungal disease, immunocompromised or diabetic patient with possible invasive fungal disease, suspected complication of sinusitis, suspected underlying mass.
Screening sinus CT: uncertainty of diagnosis.
Full or screening CT: indicated in cases of frequent acute sinusitis or failure to respond.

Other investigations based on clinical findings

Chest radiography: if suspected associated pneumonia or systemic illness such as Churg-Strauss syndrome, Wegener's disease, sarcoidosis.
ESR, urinalysis and sediment; antineutrophilic cytoplasmic antibody: to screen for Wegener's disease or (less commonly) Churg-Strauss syndrome or other systemic vasculitis.
Immunoglobulin levels (IgA, IgM, IgG, and IgG subclasses): for patients with unusually frequent bacterial respiratory infections.
Nasal smear: most commonly performed by allergist to identify bacteria as well as lymphocytes, neutrophils, or eosinophils as predominant cell type.
• Cultures (sinus tap vs. endoscopic middle meatus culture) are usually performed by an otolaryngologist.

Complications

General: exacerbation of asthma, pneumonia, pharyngitis, otitis media, mucocele.
Ophthalmologic: periorbital or preseptal cellulitis (lid only); subperiosteal abscess; orbital cellulitis; orbital abscess; cavernous sinus thrombosis.
Intracranial complications: higher risk with sphenoid and frontal sinusitis; subdural empyema; epidural empyema; cerebral abscess; meningitis.
Invasive fungal disease: extension into orbit, brain, soft tissues of face, nasal cavity, and palate with tissue ischemia and necrosis.

Differential diagnosis

Allergic rhinitis with headache.
Nasal dryness and crusting (bacterial rhinitis).
Headache (migraine, tension, or ophthalmologic).
Temporomandibular joint or dental pain.
Gastroesophageal reflux laryngitis/pharyngitis (manifested as postnasal drip, hoarseness, cough).
Systemic diseases (Wegener's granulomatosis, sarcoidosis, Churg-Strauss syndrome).
Neuralgia and other neurological disorders.
Temporal arteritis.

Etiology and predisposing conditions

• The most common precipitating event is a bacterial or viral upper respiratory infection (URI).
• Common predisposing conditions include: mucosal edema (rhinitis: allergic, vasomotor, bacterial, or viral).
Mechanical obstruction (polyps, septal deviation, trauma, tumor, foreign body).
Impaired ciliary motility or mucosal disease (Wegener's disease, sarcoidosis, cystic fibrosis, bacterial rhinitis/crusting).
Rapid change in altitude or pressure.
Dental infection.
Bacterial rhinitis secondary to dryness and crusting.

Epidemiology

• Estimates are that 0.5%–5% of URIs in children will be associated with sinusitis.
• ~35 million adults in the United States suffer from "chronic sinusitis."
• Increasing incidence of bacterial resistance is expected.

Pathophysiology

URI.
Osteomeatal complex obstruction.
Sinus hypoxia, ciliary dysfunction, retained secretions, and cycle of infection.

Treatment

Diet and lifestyle

- Patients should avoid seasonal (pollens, grasses, trees) and perennial (dust, mold, danders) allergens.
- Patients should stop smoking.
- Saline sprays and/or saline bulb syringe irrigations are recommended.

Pharmacological treatment

Decongestants

Standard dosage Oxymetazalone spray twice daily for 3–5 days (beware of rebound rhinitis medicamentosa if used >5 days).
Pseudoephedrine, short- or long-acting preparations (may elevate blood pressure or exacerbate urinary retention).

Antibiotics (acute rhinosinusitis)

- Standard length of therapy is 10 days.

Standard dosage First-line therapy: amoxicillin, 500 mg orally 3 times daily.
Bactrim DS, twice daily.
Alternative or second-line therapies (14–21 days' duration):
Clarithromycin, 500 mg twice daily.
Ceftin, 250–500 mg twice daily.
Augmentin, 875 mg twice daily or 500 mg every 8 hours (with food).
Levofluxacin, 500 mg once daily.

Antibiotics (chronic rhinosinusitis)

- Standard course of therapy is 3–6 weeks based on underlying comorbidities.

Standard dosage Ceftin, 500 mg twice daily.
Augmentin, 500 mg every 8 hours (with food).
Biaxin, 500 mg twice daily.
Loracarbef, 400 mg twice daily.
Levofluxacin, 500 mg once daily (± flagyl, 500 mg 3 times daily).

Special points Prescription for antibiotics should avoid known allergies; consider compliance with dosing; and account for underlying comorbid conditions, such as severe allergies or polyps, for which longer courses may be appropriate.
Patients with acute infections should be told to call their physician if symptoms, particularly pain and fever, are not responding to therapy after 48–72 hours.

For allergies

- Steroids sprays, antihistamine decongestants, immunotherapy are recommended.

When to refer for otolaryngologic evaluation and/or sinus surgery

Recurrent acute sinusitis 3–4 times a year documented by a screening CT.

Chronic sinusitis refractory to maximal medical treatment as evidenced by persistent obstruction of the sinuses or osteomeatal complex after 3–6 weeks of therapy.

Complication or impending complication of sinusitis.

Suspected fungal sinusitis (mycetoma, allergic fungal sinusitis, or invasive disease).

Immunocompromised patient not responding to therapy.

Bony erosive or destructive process on CT scan suggestive of more aggressive disease.

Nasal mass, tumor, or extension into other sinus.

Treatment aims

Treatment

To minimize symptoms of pain and rhinorrhea.

To avoid development of complications.

Surgery

To widely open the osteomeatal complex, ethmoid, maxillary, and other sinuses to allow aeration of the cavity, restore mucociliary clearance of the sinuses, and thereby reduce the frequency and severity of infections.

Other treatments

Allergy testing and immunotherapy.

Skin testing appropriate for patients with allergic rhinitis refractory to avoidance, steroid sprays, antihistamines, and decongestants, or when allergens not readily identified; this may be followed by immunotherapy.

- Ideally, allergies should be maximally treated prior to sinus surgery (if required) to enhance mucosal healing.

Prognosis

- Majority of patients with sinusitis for several months will have such extensive irreversible mucosal disease that surgery may be necessary to establish drainage to allow resolution of the infection.
- 85%–90% of patients will be substantially improved by endoscopic sinus surgery.

Follow-up and management after surgery

Maintain or enhance mucociliary clearance with over-the-counter nasal saline sprays or salt water bulb syringe irrigations.

For patients with allergies and/or polyps: consider long-term daily steroid sprays.

Aggressive treatment of infections, especially in the first 3–6 months after surgery during which time mucociliary function is still compromised.

General references

Benninger MS, Sedory Holzer SE, Lau J: Diagnosis and treatment of uncomplicated acute bacterial rhinosinusitis: summary of the Agency for Health Care Policy and Research evidence-based report. *Otolaryngol Head Neck Surg* 2000, **122**:1–7.

Osguthorpe JD, Hadley JA: Rhinosinusitis: current concepts in evaulation and management. *Med Clin North Am* 1999, **83**:27–41.

Poole MD: A focus on acute sinusitis in adults: changes in disease management. *Am J Med* 1999, **106**:38S–47S.

Rubella (German measles)

Diagnosis

Symptoms

• Symptoms are mostly trivial; patients are systemically well.

Mild fever.

Rash: in ~50% of infected patients.

Signs

Rash: fine, erythematous pink macules, almost confluent on trunk on second day, rarely lasts >3 days.

Reddened throat: sometimes with tonsillar exudates.

Enlarged lymph nodes: notably occipital, sometimes splenomegaly.

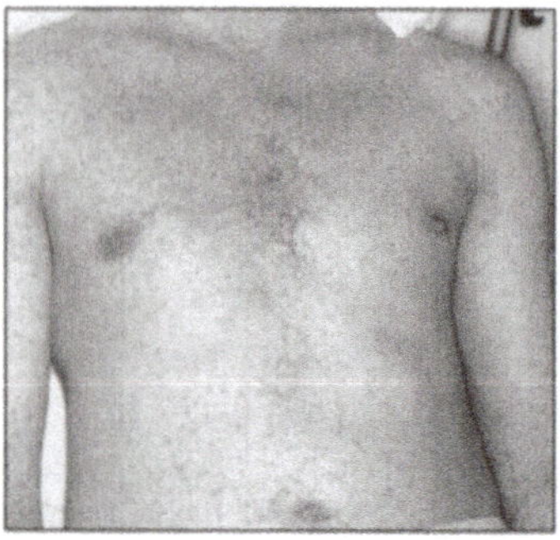

Fine nonblotchy rash of rubella. (See Color Plate.)

Investigations

• The diagnosis of rubella is established serologically.

• A patient's unconfirmed history of rubella should be discounted.

Serology: IgM detectable in serum within 1–2 days of rash; hemagglutination-inhibiting antibodies rise within 1–2 days of rash, peak in 6–12 days, and thereafter fade but remain detectable at lower levels.

Complications

General

Arthralgia or arthritis of fingers, wrists, and knees: usually in young women.

Encephalitis.

Thrombocytopenia.

Neuritis.

Congenital rubella

Cataract, retinopathy, microphthalmos, glaucoma.

Patent ductus arteriosus, ventricular septal defect, pulmonary stenosis.

Deafness.

Thrombocytopenic purpura, hepatosplenomegaly, hepatitis, CNS defects, bone lesions.

Differential diagnosis

• Patients with rubella are usually well and the rash is not blotchy.

Measles: marked prodrome, malaise, dusky-red maculopapular erythematous rash that travels down body over 3 days.

Adenovirus or enterovirus infections, mild scarlet fever, cytomegalovirus or Epstein–Barr virus infection, toxoplasmosis.

Etiology

• Infection is by rubella virus, an RNA virus.

• Transmission is by respiratory droplets.

• Fetal infection occurs secondary to maternal viremia; the incidence and type of defect are related to the age of the fetus at the time of infection.

• Significant defects are found with early infection.

Epidemiology

• Rubella occurs worldwide.

Infectivity

• ~16% of affected infants have major defects at birth after maternal rubella in the first trimester.

• Rubella is moderately infectious: patients are infectious during the rash and probably for ~7 days before and up to 5 days after illness, although the virus is detectable in throat secretions up to 10 days before and until 16 days after the rash.

• Babies with congenital rubella excrete the virus in throat and urine for prolonged periods.

Mean incubation period

~18 days.

Treatment

Diet and lifestyle

• No special diet is necessary.

• Affected patients should keep away from pregnant women.

Pharmacological treatment

Symptomatic

Analgesics, *e.g.*, acetaminophen.

Prophylactic

• Vaccination is by live attenuated virus: this may produce a mild rubella-like illness; women should not be pregnant or become so within 8–12 weeks of vaccination.

• It is routinely recommended in the second year of life as part of MMR, for girls aged 10–14 years at present, and any identified susceptible adult women of childbearing potential.

• Prompt serological testing of pregnant contacts of a patient with rubella is essential to assess susceptibility.

• The use of hyperimmune globulin should be considered if the risk is significant and if therapeutic abortion would not be considered should rubella develop later.

Treatment aims

To relieve symptoms.

To prevent congenital rubella.

Prognosis

• The prognosis in rubella is excellent.

• Deaths are rare and usually associated with encephalitis.

Follow-up and management

• Follow-up and management are not needed except in pregnancy, when risks and discussion of termination should be considered.

General references

Anonymous: *Immunization Against Infectious Diseases.* London: HMSO; 1992

Hall AJ, Peckham CS: Infections in childhood and pregnancy as a cause of adult disease: methods and examples. *Br Med Bull* 1997, **53**:10–23.

Miller E, *et al.*: Rubella surveillance to June 1994. *Comm Dis Rep* 1994, **4**:R146–R152.

Morgan-Capner P. Diagnosing rubella. *BMJ* 1989; **229**:338–339.

Diagnosis

Symptoms

• Patients may have no respiratory symptoms.

Dyspnea.

Cough: usually unproductive.

Chest discomfort: vague intermittent ache.

Fatigue, malaise, weight loss, fever, anorexia.

Symptoms of the complications of sarcoidosis.

Signs

Fine inspiratory crackles and wheezes: rarely.

Lymphadenopathy.

Uveitis, keratoconjunctivitis sicca, retinopathy.

Erythema nodosum, skin nodules, maculopapular rash, lupus pernio.

Hepatomegaly, splenomegaly, portal hypertension.

Bone cysts, polyarthralgia, myopathy.

Investigations [1,3]

Chest radiography: 90% of patients have abnormal radiographs, which show a wide variety of appearances (*see* Clinical staging).

Pulmonary function tests: may be entirely within normal limits, despite extensive radiographic shadows, or may show significant physiological dysfunction with clear radiographical lung fields. A restrictive defect is most common.

Skin test: anergy in two-thirds of patients.

Blood tests: leukocyte count may show lymphopenia; ESR may be raised; serum immunoglobulins and electrophoresis may show panhyperglobulinemia; serum angiotensin-converting enzyme increased in two-thirds of acute patients; hypercalcemia in ~18% of patients; liver function indices in a few may show intrahepatic cholestasis.

24-hour urine collection: hypercalciuria may be present despite normal serum calcium concentration.

ECG: arrhythmias, bundle branch block pattern in some patients.

Biopsy of lymph node, lung tissue, skin, liver, or other tissue: shows noncaseating epithelioid granulomata.

Fiberoptic bronchoscopy with transbronchial biopsy: the procedure of choice in patients with suspected pulmonary involvement.

Bronchoalveolar lavage: may be helpful adjunct to diagnosis; many patients with "active" sarcoidosis show increased percentage of lymphocytes and a high CD4/CD8 cell ratio.

• Ophthalmological assessment, including slit lamp examination and fluorescein angiography (needed in patients with associated occular symptoms).

Complications

Peripheral neuropathy, facial-nerve palsy, other cranial-nerve palsies, papilledema, meningitis, space-occupying lesions, epilepsy, cerebellar ataxia, hypopituitarism, diabetes insipidus.

Bundle branch block, arrhythmias, congestive cardiac failure, pericarditis, cardiomyopathy, cor pulmonale.

Disordered calcium metabolism, hypercalcemia, hypercalciuria, nephrocalcinosis.

Enlarged parotid and lacrimal glands.

Glaucoma, cataract: complication of chronic uveitis.

Differential diagnosis

Hilar lymphadenopathy
Tuberculosis, Hodgkin's lymphoma, infectious mononucleosis, metastases, enlarged pulmonary arteries.

Hilar lymphadenopathy with pulmonary infiltration
Tuberculosis, pneumoconiosis, lymphangitic carcinoma, idiopathic hemosiderosis, pulmonary eosinophilia, alveolar-cell carcinoma, histiocytosis X.

Diffuse pulmonary infiltration
The above and also chronic beryllium disease, honeycomb lung, rheumatoid lung, Sjögren's syndrome, interstitial lung disease, cystic fibrosis, hypersensitivity pneumonitis.

Noncaseating granulomata
Tuberculosis and other mycobacterial infections, fungal infections, leprosy, syphilis, cat-scratch disease, berylliosis, hypersensitivity pneumonitis, foreign-body reactions, lymphoma, carcinoma, biliary cirrhosis, Crohn's disease, hypogammaglobulinemia, granulomatous vasculitides, parasitic infection.

Etiology

• The cause is unknown, but alterations in the immune system is involved in its pathogenesis.

Epidemiology

• Sarcoidosis is usually manifest in the 20–40-year age group.

• It is more usual in temperate than in tropical climates.

• The prevalence rates are difficult to establish because the disease is often asymptomatic; in the United States, the incidence is 40 in 100 000 population.

• Sarcoidosis is more prevalent and tends to be more chronic in blacks, who have higher risk of nonrespiratory manifestations.

Clinical staging

Stage 0: normal chest (5%–10% of patients).

Stage I: bilateral hilar adenopathy (50%).

Stage II: bilateral hilar adenopathy and peripheral pulmonary infiltration; paratracheal nodes may also be enlarged (25%).

Stage III: parenchymal infiltration only (15%).

Treatment

Diet and lifestyle

• No special precautions are necessary.

Pharmacological treatment [2–4]

• Treatment is not needed in many patients because the disability is mild and remission is usual. Spontaneous total remissions occur in many. Constitutional symptoms or CNS involvement are some of the indications for systemic treatment.

Corticosteroids—drug of first choice

• These can suppress the manifestations of acute sarcoidosis, with rapid clearing of radiographic lesions; whether they alter the long-term outcome or prevent development of late fibrosis if started early remains unproven.

Standard dosage	Prednisone, 30–40 mg daily for 4–6 weeks; with rapid tapering to 15 mg daily for 3 months.
Contraindications	Uncontrolled hypertension, diabetes mellitus, infection, severe osteoporosis.
Special points	Relapses treated by increased dose; some patients with objective evidence of relapse on >3 occasions may need long-term low-dose maintenance prednisone.
Main drug interactions	Antihypertensive drugs.
Main side effects	Weight gain, edema, bruising, purple striae in skin (particularly abdomen), moon face, osteoporosis, collapse of vertebrae, diabetes mellitus, hypertension, myopathy (especially proximal girdle muscles), hirsutism, menstrual disturbances, psychotic reactions, cataracts, withdrawal phenomena.

Immunosuppressants

• Treatment should be given under specialist supervision.

• In resistant cases, immunosuppressants are sometimes partially effective (*e.g.*, methotrexate, azathioprine). Other agents rarely tried include cyclophosphamide, chlorambucil, and chloroquine.

Standard dosage	Methotrexate, 10 mg once weekly for 3 months; repeated courses every 6 months, possibly with oral steroids. Azathioprine, 100–200 mg daily.
Contraindications	Hepatic and renal impairment.
Main drug interactions	Alcohol, NSAIDs, antacids.
Main side effects	*Methotrexate:* hepatic fibrosis, acute bone-marrow suppression. *Azathioprine:* bone-marrow toxicity, gastrointestinal symptoms, rash, fever.

NSAIDs

• Anti-inflammatory agents are occasionally used in acute arthritic manifestations of sarcoidosis.

Standard dosage	Indomethacin, 50–200 mg daily in divided doses, with food.
Contraindications	Active peptic ulceration; severe renal, cardiac, and hepatic failure.
Main drug interactions	Angiotensin-converting enzyme inhibitors, anticoagulants, antidiabetics, antidepressants, 4-quinolones.
Main side effects	Gastrointestinal disturbances, ulceration, and bleeding, blood disorders (thrombocytopenia), headache, dizziness.

Treatment aims

To prevent development of irreversible pulmonary fibrosis.

Other treatments

• Lung transplantation or heart-lung transplantation has been done with end-stage disease.

Prognosis [2]

• 50% of patients remit spontaneously.

• Accompanying hilar adenopathy usually regresses within ~1 year.

• ~10% of patients develop parenchymal lesions, of which many resolve within 1 year.

• ~40% of patients resolve spontaneously within 1 year; the rest may progress with varying speed to irreversible fibrosis, which, in severely ill patients, may be complicated by upper-zone bullous disease and aspergillomas, with recurrent infection and haemoptysis.

Follow-up and management

• Regular clinical review is needed for patients being treated by steroids or immunosuppressants.

Key references

1. Winterbauer R, Belic N, Moores K: A clinical interpretation of bilateral hilar adenopathy. *Ann Intern Med* 1973, **78**:65–71.
2. Hunninghake G, *et al.*: Outcome of the treatment for sarcoidosis. *Am J Respir Crit Care Med* 1994, **149**:893–898.
3. American Thoracic Society. Statement on sarcoidosis. *Am J Respir Crit Care Med* 1999, **160**:736–755.
4. Lynch JP III: Pulmonary sarcoidosis: current concepts and controversies. *Compr Ther* 1997, **23**:197–210.

Shock, acute hypotensive

Diagnosis

Symptoms

• Symptoms of hypotensive shock are nonspecific; they include the following:

Restlessness.

Confusion or stupor.

Breathlessness.

Chest pain.

• Symptoms of the underlying cause may predominate.

Signs

Hypotension: a useful definition is systolic blood pressure <90 mm Hg.

Oliguria.

Cyanosis.

Confusion.

Peripheral vasoconstriction or vasodilatation: may indicate high or low systemic vascular resistance, respectively.

Tachycardia and third heart sound.

Investigations

Initial investigations

Complete blood count, hematocrit, urine and electrolytes, toxicology screen, and creatinine analysis.

Cardiac enzyme analysis: if myocardial injury suspected.

Blood culture: if any infective process known or suspected.

Arterial blood gas analysis: to assess hypoxemia and acidosis.

ECG and chest radiography: mandatory.

Circulatory assessment

• This should ideally be done in an intensive care unit.

Central venous cannulation: to measure central venous pressure.

Arterial cannulation: sphygmomanometry may be unreliable in shock.

Pulmonary artery catheterization: for pulmonary artery pressure, pulmonary capillary wedge pressure, and thermodilution cardiac output.

Echocardiography: for left ventricular function or if valve lesion, ventricular septal defect, or tamponade suspected.

Complications

Myocardial ischemia or infarction.

Acute renal failure.

Ischemic stroke.

Hepatic dysfunction.

Paralytic ileus.

Lactic acidosis: an indicator of tissue hypoxia.

Differential diagnosis

Not applicable.

Etiology

Low central venous pressure

Indicates hypovolemia.

Warm peripheries (low systemic vascular resistance): vasodilatation due to septicemia or drug overdose.

Cool peripheries (high systemic resistance): normal hemoglobin or hematocrit indicates hemorrhage; high hemoglobin indicates salt and water loss, *e.g.*, from peritonitis, pancreatitis, diabetic ketoacidosis, burns, polyuric phase of acute tubular necrosis.

Elevated central venous pressure

Indicates "pump failure."

Tension pneumothorax.

Pulmonary embolism.

Impaired myocardial contractility due to acute myocardial infarction or ischemia, sepsis, acidemia, electrolyte disturbance, negatively inotropic agents (*e.g.*, beta-antagonists, antiarrhythmic agents).

Arrhythmia.

Cardiac tamponade.

Ruptured interventricular septum.

Acute mitral or aortic valve regurgitation.

Aortic stenosis.

Epidemiology

Not applicable.

Septicemia and hypotensive shock

• The circulatory hallmark of sepsis is an unpredictable derangement of regional blood flow. Inappropriate vasodilatation of muscle and skin arterioles may coexist with profound vasoconstriction of the renal and splanchnic vascular beds.

• The hypotension has many causes, *e.g.*, a fall in systemic vascular resistance to <25% of normal, depression of myocardial contractility by hypoxemia and acidemia, dilatation of venous capacitance vessels resulting in low central venous pressure, and disruption of capillary function causing leakage of intravascular fluid and plasma proteins into alveoli, gastrointestinal tract, peritoneal cavity, and other tissues.

• The combination of myocardial impairment and damage to alveolar capillary basement membranes means that attempts to restore the blood pressure by rapid i.v. infusion of fluid will probably result in pulmonary edema.

Treatment

Diet and lifestyle

• No special precautions are necessary.

Pharmacological treatment

• Whenever possible, the underlying cause should be treated.

• Immediate measures include the following:

Provision of oxygen: hypoxemia contributes to lactic acid production.
Treatment of arrhythmias: cardioversion preferable to negatively inotropic antiarrhythmic drugs.
Plasma expander administration, if central venous pressure is reduced.
Correction of any electrolyte disturbance.
Broad-spectrum antibiotic treatment, if sepsis suspected.
Inotropic support for hypotension without hypovolemia, as follows:

For oliguria

• Dopamine is the first choice in oliguria; it enhances renal blood flow at a low dose (3–5 mg/kg/min), inotropic and vasoconstrictor at doses >5 μg/kg/min (beta$_1$-, alpha-agonism). It must be administered centrally.

After myocardial infarction

• Dobutamine (5–20 μg/kg/min) is the first choice after myocardial infarction; it is predominantly a beta$_1$-agonist; it improves myocardial oxygen supply:demand ratio and causes peripheral vasodilatation (hence its use if the systemic vascular resistance is high).

For severe hypotension

• Epinephrine (2–40 μg/min) is the most positively inotropic catecholamine; it acts as a beta-agonist at low dose, and an alpha-agonist at doses >10 μg/min and causes peripheral vasoconstriction (hence its use if systemic vascular resistance is low).

For bradycardia, atrioventricular block, and right heart failure

• Isoproterenol (1–10 μg/min) is used in bradycardia, atrioventricular block, and right heart failure; it causes pulmonary and systemic vasodilatation; it worsens myocardial supply:demand ratio and ventilation/perfusion mismatch.

If systemic vascular resistance is profoundly low

• Norepinephrine is used if the systemic vascular resistance is profoundly low; its alpha agonism causes vasoconstriction; a rise in blood pressure occurs at the expense of a fall in cardiac output.

Nonpharmacologic treatments

Mechanical ventilation:

• This allows effective correction of hypoxemia and eliminates the work of breathing.

Intra-aortic balloon pump:

• A temporary measure while spontaneous improvement or definitive treatment is awaited.

• Useful in cardiac surgery and refractory unstable angina.

• Complications, in 20% of patients, include leg ischemia, aortic dissection, hemolysis, thrombocytopenia, infection.

Extracorporeal membrane oxygenation (ECMO):

• This traditionally involves withdrawing venous blood, passing it through a membrane oxygenator, and returning it to the arterial circulation. More recently, a veno-venous circuit has been used; it may be associated with lower complications. In expert centers, ECMO has been used as a bridge to heart transplantation or insertion of left ventricular assist device.

Surgery:

• Surgery is indicated early in rupture of interventricular septum or papillary muscle, aortic dissection, and subacute myocardial rupture causing tamponade.

• In patients with cardiogenic shock, emergency revascularization did not significantly reduce overall mortality at 30 days. However, after 6 months a significant survival benefit was seen. Early revascularization should be strongly considered for patients with acute myocardial infarction complicated by cardiogenic shock.

Treatment aims

To increase cardiac output, blood pressure, and tissue oxygen delivery to a level that avoids the detrimental end-organ effects of anaerobic metabolism and lactic acid production.

Prognosis

• The main determinant of outcome is the underlying disorder: for example, hypotension due to diabetic ketoacidosis in a young person has a favorable prognosis, whereas cardiogenic shock resulting from acute anterior myocardial infarction has a mortality of 80%–90%.

Follow-up and management

• No follow-up is needed.

General reference

Hochman JS: Early revascularization in acute myocardial infarction complicated by cardiogenic shock. The SHOCK Investigators. *N Engl J Med* 1999, **341**:625634.

Pranikoff T, *et al.*: Venovenous extracorporeal life support via percutaneous cannulation in 94 patients. *Chest* 1999, **115**:818–822.

Diagnosis

Symptoms

Pain (supraspinatus tendinitis, deltoid, bicipital tendinitis, posterior, anterior, referred).

Functional impairment.

Sleep disturbance.

Diminished range of motion.

Weakness.

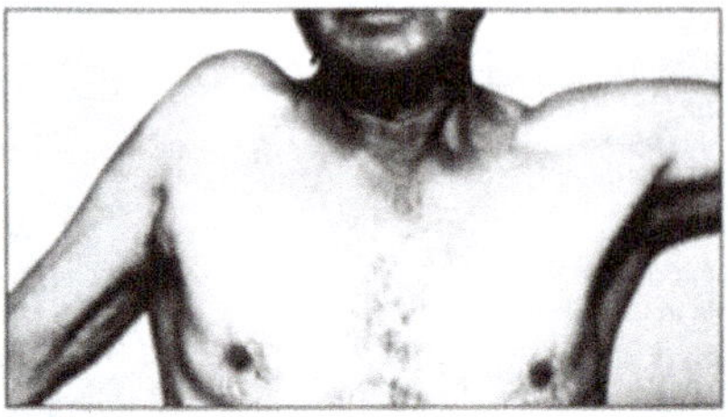

Shoulder rotator cuff tear

Signs

Atrophy.

Frozen shoulder.

Diminished range of motion.

Point tenderness.

Effusion.

Weakness.

Painful arc.

Yergason's drop-arm test.

Investigations

Radiography.

Electromyolography.

Ultrasonography.

Magnetic resonance imaging.

Arthrography.

Arthroscopy.

• Sophisticated imaging studies are not generally required, unless there is failure of conservative initial management or compelling physical examination evidence or radiographical indication of rotator cuff tear.

Complications

Frozen shoulder.

Functional impairment.

Sleep disturbance.

Chronic pain.

Work impairment.

Differential diagnosis

Periarticular disorders

Impingement syndromes.

Rotator cuff tendinitis.

Rotator cuff tears.

Adhesive capsulitis.

Cervical radiculopathy.

Reflex sympathetic dystrophy.

Fibromyalgia.

Diabetes mellitus.

Glenohumeral disorders

Osteoarthritis.

Osteonecrosis.

Septic arthritis.

Glenoid labral tears.

Adhesive capsulitis.

Regional disorders

Cervical radiculopathy.

Brachial neuritis.

Nerve entrapment syndrome.

Reflex sympathetic dystrophy.

Fibromyalgia.

Neoplasia.

Miscellaneous

Cholecystitis.

Splenic trauma.

Subphrenic abscess.

Myocardial infarction.

Diabetes mellitus.

Renal osteodystrophy.

Thyroid disease.

Hemarthrosis.

Etiology

Traumatic (acute injuries vs. chronic overuse).

Degenerative osteoarthritis.

Inflammatory.

Crystalline (hydroxyapatite).

Infectious.

Viscerogenic.

Hemorrhagic.

Infiltrative.

Neoplastic.

Epidemiology

• Shoulder disorders are among the most common presenting complaints in primary care.

• Duration of impairment may be 3–18 months.

• Risk factors include overhead work (*e.g.*, filing, reaching, painting), throwing sports, collision and contact sports.

Other information

• There is considerable overlap in the presentation and localizing symptoms and signs for many of the disorders listed above. An important concept to understand is the final common pathway of adhesive capsulitis (frozen shoulder).

Treatment

Diet and lifestyle

- Modification of work requirements may be necessary.
- Modification of exercise activities may be essential to recovery.

Pharmacological treatment

Acetaminophen.

Nonsteroidal anti inflammatory drugs.

Intra-articular corticosteroid administration.

- Intra-articular steroids are within the scope of the primary care physician.
- Standard procedure manuals outline the technique.

Nonpharmacological treatment

RICE—*R*est, *I*ce, *C*ompression, *E*xercise.

- Physical therapy modalities indicate the following:

Heat/cold.

Mobilization techniques.

Ultrasound.

Phonopheresis.

Iontophoresis.

- Other therapeutic options include arthroscopy, orthopedic surgery, and arthroplasty.
- Referral to musculoskeletal specialist may be needed early for surgical repair candidates (*i.e.,* return to work or to elite competition).

Treatment aims

- The goals of physical therapy are:

To relieve pain.

To restore normal range of motion.

To restore strength.

To restore function.

To strengthen to prevent recurrence.

Prognosis

- With accurate, prompt diagnosis, most patients show improvement.
- Early institution of range-of-motion exercises prevents frozen shoulder.
- Long duration of symptoms must be met by support from physician and rehabilitation personnel, because encouragement enables patients to persist and ultimately improve.

Follow-up and management

- At the time of diagnosis, patients should be instructed on home exercises for the shoulder.
- Medications may be helpful adjunctive therapy.
- Physical therapy supervision may be necessary for refractory cases.
- Intra-articular steroids may be necessary for physical therapy failures or severely frozen shoulder.
- Patient expectations regarding the time course for improvement need to be reviewed at outset.

General references

Birrer RB (ed.): *Sports Medicine for the Primary Care Physician*, edn 2. Boca Raton, FL: CRC Press; 1994.

Garrick JG, Webb DR: *Sports Injuries: Diagnosis and Management*. Edited by Wickland E Jr. Philadelphia: WB Saunders; 1990.

Jahnke AH, *et al.*: A prospective comparison of computerized arthrotomography and magnetic resonance imaging of the glenohumeral joint. *Am J Sports Med* 1992, **20**:695–701.

Petri M, *et al.*: Randomized, double-blind, placebo-controlled study of the treatment of the painful shoulder. *Arthritis Rheum* 1987, **30**:1040–1046.

Warren RF: Shoulder pain. In *Manual of Rheumatology and Outpatient Orthopedic Disorders*, edn 2. Edited by Beary JF, *et al.* Boston: Little, Brown and Company; 1987:81–86.

Diagnosis

Symptoms

• Patients with SS and Sβ° thalassemia are generally more severely affected than those with SC; Sβ⁺ is the mildest disorder.

Acute painful vaso-occlusive crisis: causes >90% of hospital admissions affecting bones, joints, and muscles; initial presentation in one-third is the "hand foot" syndrome from age of 4 months; limb pain in older children, more central pain distribution in adolescents and adults.
Chronic pain: in hip or shoulders, caused by avascular necrosis.

Signs

• Often patients present with no signs in mild crisis.

Constitutional upset mimicking septicemia: in severe crisis (infection can precipitate crisis).
Localized swelling, tenderness, and redness of bone, joint, or muscle.
Abdominal pain mimicking more severe disease.
Limited range of hip or shoulder movement: with active avascular necrosis.

Investigations

For diagnosis

• Investigations should be made preferably when the patient is in a stable state.

Complete blood count: to establish degree of anemia.
Reticulocyte count: to establish degree of hemolysis.
Hemoglobin electrophoresis: to determine variant hemoglobins.
"Sickle test": to confirm presence of hemoglobin S.
Hemoglobin F estimation: high concentrations diminish severity.
Extended erythrocyte grouping: to ensure appropriate erythrocytes for transfusion.
Plasma blood urea nitrogen, creatinine, electrolytes analysis: to monitor renal function.
Liver function tests: to monitor hemolysis and exclude hepatitis.

In crisis

• The results should be compared with those from the stable state.

Complete blood count: hemoglobin raised with dehydration; falls in sequestration and aplasia.
Blood urea nitrogen, creatinine, electrolytes analysis: to detect dehydration.
Liver function tests: to measure dysfunction.
Cultures and viral screening: urine, blood, sputum, throat swab; to exclude infection (before antibiotic treatment); screening for parvovirus (not routine unless severely anemic).
Reticulocyte count.
Viral screen, chest radiography, blood gas and arterial oxygen saturation measurement: if patient has chest pain or signs.

Complications

Stroke: in 8% of patients, median age 7 years.
Sequestration syndromes: common cause of death; erythrocytes pooled in the organ, causing hemoglobin to fall by ≤2 g/dL, leading to dysfunction of the following organs: spleen (in infants; high risk of recurrence), liver (in children and adults), chest (a medical emergency, exchange transfusion if partial arterial oxygen pressure <60 mm Hg), splanchnic circulation (in adults, clinical picture of paralytic ileus that resolves spontaneously).
Infection: common and serious or life-threatening because of autosplenectomy, therefore susceptible to encapsulated bacteria, especially *Streptococcus pneumoniae* and *Salmonella* spp.; gram-negative infections, particularly *Escherichia coli*, account for 10% of deaths in adults; *Yersinia enterocolitica* infections in iron overloaded patients; aplastic crisis due to parvovirus B19.
Priapism, proliferative retinopathy, cholecystitis and cholelithiasis secondary to hemolysis.

Differential diagnosis

• It can be difficult to distinguish simple vaso-occlusive crisis from that associated with infection.
• Other diseases may also manifest (*e.g.*, appendicitis) or coexist.

Etiology

• Sickle cell disease is inherited in a Mendelian recessive manner.
• Clinical problems also occur when hemoglobin S interacts with other variant hemoglobins (*e.g.*, SC) and with a β-thalassemia gene (β° or β⁺).

Epidemiology

• It is rarely manifest before the age of 4–6 months; production of fetal hemoglobin continues until that age because of the late switching off of the fetal hemoglobin gene.

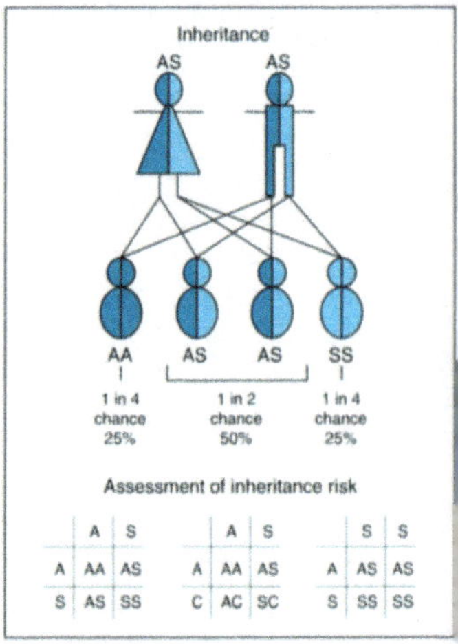

Assessment of inheritance risk. Among Jamaican and American sickle cell patients of African heritage, 50%–70% are Benin, 15%–30% are Bantu-CAR, and 5%–15% are Senegal haplotypes.

Treatment

Diet and lifestyle

• Patients should avoid factors that precipitate painful crisis, *e.g.*, infection, dehydration, exhaustion, cold, marked temperature changes, smoking, high altitude, and unpressurized aircraft; in some patients, stress is reported to be a precipitant.

Pharmacological treatment [1–3]

Analgesia

Standard dosage	*For mild to moderate pain:* acetaminophen, 12–15 mg/kg every 8 hours, codeine phosphate, 1–2 mg/kg every 6 hours (up to 3 mg/kg in 24 hours), or NSAIDs, all orally. *For severe pain:* morphine, 0.1 mg/kg i.v. loading dose, then 1–2 mg/kg i.v. infusion over 24 hours using patient-controlled analgesia system, or equivalent with other narcotic analgesics, in adults.
Contraindications	*Oral drugs:* hepatic and renal impairment, peptic ulceration, asthma. *Parenteral drugs:* raised intracranial pressure.
Special points	*Meperidine:* respiratory rate must be monitored hourly, risk of seizures.
Main drug interactions	*Codeine and morphine:* alcohol, anxiolytics and hypnotics, dompetidone and metoclopramide, cimetidine. *Diclofenac:* caution with other analgesics, anticoagulants, antihypertensives, β-blockers, and cardiac glycosides.
Main side effects	*Oral drugs:* rashes, blood dyscrasias, acute pancreatitis, constipation, respiratory depression. *Morphine:* respiratory depression, nausea, bronchospasm, severe pruritus, constipation, somnolence. *Meperidine:* seizures.

Antibiotics

• Antibiotics are indicated for patients in severe crisis or when infection is suspected.

Standard dosage	Amoxicillin, 500 mg 3 times daily.
Contraindications	Penicillin allergy.
Special points	If pneumococcal infection is suspected, penicillin should be added.
Main drug interactions	Anticoagulants, antacids, oral contraceptives.
Main side effects	Nausea, diarrhea, rashes, pseudomembranous colitis.

Pharmacological augmentation of fetal hemoglobin production with hydroxyurea or 5-azacytidine [4,5]

• Reduces frequency of sickle cell crisis.

• Should not be administered without supervision of a hematologist.

Nonpharmacological treatment [3]

Rehydration

Oral fluids increased in patients with mild pain; i.v. clear fluids in patients with severe pain at 80 mL/kg/24 h.

Oxygen treatment

60% oxygen if partial arterial oxygen pressure on air is <60 mm Hg; 35% if 60–70 mm Hg; 28% if 70–80 mm Hg.

Blood transfusion

See Transfusion medicine *for further details.*

Additive: when hemoglobin <5 g/dL and patient symptomatic from anemia; for aplastic crisis, sequestration, bleeding (*e.g.*, renal papillary necrosis).

Exchange: when hemoglobin >5 g/dL but improved oxygen transport needed.
Overall aim: hemoglobin S <20%, total hemoglobin 11–14.5 g/dL (possibly 3–4 procedures); for chest syndrome (if partial arterial oxygen pressure <60 mm Hg), priapism (if >4 hours), acute neurological deficit or splanchnic sequestration, severe or protracted crisis (occasionally), preoperatively in selected patients.

Long-term transfusion: to maintain hemoglobin at 11–14.5 g/dL, with hemoglobin S <25%; for neurological deficit, sickle chronic lung disease, prevention of pain (occasionally), pregnant women (selected).

Treatment aims

To provide early and effective relief of pain.

To treat infection.

To maintain hydration.

To maintain tissue oxygenation.

Prognosis

• All types of sickle cell disease are variable in clinical manifestations; no markers exist to predict severity for a particular patient.

• 87% of patients are alive at 20 years, 50% at 50 years.

• Deaths in childhood are most commonly due to infection.

• Deaths in adolescents and young adults are most commonly due to neurological and lung complications.

• Deaths in middle age are most commonly due to chronic organ failure.

• Successful outcome after bone-marrow transplantation has now been recorded and drugs that raise hemoglobin F levels look promising [5].

Follow-up and management

• Full education and counseling must be ensured, with family screening and genetic advice.

• Penicillin prophylaxis must be ensured for children, and antipneumococcal and hemophilus B vaccination should be considered.

• Children should be checked for upper airways obstruction.

Key references

1. Davies SC, Wonke B: The management of haemoglobinopathies. *Baillières Clin Haematol* 1991, **4**:361–389.
2. Embury SH, *et al.*: *Sickle Cell Disease: Basic Principles and Clinical Practice.* New York: Raven Press; 1994.
3. Ballas SK: Complications of sickle cell anemia in adults: guidelines for effective management. *Cleve Clin J Med* 1999, **66**:48–58.
4. Steinberg MH, Lu ZH, Barton FB, *et al.*: Fetal hemoglobin in sickle cell anemia: determinants of response to hydroxyurea. Multicenter study of hydroxyurea. *Blood* 1997, **89**:1078–1088.
5. Steinberg MH: Management of sickle cell disease. *N Engl J Med* 1999, **340**:1021–1030.

Diagnosis

Symptoms and signs

Impetigo

Isolated lesions or multiple small areas of golden yellow crusts, pustules or erosions.

Erysipelas

Inflammation of the skin with marked lymphatic involvement; erythema with well-defined and palpable margins, swelling, heat, pain, fever and malaise.

Cellulitis

Inflammation of the skin involving deep subcutaneous tissues; swelling, ill-defined erythema, heat, pain, fever, malaise.

Furuncle or abscess: focal area of pus formation, often painful, abscesses may be enlarged and pointing.

Carbuncle: a more extensive, deeper lesion than a furuncle.

Methicillin-resistant *Staphylococcus aureus (MRSA)* infections

• Patients may be colonized, develop local infection, or become septic.

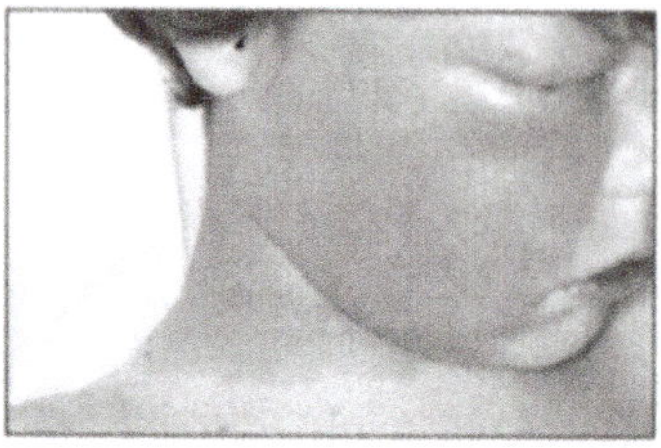

Erysipelas. (*See* Color Plate.)

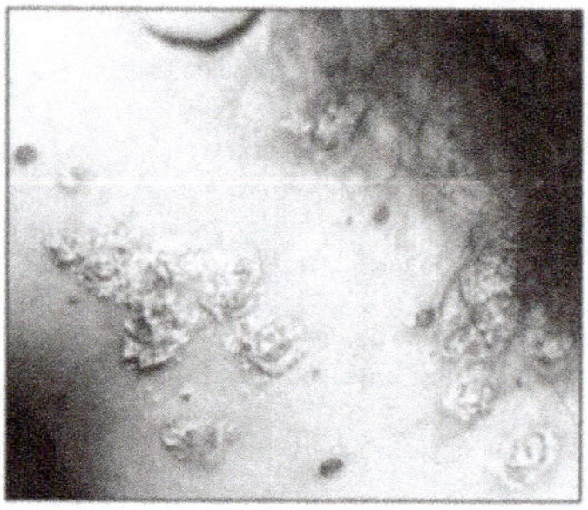

Impetigo. (*See* Color Plate.)

Investigations

Cultures

• Impetigo should be cultured because MRSA infection cannot be diagnosed clinically.

• Culture of tissue aspirate may be done for erysipelas or cellulitis, although yield may be low.

• Pus from abscesses should be sent for culture.

• Blood cultures should be obtained in cellulitis.

Complications

Poststreptococcal glomerulonephritis.

Lymphangitis.

Sepsis.

Differential diagnosis

Contact dermatitis.

Herpes zoster/herpes simplex.

Panniculitis.

Venous stasis.

It is important to distinguish periorbital cellulitis from orbital cellulitis, an uncommon but serious process characterized by orbital pain, proptosis, and visual disturbances.

Etiology

• Impetigo is usually caused by *S. aureus*, (especially when bullous) or group A *Streptococcus*.

• Erysipelas is most commonly caused by group A *Streptococcus*.

• Cellulitis is usually caused by group A *Streptococcus* or *Staphylococcus aureus*, although other bacteria may be causative; coexistent tinea pedis (athlete's foot) should be suspected in cases of lower-extremity cellulitis.

Epidemiology

• Impetigo is most common in children aged 2–5 years in warm climates and with poor hygiene; the incidence increases in summer.

• Pharyngeal carriage of group A *Streptococcus* is more common in younger age groups and can reach 15%–20% in crowded conditions, especially in winter.

• Frequency of nasal carriage of *S. aureus* varies; up to 50% of military trainees are carriers.

• The frequency and severity of invasive streptococcal disease have been increasing in the United States and Europe since the late 1980s.

• Where antibiotic use is intense, *e.g.*, hospitals, most staphylococci are resistant to penicillin.

• Outbreaks of methicillin-resistant *S. aureus*, usually in hospitals, have been reported since 1960; some strains are virulent, whereas others are harmless unless they infect vulnerable patients.

Treatment

Diet and lifestyle

•Patients should pay strict attention to hygiene and control of complicating factors such as diabetes.

•Body piercing is associated with a high incidence of localized skin infections.

Pharmacological treatment

For impetigo

• Topical mupirocin is effective in 90% of cases.

• Oral antibiotics with gram-positive coverage may be used.

For erysipelas or cellulitis

• Oral or i.v. antibiotics may be used according to severity.

• Antibiotics with good coverage of *Staphalococcus* and *Streptococcus* should be used. The choice of antibiotic should be based on culture results (if available), geographic pattern of antimicrobial susceptibilities, and comorbid conditions.

• For oral therapy, consider dicloxacillin, cephalexin, trimethoprim-sulfamethoxazole, ciprofloxacin, erythromycin, azithromycin.

• For parenteral therapy, consider nafcillin, cefazolin.

• If cultures demonstrate MRSA, treatment should be based on susceptibility; parenteral vancomycin may be necessary.

• Surgical exploration may be necessary to treat or define the extent of anaerobic cellulitis.

For furuncles and abscesses

• Incision and drainage is indicated to release pus.

• Oral antibiotic with gram-positive coverage.

Treatment aims

To eradicate infection.

To avoid spread of MRSA infection.

Prognosis

• Further attacks of erysipelas are common at the same site; patients should report promptly for antibiotic treatment.

Follow-up and management

• Patients should be followed up 24 hours after initiation of therapy, with individualized management thereafter depending on severity.

Prevention of spread of MRSA

• The patient must be isolated and infectious precautions used (*i.e.*, gloves, masks, hand washing)..

• The Infection Control Team must be contacted immediately.

• The source of the MRSA must be sought.

• The patient can be discharged unless contacts are vulnerable; if discharge is not possible, infected individuals must be isolated (even if asymptomatic).

General references

Danik SB, *et al.*: Cellulitis. *Cutis* 1999, **64**: 157–164.

Duckworth DJ: Diagnosis and management of methicillin resistant *Staphylococcus aureus* infection. *BMJ* 1993, **307**:1049–1052.

O'Dell ML: Skin and wound infections: an overview. *Am Fam Physician* 1998, **57**: 2424–2432.

Semel JD, Goldin H: Association of athlete's foot with cellulitis of the lower extremities: diagnostic value of bacterial cultures of ipsilateral interdigital space samples. *Clin Infect Dis* 1996, **23**:1162–1164.

Sleep apnea, central hypoventilation, periodic breathing

Diagnosis

Definition

• Central sleep apnea is a clinical syndrome with a range of causes.

Neuromuscular weakness or chest-wall disease: the primary problem is inefficiency of the respiratory pump; patients may develop daytime ventilatory failure.

Periodic respiration (Cheyne–Stokes breathing): the primary problem is disordered respiratory feedback control; patients do not develop daytime ventilatory failure.

Pure central sleep apnea: characterized by hypoventilation despite normal airway, lungs, chest wall, and muscles; occurs in lesions of brainstem and with primary alveolar hypoventilation (Ondine's curse).

Symptoms

Daytime sleepiness, restless sleep, transient breathlessness: during the arousal and tachypnea that follow an apnea; symptoms of sleep disturbance.

Morning headache and nausea, poor exercise tolerance, ankle swelling, daytime breathlessness: only with neuromuscular or chest-wall disease; symptoms of respiratory failure.

Symptoms of primary causative disease.

Signs

Cyanosis, peripheral edema, raised venous pressure, signs of pulmonary hypertension or right ventricular hypertrophy: signs of ventilatory failure and cor pulmonale.

Raised venous pressure and edema: signs of heart failure.

Muscle fasciculation, weakness, loss of tendon reflex: signs of myopathy, dystrophy, motor neuron disease, postpoliomyelitis syndrome.

Supine breathlessness and paradoxical abdominal movement on sniffing: signs of diaphragm weakness due to bilateral phrenic palsy, acid maltase deficiency, or other muscular disease.

Upper motor neuron and brain stem signs: signs of stroke.

Chest-wall deformity: signs of scoliosis, thoracoplasty.

Investigations

Initial

Awake arterial oxygen saturation and blood gas analysis: for possible hypercapnia; alveolar-arterial oxygen gradient often normal.

Spirometry: to exclude chronic obstructive pulmonary disease and assess lung volume; daytime ventilatory failure with central sleep apnea rare if vital capacity >1.5 L standing; supine fall in forced vital capacity of >20% suggests marked diaphragm weakness.

Hemoglobin analysis: for polycythemia.

Nerve physiology, muscle biopsy, ECG, echocardiography: can also be considered.

Sleep studies [1]

• These are used to exclude obstructive sleep apnea, show characteristic apneas without continuing respiratory effort, show worsening hypoventilation during rapid eye movement sleep, and quantify the severity of the abnormality present.

• Complete study should include electroencephalography, electro-oculography, electromyography, oximetry, measurement of respiratory effort and airflow.

• Interpretation can be difficult because some patients with apnea due to pharyngeal collapse make little respiratory effort and some patients with a primary failure of respiratory drive have secondary airway collapse.

Complications

Ventilatory failure, cor pulmonale, pneumonia: in patients with neuromuscular or chest-wall disease.

Accidents: particularly motor vehicle accidents, due to poor daytime vigilance.

Differential diagnosis

Daytime sleepiness

Obstructive sleep apnea.

Narcolepsy.

Idiopathic hypersomnolence.

Periodic movements of legs during sleep.

Inadequate sleep.

Respiratory failure

Chronic obstructive lung disease.

Obstructive sleep apnea.

Etiology [2,3]

Neuromuscular or chest-wall disease

• Patients just able to sustain normal ventilation while awake hypoventilate as respiratory drive falls at onset of sleep.

• This worsens further with the muscle atonia of rapid eye movement sleep.

• How this contributes to the daytime ventilatory failure is not clear.

• The sleeping hypoxemia probably accelerates blunting of ventilatory drive, which allows further daytime ventilatory deterioration.

• Thoracic wall stiffness and respiratory muscle fatigue are probably also important.

Periodic respiration

• This develops when the feedback loop controlling respiration has an excessive feedback gain or delay.

• Contributing factors include excessive central drive levels (CNS disease), circulatory delay (heart failure), hypoxemia, hypocapnia, and arousal from sleep (high altitude).

Epidemiology [4]

• Neuromuscular causes of central sleep apnea are unusual.

• Sleeping periodic respiration affects >50% of patients with severe chronic heart failure and >20% of inpatients with neurological disease.

Treatment

Diet and lifestyle

• Changing diet and lifestyle do not alter central sleep apnea.

• Patients should not smoke: concurrent lung disease worsens respiratory failure.

Pharmacological treatment

• Patients with hypoventilation syndromes should be cautioned against the use of sedative medications, which may induce acute respiratory failure.

For neuromuscular or chest-wall disease [2]

• The mainstay of treatment for these conditions is nocturnal ventilatory support.

• Respiratory stimulants may be tried (*e.g.*, theophylline, acetazolamide, medroxyprogesterone), but their long-term efficacy has been disappointing..

For periodic respiration [3,4]

• Many patients with periodic respiration are asymptomatic and need no treatment; treatment of symptomatic periodic respiration remains experimental.

• Underlying heart failure or chronic obstructive pulmonary disease should be controlled.

• Oxygen, low-dose carbon dioxide, positive airway pressure, or acetazolamide may have a role.

Nonpharmacological treatment [3,5–7]

Nocturnal ventilatory support

• This is indicated for patients with central sleep apnea, daytime ventilatory failure and an otherwise good quality of life.

• It improves daytime symptoms, respiratory failure, and cor pulmonale, thereby improving prognosis.

• The first approach should be nasal continuous positive airway pressure. This allows for adequate ventilation in most patients.

• Older techniques include the rocking bed and tank and cuirass ventilators.

Advantages: corrects sleep disruption, daytime sleepiness, and respiratory failure.

Disadvantages: need for specialist care to acclimatize patient to ventilator and for follow-up.

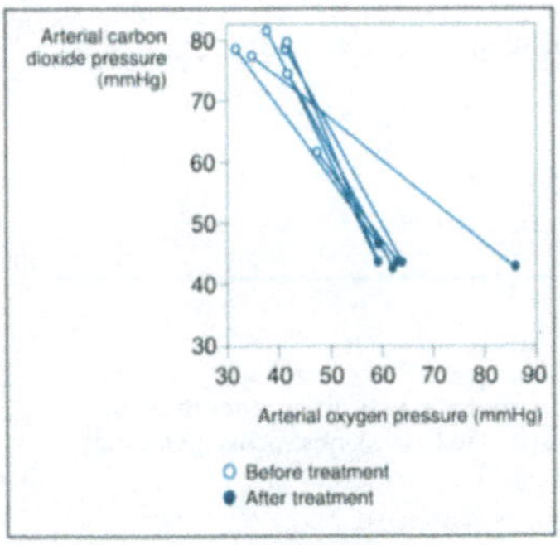

Improvements in awake arterial blood gases in seven patients with neuromuscular or chest wall disease and ventilatory failure after overnight support ventilation.

Causes of treatment failure: ventilator or mask failure due to mechanical failure or air leaks, poor compliance due to mouth air leak, nasal obstruction, claustrophobia, inadequate patient education, or poor mask fit, upper airway collapse secondary to extrathoracic negative-pressure (tank or cuirass) ventilation, incorrect diagnosis (respiratory failure due to obstructive lung disease).

Oxygen

• Overnight oxygen (24%–28%) may improve symptoms of patients in whom ventilatory support is not appropriate; it has not been shown to improve prognosis in this group and may worsen daytime ventilatory failure.

Treatment aims

Neuromuscular or chest-wall disease

To improve symptoms and quality of life.

To correct respiratory failure and cor pulmonale.

To improve mortality and morbidity.

Periodic respiration

To improve sleep disturbance symptoms.

Prognosis

Neuromuscular or chest-wall disease

• Untreated patients with significant daytime respiratory failure and central sleep apnea have a limited life expectancy (usually only a few months).

• With successful nocturnal ventilatory support, the prognosis approaches that of the underlying condition.

Periodic respiration

• Cheyne–Stokes breathing is not now thought to predict mortality independently of the severity of the underlying disease.

Follow-up and management

• Patients with neuromuscular or chest-wall disease and an otherwise good prognosis, but not in daytime ventilatory failure, need review so that overnight ventilation can be started with onset of daytime hypercapnia.

• Patients on domiciliary nocturnal ventilation need long-term support.

Key references

1. Bradley TD, Phillipson EA: Central sleep apnea. *Clin Chest Med* 1992, **13**:493–505.
2. Goldstein RS: Hypoventilation: neuromuscular and chest wall disorders. *Clin Chest Med* 1992, **13**:507–521.
3. De Backer WA: Central sleep apnoea, pathogenesis and treatment: an overview and perspective. *Eur Respir J* 1995, **8**:1372–1383.
4. Martin TJ, Sanders MH: Chronic alveolar hypoventilation: a review for the clinician. *Sleep* 1995, **18**:617–634.
5. Hill NS: Noninvasive ventilation. *Am Rev Respir Dis* 1993, **147**:1050–1055.
6. Meyer TJ, Hill NS: Noninvasive positive pressure ventilation to treat respiratory failure. *Ann Intern Med* 1994, **120**:760–770.
7. American Thoracic Society: Indications and standards for use of nasal continuous positive airway pressure (CPAP) in sleep apnea syndromes. *Am J Respir Crit Care Med* 1994, **150**:1738–1745.

Sleep apnea, obstructive

Diagnosis

Definition

• Obstructive sleep apnea is a recurrent obstruction to breathing due to upper-airway narrowing or collapse during sleep.

• A mixed obstructive and central sleep apnea syndrome is often seen.

Symptoms [1]

• Symptoms are often manifest for several years before diagnosis.

Loud snoring, thrashing, restless sleep: usual adult presentation, often with history of witnessed apneas from partner.

Daytime somnolence, morning sluggishness, headaches, fatigue.

Nocturnal choking or panic attacks, irritability, nocturia, enuresis, impotence, cognitive dysfunction, memory loss, social disharmony, emotional disturbances: less common.

Behavioral disturbance, failure to thrive: nonspecific features in children, in addition to adult symptoms.

Signs

Obesity: particularly neck; characteristic but not invariable.

Small crowded pharynx with mucosal edema.

Retrognathia.

Tonsil hypertrophy: usual cause of obstructive sleep apnea in children.

Nasal obstruction.

Cyanosis.

Respiratory failure or cor pulmonale: in 10% of patients.

Features of hypothyroidism or acromegaly: rare.

Investigations

Initial

Awake arterial oxygen saturation or blood gas analysis, spirometry, hemoglobin analysis: for ventilatory failure (arterial oxygen and blood gases), obstructive pulmonary disease (spirometry), and polycythemia (hemoglobin).

Thyroid or growth hormone estimations: can be considered.

Sleep studies

• Sleep studies are needed to establish the diagnosis by showing upper-airway obstruction with continuing respiratory efforts; no ideal combination of physiological signals exists, but markers of respiratory effort, apnea, and sleep disturbances are needed.

Polysomnography: gold standard; includes EEG sleep staging, monitoring of ocular movements, oronasal airflow assessment, and measurement of thoracoabdominal movement or esophageal pressure; accurately identifies obstructive apneas but time-consuming and expensive and disturbs patient's sleep [2].

Complications

Respiratory failure, cor pulmonale: usually in patients with peripheral airways obstruction (often mild).

Accidents: particularly motor accidents, due to poor daytime vigilance.

Cardiovascular disease: increased vascular mortality (improves with effective treatment).

Differential diagnosis

Daytime sleepiness

Narcolepsy.

Idiopathic hypersomnolence.

Central sleep apnea.

Periodic breathing.

Periodic movements of legs during sleep.

Inadequate sleep.

Respiratory failure

Chronic obstructive pulmonary disease.

Neuromuscular weakness.

Scoliosis.

Congestive heart failure.

Etiology [2]

Pharyngeal narrowing due to obesity, endopharyngeal masses (including tonsils), retrognathia, micrognathia, hypothyroidism, acromegaly.

Reduced pharyngeal muscle activity due to alcohol, sedative drugs, neuromuscular disorders.

Nasal obstruction.

Epidemiology

• The peak age of presentation is 40–60 years.

• The male:female ratio is 4–10:1.

• The sleep apnea/hypopnea syndrome may affect 1%–4% of men >40 years of age.

Variants of obstructive sleep apnea

Simple snoring: in 20% of men.

Snoring with arousals from sleep: severe sleep fragmentation and daytime sleepiness after heavy snoring without apneas or hypoxemia.

Obstructive sleep hypopnea: airflow does not entirely cease.

Central variant: patients do not make efforts to breathe during the apneas, particularly while lying supine; snoring or typical obstructive sleep apnea usually occurs in other postures.

Laryngeal sleep apnea: sleeping stridor due to laryngeal disease or denervation or Shy–Drager syndrome.

Treatment

Diet and lifestyle

• Weight loss can correct obstructive sleep apnea, but most patients also need other treatment.
• Reduced alcohol intake helps simple snoring and mild obstructive sleep apnea.
• Obstructive sleep apnea present only when patient is supine is improved by avoiding this posture.

Pharmacological treatment [3–5]

• Avoidance of alcohol and sedatives before bedtime is an important part of therapy.
• Drug treatment is secondary to continuous airways pressure.
• Hypothyroidism should be evaluated and treated.

Nasal steroids and decongestants

• These reduce simple snoring but have little effect on obstructive sleep apnea; they may be needed during continuous positive airway pressure therapy.

Standard dosage Beclomethasone, 42–84 µg; or budesonide, 64 µg, twice daily in each nostril.

Contraindications None.

Special points Vasoconstrictor decongestants worsen nasal obstruction with sustained use and should be avoided.

Main drug interactions None.

Main side effects Nasal dryness.

Tricyclic antidepressants

• Antidepressants have a minor role in mild obstructive sleep apnea by suppressing rapid eye movement sleep, when sleep apnea often worsens.

Standard dosage Protriptyline, 10–20 mg orally at night.

Contraindications Cardiac disease, epilepsy, mania, liver disease, glaucoma.

Main drug interactions Alcohol, monoamine oxidase inhibitors, antihistamines, anticonvulsants.

Main side effects Anticholinergic effects, arrhythmias, impotence, urinary retention.

Nonpharmacological treatment [4–6]

Nasal continuous positive airways pressure (CPAP) (usually 5–15 cm H_2O)

• This is the main treatment in most patients with substantial daytime sleepiness.
Advantages: dramatic correction of sleep disruption, daytime sleepiness, snoring, and apneas.
Disadvantages: unsightly, mask may be claustrophobic or cause nasal ulceration if badly fitted.
Causes of treatment failure: machine or mask failure; poor compliance due to nasal obstruction, claustrophobia, inadequate patient education, poor mask fit (air leaks or nasal ulceration), mouth air leak; incorrect diagnosis (central sleep apnea, narcolepsy, respiratory failure from another cause).

Surgery

• Surgery is indicated for patients with the following:
Structural nasal obstruction (*e.g.*, polyps, deviated septum).
Tonsil hypertrophy.
Facial maldevelopment.
Severe obstructive sleep apnea with continuous positive airways pressure failure.
• Tracheostomy is rarely indicated.
• Surgery (uvulopalatopharyngoplasty) should be attempted only in established centers.
• Soft-palette resection is not consistently curative.

Treatment aims

To relieve symptoms.
To correct respiratory failure.
To reduce excess vascular mortality.

Prognosis

• After effective treatment, patients are symptom-free and have a similar prognosis to weight-matched controls.
• Few patients reduce their weight sufficiently to stop CPAP.

Follow-up and management

• Patients on CPAP treatment need review, including maintenance of their equipment, replacement of masks, and consideration of reducing their airway pressure or stopping treatment after weight loss.

Key references

1. Findley LJ, Weiss J, Jabour EP: Drivers with untreated sleep apnoea. *Arch Intern Med* 1991, **151**:1451–1452.
2. McNamara SG, Grunstein RR, Sullivan CE: Obstructive sleep apnoea. *Thorax* 1993, **48**:754–764.
3. Kryger MH: Management of obstructive sleep apnea. *Clin Chest Med* 1992, **13**:481–492.
4. American Thoracic Society: Indications and standards for use of nasal continuous positive airway pressure (CPAP) in sleep apnea syndromes. *Am J Respir Crit Care Med* 1994, **150**:1738–1745.
5. Strollo PJ Jr, Rogers RM: Obstructive sleep apnea. *N Engl J Med* 1996, **334**:99–104.
6. Hudgel DW: Treatment of obstructive sleep apnea. *Chest* 1996, **109**:1346–1358.

Diagnosis

Symptoms

Insomnia
Daytime fatigue, sleepiness.

Depression.

Obstructive sleep apnea [1]
Habitual snoring, witnessed apnea.

Breath holding.

Partial arousal.

Excessive daytime sleepiness.

Narcoleptic syndrome
Excessive daytime sleepiness.

Sudden weakness: with emotion or expectation of sudden event (cataplexy).

Short night sleep latency.

Excessive motor activity during sleep: leg kicking and sleep-walking.

Sleep paralysis (loss of muscle tone).

Hypnopompic or hyponagogic hallucinations.

Parasomnias
Somnambulism, confusional arousals, and night terrors: 60–90 minutes after sleep onset, during non–rapid eye movement (REM) sleep.

Acting out dream content (REM behavior disorder), cluster headache, nightmares: during REM sleep; accompanied by dreaming.

Other
Enuresis, sleep-talking, leg-kicking: common.

Bruxism, head-banging: less common.

Circadian sleep disorders
Sleep phase disturbance (lag or lead).

Signs
• No abnormal physical signs are manifest in most sleep disorders, although obstructive apneas are associated with retrognathia, micrognathia, macroglossia, or enlarged tonsils or soft palate.

Investigations
Polysomnography: necessary in most sleep–wake disorders, including the narcoleptic syndrome; allows detailed scientific sleep study and may occasionally clarify diagnosis of sleep disorder, particularly when combined with video monitoring [2].

Sleep oximetry: useful in evaluation of sleep apnea and review of treatment.

Multiple sleep latency test: in narcoleptic syndrome and other forms of daytime sleepiness; in narcolepsy, sleep latency is short and REM often begins within 15 minutes of sleep onset; ≥2 of 5 naps containing REM sleep is suggestive of narcolepsy.

Plasma and urinary screen: for hypnotic or CNS stimulant drugs, occasionally useful in suspected drug abuse or poor drug compliance.

Complications
• Sleep disorders may be as disabling as epilepsy.

Daytime sleepiness, depression, sleep "attacks."

Work and social problems: major cause of traffic accidents.

Differential diagnosis
Not applicable.

Etiology
• Insomnia is often multifactorial, with abnormal lifestyle, physical and psychological factors and sometimes hypnotic-stimulant drug or alcohol misuse.

• Familial insomnia is not uncommon.

• The narcoleptic syndrome has 99% association with HLA DR2 and DQw1; only 1 in 500 HLA DR2–positive patients, however, has the narcoleptic syndrome.

• Circadian sleep disorders are often due to shift work and/or psychological factors.

Epidemiology
• Chronic insomnia occurs in up to 20% of adults; it is more common in women than in men.

• Persistent excessive daytime sleepiness is usually caused by obstructive sleep apnea, the narcoleptic syndrome, or periodic leg movements with frequent arousals.

• Parasomnias, including bed wetting and sleep walking, are common, most frequently in childhood.

• Circadian sleep disorders caused by shift work occur in one-third of the workforce; shift work is tolerated better by younger people.

• The delayed sleep phase syndrome has an incidence of 1 in 10 000 people.

Treatment

Diet and lifestyle

• Good "sleep hygiene" with regular sleep and wake times, avoidance of books and TV while in bed, and finding another time for review of the day can improve insomnia. In some cases, initial sleep restriction is needed.

• In the narcoleptic syndrome, 2–3 planned short naps during the day may improve alertness.

• Sleep regularity with fixed stable bedtime and waketime is useful in the management of many parasomnias.

Pharmacological treatment

For insomnia

Standard dosage	Short-term (2–4 weeks) benzodiazepine or nonbenzodiazepine hypnotic, *e.g.*, temazepam, 2–3 times weekly, can be considered.
Contraindications	Pregnancy, psychiatric illness, sleep apnea.
Special points	Long-term nightly use to be avoided; can be combined with psychological support, although hypnotics not main-line treatment for most forms of chronic insomnia.
Main drug interactions	Enhanced sedative effect with many other drugs; metabolic interactions.
Main side effects	Waking sedation, tolerance.

For narcoleptic syndrome: daytime sleepiness [3]

Standard dosage	Methylphenidate, maximum 60 mg daily, pemoline, modafenil, mazindol, dextroamphetamine; exact dose titration and timing essential.
Contraindications	Vascular disease, hypertension, pregnancy, prostatism, breast-feeding.
Special points	Stimulants ineffective for cataplexy. Regular monitoring of patients on long-term treatment needed.
Main drug interactions	Sympathomimetics, monoamine oxidase inhibitors.
Main side effects	Talkativeness, euphoria, gastrointestinal irritation, sweating, constipation.

For narcoleptic syndrome: cataplexy

Standard dosage	Clomipramine or imipramine, 10–50 mg once daily.
Contraindications	Recent myocardial infarction, heart block.
Special points	Cataplexy does not respond to stimulants, but these can be used in combination with clomipramine.
Main drug interactions	As for tricyclic antidepressants.
Main side effects	Appetite changes, sexual malfunction, or orthostasis.

Treatment aims

To restore normal waking alertness and mood.

To prevent sleep hypoxia, arousal, and cor pulmonale.

To alleviate symptoms of narcolepsy.

Other treatments

Continuous positive airways pressure: effective in patients with obstructive sleep apnea.

Consideration of surgery.

Prognosis

• The prognosis varies widely among the different sleep disorders.

• The narcoleptic syndrome does not remit.

• In many forms of insomnia, the prognosis is poor.

Follow-up and management

• Assessment of insomnia requires medical, psychiatric, and psychological review; a written treatment plan should be drawn up with the patient, aiming for sustained benefit in 3–6 months of treatment.

• In patients with the narcoleptic syndrome, progress should be monitored using a sleep–wake diary; drug compliance can be ensured by monitoring plasma and urine concentrations.

Patient support

American Sleep Disorders Association,
1610 14th St NW, Suite 300,
Rochester, MN 55901-2205;
phone (507) 287-6006.

Driving regulations

• The general guideline is that driving ability with excessive daytime sleepiness depends on the success of and degree of compliance with treatment.

Key references

1. Hill NS: Noninvasive ventilation. *Am Rev Respir Dis* 1993, **147**:1050–1055.
2. Douglas NJ, Thomas S, Jan MA: Clinical value of polysomnography. *Lancet* 1992, **339**:347–350.
3. Thorpy MJ: *Handbook of Sleep Disorders*. New York: Marcel Dekker; 1990.

Spinal cord & cauda equina compression

Diagnosis

Symptoms

• The neurological symptoms are progressive.

Localized back pain.

Radicular pain.

Numbness or paresthesia, weakness: below level of lesion; may be asymmetrical.

Loss of control of sphincters.

Signs

At level of lesion

Spinal tenderness or deformity: depending on the disease.

Weakness, wasting, reflex loss: root lesion.

Below level of lesion

• Signs may be asymmetrical, *e.g.*, Brown–Sequard's syndrome.

• With spinal cord lesions, sacral sensation may be relatively "spared," whereas perineal sensation is lost early in conus lesions.

Weakness.

Sensory loss.

Spasticity, clonus, hyperreflexia, extensor plantars: if above L1, *i.e.*, spinal cord.

Flaccidity, areflexia: if below L1, *i.e.*, cauda equina.

Investigations

• Laboratory investigations may indicate cause, suggest alternative diagnosis, or help in preparation for surgery.

Complete blood count and ESR measurement: may identify anemia or suggest infection.

Serum vitamin B_{12}, syphilis serology, serum acid phosphatase measurement, plasma protein electropheresis: may be helpful in some patients.

Chest radiography: may show mass or infection.

Plain radiography of spine: may show loss of pedicle or vertebral collapse.

MRI, CT myelography: often needed urgently.

Plain CT: in some patients.

Spinal fluid: if a compressive lesion is not identified.

Complications

Irreversible neurological damage: due to infarction of cord or roots.

Urinary infection: due to neurogenic bladder.

Deep venous thrombosis and pressure sores: from immobility.

Differential diagnosis

Spastic paraparesis

Inflammatory myelopathies: acute transverse myelitis, multiple sclerosis, HIV infection, tropical spastic paraparesis, sarcoidosis (human T-cell leukemic virus I).

Vascular myelopathies: spinal stroke (anterior spinal artery distribution), vascular malformation.

Malformations: Arnold–Chiari (possible lower brain stem or cerebellar signs), syringomyelia (absent arm reflexes and suspended sensory loss).

Cerebral lesions: bilateral strokes, parasagittal tumor.

Flaccid paraparesis

Flaccidity and absent reflexes (spinal shock) caused by acute spinal cord lesions; rare in compression.

Acute Guillain–Barré syndrome: symmetrical, distal sensory loss, areflexia.

Etiology

Extradural tumors: secondary carcinoma, lymphoma, myeloma [1].

Intradural–extramedullary tumors: meningioma, neurofibroma.

Intramedullary tumors: glioma, ependymoma, lipoma.

Disk protrusions: usually cervical or lumbar, usually spontaneous, often sudden onset.

Osteophytic ridges: may combine with narrow spinal canal, *i.e.*, cervical or lumbar canal stenosis.

Infection: pyogenic epidural abscess, tuberculosis.

Trauma: fractures or dislocations of vertebrae.

Hematomas: epidural and subdural (rare).

Epidemiology

Occurs in 5% of patients with systemic malignancy.

Treatment

Diet and lifestyle

• No special precautions are necessary.

Pharmacological treatment

Chemotherapy or radiotherapy: after decompression or biopsy of malignant lesion.

Steroids: before and after surgery to minimize spinal-cord edema (*e.g.*, dexamethasone, 24–100 mg daily in divided doses).

Nonpharmacological treatment

• If acute spinal cord compression is suspected, the patient must be referred to a neurosurgical unit immediately.

• Any delay may lessen the chance of recovery.

Decompression

• Lesions lying posterior to the spinal cord or within the dura mater should be removed from behind through a laminectomy.

• Lesions lying anterior to the dura mater, with the exception of lumbar disk protrusions, should be removed from the front.

Spinal stabilization

• Lesions that cause collapse of the vertebral bodies cause forward angulation; stabilization should be by insertion of a graft from the front or instrumental stabilization attached to laminae in extension, *e.g.*, Hartshill rectangle.

Radiotherapy

• Radiotherapy is useful alone or after surgery for metastatic lesions.

Treatment aims

To establish the diagnosis.

To reverse neurological deficit while preserving spinal stability, if lesion removable.

To prevent progression or recurrence, if lesion not removable.

Prognosis

• The prognosis depends on the underlying cause, the rate rather than degree of compression, and the delay in decompression.

• Patients with long-established myelopathy due to hard disk material or osteophytic bars have poor prognosis; those with soft disk protrusions do well.

• Myelopathies due to prostatic metastases have a relatively good prognosis.

• Metastases from breast or bronchus have a poor prognosis; direct invasion from bronchus has a very poor prognosis.

• Good recovery even from severe neurological deficit may follow successful surgical removal of benign tumors.

• Prognosis is good if decompression occurs before the onset of severe paraparesis.

Follow-up and management

• Patients need subsequent physical therapy, rehabilitation, surgical appliances (*e.g.*, walking aids, orthoses, wheelchair), occupational therapy, and home assessment.

• Patients should be referred to a spinal unit if the residual deficit is severe.

• Complications can be prevented by anti-embolism stockings, low-dose s.c. heparin, prevention of pressure sores, bladder care, and early treatment of intercurrent infection.

Key reference

1. Portenoy RK, *et al.*: Back pain in the cancer patient: an algorithm for evaluation and management. *Neurology* 1987, **37**:134–138.

Diagnosis

Definition

- Stroke is defined as rapidly developing (usually over minutes) clinical symptoms or signs of cerebral dysfunction lasting >24 hours, with no apparent cause other than that of vascular origin.

Symptoms

- Symptoms depend on the vascular territory involved.

Anterior (carotid) circulation

Combination of aphasia, unilateral, visuospatial, motor, or sensory loss: more common with cortical lesions.

Isolated contralateral sensory or motor loss: may indicate deeper hemispheric lesions.

- Extensive hemispheric involvement may eventually lead to altered consciousness due to cerebral edema.

Posterior circulation

Homonymous hemianopia or brain stem disturbance: *e.g.*, diplopia, vertigo, ataxia, gait imbalance, altered consciousness.

- Headache, loss of consciousness, and seizures are more common presenting features in subarachnoid or primary intracerebral hemorrhage than in cerebral infarction.

Signs

- Signs range from none or very subtle (*e.g.*, subjective sensory disturbance) to brain death.

Investigations

Serological

Prothrombin time/partial thromboplastin time, fibrinogen, platelet count, complete blood count, renal and hepatic function tests, sedimentation rates, cholesterol profile.

- In patients aged ≤50 years, add protein S & C, antithrombin III, anticardiolipin and antiphospholipid antibodies, homocystine levels, lactate/pyruvate, adrenoleukodystrophy and metachromatic leukodystrophy screen, where indicated.

Structural and etiological

CT or MRI of brain (MRI required for posterior circulation event).

MR angiography: for large- and medium-vessel disease.

Carotid ultrasonography.

ECG.

Transesophageal echocardiography.

Angiography: for all patients with hemorrhage and needed for many without clear stroke etiology; often necessary to exclude vasculitis or dissection in young adults.

Temporary artery biopsy: if indicated.

Lumbar puncture: for hemorrhage or suspected vasculitis.

Complications

Infections (*e.g.*, aspiration pneumonia, urinary tract infection).

Venous thromboembolism.

Cardiac arrhythmias, cardiac failure, myocardial infarction.

Pressure sores.

Spasticity, contractures.

Mood disorders.

Seizures.

Falls, fractures.

Differential diagnosis

Intracranial tumor.

Subdural hematoma.

Etiology

Cerebral infarction

As for transient ischemic attacks (see Transient ischemic attacks).

Hypercoagulability.

Cerebral vasculitis.

Intracranial hemorrhage

Hypertension.

Aneurysm or arteriovenous malformation.

Epidemiology

- Stroke is the third most common cause of death in industrialized countries.
- It is the largest single cause of severe disability in people living at home.

Classification

- Stroke can be classified as follows:

Cerebral infarction: in 80% of patients.

Primary intracerebral hemorrhage: in 10%.

Subarachnoid hemorrhage: in 5%.

Uncertain: in 5%.

- Cerebral infarction may be further classified on clinical criteria, as follows:

Total anterior circulation infarction: hemiplegia, hemianopia, new cortical deficit.

Partial anterior circulation infarction: two of the above three, new cortical deficit alone, or motor or sensory deficit more restricted than lacunar infarction.

Lacunar infarction: pure motor or sensory stroke, sensorimotor stroke, or ataxic hemiparesis; thought to be caused by intrinsic disease of single perforating artery.

Posterior circulation infarction: evidence of brain stem lesion or homonymous hemianopia.

Treatment

Diet and lifestyle

• Attention to controlling hypertension, hyperlipidemia, and cessation of smoking are very important preventive measures.

Pharmacological treatment

• In acute stroke (≤180 minutes from initial symptoms), tissue plasminogen activator is recommended if patient meets inclusion criteria [1].

Standard dosage	0.9 mg/kg (up to 90 mg) given over 1 hour.
Inclusion criteria	No hemorrhage by CT, clearly defined onset.
Exclusion criteria	Improving or minor symptoms (2 weeks); blood pressure >185/110 (21 days); recent hemorrhage, surgery, head trauma (3 months); seizure; anticoagulant use.
Special points	Intensive care unit monitoring for BP and intracranial hemorrhage required.

Heparin: is currently indicated for posterior circulation ischemic stroke, cardiogenic emboli, and in many cases, for crescendo transient ischemic attacks and stroke in progression.

Aspirin: has been proved to be beneficial in reducing long-term risk after transient ischemic attacks in undifferentiated groups at risk.

Warfacin: is useful for most patients with embolic sources, atrial fibrillation, or nonoperable critical stenosis; broader use is under investigation.

Ticlopidine: 500 mg daily, is useful in some patients with small-vessel or posterior circulation disease but is associated with occasional neutropenia and requires close monitoring [2].

• The role of acute thrombolytic therapy is under investigation.

Nonpharmacological treatment

Surgery [3]

• Some patients with intracerebral hematomas may benefit from surgical drainage, although no universally acceptable selection criteria exist.

• Patients with subarachnoid hemorrhages should be managed in an intensive care unit and may require aneurysm repair.

• Carotid endarterectomy is indicated in symptomatic patients with stenosis >70% and in selected asymptomatic patients.

• Interventional cerebral angiography is increasingly used in acute stroke for intra-arterial thrombolysis or embolectomy.

Rehabilitation

• Stroke units combining physical, occupational, and speech therapy save lives.

• Immobilized patients should wear antiembolism stockings.

• Support from the social services is an important but often neglected element in a patient's recovery.

• Physical, speech, and occupational therapy are vital to recovery.

Treatment aims

To prevent further cerebral damage or secondary complications.

To treat the cause of the stroke, where possible.

To enable survivors to achieve independence.

Prognosis

• For cerebral infarction, the overall 30-day case fatality is 10%.

• ~50% of survivors remain dependent.

• Important prognostic indicators include type and extent of stroke, age, and presenting level of consciousness.

• Intracranial hemorrhage carries a notably worse prognosis.

Follow-up and management

• The key aim is to identify and modify treatable risk factors (*e.g.*, hypertension, smoking).

• Lifelong antiplatelet treatment is indicated (aspirin, 75–150 mg daily) after cerebral infarction.

• Anticoagulation is effective as primary and secondary prophylaxis for cerebral infarction when atrial fibrillation is present.

• For patients who recover well from a limited carotid distribution stroke, endarterectomy may be indicated.

Key references

1. NINDS Stroke and PA Study Group: Tissue plasminogen activator for acute ischemic stroke. *N Engl J Med* 1995, **333**:1581–1587.

2. Hass WK, *et al.*: A randomized trial comparing ticlopidine with aspirin. *N Engl J Med* 1989, **321**:501–507.

3. ACAS Group: Endarterectomy for asymptomatic carotid artery stenosis. *JAMA* 1995, **273**:1421–1459.

General references

Baumlin KM, Richardson LD: Stroke syndromes. *Emerg Med Clin North Am* 1997, **15**:551–561.

Caplan LR: *Stroke: A Clinical Approach*, edn 2. Oxford: Butterworth–Heinemann; 1993.

Suicide: risk factors & prevention

Diagnosis

Symptoms and signs

• Because of the low rate of suicide (11 per 100 000), predicting an individual suicide is very difficult; nonetheless, patients who attempt or commit suicide frequently consult their physician shortly before their attempt or death.

Risk factors [1]

Major depression (10-fold increased risk) or panic disorder (5-fold increased risk) within the previous year.

History of attempted suicide.

Current or recent alcohol or illicit substance abuse.

Lifetime history of any major psychiatric disorder.

Chronic debilitating medical illness.

Being separated or divorced.

Medical hospitalization within the past year.

Screening for suicidal behavior [1,2]

• Patients who have one or more risk factors for suicide should be asked: "Have you ever felt like hurting yourself or committing suicide?" or "Have you ever felt you wanted to die?"

• Answering "yes" to two or more questions on the Suicidal Ideation Screening Questionnaire may identify patients at high risk of suicide, but who may deny suicidal ideation on direct questioning [1].

Suicidal ideation screening questionnaire

1. Sleep disturbance: have you ever had a period of 2 weeks or more when you had trouble falling asleep, staying asleep, waking up too early, or sleeping too much?
2. Mood disturbance: have you ever had 2 weeks or more during which you felt sad, blue, depressed, or when you lost interest and pleasure in things that you usually cared about or enjoyed?
3. Guilt: has there ever been a period of 2 weeks or more when you felt worthless, sinful, or guilty?
4. Hopelessness: has there ever been a period of time when you felt that life was hopeless?

Investigations

• With patient's consent, further history should be obtained from available informants.

• Available databases should be checked for evidence of previous or current psychiatric care.

Complications

• Suicidal patients are at risk for social or occupational dysfunction, with resulting relational and/or financial stress on patient, spouse, and children.

• Unsuccessful suicide attempts can result in permanent injury (*e.g.*, vascular trauma) or functional impairment (*e.g.*, anoxic brain injury).

• Successful suicide creates tragic and long-lived consequences in the lives of family and relations.

Differential diagnosis

Threats or actual self-cutting or self-damage to relieve tension: often multiple superficial cuts on forearms.

Threats or actual self-mutilation in context of psychotic illness: especially schizophrenia.

Accidental ingestion of toxic substances: *e.g.*, tablets that look like sweets to children, weedkiller stored in a lemonade bottle.

Etiology

• Suicide has been conceptualized as a continuum, from ideation, to contemplation, to threats, to attempts, to completion [4]. Predicting the movement of an individual patient along the continuum, however, is difficult.

• One model postulates that factors from five domains—psychiatric, personality, psychosocial and environmental, genetic, and biochemical—all contribute to suicide risk. Adequate evaluation and treatment require assessment of all domains.

Epidemiology

• Suicide is the third leading cause of death in youths aged 15–24 years, and fifth leading cause of death in adults aged 25–64 years.

• ~30 000 Americans commit suicide each year.

• ~2%–3% of adults who receive care in general medical settings have had suicidal thoughts within the previous year.

• 73% of suicides in the United States are by white men.

• Suicide rates are highest among men older than 69.

Treatment

Diet and lifestyle

• High alcohol intake, social isolation, and lack of employment are all strong risk factors for suicide attempts, so efforts should be made among high-risk patients to change the lifestyle of the patients through therapeutic interventions.

• Family members of high-risk patients should be instructed to remove all potentially lethal objects (*e.g.*, guns, knives, medications) from the house.

Pharmacological treatment

• Adequate and early therapy of depressive illness (*see* Depression) and panic disorder (*see* Panic and generalized anxiety disorder) will reduce the likelihood of attempted or successful suicide.

• Antidepressants or other psychoactive medications should be prescribed in limited quantities (5–10 days) without refills to minimize risk of overdose and enhance follow-up.

• Except in emergencies, psychotropic drugs should be given only for treatment of specific mental illness, with psychiatric supervision when necessary.

• For the emergency management of violently mentally disturbed patients, a short-acting antipsychotic, *e.g.*, haloperidol in 5-mg increments i.m. every 15 minutes, should be used until symptoms are controlled, unless seizures are a risk. An antiparkinsonian drug, *e.g.*, procyclidine, 5–10 mg i.m., can be added to avoid dystonic reactions. Drugs should not be given i.v. when the cause of the mental disturbance is not known.

• When seizures are a risk, a benzodiazepine, *e.g.*, diazepam in 5-mg increments i.v. or lorazepam, 2–5 mg i.m., can be used. Benzodiazepines must be avoided in patients with severe respiratory impairment. Antipsychotic agents and benzodiazepines combined have an additive tranquilizing effect.

Nonpharmacological treatment [2,4]

Counseling

• Low-risk patients should be offered brief problem-oriented counseling, where available.

• Current or past high-risk patients should be asked about suicidal thoughts and plans at every visit.

• Patients with alcohol or substance abuse problems should be referred to the relevant specialist services.

• Relationship therapy should be offered to patients with relationship problems if both partners are agreeable.

• Open access or a telephone help-line may be offered, if available.

• Maintaining a strong therapeutic alliance is often an important "life line" for the patient.

Psychiatric referral

• Assessment and/or comanagement by a psychiatrist or experienced counselor is indicated when the primary physician needs assistance in suicide risk assessment, and for patients with recurrent or persistent suicidal ideation.

• Actively suicidal patients should be referred immediately for acute psychiatric intervention, usually on an inpatient basis. Compulsory inpatient admission must be considered in cases of psychiatric illness or serious suicide risk.

• Patients with major mental illness need urgent psychiatric treatment, usually on an inpatient basis.

• Emergency action in the patient's best interest is legally sanctioned in virtually every state; failure to act may be construed as negligence.

Treatment aims

To avoid attempted suicide by identifying and treating patients in earlier stages of the suicide continuum.

To treat any underlying mental disorder.

To help patient solve problems and to provide support through current crisis.

To strengthen the patient's future coping skills.

Prognosis

• Prognosis is largely determined by the underlying mental illness, substance abuse, or other risk factors.

• Repeat suicide attempts most often occur within the first 3 months of an episode.

• Among patients with a history of attempted suicide, long-term risk of completed suicide is ~1% at 1 year and 3% at 8 years.

• ~7% of patients with a history of attempted suicide make two or more attempts.

Follow-up and management

• Low-risk patients whose stressors and other risk factors have been addressed do not need special follow-up care.

• A telephone call should be placed to all currently or recently suicidal or high-risk patients who miss appointments.

• High-risk patients and those with mental illness need close monitoring.

Key references

1. Cooper-Patrick L, Crum RM, Ford DE: Identifying suicidal ideation in general medical patients. *JAMA* 1994, **272**:1757–1762.
2. Hirschfield RMA, Russell JM: Current concepts: assessment and treatment of suicidal patients. *N Engl J Med* 1997, **337**:910–915.
3. Gliatto MF, Rai AK: Evaluation and treatment of patients with suicidal ideation. *Am Fam Phys* 1999, **59**:1500–1513.
4. Beck A, Kovacs M, Weissman M: Assessment of suicidal ideation: the scale for suicide ideation. *J Consult Clin Psychol* 1979, **46**:559–563.

Diagnosis

Definition

• Syncope is a sudden, transient loss of consciousness and postural tone with subsequent spontaneous recovery.

Symptoms

• Symptoms are not always apparent; associations depend on the cause of syncope.

Presyncope.

Orthostatic hypotension.

Neurological (seizures, dizziness, vertigo, dysarthria, visual disturbance).

Postevent fatigue or confusion.

Chest pain.

Palpitations.

Dyspnea.

Emotional and/or physical stress.

Autonomic activation (*e.g.*, nausea, diaphoresis, pallor).

Generalized or focal weakness.

Signs

• Signs are not always apparent; findings vary depending on the cause of syncope.

Orthostatic hypotension.

Pulse deficit and asymmetric blood pressures in the arms: aortic dissection.

Murmurs or physical findings consistent with cardiovascular abnormalities.

Focal neurological deficits.

Vascular bruits.

Investigations

• History and physical examination are critical in assessment.

• Sudden onset of symptoms without a prodrome may suggest arrhythmias, whereas protracted autonomic symptoms (pallor, diaphoresis, nausea) in association with a precipitating factor such as pain, extreme heat or emotion, or prolonged standing suggest vasovagal syncope. Exertional syncope suggests possible structural heart disease. Recovery from cardiac syncope is often brief (30 seconds); neurally mediated syncope (*e.g.*, vasovagal) is often accompanied by postevent fatigue or other symptoms of longer duration.

• Neurological syncope is suggested by brainstem findings (vertigo, dysarthria, ataxia, visual disturbances); postevent confusion is associated with seizures.

• Emphasis should be placed on the circumstances surrounding the syncopal event, associated symptoms, medication/drugs, family/psychiatric history, and presence of known cardiac disease. Observations from witnesses may be helpful.

• Routine nonselective neurological testing (CT, EEG, carotid Dopplers) and laboratory evaluations rarely provide useful diagnostic information. These tests and others (*e.g.*, nuclear scans, cardiac catheterization, cerebral angiography) should be selectively performed as directed by clinical data.

Carotid sinus massage: useful in elderly patients and those with features suggestive of carotid sinus syncope if not contraindicated.

12-lead ECG and rhythm strips: abnormalities can lead to the cause of syncope and/or direct additional testing; a normal ECG suggests a more favorable prognosis and makes arrhythmias less likely.

Ambulatory ECG monitoring (AEM): helpful when arrhythmia is detected and correlates with symptom reproduction; most helpful in patients with underlying heart disease.

Intermittent loop recorders: valuable in patients with frequent episodes not detected by AEM in which an arrhythmia is still suggested. Event recorder and transtelephone ECG monitoring may be helpful in patients with intermittent presyncopal episodes. Implantable loop recorder should be considered in patients in whom other monitoring devices have not provided data.

Head-up tilt testing: detects neurally mediated syncope, the most common cause of syncope in those without cardiac disease; the sensitivity, specificity, and reproducibility are variable.

Signal average ECG: possibly useful in patients with coronary artery disease and left ventricular dysfunction.

Electrophysiologic study: diagnostic value greatest in patients with abnormal ECG or AEM and structural heart disease.

Echocardiography: if cardiac disease is suspected or is manifest based on the history, physical examination, and ECG.

Exercise stress testing: if ischemic cause is suspected or with exertional syncope.

Psychiatric assessment: in syncope of unexplained cause with frequent recurrences and nonspecific complaints.

Complications

Sudden death; recurrent syncope; falls or accidents.

Differential diagnosis

Extensive, including common benign problems to life-threatening ones with potential for sudden death.

Need to exclude cardiogenic syncope in patients with structural heart disease, especially ischemic heart disease with left ventricular dysfunction.

Etiology

• Syncope can be classified into four broad categories:

Neurally mediated syncope

Vasodepressor (vasovagal, neurocardiogenic), situational, carotid sinus syncope, psychiatric, and other causes.

Orthostatic hypotension

Drugs, autonomic insufficiency, volume depletion.

Cardiac syncope

Electrical (arrhythmic): tachyarrhythmias (ventricular tachycardia, supraventricular tachycardia, torsades de pointes, preexcitation) and bradyarrhythmias (sinus node dysfunction, atrioventricular block).

Mechanical/obstructive: valvular stenosis (aortic, mitral, pulmonic), prosthetic valve dysfunction/thrombosis, hypertrophic cardiomyopathy, aortic dissection, pulmonary embolism, pulmonary hypertension, myxoma, tamponade, subclavian steal, severe left ventricular dysfunction, myocardial infarction.

Neurological syncope

Transient ischemic attacks, seizures, vertebrobasilar syndromes.

• Unexplained etiology.

Epidemiology

• Syncope is a common problem occurring in ≥3% of patients. It is a major reason for medical evaluation and hospitalization.

Treatment

Diet and lifestyle

• Avoidance of potential precipitating events is recommended, if possible, for example in neurally mediated syncope (*e.g.*, situational) or orthostatic hypotension (*e.g.*, volume depletion).

• In general, no special dietary precautions are required unless intake potentially aggravates the situation (*e.g*, caffeine and supraventricular arrhythmias).

• Increased salt intake is occasionally used in the treatment of orthostatic hypotension or neurocardiogenic syncope.

• Alcohol intake or lack of sleep may aggravate neurally mediated syncope.

• Only eight states have specific laws regarding resumption of driving in patients with syncope, whereas 42 have laws restricting driving in patients with seizure disorders. No adequate data support restriction in patients who have not experienced symptomatic arrhythmias, although patients with frequent nonsustained ventricular tachycardia, associated heart disease, and significant left ventricular dysfunction are at high enough risk to warrant cautioning.

Pharmacological treatment

• Treatment is individualized and directed toward the documented or presumed cause of syncope.

Neurocardiogenic syncope: difficult to make conclusive recommendations, but beta-blockers are effective and commonly used.

Neurocardiogenic syncope

• Difficult to make conclusive recommendations, but the following medications have been used.

β-blockers: effective and commonly used for prevention of vasovagal syncope. Metoprolol, pindolol, and atenolol have been most frequently studied. Pindolol has gained favor because of its intrinsic sympathetic activity, which diminishes the severity of resting bradycardia in treated patients. Overall, no compelling evidence suggests that any β-adrenergic blocker is superior to others.

Disospyramide: a class I anti-arrhythmic agent with prominent vasolytic effects and a disconcerting degree of negative inotropic effect. The required dosage has been a source of controversy, ranging from 200 to >700 mg/d. Currently, controversy regarding its effectiveness aside, disopyramide is best chosen for the young, active patient without structural heart disease or QT-interval prolongation. In this setting, it may be more tolerable than a β-adrenergic blocker.

Scopalmine patch: 1 patch every 3 days.

Serotonin reuptake inhibitors (sertraline hydrochloride, fluoxetine): have anecdotally been used to manage vasovagal syncope and carotid sinus syncope.

Midodrine: an a-agonist; promising agent for managing orthostatic hypotension and neurally mediated syncope. It is hoped that tachyphylaxis does not hamper its continued effectiveness.

Fludrocortisone: has been used if expansion of central volume is a therapeutic goal.

Orthostatic hypotension: fludrocortisone combined with increased salt intake and nonpharmacological measures may be effective.

Cardiac syncope: antiarrhythmic therapy if clinically indicated for electrical cause.

Nonpharmacological treatment

• Implantable defibrillators should be considered in patients with cardiac syncope secondary to or at high risk for lethal ventricular dysrhythmias.

Dual-chamber cardiac pacing may be effective in the predominantly cardioinhibitory type of neurocardiogenic syncope. Cardiac pacing is effective for indicated bradyarrhythmias.

Compression garments/stockings have been used to help maintain central volume.

Treatment aims

To address the underlying cause of syncope and to prevent recurrent syncopal events.

• This is critical for those with cardiac syncope because the major goal is to identify and treat the underlying heart disease.

• Treatment for neurally mediated syncope should be directed toward those with frequent, bothersome, or incapacitating symptoms.

• Consider that pharmacological drugs may be contributory to the cause of syncope and that withdrawal of a medication may alleviate the problem.

Prognosis

• Prognosis depends on the underlying cause of syncope.

• Cardiac syncope is associated with a high 1-year mortality (18%–33%) and an increased risk for sudden death. Noncardiac syncope and syncope of unexplained cause are associated with a better prognosis.

• The prognosis for neurally mediated syncope and for psychiatric patients with syncope is excellent. Recurrences, however, are common, especially in the psychiatric population.

Follow-up and management

• Management should be directed toward the identification and treatment of existing heart disease, if present. Otherwise, management should be individualized based on symptoms and the frequency of syncopal events.

• Patients with suspected or documented heart disease should be considered for referral to a cardiologist.

General references

Abboud FM: Neurocardiogenic syncope. *N Engl J Med* 1993, **328**:1117–1120.

Bansch D, *et al.*: Syncope in patients with an implantable cardioverter-defibrillator: incidence, prediction and implications for driving restrictions. *J Am Coll Cardiol* 1998, **31**:608.

Benditt DG, *et al.*: Pharmacotherapy of neurally mediated syncope. *Circulation* 1999, **100**:1242–1248.

Epstein AE, *et al.*: Personal and public safety issues related to arrhythmias that may affect consciousness: implications for regulation and physician recommendations. *Circulation* 1996, **94**:1147.

Syndrome of inappropriate antidiuresis

Diagnosis

Symptoms

• Mild chronic hyponatremia (serum sodium concentration 125–135 mEq/L) may be asymptomatic.

• More profound hyponatremia (serum sodium concentration <120 mEq/L) can cause the following:*

Headache.	**Confusion.**	**Seizures.**
Malaise.	**Depression.**	**Coma.**
Nausea and vomiting.	**Cramps.**	**Death.**
Irritability.	**Drowsiness.**	

*The severity of symptoms depends on the rate of fall of serum sodium as much as on the absolute value.

Signs [1]

• Mild chronic hyponatremia usually has no specific signs.

• Severe hyponatremia may cause the following:

Diminished reflexes.

Extensor plantar responses.

Cardinal features

Dilutional hyponatremia: plasma osmolality appropriately low for serum sodium.

Urine osmolality greater than plasma osmolality.

Persistent renal sodium excretion.

Absence of hypotension, hypovolemia, or edema-forming states.

Normal thyroid, renal, and adrenal function.

Investigations [1]

• Laboratory tests are not specific for the diagnosis but help to exclude other causes of hyponatremia and to identify underlying causes.

Chest radiography: to rule out a pulmonary process.

Serum sodium measurement: low concentration.

Plasma osmolality measurement: <270 mOsm/kg.

Blood glucose measurement: to exclude spurious hyponatremia in hyperglycemia.

Serum protein and lipoprotein measurement: to exclude pseudohyponatremia.

Serum uric acid measurement: low concentration.

Urine osmolality measurement: usually >300 mOsm/kg.

Renal function tests: creatinine clearance rate or serum creatinine concentration.

Thyroid function tests: free thyroxine, thyroid-stimulating hormone; to exclude hypothyroidism.

Adrenocortical tests: short cosyntropin test; to exclude cortisol deficiency.

Plasma vasopressin measurement: rarely checked.

Pituitary function tests: to exclude corticotropic hormone deficiency.

Complications

Permanent neurological deficit, high neurological morbidity and mortality: caused by prolonged profound hyponatremia or overly aggressive treatment leading to rapid rise in serum sodium concentration.

Differential diagnosis [2]

Hyponatremia associated with hypervolemia

Cardiac failure.

Cirrhosis.

Nephrotic syndrome.

Renal failure.

Hyponatremia associated with hypovolemia

Gastrointestinal fluid loss.

Severe burns.

Mineralocorticoid deficiency (*i.e.*, Addison's disease).

Salt-losing nephritis.

Etiology [2–4]

Neoplastic disease: *e.g.*, lung cancer, pancreatic cancer, lymphoma.

Chest disorders: *e.g.*, pneumonia, tuberculosis, abscess.

Neurological disorders: *e.g.*, head injury, infections, hemorrhage.

Drugs: *e.g.*, thiazides, cytotoxic agents, carbamazepine.

Epidemiology

• Hyponatremia is the most common electrolyte disturbance seen in hospitals (~10% of patients have serum sodium concentrations of <130 mEq/L).

• ~50% of all hyponatremia is due to the syndrome of inappropriate antidiuresis.

Treatment

Diet and lifestyle

• Fluid should be restricted to 0.5–1.0 L daily.

• Patients must eat a well-balanced diet.

Pharmacological treatment [1,5]

• The underlying cause of the syndrome should be treated (*e.g.*, cancer of the bronchus).

• **Fluid restriction is the mainstay of therapy.**

• Specific V_2-receptor antagonists to block the antidiuretic effect of vasopressin have been tested in humans.

• Treatment of severe hyponatremia is covered elsewhere (*see* Hyponatremia and Hyponatremia).

Induction of partial nephrogenic diabetes insipidus

Standard dosage	Demeclocycline, 1.2 g in divided doses. Lithium carbonate 0.4–1.2 g daily.
Contraindications	*Demeclocycline*: renal failure, pregnancy, children. *Lithium carbonate:* renal and cardiac disease.
Special points	*Demeclocycline:* full effect may need up to 3 weeks of treatment. *Lithium carbonate:* narrow therapeutic level; plasma concentrations must be measured.
Main drug interactions	*Demeclocycline:* warfarin. *Lithium carbonate:* diuretics, antibiotics, antihypertensives, sumatriptan.
Main side effects	*Demeclocycline:* nausea, diarrhea, photosensitivity. *Lithium carbonate:* gastrointestinal disturbances, goiter, CNS dysfunction.

Inhibition of neurohypophysial vasopressin secretion

Standard dosage	Phenytoin, 300 mg daily.
Contraindications	Renal and hepatic dysfunction, porphyria.
Main drug interactions	Antibacterials, anxiolytics, hypnotics, calcium antagonists.
Main side effects	Drowsiness, ataxia.

Induction of diuresis and natriuresis

Standard dosage	Furosemide, 40–80 mg daily, and sodium chloride, 3 g orally daily.
Contraindications	Decompensated liver cirrhosis; caution in prostatism.
Main drug interactions	Antifungals, potassium-losing drugs.
Main side effects	Hypokalemia, gastrointestinal disturbances.

Treatment aims

To relieve symptoms of hyponatremia.

To increase serum sodium concentration to 125–140 mEq/L.

Prognosis

• Prognosis depends on the underlying cause.

• Patients with serum sodium concentrations <110 mEq/L have high morbidity and mortality (~50%).

• Development of osmotic demyelination syndrome indicates poor prognosis (~50% mortality).

Follow-up and management [1]

• Depending on the underlying condition, fluid restriction or drug treatment may be needed indefinitely.

• Serum sodium concentrations must be checked regularly.

Osmotic demyelination syndrome [6]

• This occurs after rapid correction of chronic severe hyponatremia, irrespective of the means of increasing serum sodium concentrations.

• It is found in central pontine and intracerebral structures.

• It is clinically evident 2–4 days after correction of serum sodium concentrations.

• It occurs rarely and predominantly when serum sodium is rapidly connected (>1 mEq/L/hr).

Key references

1. Robertson GL: Syndrome of inappropriate antidiuresis. *N Engl J Med* 1989, **321**:538–539.
2. Ayus JC, Arieff AI: Pathogenesis and prevention of hyponatremic encephalopathy. *Endocrinol Metab Clin North Am* 1993, **22**:425–446.
3. Baylis PH, Thompson CJ: Osmoregulation of vasopressin and thirst in health and disease. *Clin Endocrinol* 1988, **29**:549–576.
4. Berl T, *et al.*: Clinical disorders of water metabolism. *Kidney Int* 1976, **10**:117–132.
5. Arieff AI: Management of hyponatraemia. *BMJ* 1993, **307**:307–308.
6. Sterns RH, Riggs, J, Achochet SS: Osmotic demyelination syndrome following correction of hyponatremia. *N Engl J Med* 1986, **314**:1535–1542.

Syndrome X

Diagnosis

Definition

• Cardiac syndrome X is the presence of classic angina with normal or near-normal findings on coronary angiography (in patients who do not have cardiomyopathy or coronary-artery spasm). It is more common in women and has been ascribed to coronary microvascular disease.

Symptoms

Anginal chest pain.

Anxiety.

Signs

Normal clinical examination.

Investigation

• Treadmill exercise test or dobutamine stress test usually shows ischemic-appearing ST-segment depression.

• Coronary angiography has to be done to exclude underlying coronary artery disease. Slow flow of dye in the normal epicardial coronary arteries has been described in some patients.

• Phosphorus-31 nuclear magnetic resonance spectroscopy may show abnormal metabolic response to handgrip exercise in a subgroup of women who have chest pain but normal coronary angiograms.

• Cerebral positron-emission tomography has suggested that abnormal central processing of afferent pain messages from the heart may play a determining role in perception of pain in these patients.

Complications

Psychological.

Differential diagnosis

• Endocrine syndrome X or Reaven's syndrome is a cluster of metabolic abnormalities including high blood glucose level, high blood pressure, increased very-low-density lipoprotein (VLDL) cholesterol levels, low high-density lipoprotein (HDL) cholesterol levels, high triglyceride levels, and insulin resistance.

Epidemiology

• According to data from the Coronary Artery Surgery Study (CASS), more than half of all women with chest pain who are referred for coronary angiography do not have angiographically significant coronary stenosis, compared to only 17% of men.

Treatment

Diet and lifestyle

• Treatment is entirely empirical. A sympathetic appreciation by the physician of the deleterious impact of chronic pain on the patient's quality of life can go a long way toward reassuring the patient that an earnest attempt is being made to help alleviate symptoms.

• All patients should be started on a regular exercise program to improve their stamina (many patients are severely deconditioned) and to encourage a positive attitude regarding their state of health. This effort is assisted by discontinuing all unnecessary medications. In some patients, this approach will suffice and alleviate symptoms; thus, no further evaluation will be necessary.

Pharmacological treatment

• If dobutamine stress or exercise stress echocardiography shows wall-motion abnormalities or diminished transmural contractility, then a trial of anti-ischemic therapy should be considered. Calcium-channel antagonists are sometimes effective; other anti-anginal agents may be used, but efficacy is uncertain.

• If dobutamine infusion is associated with chest pain despite a uniform increase in contractility, myocardial ischemia alone is unlikely to account for symptoms and a trial of tricyclic antidepressants (imipramine, 50 mg/d) coupled with beta-blockers (to block anticholinergic effects of this therapy) may relieve symptoms by reducing visceral pain sensitivity.

• If chest pain persists despite these therapeutic trials, gastrointestinal evaluation with endoscopy may be necessary to rule out chronic inflammatory disease, perhaps of an infectious cause (*e.g.*, *Helicobacter pylori* infection or reflux esophagitis).

• The value of aspirin has not been proven.

• Treatment with trimetazidine, a metabolic modulator, is promising because it decreases signs of angina during exercise and improves tolerance of exercise of patients with syndrome X.

• Should therapeutic trials fail to control chest pain, referral to pain clinic may be necessary for a multidisciplinary approach to pain management.

Other treatments

• Neurostimulation with transcutaneous electrical nerve stimulation (TENS) and spinal cord stimulation (SCS) may be useful in refractory cases.

Treatment aims

To relieve pain and anxiety.

Prognosis

• Although the symptoms are difficult to treat, myocardial ischemia in patients with normal coronary arteries is associated with excellent prognosis.

General references

Buchthal SD, *et al.*: Abnormal myocardial phosphorus-31 nuclear magnetic resonance spectroscopy in women with chest pain but normal coronary angiograms. *N Engl J Med* 2000, **342**:829–835.

Cannon RO III, Balban RS: Chest pain in women with normal coronary angiograms. *N Engl J Med* 2000, **342**:.

Cannon RO III, Camici PG, Epstein SE: Pathophysiological dilemma of syndrome X. *Circulation* 1992, **85**:883–892.

Cannon RO III, *et al.*: Imipramine in patients with chest pain despite normal coronary angiograms. *N Engl J Med* 1994, **330**:1411.

Davis KB, *et al.*: Comparison of 15-year survival for men and women after initial medical or surgical treatment for coronary artery disease: a CASS Registry Study. *J Am Coll Cardiol* 1995, **25**:1000–1009.

Systemic lupus erythematosus

Diagnosis

Symptoms and signs

Tiredness: indicating anemia; one of the most difficult and resistant symptoms in systemic lupus erythematosus (SLE).

Polyarthralgias and nonerosive symmetric arthritis: involving predominantly small joints (rarely deforming) [1,2].

Rashes: photosensitive, discoid, and, less often, classic facial butterfly rash [1].

Vasculitic lesions of extremities: leading to gangrene of digits (rare).

Oral or pharyngeal ulcers.

Myalgia.

Pleuritic or pericardial pain: indicating serositis.

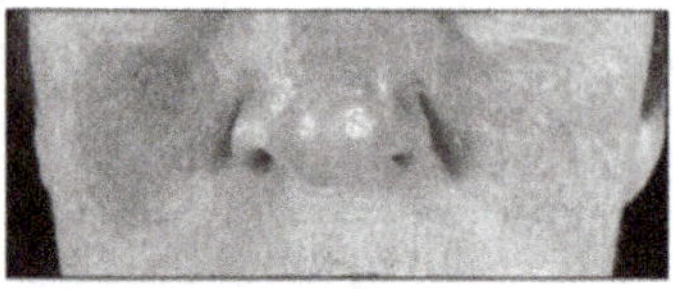

Classic butterfly rash. (*See* Color Plate.)

Epistaxis, bleeding gums, menorrhagia, purpura: symptoms of thrombocytopenia.

Visual and auditory hallucinations or epilepsy.

Edema or hypertension: *e.g.*, nephrotic syndrome or acute nephritic illness.

Alopecia [1].

Raynaud's phenomenon.

Lymphadenopathy.

Fever.

Livedo reticularis.

Investigations

Laboratory tests

• These are useful in the diagnosis of SLE, but no single diagnostic test is available [3].

Complete blood count: may reveal anemia, leukopenia, neutropenia, lymphopenia, or thrombocytopenia; raised ESR common in active disease; evidence of hemolytic anemia requires further investigation, *e.g.*, a Coombs' test [1].

Antinuclear antibody analysis: antibodies found in at least 95% of SLE patients but not disease-specific; antibodies to double-stranded DNA and Sm are relatively disease-specific but do not occur in all patients (~50% and ~5%, respectively); antibodies to Ro, La, and U1 ribonucleoprotein helpful in defining disease subsets and overlap syndromes; positive antiphospholipid antibodies and lupus anticoagulant define patients at risk from major arterial and venous thromboses [1].

For markers of disease activity or organ involvement

ESR measurement: raised ESR with normal CRP usual except when bacterial infection coexists [1,4].

Plasma-complement analysis: low C3, C4, and CH50 indicate activity.

Anti–double-stranded DNA antibody analysis: antibodies can rise with disease flares, especially those involving the kidney.

Dipstick testing of urine: for proteinuria and hematuria.

Microscopic examination: for red cell casts, leukocyte casts.

Measurements of renal function and 24-hour urine protein loss.

Complications

Severe renal involvement [4].

Cerebral involvement: infarcts or neuropsychiatric disease [4].

Infections secondary to immunosuppression.

Major thrombotic events: especially when high-titer antiphospholipid antibodies are present [5].

Differential diagnosis

Other connective tissue diseases: *e.g.*, rheumatoid arthritis, progressive systemic sclerosis.

Infection.

Malignancy.

Etiology

• Causes include the following:

Genetic factors and inherited defects of the early components of the classic complement pathway.

Environmental factors: *e.g.*, sunlight.

Drugs: *e.g.*, hydralazine, procainamide, phenytoin.

Epidemiology

• The prevalence of SLE in the United States is 45 in 100 000 women, 3.7 in 100 000 men [6].

• The highest incidence is in the 20–40 year age group.

• SLE is unusual in children.

Treatment

Diet and lifestyle

• Patients, especially those with photosensitivity, should avoid sunlight and should use high-factor sunscreen (ultraviolet A and B).

Pharmacological treatment

Indications

Discoid lupus erythematosus rashes: topical steroids.

Joint and skin involvement: hydroxychloroquine.

Systemic involvement: acute treatment by corticosteriods, introduction of cytotoxic agents, *e.g.*, azathioprine, chlorambucil, methotrexate.

Severe vasculitis (including cerebral and renal involvement): pulse cyclophosphamide and methylprednisolone [7,8].

Systemic treatment

Standard dosage

Hydroxychloroquine, 200 mg once or twice daily.
Prednisone, 10–40 mg daily and azathioprine, 1–2.5 mg/kg daily to allow subsequent steroid reduction.
Pulse methylprednisolone, 1 g i.v. daily for 3 days and pulse cyclophosphamide, 500–750 mg/m², adjusted downward for creatinine clearance <35 mL/min or myelosuppression.
Cyclophosphamide is given i.v. monthly for 6 months, then i.v. every 3 months until clinical improvement or toxicity occurs.
Cyclophosphamide dosing is complex and should be supervised by a specialist (*e.g.*, rheumatologist, nephrologist, pulmonologist).

Contraindications

Known hypersensitivity, systemic infections.

Special points

Cyclophosphamide: infusions must be preceded by a complete blood count to check for bone-marrow toxicity, in particular evidence of neutropenia.

Main drug interactions

Cyclophosphamide: concurrent allopurinol should be avoided because of enhanced toxicity.

Main side effects

Hydroxychloroquine: retinopathy, skin rashes.
Azathioprine: bone-marrow suppression, gastrointestinal disturbances, liver toxicity.
Cyclophosphamide: nausea and vomiting, hair loss, hemorrhagic cystitis, premature menopause [7].
All cytotoxic agents: teratogenicity (adequate contraception essential) [7,9].

Treatment aims

To alleviate disease flares.

Prognosis

• Renal and cerebral involvement and the complications of treatment, especially infection, are the major contributors to mortality.

• The survival rate has improved in the past 2 decades and is now ~95% at 5 years.

Follow-up and management

• Prompt treatment of lupus flares is mandatory.

• The use of oral cytotoxic drugs requires monthly blood counts to check for bone-marrow suppression and liver function tests with methotrexate.

Key references

1. Tan E, *et al.*: The 1982 revised criteria for the classification of systemic lupus erythematosus. *Arthritis Rheum* 1982, **25**:1271–1277.
2. Mills JA: Systemic lupus erythematosus. *N Engl J Med* 1994, **330**:1871–1879.
4. Boumpas DT, *et al.*: Systemic lupus erythematosus: emerging concepts. Part 1. Renal, neuropsychiatric, cardiovascular, pulmonary and hematologic disease. *Ann Intern Med* 1995, **122**:940–950.
3. Egner W: The use of laboratory tests in the diagnosis of SLE. *J Clin Pathol* 2000, **53(6)**:424–432.
5. Petri M: Systemic lupus erythematosus and pregnancy. *Rheum Dis Clin North Am* 1994, **20**:87–118.
6. Tench CM, Isenberg DA: The variation in anti-ENA characteristics between different ethnic populations with systemic lupus erythematosus over a 10-year period. *Lupus* 2000, **9(5)**:374–376.
7. Rothfield NF: Clinical features of SLE. In *Textbook of Rheumatology*. Edited by Kelley NN, *et al.* Philadelphia: WB Saunders; 1988.
8. Fox DA, McCune WJ: Immunosuppressive drug therapy of systemic lupus erythematosus. *Rheum Dis Clin North Am* 1994, **20**:265–291.
9. Pisetsky DS, Gilkeson G, St. Clair EW: Systemic lupus erythematosus: diagnosis and treatment. *Med Clin North Am* 1997, **81**:113–128.

Systemic sclerosis

Diagnosis

Symptoms

- Scleroderma is unlikely in the absence of Raynaud's phenomenon.
- It has two major subgroups of prognostic and therapeutic importance, as follows:

Limited cutaneous disease

- This occurs in 60% of patients.
- It was previously called CREST syndrome [1].

Swollen painful fingers: ulcers possible.

Thick skin on hands.

Calcium deposits.

Swallowing difficulty.

Diffuse cutaneous disease

- This occurs in 40% of patients.

Puffy hands, feet, arms, legs, tight skin.

Weight loss, fatigue.

Muscle and joint pain.

Breathlessness, dry cough, palpitations.

Indigestion, bloating, diarrhea [2,3].

Signs

Limited cutaneous disease

Early (<10 years)

- Distribution is limited to hands, feet, and face.

Sclerodactyly, swollen fingers, microstomia.

Pitting scars, pulp atrophy.

Digital ulcers.

Telangiectasia.

Calcinosis.

Late (>10 years)

Loud pulmonary second sound.

Right heart failure.

Abdominal bloating.

Wasting and other signs of malabsorption.

Diffuse cutaneous disease

Early (<5 years)

Diffusely puffy or sclerosed skin, including truncal changes.

Friction rubs.

Joint contractures.

Muscle weakness.

Digital pits and ulcers.

Basal crepitations, pericardial rub, arrhythmia.

Late (>5 years)

Dry, shiny skin.

Ulcers: atrophic, on fingers or elbows.

Muscle wasting.

Joint contractures.

Cardiac or respiratory failure.

Investigations

Complete blood count: to detect anemia of chronic disease.

Creatinine clearance measurement: to assess renal function.

Autoantibody tests: antinuclear antibodies are positive in 90% of patients; full screen useful to mark subsets of systemic sclerosis or overlap with other disorders.

Nailfold capillary tests (ophthalmoscope or microscopic): useful in "prescleroderma" and early disease; abnormal pattern of vessel drop-out and distortion.

Esophageal scintiscanning: to detect dysmotility (other "gut" tests as indicated).

ECG, echocardiography, Doppler ultrasonography: to detect cardiac involvement and to estimate pulmonary artery pressure.

Chest radiography, pulmonary function tests, high-resolution CT: to detect lung involvement; CT best test for presence and extent of early fibrosis.

Electromyography, biopsy: to diagnose inflammatory muscle disease in overlap disorders.

Joint radiography: to detect acro-osteolysis, calcinosis.

Skin biopsy: usually not needed in established disease, best used in early puffy stage for diagnosis or to differentiate systemic sclerosis from eosinophillic fasciitis, which is steroid-responsive.

Complications

Hypertensive renal crisis: in diffuse cutaneous disease, usually within first 5 years of disease; in 7%–10% of patients.

Interstitial pseudo-obstruction: late complication often of limited cutaneous disease; in <5%.

Carcinoma of lung: associated with pulmonary fibrosis.

Differential diagnosis

Eosinophilic fasciitis.

Mixed connective tissue disease.

Overlap syndromes.

Chronic graft-versus-host disease.

Eosinophilia-myalgia syndrome.

Vinyl chloride disease.

Toxic-oil syndrome.

Scleromyxedema.

Scleredema of Buschke.

Carcinoid syndrome.

Insulin-dependent diabetes mellitus skin changes.

Chronic reflex sympathetic dystrophy.

Idiopathic pulmonary fibrosis.

Primary pulmonary hypertension.

Cardiomyopathies.

Intestinal hypomotility syndromes.

Etiology

- In most cases, the cause is unknown, but the following may play a role:

Genetic: HLA classes II and III genes (weak association).

Environmental: organic chemicals (*e.g.*, vinyl chloride), epoxy resins, silica, rapeseed oil, drugs (*e.g.*, bleomycin).

Epidemiology

- Systemic sclerosis occurs worldwide.
- 12–20 in one million people are affected annually.
- The female:male ratio is 3:1 overall and 10:1 in people of child-bearing age.
- The disease is more severe in nonwhites.
- 30–60 years is the usual age of onset.

Treatment

Diet and lifestyle

• Patients should avoid cold and sudden drops in temperature.

• Patients should stop smoking.

• Skin care involves protection and moisturizers (cosmetic cover for telangiectasia).

• Patients should follow a daily exercise program to prevent, reduce, or delay contractures and to maintain strength and function.

Pharmacological treatment

For Raynaud's phenomenon and vascular insufficiency [4–7]

• Response can be variable, so more than one drug within a class is worth trying.

Standard dosage	Calcium antagonists: *e.g.*, nifedipine, 10–40 mg slow release twice daily. Angiotensin-converting enzyme (ACE) inhibitors: captopril, 6.25–18.75 mg daily; enalapril, 5–15 mg daily.
Contraindications	*Calcium antagonists:* pregnancy; caution in hepatic or renal disease. *ACE inhibitors:* pregnancy.
Special points	*ACE inhibitors:* may cause rapid fall in blood pressure.
Main drug interactions	*Calcium antagonists:* antiepileptics, antiarrhythmics. *ACE inhibitors:* must not be given with potassium-sparing diuretics.
Main side effects	*Calcium antagonists:* flushing, headache, edema. *ACE inhibitors:* dry cough, voice change, rashes.

For early diffuse disease

• No drug is of proven efficacy [5–7].

Standard dosage	D-Penicillamine, 750–1000 mg daily; methotrexate, 7.5–15 mg orally weekly; cyclosporine, 2.5–5 mg/kg orally daily; prednisolone, 20 mg on alternate days.
Contraindications	Pregnancy, existing liver and renal disease.
Main drug interactions	Cyclophosphamide with allopurinol, cyclosporine with ACE inhibitors.
Main side effects	Bone-marrow toxicity, renal and liver impairment, alopecia, rashes.

For esophageal involvement [5–7]

Standard dosage	Proton-pump inhibitor: omeprazole, 20 mg/d. Prokinetic drug: (controversial) cisapride, 10 mg 3–4 times/d for 12 weeks, taken 30 min before meal or at bedtime. Others include metoclopramide anad erythromycin. Propulsid (Janssen, Titusville, NJ) has been withdrawn.
Contraindications	Pregnancy, breast-feeding.
Special points	*Omeprazole:* can increase bowel colonization.
Main drug interactions	Oral anticoagulants, phenytoin, theophylline.
Main side effects	*Omeprazole:* constipation, headache, diarrhea. *Cisapride:* abdominal cramps, diarrhea, cardiac arrythmias.

For mid-gut involvement: bacterial overgrowth

• Rotation antibiotics can be used in various combinations, *e.g.*, metronidazole, 400–600 mg twice daily, tetracycline, 250 mg 3 times daily; erythromycin, 250 mg 4 times daily, or ciprofloxacin, 500 mg twice daily.

• These should be given for short periods, *e.g.*, 3–4 weeks, with "holidays" of 1–2 weeks.

Nonpharmacological treatment

Lumbar or digital sympathectomy for severe Raynaud's phenomenon with critical ischemia.

Selective removal of calcinosis.

Treatment aims

To reduce symptoms.
To halt disease.
To treat complications.
• Systemic sclerosis has no cure.

Prognosis

5-year cumulative survival rate is 34%–73%.

Factors adversely affecting outcome: increasing age; male sex; extent of skin involvement; lung, heart, and kidney disease.

• For patients with diffuse cutaneous disease, the first 5 years are the most dangerous; with limited cutaneous disease, the most dangerous period is after 10 years, with a risk of pulmonary hypertension and widespread gut disease.

Follow-up and management

• Diffuse disease needs frequent follow-up in the first 4 years, *i.e.*, 3-monthly or more frequently if necessary; hypertensive renal crisis is the greatest risk.

• Limited disease needs yearly follow-up, with attention to late disease complications, *i.e.*, pulmonary hypertension, malabsorption.

• Attention to vascular insufficiency, possible superimposed infections, and changing internal organ involvement permits therapeutic adjustments that can improve quality of life for patients.

Key references

1. Medsger TA Jr: Systemic sclerosis (scleroderma), localized forms of scleroderma and calcinosis. *Arthritis and Allied Conditions* 1993, **2**:1253–1292.
2. Mitchell M, Bolster MB, LeRoy EC: Scleroderma and related conditions. *Med Clin North Am* 1997, **81**:129–149.
3. Penez M, Kohn SR: Systemic sclerosis. *J Am Acad Dermatol* 1993, **28**:525–547.
4. Kahaleh MB: Raynaud's phenomenon and vascular disease and scleroderma. *Curr Opin Rheumatol* 1994, **6**:621–627.
5. Medsger TA Jr: Treatment of systemic sclerosis. *Ann Rheum Dis* 1991, **50(suppl)**:877–886.
6. Van-den Hoogen FH, *et al.*: Treatment of systemic sclerosis. *Curr Opin Rheumatol* 1994, **6**:637–641.
7. Pope JE: Treatment of systemic sclerosis. *Rheum Dis Clin North Am* 1996, **22**:893–907.

Tachycardia, supraventricular

Diagnosis

Definition

• Supraventricular tachycardias include the following:

Sinus tachycardia.

Atrial fibrillation.

Atrial flutter.

Atrial tachycardia.

Atrioventricular re-entrant tachycardia.

Atrioventricular nodal re-entrant tachycardia.

• Atrioventricular re-entrant and nodal re-entrant tachycardias, the two common supraventricular tachycardias arising from the atrioventricular junction, are discussed here.

Symptoms

Palpitation: paroxysms of regular palpitation at 140–240 beats/min, with sudden onset and offset.

Syncope: palpitation may be associated with syncope or presyncope at onset of attack, when blood pressure is probably at its lowest.

Chest pain: unusual but may occur during attacks, particularly in presence of ischemic heart disease.

Paroxysmal attacks: occasionally precipitated by postural changes or may be associated with particular times in menstrual cycle.

Diaphoresis, lightheadedness, and dyspnea.

Signs

Pulse

Fast, regular pulse.

Jugular venous pulse

• In atrioventricular nodal re-entrant tachycardia, prominent jugular venous pulsations that match the rate of tachycardia, a feature referred to as the frog sign.

Heart

Signs of left ventricular failure: unusual unless structural heart disease is coexistent.

• Atrioventricular dissociation is not evident (no cannon waves in neck).

• Blood pressure is usually well maintained after the first few seconds of an attack.

Investigations

ECG: regular rhythm present, usually with narrow QRS complexes; occasionally, pre-existing or rate-related bundle branch block leads to broad QRS complexes.

Atrioventricular nodal re-entrant tachycardia: Usually the P waves are superimposed in the QRS complex in II, III, and aVF. In about 10% of the patients, clearly visible inverted P waves are seen in II, III, and aVF and an RP interval during tachycardia that is much longer than the PR interval.

Chest radiography: usually normal unless structural heart disease coexistent.

Electrophysiology: indicated if catheter ablation contemplated or for risk assessment in symptomatic patients with Wolff–Parkinson–White syndrome.

Complications

Left ventricular failure: caused by coexistent structural heart disease; supraventricular tachycardia may cause ventricular failure in the absence of pre-existing structural heart disease only if tachycardia is incessant and has continued uninterrupted for months or years.

Differential diagnosis

Atrial tachycardia or atrial flutter.

Ventricular tachycardia: if atrioventricular re-entrant tachycardia is conducted with bundle branch block.

• When the history is being taken, establishing the presence or absence of structural heart disease, *e.g.*, cardiomyopathy or previous myocardial infarction, is important. A history or known diagnosis of either of these conditions makes a diagnosis of ventricular tachycardia much more probable than atrioventricular re-entrant or nodal re-entrant tachycardia. If the QRS complex is broad and has a pattern unlike that of classic left or right bundle branch block, then diagnosis is probably ventricular tachycardia.

Etiology

Atrioventricular re-entrant tachycardia

• The structural substrate is a congenital abnormality of the conducting system of the heart, whereby an extra electrical connection exists between the atria and the ventricles.

• Tachycardia arises when an electrical impulse passes from the atrium to the ventricle through the normal atrioventricular node but returns to the atria by the accessory pathway.

Atrioventricular nodal re-entrant tachycardia

• Patients have two functionally separate pathways within or close to the atrioventricular node.

• Tachycardia arises in a similar way to that arising in patients with atrioventricular reentrant tachycardia.

Epidemiology

• These arrhythmias occur frequently and form most of the tachycardias in patients with structurally normal hearts.

• Men are more likely to have atrioventricular re-entrant tachycardia, and women atrioventricular nodal re-entrant tachycardia.

• Paroxysms of palpitation may start in infancy but more usual in teenage years or twenties.

• Although AVNRT may appear at any age, most patients seek medical attention during the fourth or fifth decade of life.

Treatment

Diet and lifestyle

- If the tachycardias are initiated by atrial premature beats, abstinence from caffeine may help.
- Otherwise, no special precautions are necessary.

Pharmacological treatment

Acute treatment

Standard dosage Adenosine, i.v. bolus dose followed by saline flush, starting at 3 mg, with a second dose of 6 mg if tachycardia does not terminate after 60 seconds; a further dose of 12 mg is given if tachycardia does not terminate after another 60 seconds. Verapamil, 5 mg i.v. slowly (30 seconds); if tachycardia has not terminated after 5 minutes, a second 5-mg dose may be given, if hypotension has not occurred.

Contraindications *Adenosine:* asthma.
Verapamil: poor ventricular function.

Special points *Adenosine:* although 12 mg is maximum adult dose recommended in product license, bolus doses of 18 mg may occasionally be need to terminate tachycardia; may exacerbate bronchoconstriction.
Verapamil: negatively inotropic and should not be given to patients with known abnormal ventricular function or with signs of cardiomegaly on chest radiography; best not given to patients with a broad complex tachycardia because it may cause cardiovascular collapse if erroneously given to patients with ventricular tachycardia; i.v. verapamil should not be given to patient taking oral beta-blockers because sinus arrest or dramatic hypotension may occur.

Main drug interactions *Adenosine:* increased effect with dipyridamole; decreased effect with theophylline.

Main side effects *Adenosine:* flushing and chest tightness (transient).

Prophylaxis

- Beta-blockade (*e.g.*, atenolol, 50–100 mg) is often effective in this role, particularly if the attacks are exercise-induced.
- Digoxin, 0.125 mg, and verapamil, 180–360 mg, may be effective but are contraindicated in the presence of a delta wave because they may increase the ventricular rate if atrial fibrillation complicates the Wolff–Parkinson–White syndrome.

Treatment aims

To terminate an acute paroxysm of tachycardia.
To suppress tachycardia.
To cure tachycardia.

Other treatments

Vagal maneuvers
- Deep breathing or the Valsalva maneuver, with straining for at least 15 seconds.

Cardioversion
- When adenosine and verapamil are contraindicated or ineffective, synchronized electrical cardioversion is almost always effective in restoring sinus rhythm. When digitalis toxicity is suspected or present, electrical cardioversion should be avoided.

Radiofrequency catheter ablation
- The treatment of choice for patients with recurrent symptomatic junctional tachycardias that do not respond to prophylactic drug treatment or as an alternative to chronic pharmacologic therapy. Ablation is also extremely effective in atrioventricular tachycardia owing to an accessory pathway. More recent advances include ablation of atrial flutter and modification techniques in atrial fibrillation.

Prognosis

- Prognosis is generally excellent, and life expectancy does not differ from that of the normal population.
- Symptomatic patients with the Wolff–Parkinson–White pattern on the ECG during sinus rhythm have a small risk of sudden death, associated with the development of atrial fibrillation. Symptomatic patients should undergo ablation.

Follow-up and management

- Oral aspirin is advisable for 6 weeks after catheter ablation.
- Patients should be assessed for recurrence of symptoms or re-emergence of the Wolff–Parkinson–White pattern on the ECG.

General references

Ganz LI, Friedman PL: Supraventricular tachycardia. *N Engl J Med* 1995, **332**:162.

Morady F: Radio-frequency ablation as treatment for cardiac arrhythmias. *N Engl J Med* 1999, **340**:534.

Tachycardia, ventricular

Diagnosis

Symptoms

• Symptoms are not always manifest.

Palpitations.

Sudden shortness of breath.

Dizzy spells.

Blackouts.

Cardiac arrest.

Sudden death.

Signs

• Signs are not always manifest.

Tachycardia: 100–300 beats/min.

Hypotension and associated signs.

Cannon waves in jugular venous pressure, variable blood pressure, variation in intensity of first heart sound: signs of atrioventricular dissociation.

Investigations

12-lead ECG: initially, to confirm diagnosis, after treatment, for comparison of sinus rhythm; reveals tachycardia with QRS complexes 140 ms duration, evidence of atrioventricular dissociation (independent P waves, fusion beats, capture beats, second-degree ventriculo-atrial block), marked left or right axis deviation during tachycardia, absence of RS complexes in chest leads during tachycardia.

Adenosine test: initially, to distinguish from junctional or atrial tachycardia; if patient presents with stable tachycardia and if 12-lead ECG cannot be interpreted as showing ventricular tachycardia, incremental boluses of adenosine 0.05–0.20 mg/kg i.v. should be given, which terminates almost all junctional tachycardias, slows most atrial tachycardias, but affects almost no ventricular tachycardias except those arising in the right ventricular outflow tract.

Cardiac enzyme analysis: after treatment, if history suggests infarction.

Echocardiogram: to determine underlying cardiomyopathy or valvular disease, to assess left and right ventricular function.

Exercise test: under supervision of arrhythmia specialist to look for coronary disease, to provoke arrhythmia, and to assess drug efficacy.

24-hour ambulatory ECG recording: to quantify frequency of ventricular arrhythmia and associated arrhythmias (*e.g.*, ventricular premature beat).

Left ventricular and coronary angiography.

Programmed electrophysiologic testing: to determine inducibility, morphology, and suppressibility of symptoms and to guide decisions among drug, ablative, or ICD therapy.

Complications

Cardiac arrest.

Sudden death.

Cardiogenic shock.

Pulmonary edema.

Differential diagnosis

Supraventricular tachycardia: either atrial or junctional, with either right or left bundle branch block.

• All wide-complex tachycardias should be considered ventricular in origin until proved otherwise.

Etiology

Acute ischemia: coronary obstruction by thrombus.

Large scar old infarction: previous surgery, dysplasias.

Microscopic scar infiltration: fibrosis.

No clinical disease: *e.g.*, right ventricular outflow tachycardia.

• Right ventricular dysplasia (where the right ventricular muscle is replaced by fibrofatty tissue and dilated RV can be determined by echocardiography).

• Hypertrophic cardiomyopathy (Sustained VT in these patients carries a high risk of sudden death).

Viral myocarditis.

Functional disease: "fascicular" tachycardia.

• Fallot Tetralogy or VSD when successfully corrected at risk for late development of VT.

Tumors, malformations, other causes (rare).

Epidemiology

• 2%–10% of patients suffering a myocardial infarction have a sustained ventricular tachycardia or cardiac arrest within 12 months.

Treatment

Diet and lifestyle

• Avoid strenuous exercise and eat a normal diet unless evidence of coronary disease.

Pharmacological treatment

• The underlying disease process or associated cardiogenic fluid retention must be treated.

Emergency

Cardiopulmonary resuscitation if necessary.

Lidocaine 1 to 1.5 mg/kg intravenously, followed by infusion at 1 to 4 mg/min, supplemented by boluses of 0.5 to 0.75 mg/kg every 5 to 10 minutes to a maximum of 3 mg/kg (in those with heart failure or liver damage and in the elderly, the infusion rate should be titrated to toxicity).

Procainamide 1 g intravenously over 30 minutes followed by 1 to 2 mg/min (decrease the infusion rates in patients with renal insufficiency).

Amiodarone 150 mg intravenously over 10 minutes followed by 360 mg intravenously over 6 hours, then 0.5 mg/min infusion.

Intravenous bretylium or lidocaine must be used with great caution and should be supervised by physicians well versed with these medications.

Direct-current cardioversion in unstable patients (synchronized and starting at 100 J) or if drug treatment fails.

A succession of drugs is unwise, especially in patients with coronary disease and impaired ventricular function.

Verapamil must not be given: it may cause profound collapse and even death.

Long-term treatment

• Drug treatment should be supervised by a cardiologist with a long-term interest in arrhythmias.

• All antiarrhythmic drugs have proarrhythmic properties especially when used in combination with other antiarrhythmic drugs.

• Whether long-term drug treatment improves prognosis is not known. Currently amiodarone holds promise in the management of non-sustained ventricular tachycardia and the results of AMIOVERT, a randomized trial, is awaited.

Implantable cardioverter defibrillator (ICD)

• Implantation of automatic defibrillator device to terminate tachycardia: this also treats ventricular tachycardia by rapid pacing.

• Two primary prevention trials MADIT (Multicenter Automatic Defibrillator Implantation Trial) and MUSTT (Multicenter UnSustained Tachycardia Trial) substantiated improved survival with ICD therapy in coronary patients with nonsustained ventricular tachycardia.

• Two secondary prevention trials that focused on patients with aborted cardiac arrest or life-threatening cardiac arrhythmias have also been completed: these are the AVID (Antiarrhythmic Versus Implantable Defibrillator) study and the CIDS (Canadian Implantable Defibrillator Study). A similar survival benefit was achieved with ICD therapy when compared with amiodarone in both these trials.

• The AVID data suggested that patients with relatively well preserved ejection fraction (≥0.35) do *not* have a better survival rate when treated with the ICD when compared with anti-arrhythmic drugs (mostly amiodarone). However, in patients with low ejection fraction, the ICD was associated with improved survival when compared with anti-arrhythmic drugs. Currently two randomized trials MADIT-II and SCD-HeFT (Sudden Cardiac Death-Heart Failure Trial) are evaluating the survival benefit of ICD therapy in patients with left ventricular dysfunction.

• ICD is not stand-alone therapy for prevention of sudden cardiac death. The reduction of sudden death with beta-blockers and angiotensin converting enzyme inhibitors in patients with heart failure is well substantiated and hypolipidemic therapy may also contribute additional benefit in patients with heart failure due to coronary disease.

Treatment aims

To suppress recurrence of tachycardia (drug treatment).

To terminate recurrence of tachycardia (device treatment).

To destroy the arrhythmia "substrate," possibly offering a cure (ablation).

To correct mechanical heart disease and refractory arrhythmias (transplantation).

Other treatments

• Alternative long-term treatments include:

Ablation of localized focus or circuit causing tachycardia: radiofrequency energy and low-energy direct current are most popular sources.

Electrophysiologically guided surgery.

Transplantation in selected patients with severe ventricular impairment.

Prognosis

• Prognosis depends on the underlying disease process and presentation.

• 1-year mortality in patients resuscitated from cardiac arrest occurring out of hospital is up to 50%; defibrillator implantation reduces this significantly.

• Long-term prognosis is excellent for ventricular tachycardia associated with a normal heart.

Follow-up and management

• Patients should be referred to a center specializing in ventricular tachycardia to allow the correct treatment to be selected.

• Long-term drug treatment can be assessed by ambulatory monitoring.

• Ventricular tachycardia is not a curable disease and needs long-term follow-up.

General references

Moss AJ and the MADIT Investigators: Improved survival with an implanted defibrillator in patients with coronary disease at high risk for ventricular arrhythmia. *N Engl J Med* 1996, **335**:1933–1940.

Buxton AE and the MUSST Investigators: A randomized study of the prevention of sudden death in patients with coronary artery disease. *N Engl J Med* 1999, **341**:1882–1890.

Connolly SJ and the CIDS Investigators: Canadian Implantable Defibrillator Study: a randomized trial of implantable cardioverter versus amiodarone. *Circulation* 2000, **101**:1297–1302.

Morady F: Radiofrequency ablation as treatment of cardiac arrhythmias. *N Engl J Med* 1999, **340**:534.

Diagnosis

Symptoms

- β-Thalassemia is manifest during the first year of life in 90% of patients; a few present at 3–4 years (late-onset β-thalassemia major).
- 10% of patients with β-thalassemia major have a mild course (independent of transfusion).
- Patients may be asymptomatic; detection is from antenatal screening and diagnosis.

Poor weight gain.

Failure to thrive.

Fever.

Diarrhea.

Increasing pallor.

Distended abdomen.

Signs

Pallor.

Heart failure.

Splenomegaly.

Jaundice.

Investigations

Blood tests: low hemoglobin, mean corpuscular hemoglobin, mean cell volume; absent or reduced hemoglobin A (β° or β^{+} thalassemia), variable hemoglobin F and A_2 (using electrophoresis).

Genetic analysis: defines specific mutations, may help to predict disease severity and prognosis and facilitate first-trimester diagnosis.

Complications

Splenomegaly leading to hypersplenism (neutropenia, thrombocytopenia, anemia).

Anemia causing severe bone changes, short stature, and heart failure.

Differential diagnosis

Iron deficiency.

Etiology

- Thalassemia is caused by defective synthesis of the α- or β-globin chain (α- and β-thalassemia, respectively).
- The disorder is inherited (Mendelian recessive).
- It occurs in Mediterranean, Asian, Arabic, and Chinese groups because of a selective advantage against *Plasmodium falciparum*.

Epidemiology [1]

- Thalassemia is one of the most common inherited disorders throughout the world.
- Among blacks, approximately 30% of the population is either heterozygous or homozygous for the α-thalassemia-2 deletion.
- In southwest Europe, it is declining because of prevention programs; in consanguineous marriages, the birth rate of β-thalassemia increases by 30%.

Treatment

Diet and lifestyle

• Patients must avoid red meat and liver, and they should be encouraged to lead a normal active lifestyle.

Pharmacological treatment

Treatment of transfusional iron overload

• Desferrioxamine is infused s.c. over 8–12 hours from a portable syringe driver pump 5–6 nights/week.

• Chelation therapy is started when ferritin is 1000 μg/L (after 12–24 transfusions).

• Initial dose of 20 mg/kg desferrioxamine is diluted in 5–10 mL water for injection. Vitamin C, 100–200 mg orally (increases urinary iron excretion), is added when the patient is receiving desferrioxamine.

• In iron-overloaded patients, the desferrioxamine dosage is 50 mg/kg daily.

• For cardiomyopathy, continuous desferrioxamine is given through an i.v. delivery device (Hickman line, Port-a-Cath).

Complications of treatment

Alloimmunization to blood group antigens (in 25% of patients), febrile and urticarial transfusion reactions (in 75% of patients), cytomegalovirus infection and immunosuppression, transfusion-transmitted hepatitis B and C viruses: due to chronic transfusion (risk of HIV, 1 in 65 000).

Cardiomyopathy (most common cause of death), reduced growth, hypoparathyroidism, diabetes, failure of puberty: due to inadequate chelation.

Short stature, bone changes (pseudorickets), visual disturbances, hypersensitivity, hearing problems, pulmonary edema: due to desferrioxamine toxicity (overchelation).

Treatment aims

To provide good quality of life.

To provide a long life.

Other treatments [2,3]

Bone-marrow transplantation: 94% success rate if patient compliant with desferrioxamine and has no liver fibrosis or enlargement; success rate affected by age and liver status.

Splenectomy for hypersplenism.

Prognosis

• Maintenance transfusion and regular iron chelation preserve excellent health, and the prognosis is now open-ended.

• Early death is generally the result of intractable heart failure secondary to iron overload and infections.

Follow-up and management [4–6]

• The patient's ferritin, liver function, and bone metabolism must be monitored 3 times yearly, with annual anti-hepatitis C virus, anti-HIV, and hepatitis B surface antigen checks.

• Evaluation for glucose intolerance must be done yearly from the age of 10 years in patients with a family history of diabetes or from the age of 16 years in those without.

• Other endocrine and cardiac investigations should be made if clinically indicated.

• Patients should have yearly audiometry and twice-yearly eye tests.

• Patients who have undergone splenectomy have higher risk of infection and may need vaccinations.

• Patients should be vaccinated against hepatitis B.

Key references

1. Davies SC, Modell B, Wonke B: *Access to Healthcare for People From Black and Ethnic Minorities*. London: Royal College of Physicians; 1993:147–168.
2. Lucarelli G: Bone marrow transplantation for thalassaemia. *J Intern Med* 1997, **242(Suppl 740)**:49–52.
3. Loukopoulos D: New therapies for the haemoglobinopathies. *J Intern Med* 1997, **242(Suppl 740)**:439–448.
4. Piomelli S: The management of patients with Cooley's anemia: transfusions and splenectomy. *Semin Hematol* 1995, **32**:262–268.
5. Davies SC, Wonke B: The management of haemoglobinopathies. *Baillières Clin Haematol* 1991, **4**:361–389.
6. Kattamis CA, Kattamis AC: Management of thalassemias: growth and development, hormone substitution, vitamin supplementation and vaccination. *Semin Hematol* 1995, **32**:269–279.

Thyroid carcinoma

Diagnosis

Symptoms

• Patients may be asymptomatic (thyroid swelling is noted by someone else).

Neck swelling: rapid increase in size raises level of concern.

Dysphagia, dyspnea, dysphonia: symptoms of local compression.

Pain in neck, radiating to jaw or ear.

Bone pain, hemoptysis, abdominal discomfort: may indicate metastases.

Symptoms of thyrotoxicosis: exceedingly rare.

Signs

Single nodule: most common presentation; often firm or hard.

Fixation of thyroid swelling to local structures.

Cervical lymphadenopathy.

Evidence of metastases (unusual): spinal cord compression, spastic paraparesis, hepatomegaly, bone swellings, tenderness.

Investigations

• No blood test of radiological study can distinguish benign from malignant thyroid lesions.

Fine-needle aspiration cytology: test of choice to diagnose malignancy in thyroid nodules.

Thyroid function tests: serum-free thyroxine and thyroid-stimulating hormone; used to diagnose hypothyroidism or hyperthyroidism.

Isotope scanning: hot nodules (suppressing surrounding thyroid tissue) are rarely malignant; nodules that are not hot should be evaluated by fine-needle aspiration.

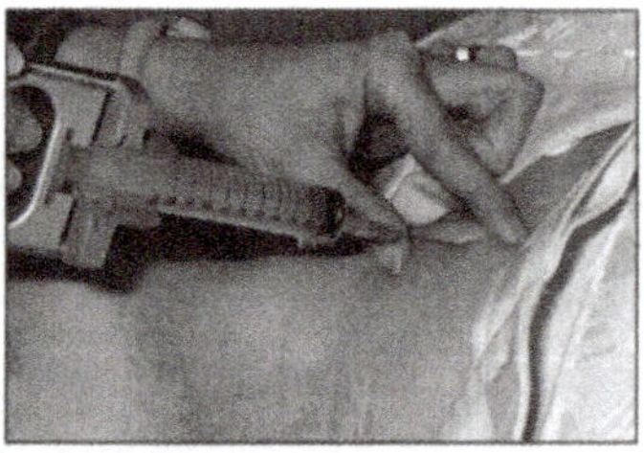

Fine-needle aspiration of a thyroid nodule, allowing rapid cytological examination of aspirated material. (*See* Color Plate.)

Ultrasonography: best for accurately measuring size of nodules in patients who are being followed; can differentiate cystic vs. solid, but either may be malignant.

Serum calcitonin measurement: should be reserved for patients with known medullary thyroid cancer (MTC) and for screening members of families with inherited forms of MTC.

Thyroglobulin evaluation: minimal value in diagnosis of thyroid nodules; extremely useful for monitoring treated patients.

Antithyroid antibody tests: of little value in evaluating thyroid nodules.

Special considerations

• Hyperthyroid patients probably should have isotope scanning. If the nodule is hot (autonomously functioning thyroid nodule), malignancy is unlikely.

• A rapidly enlarging thyroid (diffuse or nodular) should raise the possibility of lymphoma.

Complications

Local infiltration of trachea, esophagus, nerves.

Metastases of bone, liver, lung.

Differential diagnosis

Benign thyroid disease: diffuse goiter, single or multiple nodules.

Hashimoto's disease.

Other causes of lymphadenopathy.

Etiology [2]

• Causes include the following:

External irradiation of head and neck.

Genetic: medullary cancer in multiple endocrine neoplasia syndrome.

Epidemiology [2]

• Thyroid cancer accounts for <0.5% of new malignancies and <0.5% of cancer deaths.

• Goiter, including thyroid nodules, is present in up to 10% of the population.

• The female:male ratio is 3:1.

• The risk of malignancy is increased when nodules develop in children, young men, or in adults aged >60 years.

Tumor pathology

• Papillary thyroid cancer is the most frequently diagnosed malignant thyroid tumor (>80%).

• Follicular thyroid cancer is a relatively unusual malignancy (~5%–10% of all thyroid cancers).

• Medullary thyroid cancer occurs in 5%–10% of patients.

• Anaplastic thyroid cancer occurs rarely and has a very poor prognosis.

Treatment

Diet and lifestyle

• No evidence indicates that environmental factors affect the prognosis of established thyroid cancer.

• An iodine-replete diet and avoidance of external irradiation to head and neck reduce the risk of developing thyroid cancer.

Pharmacological treatment [1–4]

• After surgery, patients can be considered for radioiodine treatment.

• No consensus has been reached on ^{131}I ablation of the thyroid in patients with small solitary papillary lesions.

• Routine ablation of thyroid remnant is indicated in patients with follicular thyroid cancer.

• Radioiodine has a clear role in the management of residual disease or established metastases.

• All patients with differentiated thyroid cancer need suppressive thyroxine treatment after definitive treatment; thyroxine is necessary in all patients rendered hypothyroid after treatment.

Nonpharmacological treatment

• The extent of surgery (simple lobectomy, near-total thyroidectomy, total thyroidectomy) depends on pathology and surgical preference.

• Surgery is the primary mode of treatment for papillary, follicular, and medullary thyroid cancers.

• Surgical removal of involved lymph nodes is indicated.

Treatment aims

To cure with minimal morbidity.

To minimize morbidity of diagnostic and therapeutic interventions.

Prognosis [1,2]

• Prolonged survival is usual.

• Patients with localized papillary or follicular thyroid cancers have an excellent prognosis, (10–20-year recurrence rates of 5%–10% and death rates of 2%–5%).

• Adverse prognostic factors include older age, greater degree of invasiveness, distant metastases, and abnormal chromosomal number within tumor tissue.

Follow-up and management [1–3]

• After radioablation of the thyroid, total-body radioiodine scans can detect recurrent or metastatic disease and may be performed at 12-monthly intervals.

• Following thyroidectomy, radioactive ablation, and suppressive doses of thyroid hormone, patients with differentiated thyroid cancer should have undetectable thyroglobulin levels. Measurable thyroglobulin levels suggest residual or recurrent tumor, and rising levels frequently represent tumor growth.

Key references

1. Kaplan MM, ed: Thyroid carcinoma. *Endocrinol Metab Clin North Am* 1990, 19:741–760.
2. DeGroot LJ, *et al.*: Natural history, treatment, and course of papillary thyroid carcinoma. *J Clin Endocrinol Metabol* 1990, **71**:414–424.
3. Utiger RD: Follow-up of patients with thyroid carcinoma. *N Engl J Med* 1997, **337**:928.
4. Samaan NA, *et al.*: The results of different modalities of treatment of well differentiated thyroid carcinoma: a retrospective review of 1599 patients. *J Clin Endocrinol Metab* 1992, **75**:714–720.

Tobacco use disorder

Diagnosis

Symptoms and signs

Daily use of cigarettes for at least several weeks.

Continued smoking of cigarettes despite knowledge of health risk.

Potential for nicotine withdrawal symptoms within 24 hours of abrupt cessation of smoking: dysphoria, insomnia, irritability, anxiety, restlessness, difficulty concentrating, increased appetite.

Impairment in social or occupational functioning: may occur because of withdrawal symptoms.

Investigations

ASK [1]: must have system in place to identify all tobacco users at every visit.

• Consider tobacco status as part of vital signs (*e.g.*, tobacco use status stickers on patient charts) or inclusion of "tobacco use disorder" on active problem list.

Fagerstrom Test for Nicotine Dependence [2]: assists in establishing level of physical dependence (*see* table). Correlation exists between high level of dependence (score >6) and severity of withdrawal symptoms, difficulty with abstinence, and relapse.

Fagerstrom test for nicotine dependence

Questions		Score
1. How soon after you wake up do you smoke your first cigarette?		
	<5 minutes	3
	6-30 minutes	2
	31-60 minutes	1
	>61 minutes	0
2. Do you find it difficult to refrain from smoking in places where it is forbidden, *e.g.*, church, library, movie theater?		
	YES	1
	NO	0
3. Which cigarette would you hate most to give up?		
	The first in the morning	1
	Any other	0
4. How many cigarettes per day do you smoke?		
	>31	3
	21-30	2
	11-20	1
	<10	0
5. Do you smoke more frequently during the first hours after waking than during the rest of the day?		
	YES	1
	NO	0
6. Do you smoke if you are so ill that you are in bed most of the day?		
	YES	1
	NO	0

Complications

Cancer: causally linked to lung cancer; strong associations with cancer of oral cavity, larynx, esophagus, bladder, kidney, pancreas, stomach, and cervix.

Chronic obstructive pulmonary disease: principal risk factor for chronic obstructive pulmonary disease; current smokers have lower forced expiratory volume in 1 second (FEV_1) and accelerated decline in FEV_1 than nonsmokers.

Coronary heart disease: 2-4-fold increased incidence of coronary heart disease and sudden death.

Cerebral vascular disease: nearly 2-fold increased risk of stroke.

Pregnancy: pregnant smokers with increased incidence of low birth weight babies, spontaneous abortion, placenta previa, and placental abruption.

Differential diagnosis

Not applicable.

Etiology

• Nicotine is the agent in cigarettes responsible for addictive properties.

• Dependence occurs via increased expression of brain nicotine receptors, changes in brain glucose metabolism, and release of catecholamines.

• Positive reinforcement occurs with delivery of nicotine via cigarettes and negative reinforcement occurs via withdrawal symptoms during quit attempts.

Epidemiology

• There are 1 billion smokers worldwide.

• 25% of American adults are smokers.

• 3000 teenagers start to smoke each day; most of those who become lifelong smokers start before high school graduation.

• 440 000 deaths per year in the United States are from diseases directly linked to smoking.

Treatment

Diet and lifestyle

- The major treatment for tobacco addiction is lifestyle change: eliminate smoking.
- Patients should 1) gather support of family, friends, and coworkers; 2) remove cigarettes from daily environment; 3) anticipate difficult situations and plan a nonsmoking coping mechanism.

Pharmacological treatment

- Some form of pharmacological treatment should be offered to all patients smoking >10 cigarettes/day.
- Patient preferences, previous quit attempt experiences, cost should be weighed in choosing therapy.
- Bupropion hydrochloride is contraindicated in any patient with seizure disorder.
- No pharmacological agents well studied in pregnancy. FDA risk categories: buproprion hydrochloride, category B; nicotine gum, category C; nicotine transdermal spray and inhaler, category D.

Transdermal nicotine patch

Standard dosage 5–10 cigarettes/d, mid-range dose (10–14 mg/24 h); >10 cigarettes/d, use highest dose of brand (~21 mg/24 h). Use on hairless site, change site each day. Remove before bedtime if insomnia.

Advantages Minimal instruction, greater compliance.

Disadvantages Side effects of skin rash, pruritus, insomnia; 2–3 days to achieve maximum serum levels.

Nicotine gum

Standard dosage <20 Cigarettes/d, use 2-mg stick; >cigarettes/d, use 4-mg stick; ~1 stick gum/h; must chew and "park" between cheek and gum every 15 min; avoid acidic beverages.

Advantages May use as needed; maximum nicotine level in 20–30 min.

Disadvantages Jaw fatigue, hiccups, belching.

Nicotine nasal spray

Standard dosage 1 spray (1 mg) every 30–60 min as needed for craving. Tip head slightly back and spray mucosa; do not sniff.

Advantages Maximum nicotine levels within 5–10 min.

Disadvantages Nasal irritation common but subsides after first week.

Nicotine inhaler

Standard dosage 80 Puffs over 20–30 min, as needed or every hour. Puff frequently (3–4 puff/min); max dose, 16 cartridges/d.

Advantages Mimics tactile stimulation of smoking.

Disadvantages Cough; mouth and throat irritation.

Buproprion hydrochloride

Standard dosage 150 mg/d for 3 days, then 150 mg twice daily. Start 1 week before quit date; second daily dose before 6 pm.

Advantages Treats concomitant depression.

Disadvantages Dry mouth, insomnia.

Nonpharmacological treatment

The "4 As" of smoking cessation counseling [1]:

Step 1. ASK: identify all smokers at every visit.

Step 2. ADVISE: urge all smokers to quit with a personalized statement related to patients' health, social, or economic issues.

Step 3. ASSIST: once patient is willing to make quit attempt, set a quit date; advise total abstinence; provide nicotine replacement therapy and supplemental materials.

Step 4. ARRANGE: schedule follow-up in person or by phone, ideally during first week. Congratulate successes and review potential reasons for failures.

Physician or counselor can use the "four Rs" [1] to motivate smokers to quit:

1. RELEVANCE: to patient's age, health, family or social situation, and so on.
2. RISKS: review health risks to both individual and family members.
3. REWARDS: have patient list rewards of quitting most relevant to self.
4. REPETITION: review above as needed.

Treatment aims

To provide therapy for both the biological and psychological aspects of tobacco dependence via appropriate pharmacologic therapy and counseling.

To assist smokers in becoming lifelong nonsmokers.

Other treatments

- Single, small study shows efficacy of nortriptyline with cessation rates slightly lower than those seen with nicotine replacement therapies.
- Hypnosis and acupuncture have had disappointing results in studies. However, low-risk patients may benefit from expectation of success.
- Clonidine has not been proven effective for withdrawal symptoms or increasing cessation rates.

Prognosis

- Without physician assistance, spontaneous quit rates are 3%–4% per year.
- With pharmacologic therapy and advice, quit rates approach 20%–25%.
- Relapse is common and highest within first 3 months after quit date.

Follow-up and management

- Initial follow-up contact is best within first week of quit date.
- Second follow-up contact recommended within first month (office visit or phone call).
- Congratulate successes.
- Review reasons for failure including inadequate nicotine replacement therapy.
- Encourage patient to learn from lapse and set new quit date.
- Relapse prevention includes review of "four Rs" as well as exploration and treatment of any new problems such as weight gain or depression.

Key references

1. The Smoking Cessation Clinical Practice Guideline Panel and Staff: The Agency for Health Care Policy and Research Smoking Cessation Practice Guideline. *JAMA* 1996, **275**:1270–1280.
2. Heatherton TF, Kozlowski LT, Frecker RC, Fagerstrom KO: The Fagerstrom test for nicotine dependence: a revision of the Fagerstrom Tolerance Questionnaire. *Br J Addict* 1991, **86**:1119–1127.

Toxic shock syndrome

Diagnosis

Definition

• Definition criteria require fever, rash, hypotension, clinical or test evidence of involvement of three systems, negative results from blood (except in the case of *Staphylococcus aureus*), CSF, and throat culture, and exclusion of measles, leptospirosis, and Rocky Mountain spotted fever.

• Mild or near-miss toxic shock syndrome that does not reach the clinical severity of the full definition is almost certainly more prevalent and poorly recognized. It may resolve because of general antibiotic use or end of menstruation.

Symptoms

High temperature: often to 40°C.

Vomiting and diarrhea: usually watery.

Faintness: especially on standing.

Aching muscles.

Rash.

Signs

Hypotension: systolic blood pressure <90 mm Hg or postural drop of >15 mm Hg; below fifth percentile for age in children <16 years.

Rash: patchy erythema, likened to sunburn, especially on trunk, thighs, palms, soles.

Tender muscles.

Reddened mucosal surfaces: conjunctival, oral, vaginal.

"Red strawberry" tongue.

Confusion: without focal neurological signs.

Investigations

Hematology: thrombocytopenia usual.

Biochemistry: to assess renal function and liver inflammation; creatine kinase concentration often high.

Bacteriology: cultures of blood, stool, urine, vagina, cervix, wounds; *S. aureus* isolates to be forwarded for toxin production and phage typing.

Complications

Renal failure, coma, peripheral gangrene, acute respiratory distress: in varying combinations due to hypotension.

Marked desquamation: especially of palms, soles, and digits, 1–2 weeks after onset.

Hair loss, occasional nail loss: after 2–3 months.

Differential diagnosis

Infective gastroenteritis.
Septicemia, especially gram-negative.
Scarlatina.
Kawasaki syndrome.
Leptospirosis.

Etiology

• Toxins are produced by *S. aureus*, mostly toxic shock syndrome toxin-1, but also enterotoxin A, B, or C. (Streptococcal toxins can produce a similar illness.)

• They are absorbed into the body during menstruation (especially with tampons) or at sites of infection (wound or burn, sinusitis, empyema, postinfluenzal bronchopneumonia, conjunctivitis).

Epidemiology

• In the United States, where illness fulfilling diagnostic criteria has been notifiable, only 50% of the notifications have been menstrually related.

• Menstrual toxic shock syndrome occurs most often in high-absorbency tampon users aged 15–25 years.

• The incidence of menstrual toxic shock syndrome has declined since the early 1980s in the United States, probably as a result of increased health education, reduced tampon absorbency, and removal of acrylate fibers from tampons.

• Toxic shock syndrome has also been associated with the use of contraceptive diaphragms and sponges.

• Nonmenstrual toxic shock syndrome develops in both sexes and at any age.

• ~80% of adults have toxic shock syndrome toxin-1 antibodies, suggesting that mild or subclinical immunizing events happen frequently.

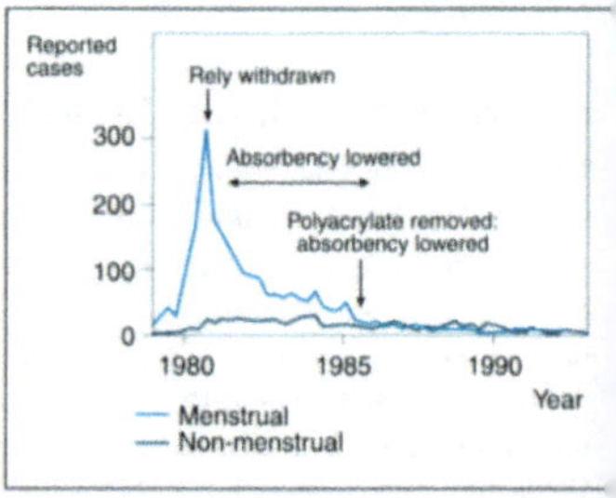

Incidence of toxic shock syndrome in the United States 1979–1993.

Treatment

Diet and lifestyle

• To reduce the likelihood of menstrually related toxic shock syndrome, women must wash hands before and after inserting tampons, use the lowest absorbency tampons that cope with their needs, change tampons regularly (at least every 4–6 hours), use pads overnight, remove and stop using tampons if acute symptoms develop during menstruation, and inform their physician of symptoms of current menstruation. Details of toxic shock syndrome are given on leaflets within tampon cartons, and a health warning is printed on the outside.

Pharmacological treatment

General resuscitation

• Severely ill patients need management and monitoring in intensive care units.

• Intravenous fluids should be used, initially with inotropic support.

• Other modalities, *e.g.*, dialysis, ventilation, should be used when indicated.

Antibiotics

• Although nafcillin does not improve case fatality rate, it reduces relapse rate.

Standard dosage	Nafcillin, 1 g i.v. every 4 hours × 10 days.
Contraindications	Hypersensitivity, porphyria.
Special points	Reduces recurrence rate in future menstrual periods. Third-generation cephalosporin can be used instead.
Main drug interactions	None.
Main side effects	Sensitivity reactions, jaundice.

Antitoxin

• The therapeutic usefulness of toxic shock syndrome toxin-1 antibodies (found in normal immunoglobulin or plasma) has not been determined.

Treatment aims

To limit hypoxic damage (prompt resuscitation).

To stop further toxin production and absorption (removal of tampons, drainage of pus, i.v. floxacillin).

To prevent subsequent relapses (floxacillin, advice on future tampon use).

Prognosis

• Mortality is 3%.

• Chronic morbidity varies and is related to acute ischemic damage to vital organs.

• The risk of recurrence during the next menstrual period is small, and symptoms tend to be milder.

• Recurrences may also follow nonmenstrual toxic shock syndrome, especially if anti-staphylococcal antibiotics are not used, and often follow subsequent skin or mucous membrane infection.

Follow-up and management

• Women should be advised against using tampons for the first few periods but can then reintroduce low-absorbency tampons, with frequent changing, and gradual return to advised standard routine thereafter.

• If further menstrual symptoms develop, tampon use must be stopped, and the patient should be given floxacillin and resuscitative measures in relation to symptoms.

General references

Kain KC, Schulzer M, Chow AW: Clinical spectrum of nonmenstrual toxic shock syndrome. *Clin Infect Dis* 1993, **16**:100–106.

Stevens DL: The toxic shock syndromes. *Infect Dis Clin North Am* 1996, **10**:727–746.

Diagnosis

Symptoms

Primary infection
Fever, neurological symptoms.

Secondary infection
Reactivation of tachyzoites: in cysts in any tissue, particularly brain, also eye, heart, and lung: symptoms are due to focal brain abscess, possibly with diffuse meningoencephalitis.

Focal symptoms
• Occur in 70% of patients.

• May be subacute in onset, evolving to persistent focal neurological deficits, including the following:

Hemiparesis, hemisensory loss, ataxia, visual field deficits, cranial nerve palsies, aphasia; cognitive changes may occur, depending on the intracranial location.

Focal and secondarily generalized seizures: in 38%.

Nonfocal symptoms
• These may predominate in up to 40% of patients; headache, fever.

Fever and malaise (variable), disorientation, psychosis, neck stiffness (in 5%), increasing confusion and coma.

Signs
• Focal signs, *e.g.*, cerebellar ataxia and hemiplegia may occur; they indicate multiple or focal CNS lesions.

• Signs of infection (fever, meningism) may be absent.

Investigations
Toxoplasma serology: IgG serology will be present in >95% of cases, representing reactivation of disease.

CT of brain with contrast: urgent; in 70%–80% of patients, shows single or multiple ring-enhancing lesions with edema (mainly in basal ganglia and bilaterally at corticomedullary junction).

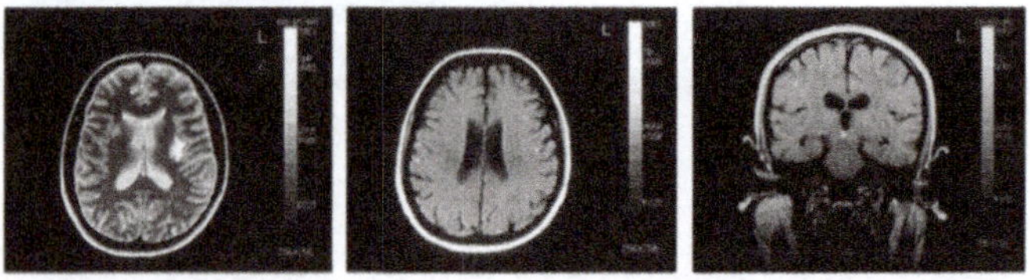

MRI scans of a patient with cerebral toxoplasmosis. Transverse section before (*left*) and after contrast (*middle*) shows multiple lesions; coronal section (*right*) shows several cortical lesions and one brain stem lesion.

MRI of brain: as alternative to CT scanning or for patients with single lesion on CT or lesions in cerebellum that do not appear on CT; demonstration of single lesion on MR strongly suggests cause other than toxoplasmosis.

Lumbar puncture: most often contraindicated because of CNS mass.

Brain biopsy: indicated for single lesions on MRI or those patients who have negative serology to *Toxoplasma gondii*.

Complications
Seizures or hydrocephalus.

Panhypopituitarism, inappropriate antidiuretic hormone secretion, encephalopathy.

Differential diagnosis

Focal neurological dysfunction
Primary CNS lymphoma, metastatic non-Hodgkin's lymphoma, progressive multifocal leukodystrophy (common).
Cytomegalovirus, herpes simplex virus, herpes zoster virus, cryptococcal meningitis, abcesses (*Tuberculosis, Nocardia, Candida* spp.), cerebrovascular disease (rare).
Pyogenic abscesses.

Diffuse encephalitis
AIDS encephalitis, AIDS dementia syndrome, cytomegalovirus or herpes simplex encephalitis.

Etiology
• Toxoplasmosis is caused by infection with *Toxoplasma gondii*; spread is by the feco-oral route.

• Silent chronic infection is characterized by tachyzoites in tissue cysts throughout the body.

• Acute reactivation involves cyst rupture, causing an encephalitis and a focal necrotizing vasculitic process.

Epidemiology
• Toxoplasmosis is ubiquitous in human populations.

• The incidence reflects the background seroprevalence in a given group: 10%–40% of adults in the United States are seropositive (90% in France).

• Up to 30% of HIV-infected people who are seropositive for *T. gondii* develop cerebral toxoplasmosis, usually with CD4 counts <100 × 10^6/L.

• Overall, toxoplasma accounts for 40% of known CNS infection and 33% of intracerebral lesions in AIDS patients.

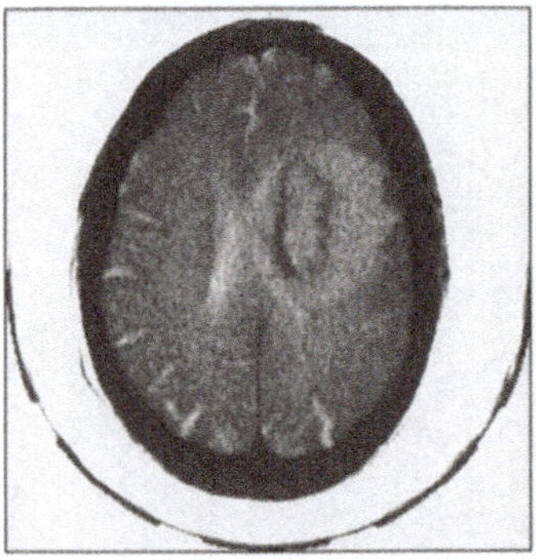

Contrast-enhanced CT scan of the same patient shows a single lesion in the left temporal lobe.

Toxoplasmosis in AIDS

Treatment

Diet and lifestyle

• No special precautions are necessary.

Pharmacological treatment

• Treatment is begun empirically for a presumptive diagnosis of toxoplasma encephalitis based on clinical presentation and CT or MRI evidence (usually) of multifocal rung-enhancing lesions in a person who has positive serology to *T. gondii*. A brain biopsy is not indicated before initiation of therapy in this patient group.

• The main regimen is pyrimethamine and folinic acid with sulfadiazine. Clindamycin or atovaquone is used in sulfa-intolerant patients.

Standard dosage	Pyrimethamine, 75 mg to load (or 100–200 mg), then 50 mg orally daily. Folinic acid, 15 mg daily to prevent myelosuppression. Sulfadiazine, 4–6 g daily in divided doses. Clindamycin, 2400 mg daily in divided doses, if sulfa-intolerant. Atovaquone, 750 mg 4 times daily if cannot tolerate clindamycin.
Contraindications	*Pyrimethamine:* hepatic or renal impairment. *Sulfadiazine:* pregnancy, renal or hepatic failure, jaundice, porphyria. *Clindamycin:* diarrheal states.
Special points	Careful monitoring of neurological condition and repeat CT or MRI to check for improvement within 3 weeks. With clinical and radiographic improvement, treatment is normally continued for 4–6 weeks; if no improvement occurs in the first 14–21 days, stereotactic brain biopsy should be performed. *Pyrimethamine, sulfadiazine:* disrupt folic acid metabolism; blood count must be monitored weekly. *Clindamycin:* liver function and blood count must be monitored.
Main drug interactions	*Pyrimethamine:* increased antifolate effect with phenytoin and trimethoprim. *Sulfadiazine:* warfarin, phenytoin, pyrimethamine, cyclosporine. *Clindamycin:* neostigmine, tubocurarine.
Main side effects	*Pyrimethamine:* nausea, vomiting, myelosuppression (folate). *Folinic acid:* pyrexia. *Sulfadiazine:* nausea, vomiting, rashes, blood dyscrasias (treatment must be stopped immediately), nephrotoxicity, headache, hepatitis (rare); adverse reaction rate 40%. *Clindamycin:* nausea, vomiting, rash, diarrhea (rare but serious pseudomembranous colitis; treatment must be stopped immediately). *Atovaquone:* diarrhea, rash.

• In patients with significant mass effect or decreased consciousness level, steroids are indicated, *e.g.*, high-dose dexamethasone, 8 mg orally or i.v. 4 times daily.

• Steroids may complicate the interpretation of clinical improvement and CT or MRI resolution during empirical antitoxoplasma treatment.

• They should be reduced and withdrawn as soon as is reasonable and repeat scans performed to check for exacerbation.

Treatment aims

To cure acute illness.

To prevent relapse.

Prognosis

• 90% of patients, including those in coma, respond to antitoxoplasma chemotherapy in 14–21 days, often sooner, but one-third have residual neurological defect.

Follow-up and management

• Maintenance treatment must be lifelong because of the presence of cysts, against which chemotherapy is ineffective.

• Pyrimethamine, 25–50 mg daily, sulfadiazine, 2–4 g daily (or clindamycin), and folinic acid, 10 mg on alternate days, must be continued indefinitely.

General references

Minkoff H, Remington JS, Holman S, *et al.*: Vertical transmission of toxoplasma by human immunodeficiency virus–infected women. *Am J Obstet Gynecol* 1997, **176**:555–559.

Porter SB, Sande MA: Toxoplasmosis of the central nervous system in the acquired immune deficiency syndrome. *N Engl J Med* 1992, **327**:1643–1647.

Wong S, Israelski D, Remington J: AIDS-associated toxoplasmosis. In *The Medical Management of AIDS*. Edited by Sande M, Volberding P. Philadelphia: WB Saunders; 1995.

Transfusion medicine

Indications

Erythrocytes

• A low hemoglobin level per se is not an indication for transfusion. Factors such as the patient's condition, the rate of fall of hemoglobin, and the cause of anemia must be considered to determine the correct treatment.

Whole blood

For acute massive blood loss.

For exchange transfusion of infants to avoid multiple donors.

Erythrocyte concentrates

For chronic blood loss or anemia.

For blood loss <1 blood volume in elective surgery (in additive solution).

Filtered blood

To prevent or delay nonhemolytic febrile transfusion reactions in patients who are erythrocyte dependent.

For patients with newly diagnosed aplastic anemia who are potential bone-marrow transplant recipients.

When cytomegalovirus-antibody–negative blood is indicated but not readily available.

For intrauterine transfusion.

Washed cells

For patients with proven hypersensitivity reactions to plasma proteins.

For neonates who have necrotizing enterocolitis.

Cryopreserved erythrocytes

For patients needing blood of rare phenotypes or blood compatible with multiple erythrocyte alloantibodies.

For patients with anti-IgA in the absence of IgA-negative blood.

Irradiated erythrocytes

For recipients at risk of graft-versus-host disease: in utero transfusion, after bone-marrow transplantation.

For rare cases of transfusions from relatives.

Platelets [1]

To prevent or treat bleeding in patients with thrombocytopenia and rarely to treat bleeding in patients with platelet function defects: the cause of thrombocytopenia and significance of hemorrhage influence the use of platelet transfusions.

For acute bone-marrow failure (*e.g.*, due to aplasia, chemotherapy): if platelet count $10–50 \times 10^9$/L, serious spontaneous bleeding is unlikely, although minor bleeding (purpura, epistaxis) may occur; prophylactic platelet transfusions to maintain count $>10 \times 10^9$/L reduces risk of hemorrhage as effectively as keeping count higher and reduces morbidity but not mortality; patients with fever, infection, coagulopathy, or rapid fall in platelet count should be transfused to maintain platelets $>20 \times 10^9$/L.

For acute disseminated intravascular coagulation: when thrombocytopenia is associated with bleeding (not indicated in chronic disseminated intravascular coagulation without bleeding).

For massive blood loss: to maintain platelets $>50 \times 10^9$/L.

Prophylaxis for surgery: to maintain platelets $>50 \times 10^9$/L or $>100 \times 10^9$/L for surgery in a critical site, *e.g.*, brain or eye (not routinely with cardiopulmonary bypass).

For autoimmune thrombocytopenia: platelet transfusions rarely used.

Fresh frozen plasma [2]

To replace single coagulation factor deficiencies when a specific or combined factor concentrate is unavailable.

For immediate reversal of warfarin effect.

For acute disseminated intravascular coagulation.

For thrombotic thrombocytopenic purpura.

For bleeding or disturbed coagulation associated with massive transfusion, liver disease, or cardiopulmonary bypass surgery.

Autologous transfusion [3,4]

Advantages

• The possibilities of alloimmunization, immunosuppression, and transfusion-transmitted infection are avoided.

Disadvantages

• Not all patients are eligible.

• Predeposited blood may be unused, *e.g.*, if surgery is cancelled, or may be insufficient to meet the patient's needs.

• Collecting predeposited autologous blood is more expensive than using standard units.

Options

Autologous predeposit: up to 5 U of blood collected and stored during the weeks before surgery.

Acute normovolemic hemodilution: blood drawn from patient under anesthetic and replaced by crystalloid so that blood lost during surgery has a lower hematocrit; when blood loss starts or at end of procedure, patient's whole blood is returned.

Erythrocyte salvage: blood lost at operating site recovered and processed for transfusion.

Directed blood donations

• Blood donations from relatives or friends should be discouraged unless needed on medical grounds.

• Evidence suggests that "directed" donations are generally less safe than blood supplied by the American Red Cross.

Treatment

Erythrocytes

Whole blood: packed cell volume (PCV) 0.35–0.45, 1 U = 510 mL ± 10%; if blood loss and replacement exceed twice the blood volume, thrombocytopenia and abnormalities of hemostasis may develop.

Fresh blood (<24 hours): blood that has not been microbiologically tested must not be transfused.

Erythrocyte concentrates: PCV 0.55–0.75, 1 U = 220–340 mL.

Erythrocyte concentrates in additive solution: PCV 0.5–0.7, 1 U = 280–420 mL; not to be used for exchange or large-volume transfusion in neonates.

Filtered blood (leukodepleted <5×10^6 leukocytes/U): PCV and quantity variable; rigorous validation of blood processing and component preparation needed [5].

Washed cells (residual protein <0.5 g/U): must be used within 24 hours of preparation.

Cryopreserved erythrocytes (thawed and washed): volume usually <200 mL; must be used within 24 hours of preparation.

Irradiated erythrocytes (minimum dose, 25 Gy): must be used within 1 day if for intrauterine transfusion because of increased potassium.

Platelets [6]

Administration

- Platelets for transfusion should preferably be of the recipient ABO and RhD group.
- If RhD-positive platelets are transfused to a RhD-negative woman potentially capable of childbearing, 250 IU anti-D immunoglobulin should be given subcutaneously with each dose of platelets.

Dose and response

- A standard dose of 300×10^9 may be issued as pooled or single platelet concentrates derived from individual donations or as a single apheresis donation, respectively, to raise the platelet count (adult) by ~40×10^9/L.
- Patient factors, including sepsis, certain drugs, disseminated intravascular coagulation, splenomegaly, uremia, and platelet antibodies, can reduce the expected platelet increment.
- Patients who repeatedly under go transfusion with platelets may develop immunological refractoriness because of HLA alloimmunization and should receive platelets from HLA-matched donors.
- In some cases, platelet-specific alloantibodies develop, requiring type-specific platelet transfusions.

Fresh frozen plasma [2]

Administration

- Fresh frozen plasma (FFP) should be ABO and RhD compatible, although compatibility testing is not required.
- Group O FFP should be transfused only to group O recipients.
- If an RhD-negative woman potentially capable of childbearing has transfusion with RhD-positive FFP, 50 IU anti-D immunoglobulin should be given per unit of FFP transfused.

Dose

- A generally accepted starting dose is 12–15 mL/kg.
- The clinical and laboratory responses should be monitored to assess response and plan further management.

Management of adverse effects of transfusion [3]

Hemolytic transfusion reactions (ABO incompatibility most severe)
Safe documentation and checking of systems for compatibility testing and blood administration; treatment for acute renal failure and disseminated intravascular coagulation may be needed.

Febrile nonhemolytic transfusion reactions
Treatment by antipyretics and use of leuko-depleted cellular components if recurrent.

Allergic reactions to foreign proteins
Cessation of infusion; treatment of urticarial reactions by diphenhydramine; emergency treatment needed if anaphylaxis has developed; IgA-deficient patients who have anti-IgA should receive components from IgA-deficient donors.

Alloimmunization
Provision of antigen-negative units to transfusion-dependent patients.

Iron overload
Consideration of iron-chelation treatment in transfusion-dependent patients.

Transfusion-transmitted infection
Use of blood components from volunteer unpaid donors who have been screened by sensitive techniques for relevant viral markers; consideration of hepatitis A and B vaccination of transfusion-dependent patients.

Key references

1. Murphy MF, *et al.*: Guidelines for platelet transfusion. *Transfusion Med* 1992, **2**:311–318.
2. Contreras M, *et al.*: Guidelines for the use of fresh frozen plasma. *Transfusion Med* 1992, **2**:57–63.
3. Contreras M: *ABC of Transfusion*, edn 2. London: British Medical Association; 1992.
4. Au Buchon JP: Blood transfusion options: improving outcomes and reducing costs. *Arch Pathol Lab Med* 1997, **121**:40–47.
5. Lumadue J, Ness PM: Current approaches to red blood cell transfusion. *Semin Hematol* 1996, **33**:277–289.
6. Mollision PL, Engelfriet CP, Contreras M: *Blood Transfusion in Clinical Medicine*, edn 9. Oxford: Blackwell Scientific Publications; 1993.

General references

Goodnough LT, Brecher ME, Kanter MH, AuBuchon JP: Transfusion medicine. Part 1. *N Engl J Med* 1999, 438–447.

Goodnough LT, Brecher ME, Kanter MH, AuBuchon JP: Transfusion medicine. Part 2. *N Engl J Med* 1999, 525–533.

Transient ischemic attacks

Diagnosis

Definition

• A transient ischemic attack is abrupt loss of focal cerebral or monocular function with symptoms lasting <24 hours, which, after adequate investigations, is presumed to be due to embolic or thrombotic vascular disease.

Symptoms

• Symptoms such as syncope, confusion, convulsions, incontinence, and isolated dizziness are not acceptable for transient ischemic attacks.

Carotid territory

• This is the site of 80% of transient ischemic attacks.

Unilateral paresis: weakness, heaviness, or clumsiness.

Unilateral sensory loss.

Aphasia.

Transient monocular visual loss: amaurosis fugax.

Vertebrobasilar territory

• This is the site of 20% of transient ischemic attacks.

Bilateral or alternating weakness or sensory symptoms.

Vertigo, diplopia, dysphagia, ataxia: patients must have two or more simultaneously.

Sudden bilateral blindness: in patients aged >40 years.

Uncertain arterial distribution

Hemianopia alone.

Dysarthria alone.

Investigations [1]

• Investigations are of little help in the recognition of transient ischemic attacks; they are directed at determining the cause of the attack.

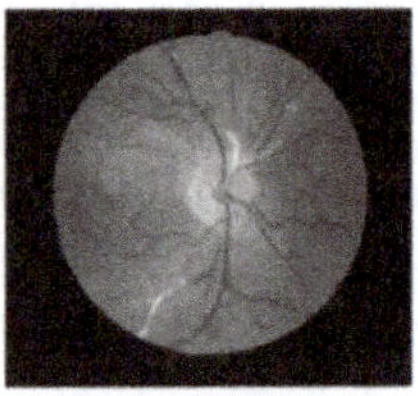

Cholesterol emboli seen on fundoscopy in a patient with amaurosis fugax. (*See* Color Plate.)

Serological

Prothrombin time/partial thromboplastin time, fibrinogen, platelet count, renal and hepatic function tests, sedimentation rates, cholesterol profile.

• In patients aged ≤50 years, add protein S & C, antithrombin III, anticardiolipin and antiphospholipid antibodies, homocystine levels, lactate/pyruvate, adrenoleukodystrophy and metachromatic leukodystrophy screen, where indicated.

Structural and etiological

CT or MRI of brain (MRI required for posterior circulation event).

MR angiography: for large- and medium-vessel disease.

Carotid ultrasonography.

ECG.

Transesophageal echocardiogram.

Angiography: for all patients with hemorrhage and needed for many without clear stroke etiology; often necessary to exclude vasculitis or dissection in young adults.

Temporal artery biopsy: if indicated.

Lumbar puncture: for hemorrhage or suspected vasculitis.

Complications

None, by definition.

Differential diagnosis

Migraine with aura.

Partial epileptic seizures.

Structural intracranial lesions: tumor, vascular malformation, chronic subdural hematoma, giant aneurysm.

Multiple sclerosis: in patients aged <40 years.

Labyrinthine disorders: *e.g.*, Ménière's disease, benign positional vertigo.

Peripheral nerve or root or spinal lesion.

Metabolic disorders: *e.g.*, hypoglycemia.

Etiology

Causes

Embolism complicating atherosclerosis of arteries to brain (50% of attacks).

Intracranial small-vessel disease (lipohyalinosis) (20%).

Embolism from the heart (20%).

Inflammatory arterial disease (*e.g.*, giant-cell arteritis).

Arterial dissections.

Hematological disorders (*e.g.*, polycythemia).

Risk factors

• Factors that increase the risk of degenerative arterial disease in general include the following:

Age, hypertension, diabetes mellitus, cigarette smoking, plasma cholesterol, plasma fibrinogen.

• Markers for arterial disease include the following:

Ischemic heart disease, peripheral vascular disease, cervical arterial bruit, left ventricular hypertrophy.

• Evidence of cardiac embolic source includes the following:

Atrial fibrillation, recent myocardial infarction, valvular disease, prosthetic heart valves.

Epidemiology [2]

• 15% of patients suffering their first stroke have had preceding transient ischemic attacks; only half of these attacks will have been seen or recognized by a doctor.

• The annual incidence of patients with attacks who present for further investigation and treatment is about 0.5 in 1000.

• The incidence increases with age.

• More men are affected than women.

Treatment

Diet and lifestyle

• Treating raised blood pressure reduces the risk of stroke by 50%, even after only a few years; the effect on coronary events is less impressive. Targets should be a systolic and diastolic pressure of below about 180 mm Hg and 100 mm Hg, respectively.

• The effect of stopping smoking is most marked on reducing cardiac events, and all patients should be encouraged vigorously to stop.

• Reducing serum cholesterol leads to a reduced risk of cardiac events, but no reliable data for stroke are available. A diet low in saturated fats should be advised.

• Physical exercise should be encouraged and probably helps by facilitating weight, cholesterol, and blood pressure control.

Pharmacological treatment

Antiplatelet drugs

• Antiplatelet drugs have shown clear evidence of benefit in a meta-analysis of all trials: the risk of nonfatal myocardial infarction and stroke is reduced by one-third; the risk of all fatal vascular events is reduced by one-sixth.

• Aspirin is the most widely used agent.

Standard dosage	Aspirin, 75–325 mg.
Contraindications	Active peptic ulceration.
Main drug interactions	Increased risk of bleeding with warfarin.
Main side effects	Gastrointestinal hemorrhage.

• Ticlopidine or clopidogrel is useful in patients with small-vessel or posterior circulation disease, and often is used if aspirin fails.

Standard dosage	Ticlopidine, 250 mg orally twice daily; clopidogrel, 75 mg daily.
Contraindications	Bone-marrow disease.
Special points	Requires regular complete blood count analysis to exclude neutropenia.
Main side effects	Nausea/gastrointestinal upset, neutropenia.

Anticoagulants

• Anticoagulants are indicated when a definite cardiac source of emboli has been identified (*e.g.*, mitral valve disease with atrial fibrillation, prosthetic heart valve, recent myocardial infarction, dilated cardiomyopathy).

• In nonrheumatic atrial fibrillation, warfarin is superior to aspirin.

• Short-term warfarin may be used empirically for symptomatic treatment of frequent attacks resistant to aspirin. Warfarin may also be useful for intracranial stenosis and posterior circulation disease.

• Possible benefits of warfarin must always be weighed against definite side effects in individual patients.

Standard dosage	Warfarin sufficient to maintain INR at 2–4.
Contraindications	Bleeding diathesis, active peptic ulceration.
Special points	Requires regular blood monitoring.
Main drug interactions	Alcohol, NSAIDs, antiepileptics, antidepressants.
Main side effects	Hemorrhage.

Treatment aims

To prevent stroke or other serious vascular events (secondary prevention).

Other treatments

Carotid endarterectomy: for symptomatic carotid stenoses >70% only [3].

Prognosis

• The risk of stroke in the first year after a transient ischemic attack is 12%.

• Thereafter, the risk is 7% each year (seven times the risk in the normal population).

• The greatest risk occurs in the first month after the attack.

• Cardiac death occurs more often than stroke death after an attack.

• The combined risk of all serious vascular events (stroke, myocardial infarction, other vascular death) is ~9% annually.

Follow-up and management

• Risk factors (*e.g.*, hypertension) must be adequately controlled and antiplatelet therapy maintained.

Key references

1. Hankey GJ, Warlow CP: *Transient Ischaemic Attacks of the Brain and Eye*. London: WB Saunders; 1994. [Major Problems in Neurology 27.]

2. Dennis M, *et al.*: The prognosis of transient ischemic attacks in the Oxfordshire community stroke project. *Stroke* 1990, **21**:848–853.

3. European Carotid Surgery Trialist's Collaborative Group: MRC European Carotid Surgery Trial: interim results for symptomatic patients with severe (70–99%) or with mild (0–29%) carotid stenosis. *Lancet* 1991, **337**:1235–1243.

Diagnosis

Definition

• Tremor is an involuntary, rhythmic, smooth, sinusoidal oscillation of a body part. Faster tremors (6–12 Hz) are usually of fine amplitude; slower tremors (2–5 Hz) are coarse and of large amplitude. Tremors may be described according to the following:
Cause or underlying diagnosis.
Clinical circumstances of occurrence: rest (limb supported), postural (limb outstretched), kinetic (during voluntary movement), task-specific action (*e.g.*, during writing), intention (in terminal stages of movement).
Affected body part: *e.g.*, head, voice, hand, leg.
Frequency (cycles/s or Hz, considerable overlap).

Symptoms

Rhythmic shaking of hands, legs, trunk, or head: often resulting in clumsiness and loss of manual dexterity.
Slow voluntary movement (with rest tremor): suggesting Parkinson's disease.
Unsteadiness when standing (shaking legs), relieved by walking or sitting: suggesting primary orthostatic tremor.

Signs [1]

Parkinsonian
Rest ("pill-rolling"), possibly with postural tremor: 4–5 and 5–6 Hz, respectively; arms affected more than legs, which are affected more than jaws or lips.

Midbrain (rubral)
Rest, postural, intention tremor: 2–5 Hz; particularly affecting proximal arms.

Cerebellar
Postural, intention, kinetic tremor: 3–6 Hz; arms and trunk more than legs; titubation (head and truncal tremor).

Essential
Postural, kinetic tremor: 5–8 Hz; arms more than head more than legs; isolated.

Neuropathic
Postural, kinetic tremor: 4–6 Hz; arms more than legs.

Dystonic
Postural, kinetic tremor: 2–6 Hz; arms more than legs; exacerbated in certain postures.

Primary orthostatic
Tremor of legs and trunk when standing: 14–16 Hz.

Physiological
Postural tremor: 8–12 Hz; affecting arms; normal finding.

Exaggerated physiological
Postural tremor: 8–12 Hz; affecting arms; larger amplitude than physiological tremor.

Focal
Postural tremor: 4–8 Hz; affecting head, face, jaw, chin, tongue, voice, trunk (alone).

Task-specific action
Kinetic tremor during specific tasks: ~6 Hz; affecting arms, lips, and head.

Investigations

• Investigations are needed to exclude symptomatic tremor or identify the cause.
Serum ceruloplasmin, thyroid function, blood glucose measurement: for Wilson's disease, thyrotoxicosis, and hypoglycemia, respectively.
Nerve conduction studies, electromyography, serum immunoglobulin measurement: in patients with suspected neuropathy.
Brain imaging: if clinical suspicion of structural lesion, *e.g.*, hemitremor, focal neurological signs, midbrain or cerebellar tremor.

Complications

Clumsiness, loss of manual dexterity, difficulty writing, embarrassment.

Differential diagnosis

Repetitive myoclonus: brisk, abrupt jerks.
Chorea: flowing random variable movements.
Dystonia: intermittent fixed postures.

Etiology [2,3]

Hereditary
Essential tremor (50% of cases inherited autosomal-dominant).

Idiopathic
Physiological tremor.
Primary orthostatic tremor.
Task-specific action tremors.

Symptomatic
Parkinson's disease.
Akinetic rigid syndromes.
Dystonic tremor.
Thyrotoxicosis.
Cerebellar disease: multiple sclerosis, degenerative ataxias.
Midbrain lesions: multiple sclerosis, vascular.
Wilson's disease.
Peripheral neuropathy (especially demyelinating).
Exaggerated physiological tremor.
Drug-induced tremor.
Toxins.

Epidemiology

• Essential tremor occurs in 300 in 100 000 population.
• Parkinson's disease occurs in 200 in 100 000 population (increasing with age).

Diagnostic difficulties [4]

Drug-induced tremor
Beta-2 agonists, caffeine, theophylline, tricyclic antidepressants, 5-HT reuptake inhibitors, lithium, neuroleptics, amphetamines, valproate, steroids, thyroxine.

Toxin-induced tremor
MPTP (1-methyl-4-phenyl-1,2,3,6-tetrahydropyridine), mercury.

Drug-withdrawal tremor
Alcohol, barbiturates, benzodiazepines, opiates.

Exaggerated physiological tremor
Drugs (as above), drug withdrawal (as above), metabolic disease: thyrotoxicosis, hypoglycemia, pheochromocytoma, anxiety, fatigue.

Treatment

Diet and lifestyle

• Caffeine and fatigue may exacerbate tremor.

• Alcohol may help essential tremor, but addiction is a possibility.

• Aids for stability when standing (*e.g.*, shooting stick) help orthostatic tremor.

Pharmacological treatment

For essential tremor

Standard dosage	Propranolol, 60–180 mg long-acting preparation daily. Primidone, up to 50 mg 2 times daily.
Contraindications	*Propranolol:* obstructive airways disease, heart failure.
Main drug interactions	None.
Main side effects	*Propranolol:* hypotension, bradycardia, bronchospasm. *Primidone:* fatigue.

• Sometimes amantadine or anticholinergics are useful.

For parkinsonian tremor

L-Dopa, anticholinergics, amantadine, dopamine agonists in doses as for Parkinson's disease (*see* Parkinson's disease *for details*).

Treatment aims

To identify and remove causes of exaggerated physiological tremor.

To identify and treat causes of symptomatic tremor.

Other treatments

Thalamotomy or thalamic stimulation: in severe tremors refractory to drugs.

Prognosis

• The prognosis depends on the cause of the tremor.

Follow-up and management

• Follow-up depends on the cause of the tremor.

Key references

1. Weiner WJ, Land AE: *Movement Disorders*. New York: Futura Publishing Company; 1989:221–256.
2. Cleeves L, Findley LJ, Marsden CD: Odd tremors. In *Movement Disorders*, edn 3. Edited by Marsden CD, Fahn S. Oxford: Butterworth–Heinemann; 1994:434–498.
3. Elble RJ: Central mechanisms of tremor. *J Clin Neurophysiol* 1996, **13**:133–144.
4. Findley LJ: Tremors: differential diagnosis and pharmacology. In *Parkinson's Disease and Movement Disorders*. Edited by Jankovic J, Tolosa E. Baltimore: Williams & Wilkins; 1993:293–313.

Tuberculosis, extrapulmonary

Diagnosis

Symptoms

• Disease may be focal, disseminated, or multifocal. Proportion by site: lymphatic ~35%; genitourinary, bone, joint ~15% each; disseminated, abdominal, cerebral <10% each; cutaneous, other sites <5% each.
• Systemic symptoms usually imply more widespread disease; focal disease may be acute or insidious (more usual).

Fever, malaise, fatigue, weight loss, night sweats.
Pain: in bone or joint, abdomen, gastrointestinal tract, or meninges.
Tissue swelling: in lymph node, joint, or peritoneum.
Frequency, dysuria, loin pain: in renal disease.
Cough, fever: in disseminated disease.
Headache, vomiting, confusion: in CNS disease.

Signs

Fever, wasting: due to tuberculous toxicity.
Erythema nodosum: a hypersensitivity reaction.
Choroidal tubercles: in miliary disease.
Nontender, fluctuant lymph node: perhaps discharging (scrofula).
Hematuria.
Bone or joint deformity, cold abscess, spinal-cord signs.
Chest signs, pleural effusion, hepatosplenomegaly: in dissemination.
Ascites, abdominal distension, bowel obstruction.
Nuchal rigidity, obtundation, focal signs: indicating meningitis.

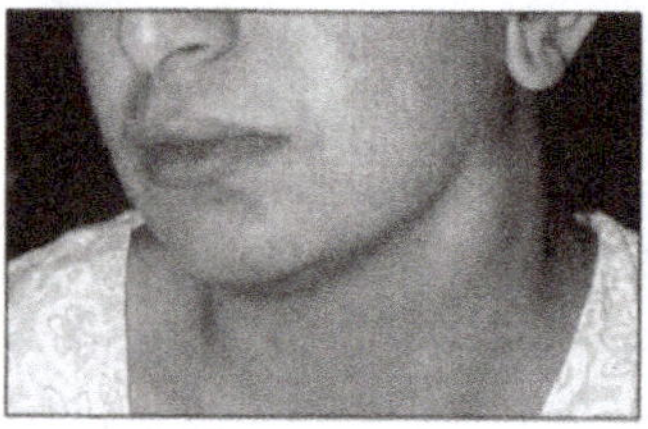

Asian woman with multiple tuberculous lymph nodes. (*See* Color Plate.)

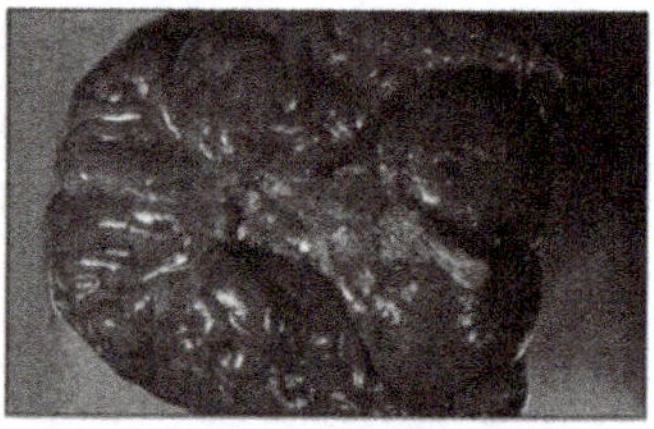

Massive cerebral edema typical of advanced tuberculous meningitis. (*See* Color Plate.)

Investigations

Chest radiography.
Blood analysis.
Tuberculin skin test.
Sputum or urine culture.
Biopsy of bone marrow, liver, lymph node, joint, or bowel.

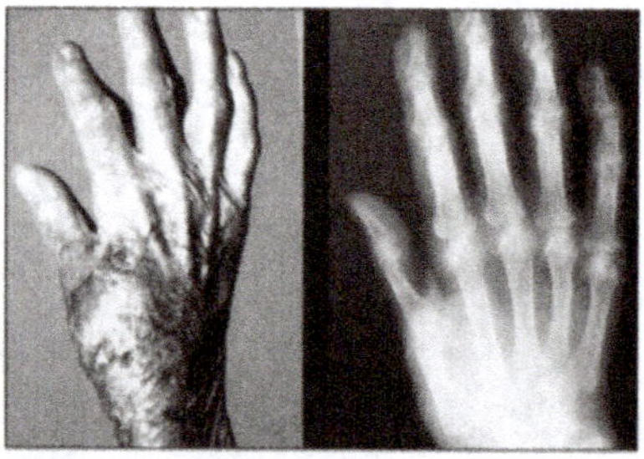

Extrapulmonary tuberculosis. (*See* Color Plate.)

Complications

Cryptic disseminated tuberculosis, acute miliary disease, or meningitis.
Focal damage.
Hydrocephalus, spinal block, cerebral vasculitis.
Acute respiratory distress syndrome.
Ureteric obstruction or renal destruction by caseation.
Spinal-cord involvement.
Bone or joint deformity.
Gastrointestinal stenosis, adhesions, obstruction.
Cutaneous cold abcesses.

Differential diagnosis

Lymphoma, toxoplasmosis, atypical mycobacterioses.
Infection: *e.g.*, endocarditis, brucellosis, pneumocystosis.
Noninfective disease: *e.g.*, lymphoma, collagenoses.
Chronic pyelonephritis.
Other arthritides, osteomyelitis, neoplasm.
Crohn's disease, starch or sarcoid peritonitis.
Viral or fungal infections or CNS neoplasm.

Etiology

• Tuberculosis is caused by infection by *Mycobacterium tuberculosis* (now rarely *M. bovis*).
• Extrapulmonary disease may be due to lymphohematogenous, contiguous, or "downstream" mucosal spread.
• Predisposing factors include genetics and race (rate in ethnic groups from Indian subcontinent 50 times European rate), immunocompromise (due to disease, drugs, alcohol), extremes of age, and HIV infection.

Epidemiology

• Extrapulmonary tuberculosis develops in ~25% of patients; pulmonary infection may coexist.
• The annual notification rate is 3–10 cases/100 000 in the United States.

Tuberculosis and HIV infection

• ~3.5 million people worldwide are co-infected.
• The infections may be mutually synergistic.
• Dissemination is much more probable.
• Many patients have extrapulmonary disease.
• Patients are more likely to be anergic on skin testing.
• Response to standard triple or quadruple treatment is usually good.

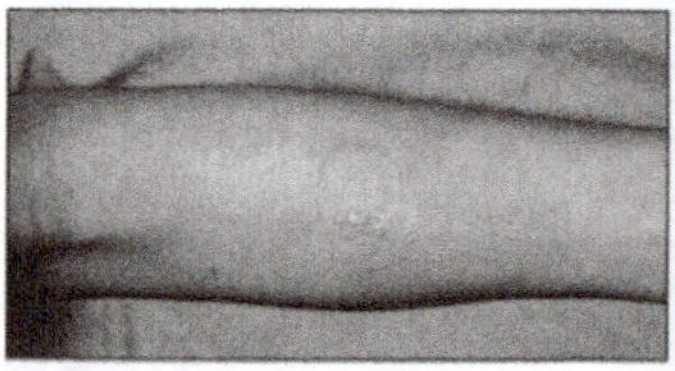

Strongly positive reaction to Mantoux test. (*See* Color Plate.)

Treatment

Diet and lifestyle

- Weight loss and malnutrition must be reversed.
- Alcohol or drug addiction should be treated.
- Social circumstances, *e.g.*, homelessness, should be improved.

Pharmacological treatment

- The advice of a tuberculosis specialist must be sought and the case reported to state authorities.
- In a seriously ill patient, empirical treatment is justified even when the diagnosis is unconfirmed; treatment is invariably instituted before sensitivities are available.
- Efforts should be made to establish diagnosis.
- Patients must comply with the drug regimen for the duration of treatment.

Standard chemotherapy

Standard dosage
Initial phase (2 months): 4 drugs, usually isoniazid, with pyridoxine, rifampin, pyrazinamide, and ethambutol.
Continuation phase (4–12 months): two drugs, usually isoniazid and rifampin.

Contraindications
Isoniazid: drug-induced liver disease, porphyria.
Rifampin: jaundice, porphyria.
Pyrazinamide: liver damage, porphyria.
Ethambutol: optic neuritis.

Special points
For suspected resistance: addition of ethambutol.
For documented resistance: drugs as indicated by sensitivities.
For cerebral, bone and joint, and drug-resistant infections: longer treatment (9 months).
For unreliable compliance: intermittent, supervised treatment 2–3 times weekly.

Main drug interactions
Rifampin: oral contraceptive.

Main side effects
Isoniazid: neuropathy (pyridoxine prophylaxis), hepatitis, hypersensitivity reactions.
Rifampin: hepatitis, gastrointestinal upset, influenza symptoms, purpura.
Pyrazinamide: hepatitis, gastrointestinal upset.

Agents to consider for treatment of multidrug-resistant tuberculosis include: ciprofloxacin, cycloserine, clofazimine, and aminosalicylic acid. These should be used after sensitivities return. Treatment is continued for 18 months for multidrug-resistant tuberculosis.

Steroids

Patients with pericarditis or meningitis should receive steroids in order to prevent obstructive hydrocephalus.

Treatment aims

To secure survival (especially in disseminated and cerebral disease).

To preserve organ function and prevent deformity.

To relieve symptoms.

To prevent relapse by eradicating infection.

To prevent drug resistance by ensuring compliance.

Other treatments

- Surgery is often done both before and after the diagnosis is confirmed.
- It is indicated for the following forms of tuberculosis:

All: for biopsy diagnosis (>35% of patients), relief of obstruction due to inflammatory response, and correction of deformity.
Lymphatic: for chronic sinus and unresponsive or marked node enlargement.
Renal: ureteric obstruction or stricture, obstinate symptoms (*e.g.*, pain).
CNS: for hydrocephalus, cerebral edema.
Spinal: for cord pressure, bone graft.
Joint: to minimize deformity.
Gut: for obstruction, adhesions, strictures.
Pericardial: to relieve constriction.
Female genital: for stricture, infertility.

Prognosis

- Prognosis is related to the precariousness of the organ involved, the stage of disease progression, and the vulnerability of host.
- Mortality is significant in cerebral disease (10%–30%) and disseminated disease (10%–25%).
- Survival can be expected in other forms, although chronic sequelae may develop.
- The prognosis in lymph-node and dermatological tuberculosis is excellent.

Follow-up and management

- Drug toxicities that may affect compliance must be identified.
- The patient must be monitored for complications and long-term sequelae.

General references

Langdale LA, *et al.*: Tuberculosis and the surgeon. *Am J Surg* 1992, **163**:505–509.

Shafer RW, *et al.*: Extrapulmonary tuberculosis in patients with human immunodeficiency virus infection. *Medicine* 1991, **70**:384–397.

Diagnosis

Symptoms

Primary infection

• 90% of patients have no symptoms; the following are seen rarely:

Malaise, fever, erythema nodosum, phlyctenular conjunctivitis.

Postprimary infection (reactivation tuberculosis)

• Often no symptoms are seen.

Malaise, weight loss, fever, night sweats, anorexia, fatigue.

Cough, mucoid or mucopurulent sputum, hemoptysis, dyspnea, dull chest ache, pleuritic chest pain.

Malaise, weight loss, fever, meningism: symptoms of miliary tuberculosis; may be nonspecific, particularly in elderly patients.

Signs

• Physical examination is often unhelpful.

Evidence of weight loss, pyrexia, erythema nodosum: in primary infection.

Signs of pulmonary collapse, consolidation, or effusion, crackles (upper zones, increased after coughing), amphoric breath sounds over a large cavity.

Investigations

Chest radiography:
Primary: normal in 70% of patients; more often abnormal in children <5 years of age; typically shows unilateral hilar lymphadenopathy; bronchial compression can produce segmental or lobar collapse or hyperinflation, particularly in lower, lingula, and middle lobes; ulceration into bronchial tree, producing distal patchy consolidation, or into pleura, producing effusion.
Postprimary: classically shows bilateral upper-zone consolidation progressing to cavitation, fibrosis, and upper-lobe contraction; chronic tuberculosis lesions often calcified.

Tuberculin skin testing: positive test implies current or past infection or previous bacille Calmette–Guérin vaccination; positivity increases with age in United States; useful in identifying primary disease in younger patients. The larger the reaction, the greater likelihood exists that infection is present. A negative test does not rule out diagnosis.

Bacteriology: sputum samples stained (fluorescent auramine or Ziehl-Neelsen) and cultured (*e.g.*, in Löwenstein-Jensen medium); useful in establishing diagnosis in postprimary disease and in guiding management; sputum smear often positive in cavitating disease; examination of two good early-morning sputum samples allows identification of 90% of smear-positive cases; smear-positive sputum implies significant risk of infection; culture and sensitivity testing takes 4–8 weeks. DNA probes for *Mycobacterium tuberculosis* assist in the identification.

Complications

Lobar or segmental collapse or consolidation, pleural effusion, pericardial involvement, tuberculoma formation: in primary tuberculosis.

Postprimary or miliary tuberculosis, later infection at distant sites: caused by blood dissemination at time of primary infection.

Differential diagnosis

• Radiographical and some clinical features can be mimicked by the following:
Lung cancer.
Sarcoidosis.
Some bacterial pneumonias.
Allergic bronchopulmonary aspergillosis.
Pneumoconiosis.
Actinomycosis.

Etiology

General disease
Inhalation of *M. tuberculosis* from the cough of a patient with sputum-positive disease.

Postprimary disease
Reactivation of dormant *M. tuberculosis* disseminated at the time of primary infection; risk increased in patients with diseases causing depressed immunity (*e.g.*, malnutrition, alcoholism, diabetes, AIDS).

Epidemiology

• The estimated annual incidence in the United States is 4–20/100 000 people.

• The annual incidence in Indian, Pakistani, and Bangladeshi ethnic groups is ~170 in 100 000.

• Recently, the overall incidence has increased slightly.

• Persons infected with HIV are at increased risk of developing tuberculosis.

Atypical tuberculosis

• The frequency of atypical tuberculosis is increasing in elderly men with pre-existing lung disease.

• It is mostly caused by *Mycobacterium kansasii, malmoense, xenopi, avium*, or *avium-intracellulare* (*M. avium-intracellulare* particularly in later stages of AIDS).

• Presentation is similar to that of *M. tuberculosis* infection: 10%–40% of patients may be asymptomatic.

• Management is complicated, involving prolonged multidrug treatment: expert advice is needed.

Treatment

Diet and lifestyle

• Smoking must be stopped, and nutrition improved.

Pharmacological treatment

• Treatment must be supervised by a physician experienced in all aspects of tuberculosis management. Drug choice depends on susceptibility.

• Patients must be educated about the disease and the importance of prolonged treatment.

• Sputum-positive patients must be advised that they remain infectious for the first 2 weeks of treatment.

Standard 6-month unsupervised regimen

• A four-drug regimen consisting of isoniazid, ritampin, pyrazinamide, and ethambutol or streptomycin is recommended. The latter may be discontinued if the organism is susceptible to isoniazid and rifampin. Pyrazinamide is stopped after 8 weeks.

Standard dosage	Isoniazid, 300 mg daily (child, 5 mg/kg daily; maximum, 300 mg) for 6 months, rifampin, 450–600 mg daily (child, 10 mg/kg daily) for 6 months, pyrazinamide, 1.5–2 g daily (child, 15–30 mg/kg daily) for 2 months, and ethambutol, 15 mg/kg daily, or streptomycin, 15 mg/kg daily.
Contraindications	*All:* previous severe adverse event. *Isoniazid:* drug-induced liver disease, porphyria; caution in liver or renal disease. *Rifampin:* jaundice, porphyria; caution in liver disease. *Pyrazinamide:* liver disease, porphyria; caution in renal impairment, gout, or diabetes.
Special points	*Isoniazid:* isoniazid-resistant *M. tuberculosis* present in 4%–6% of patients. *Rifampin:* colors urine and tears orange; may stain soft contact lenses.
Main drug interactions	*Isoniazid:* binds to pyridoxine and may produce deficiency; inhibits phenytoin metabolism. *Rifampin:* hepatic enzyme induction increases metabolism and reduces effect of anticonvulsants, oral contraceptive pill, steroids, and digoxin. *Pyrazinamide:* interferes with renal testing for ketones; reduces renal excretion of uric acid. *Streptomycin:* may potentiate neuromuscular-blocking agents.
Main side effects	*Isoniazid:* gastrointestinal intolerance, exacerbation of acne, hepatotoxicity (in 1%–2% of patients; can be severe), peripheral neuropathy (in 2%; prevented by pyridoxine supplements 10 mg daily). *Rifampin:* nausea, abnormal liver function tests (usually mild and reversible), influenza-like reaction. *Pyrazinamide:* hepatotoxicity, arthralgia, precipitation of gout, urticaria. *Streptomycin:* 8th nerve damage, nephrotoxicity.

• Longer periods are needed for meningitis and with extensive disease.

• Pyridoxine, 10 mg daily, may be added when deficiency is a possibility.

• Supervised regimen and bi- or tri-weekly therapy are available options.

Other drugs

Corticosteroids: improve outcome in pericarditis and meningitis; of value in patients with severe infection, persistent pyrexia, or weight loss; higher doses needed if rifampin used.

Streptomycin, capreomycin, cycloserine, ethionamide for multiresistant or atypical infection: specialist advice must be sought. Duration of treatment must be prolonged in these settings.

Treatment aims

To achieve bacteriological and clinical cure.

To prevent resistance (with combination treatment).

To prevent or treat disease in contacts.

Prognosis

• ~6% of adults with pulmonary tuberculosis die of it before finishing chemotherapy.

• Only ~3% relapse if the full course of chemotherapy is taken; the rate is higher if compliance is poor.

Follow-up and management

• Close supervision is necessary throughout chemotherapy.

• Compliance must be checked; urine must be checked for rifampin.

• The patient must be checked for adverse effects.

• Response must be assessed: symptoms, weight gain, radiographic changes.

Prevention

• Notification of new cases to public health authorities for communicable disease control is a legal requirement.

• Care is needed in people with close contact with sputum-positive disease: 10% develop tuberculosis, mostly identified by initial tuberculin testing or chest radiography.

General references

American Thoracic Society and Centers for Disease Control and Prevention: Diagnostic standards and classification of tuberculosis in adults and children. *Am J Respir Crit Care Med* 2000, **161**:1376–1395.

Anonymous: Prevention and treatment of tuberculosis among patients infected with human immunodeficiency virus: principles of therapy and revised recommendations. Centers for Disease Control and Prevention. *MMWR Morb Mortal Wkly Rept* 1998, **47**:1–58.

Bass JB Jr, Farer LS, Hopewell PC, *et al.*: Treatment of tuberculosis and tuberculosis infection in adults and children. American Thoracic Society and The Centers for Disease Control and Prevention. *Am J Respir Crit Care Med* 1994, **149**:1359–1374.

Drugs for tuberculosis. *Med Lett Drugs Ther* 1995, **37**:67–70.

Stead WW: Management of health care workers after inadvertent exposure to tuberculosis: a guide for the use of preventive therapy. *Ann Intern Med* 1995, **122**:906–912.

Typhoid & paratyphoid fevers

Diagnosis

Symptoms

Persistent fever: developing after recent visit to endemic country.

Mounting fever, headache, malaise, anorexia, dry cough, constipation: abdominal pain in first week of illness.

Continuing fever, mental apathy: in second week.

Abdominal distension, "pea-soup" diarrhea: in third week.

Signs

Pyrexia: in first week.

Rose spots: 2–4-mm erythematous maculopapules in crops on lower chest and upper abdomen in 30% of patients in second week.

Vagueness and withdrawal, splenomegaly, relative bradycardia: in second week.

Delirium or stupor, distended tender abdomen, dehydration, poor-volume rapid pulse, signs of complications: in third week.

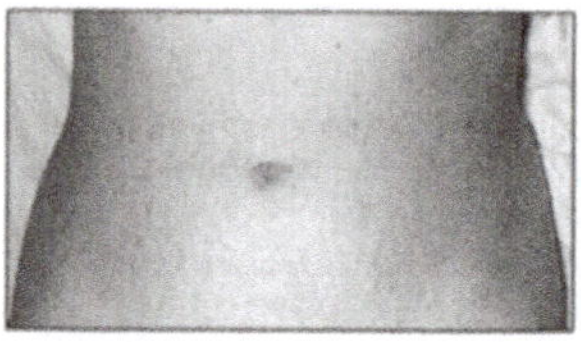

Rose spots in a patient with typhoid fever. (*See* Color Plate.)

Investigations

• Definitive diagnosis needs positive blood or bone-marrow culture.

Blood culture: highest positivity during first week (80%), declining thereafter; often negative if patient has already been given antibiotic.

Bone-marrow culture: often remains positive despite antibiotic administration.

Stool and urine culture: often positive from third week onwards; diagnostic only if clinical picture is compatible.

Widal's test: unreliable and difficult to interpret, so rarely performed.

Complete blood count: leukocyte count decreased, with relative lymphocytosis after first week.

Liver function tests: often mildly raised aspartate and alanine transaminase concentrations.

Complications

• Complications occur only in untreated patients after the second week.

Intestinal hemorrhage: indicated by sudden drop in temperature, rise in pulse rate, and rectal bleeding.

Intestinal perforation: signs of peritonitis may be difficult to detect in an already tender and distended abdomen; presence of gas under diaphragm and ascites may be the only signs.

Myocarditis: indicated by rapid, thready pulse and ECG abnormalities.

Jaundice: may be due to cholangitis, hepatitis, or hemolysis.

Typhoid abscesses: in different organs (rare).

Differential diagnosis

• Fever in a traveler returning from endemic areas may also be due to the following:

Malaria (most important).

Tropical viral infections.

Typhus.

Amebic liver abscess.

Trypanosomiasis and leishmaniasis.

Other causes of fever that are common worldwide.

Etiology

• Causes include the following:

Infection by *Salmonella typhi* or *paratyphi* A, B, or C.

Prolonged bacteremia.

Gallbladder infection.

Inflamed Peyer's patches in small intestine (may ulcerate during third week, leading to bleeding or perforation).

Epidemiology

• The disease is endemic in the Indian subcontinent, southeast Asia, the Middle East, Africa, and Central and South America; paratyphoid B also occurs in southern and eastern Europe.

• Transmission is through food or water contaminated by feces or urine of a sufferer or carrier.

Treatment

Diet and lifestyle

• Adequate nutrition and fluid replacement must be ensured.

• Chronic carriers, especially those handling foods, must practice strict hygiene because of the fecal–oral transmission of the disease; in such patients, attempts should be made to clear carriage.

Pharmacological treatment

General and supportive care

• Nutritional and fluid-electrolyte deficiencies should be corrected in patients presenting late.

Specific treatment

• Fluoroquinolones are currently the drug of choice in adults.

• Defervescence occurs in 3–5 days.

• Treatment failure, relapse, and chronic carriage are rare.

• Other drugs include third-generation cephalosporins and corticosteroids (in severe toxemia).

Standard dosage

Ciprofloxacin, 500 mg orally twice daily for 14 days (200 mg i.v. with vomiting or diarrhea).
In children (but see Special points): 10 mg/kg orally or i.v. daily in 2 divided doses.
Ceftriaxone, 3–4 g i.v. daily as single dose or 75–100 mg/kg i.v. daily in 2 divided doses for 7–10 days (shorter duration may be equally effective).
Adjunctive dexamethasone, 3 mg/kg i.v. initially, then 1 mg/kg 6-hourly for 48 hours.

Contraindications

Hypersensitivity.
Dexamethasone: caution in pregnancy, renal insufficiency, hypertension, and diabetes.

Special points

Ciprofloxacin: currently not recommended in pregnant women and children because of arthropathy in growing animals; this has not, however, been observed in children, and ciprofloxacin should not be withheld if benefits outweigh risks.
Ceftriaxone: can be used in children and pregnant women but must be given intravenously.

Main drug interactions

Ciprofloxacin: NSAIDs, oral iron, anticoagulants.
Ceftriaxone: probenecid.
Dexamethasone: phenytoin, barbiturates, ephedrine or rifampin may increase the metabolic clearance of corticosteroids.

Main side effects

Ciprofloxacin: nausea, abdominal pain, diarrhea (all unusual).
Ceftriaxone: headache, nausea, rash.
Dexamethasone: fluid and electrolyte disturbances.

Treatment of chronic carriers

• Ciprofloxacin, 750 mg, or norfloxacin, 400 mg twice daily for 28 days, is highly effective.

Drug resistance

• Chloramphenicol, cotrimoxazole, and amoxicillin are highly effective if the infecting strains are sensitive to the above drugs.

Treatment aims

To achieve clinical cure.

To prevent complications and relapse.

To prevent chronic fecal carriage after recovery.

Other treatments

• Surgery is needed for intestinal perforation (hemorrhage managed conservatively).

• Cholecystectomy should be reserved for carriers with symptomatic gallbladder disease.

Prognosis

• Untreated, typhoid and paratyphoid fevers have a mortality of up to 20%, mostly from myocarditis and intestinal hemorrhage or perforation; these complications are rarely seen in the United States.

• Recovery begins in the fourth week in the absence of complications.

Follow-up and management

• ~10% of patients relapse, and 3% become chronic fecal carriers after treatment with chloramphenicol, cotrimoxazole, or amoxicillin but rarely after ciprofloxacin treatment.

• After clinical recovery, six consecutive negative stool and urine cultures should be obtained over 3 weeks.

General references

Lassere R, Sangalang RP, Santiago L: Three day treatment of typhoid fever with two different doses of ceftriaxone, compared to 14 day therapy with chloramphenicol: a randomised trial. *J Antimicrob Chemother* 1991, **28**:765–772.

Mandal BK: Modern treatment of typhoid fever. *J Infect* 1991, **22**:1–4.

Sack RB, Rahman M, Yunus M, Khan EN: Antimicrobial resistance in organisms causing diarrheal disease. *Clin Infect Dis* 1997, **24(suppl 1)**: S102–S105.

Ulcerative colitis

Diagnosis

Symptoms

Diarrhea: often bloody and with urgency.

Abdominal pain: tenesmus often a prominent feature and should not be confused with constipation.

Anorexia, fatigue.

Fevers, weight loss: in more severe disease.

Skin, joint, or eye symptoms: in <10%.

Signs

• Signs are typically absent in mild or moderate disease (*see* Clinical patterns).

Left lower quadrant abdominal tenderness: evidence of peritoneal signs or ileus requires prompt surgical consultation for perforation or toxic megacolon.

Hematochezia on digital rectal examination.

Fever, tachycardia: in severe disease.

Perianal disease (fissures, abscess, or fistulas): distinctly unusual, consider crohn's disease.

Investigations

Stool culture: *Clostridium difficile, Entamoeba histolytica, Campylobacter* spp., and other bacterial infections should be excluded.

Complete blood count: to examine for anemia, leukocytosis.

Liver chemistry tests: to evaluate for hepatic inflammation.

Plain abdominal radiography: allows exclusion of dilatation and gives some indication of disease extent (bowel containing feces is probably not severely inflamed).

Colonoscopy with biopsies: allows accurate assessment of extent of disease and histological confirmation of inflammation or dysplasia. Inflammation almost always begins in the rectum extending proximally in a confluent pattern. Biopsies demonstrate crypt distortion, often with abscesses.

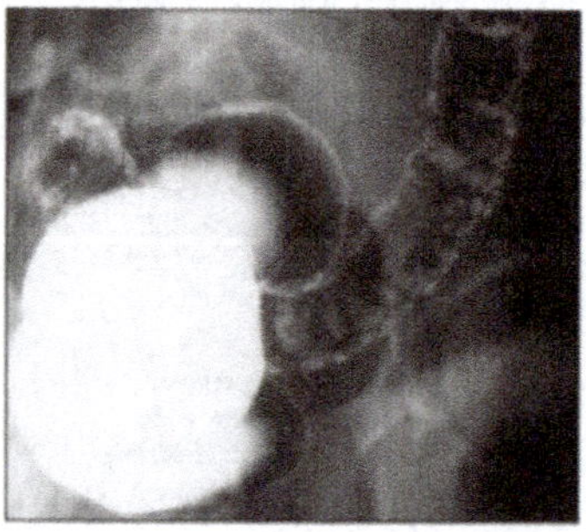

Double-contrast barium enema in severe ulcerative colitis, showing submucosal ulceration in sigmoid and descending colon.

Barium enema: less frequently used because of inability to obtain histology.

• Colonoscopy and barium enema should be avoided in an acute attack because they may cause exacerbation; limited sigmoidoscopy with rectal biopsies can often be done in these settings to exclude or confirm the disease.

Complications

Hemorrhage: chronic blood loss causing anemia common, life-threatening acute bleeding rare.

Perforation: in 5%, often a sequela of toxic megacolon; 50% mortality; avoidable with careful management and surgical referral.

Strictures: (unusual) colonoscopy and biopsy needed to exclude malignancy.

Colon cancer: risk depends on extent and duration of disease; increased risk observed after 10 years in patients with involvement of their entire colon.

Uveitis, episclera: in 5%.

Erythema nodosum, pyoderma gangrenosum: in 5%.

Arthropathy.

Sclerosis, cholangitis, cholangiocarcinoma: in <5%.

Differential diagnosis [1]

Microscopic (lymphocytic) colitis.

Collagenous colitis.

Drug-associated disorders: oral contraceptives have been associated with a Crohn's-like colitis; NSAIDs and purgatives may cause microscopic colitis.

Diversion colitis.

Crohn's colitis.

Irradiation proctitis.

Ischemic colitis.

Bacterial or amebic infection (dysentery).

Irritable bowel syndrome: should not cause bleeding or nocturnal diarrhea.

Cytomegalovirus, herpes simplex, cryptosporidia in immunosuppressed patients.

Colon cancer.

Acute self-limited colitis

Etiology [2]

Cause is unknown but is probably related to an autoimmune process in genetically susceptible individuals; no specific infectious or dietary agents have been reliably identified to date. Overall risk in first-degree relatives is 5%–10%.

Epidemiology

• Patients present at any age; the highest prevalence is in the 2nd and 3rd decades, but a second peak in the 5th and 6th decades has been reported.

• The prevalence in northwestern Europe and the United States is 1 in 1500; it is rarely diagnosed in developing countries.

• An unexplained association with non-smoking exists (95% of sufferers are nonsmokers or exsmokers).

Clinical patterns

Mild disease: diarrhea ≤4 loose stools per day with, at most, scant amounts of blood.

Moderate disease: 4–6 loose stools per day with constitutional symptoms, abdominal symptoms, and no severe bleeding.

Severe disease: >6 bowel movements per day, persistent blood loss, abdominal tenderness, fevers, tachycardia, hypoalbuminemia.

• Symptoms correlate with length of colonic involvement. Proctitis (disease limited to the rectum) is the most common pattern, with more severe disease usually found in patents with pancolitis.

Treatment

Diet and lifestyle

• Smoking (nicotine patches) often of benefit; cessation may result in flare.

• Avoid NSAIDs.

Pharmacological treatment [3,4]

For mild attacks

Standard dosage *Initially:* sulfasalazine, 2–4 g/d or one of the 5-aminosalicylic acid preparations, such as mesalamine, 2–4 g/d, or olsalazine, 1–3 g/d (divide into three doses each day). Proctitis may be managed topically with rectal corticosteroids or 5-aminosalicylic acid enemas.

Maintenance: sulfasalazine, 1.5–4 g daily, mesalamine, 1.2–2.4 g daily, or olsalazine, 1.5–3 g daily; or 5-ASA enemas for disease limited to the distal colon [3].

Contraindications *All:* salicylate intolerance, renal failure.
Sulfazalazine: sulfa allergy.

Special points Slow-acting, may require several weeks for treatment effect. Useful agents to maintain remissions. Taking with food may reduce nausea.

Main drug interactions *Sulfasalazine:* warfarin, anticonvulsants.

Main side effects Occasional nephrotoxicity.
Sulfasalazine: nausea, headaches, malaise, dyspepsia, reversible male infertility.
Mesalamine: occasional nausea, diarrhea, interstitial nephritis.
Olsalazine: diarrhea in 10%–20% of patients.

For moderate attacks

Standard dosage Prednisone, 1 mg/kg (up to 60 mg) orally once daily, with oral 5-aminosalicylic acid preparation.

Contraindications Systemic infections, hypersensitivity.

Special points Steroids most useful to achieve an acute response (some beneficial effect should be noted within 48 hours). Once symptoms resolve (usually within 1 week), begin tapering over 4–8 weeks. Steroids of no value in maintaining remission.

Main drug interactions None.

Main side effects Occasional steroid-psychosis; hyperglycemia, asceptic necrosis; osteoporosis, hyperphagia, increased energy. Steroid-related side-effects uncommon if long-term treatment avoided.

For severe attacks

• Treatment includes admission to hospital for close observation, bed rest, high-dose i.v. corticosteroids (*e.g.*, solumedrol, 15 mg every 6 hours), total parenteral nutrition if patient is vomiting or malnourished, deep venous thrombosis prophylaxis. Cyclosporine, 2–4 mg/kg/day is of benefit in patients who fail to respond to i.v. steroid therapy. However, complications of hypertension and renal insufficiency are common.

• The colonic diameter should be monitored by plain radiography daily.

For toxic dilatation

• Dilatation of the transverse colon to a diameter >7 cm accompanied by signs of fever or tachycardia may be treated conservatively for up to 48 hours with nasogastric suction and avoidance of narcotics or other agents that reduce motility. Any clinical or radiographical deterioration during this period or failure to respond to treatment necessitates immediate surgery.

Alternative medicine

Recommended use: none.

Common use: quercetin; short-chain fatty acid enemas; marshmallow (*Hibiscus mosheutos*); Slippery elm bark (*Ulmus rubra* or *U. fulva*); comfrey root (*Symphytum officinale*).

Caution: comfrey root contains pyrrolidizine alkaloids and may cause liver damage at high dosages.

Treatment aims

To achieve and maintain remission.

To avoid life-threatening complications.

Other treatments

• 20% of patients need colectomy at some time; surgery is indicated for the following:

Failed full medical treatment for severe colitis (after 1–2 weeks of hospitalization on i.v. steroids or a trial of cyclosporine).

Toxic megacolon or perforation.

Persistent colitis, with poor quality of life.

Cancer or raised dysplastic lesion.

Prognosis

• Most patients have relapses interspersed with periods of prolonged remission; 90% are capable of full-time work.

• Life expectancy is normal.

• The risk of colon cancer is significantly increased beginning 10–15 years after onset of disease in patients with pancolitis.

Follow-up and management

• Patients should continue taking 5-aminosalicylic acid preparations for 1 year or, for severe or multiple attacks, until they have been free of disease for at least 5 years.

• Patients should be screened by colonoscopy for dysplasia or early colon cancer on a yearly basis if disease present >10 years.

Patient support

Crohn's and Colitis Foundation of America, 386 Park Ave S., New York, NY 10016-7374.

Key references

1. Hanauer SB: Inflammatory bowel disease. *N Engl J Med* 1996, **334**:841–848.
2. Kirsner JB, Short RG (eds.): *Inflammatory Bowel Disease*, edn 4. Baltimore: Williams & Wilkins; 1995.
3. Kornbluth A, Sachar DB: Ulcerative colitis practice guidelines in adults. *Am J Gastroenterol* 1997, **92**:204–209.
4. Greenwald BD, *et al.*: Advances in ulcerative colitis. *Clin Perspect Gastroenterol* 1999, January/February: 25–39.

Upper gastrointestinal tract bleeding

Diagnosis (*See also* Variceal bleeding)

Differential diagnosis

Epistaxis.

Swallowed blood from hemoptysis.

Ingestion of iron or bismuth-containing preparations creating the false impression of melena.

Epidemiology

- Estimated rate of hospitalization for upper gastrointestinal bleeding has been estimated at 150 patients per 100 000 members of the population.
- It is more common in patients with chronic liver disease, renal failure, diabetes mellitus, and individuals with coagulopathies.
- Elderly patients are particularly at risk in part due to limited compensatory reserve; the widespread use of NSAIDs in this population for management of arthritis is a major predisposing factor.

Definition

Brisk or slow blood loss from the esophagus, stomach, or small intestine (*i.e.,* duodenum) proximal to the ligament of Treitz.

Symptoms

Vomiting blood: *i.e.*, hematenesis.

Passage of black, tarry stool: *i.e.,* melena.

Abdominal pain.

Syncope.

Weight loss.

Fatigue.

Signs

Hematemesis.

Melena.

Tachycardia with orthostatic hypotension.

Pallor.

Abdominal tenderness: nonspecific.

Stigmata of chronic liver disease (*i.e.,* palmar erythema, spider angiomata, gynecomastia): should be assessed in all patients with upper gastrointestinal bleeding.

Investigations

Complete blood count: evaluate anemia. Initial hemoglobin will not reflect severity of bleeding in acute presentations; presence of microcytosis (*i.e.,* mean corpuscular volume <80) suggests chronic blood loss; adequate platelets, prothrombin time, partial thromboplastin time, and iron stores should also be verified, particularly in patients with evidence of chronic liver disease. Blood urea nitrogen levels are often elevated with bleeding and may rise further in hypotensive patients.

Esophagogastroduodenoscopy: provides visualization of the proximal gastrointestinal tract to the level of the midduodenum. Allows prediction of rebleeding in patients with peptic ulcer disease (*i.e.*, rebleeding is more likely in patients with visible vessels, adherent clots, ulcers larger than 2 cm, and endoscopic evidence of portal hypertension), direct control of hemorrhage in patients with bleeding ulcers or varices, and biopsy of suspicious lesions.

Complications

Exsanguination.

Perforation.

Cardiac or cerebrovascular ischemia.

Metabolic acidosis.

Prerenal insufficiency.

Aspiration.

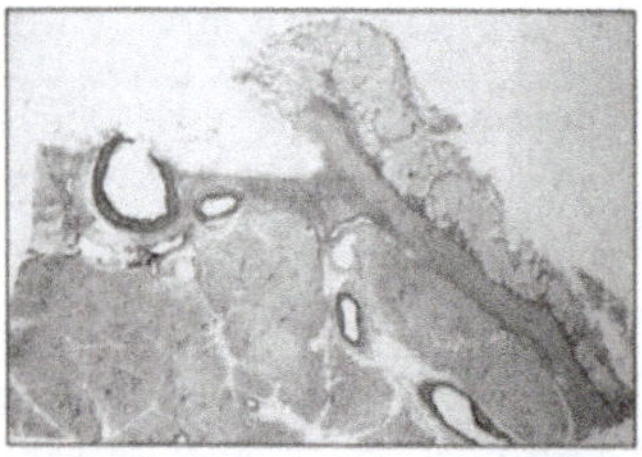

Large hole in an artery in the large duodenal ulcer in a patient who died.

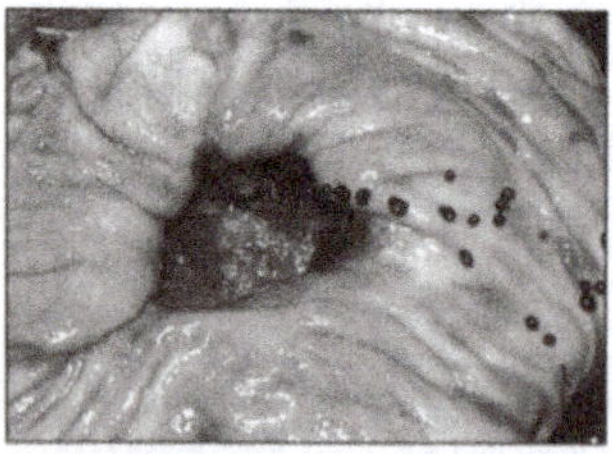

Bleeding gastric ulcer (*see* Color Plate).

Treatment

Diet and lifestyle

• Patients with a history of peptic ulcer disease should refrain from the use of NSAIDs with the exception of acetaminophen, which does not significantly contribute to erosive disease or platelet dysfunction. The new cyclooxygenase-2 inhibitors (*e.g.*, rofecoxib, celecoxib) also appear to cause little, if any, gastropathy. Enteric or buffered aspirin is no safer than regular aspirin and doses as low as 80 mg/day have been associated with gastropathy and an increased risk for bleeding.

• Patients should not eat for 8 hours before endoscopy or surgery; at other times, no evidence suggests that allowing patients to eat will increase their tendency to bleed.

Pharmacological treatment [4]

• *See* Esophagitis, Duodenal ulcer, Gastric ulcer, *and* Variceal bleeding *for specific treatment regimens.*

• Drug treatment has a relatively small role in the management of active upper gastrointestinal bleeding except in patients with bleeding from esophageal varices, in whom i.v. octreotide appears beneficial (*see* Variceal bleeding).

• Use of proton pump inhibitors (*e.g.*, omeprazole) probably provides mild to moderate risk reduction in ulcer rebleeding when used as an adjunct to endoscopy in contrast to H_2 blockers, which are unlikely to be of benefit.

• Volume expansion should be rapidly achieved with i.v. crystalloid infusions via large-bore needles in patients with evidence of brisk bleeding or hemodynamic compromise; the patient's volume status and rate of bleeding should be used in conjunction with the hematocrit to determine the need for blood transfusion.

• Transfusion with packed red blood cells should be used judiciously to minimize the chances of iatrogenic infections and complications; avoid overtransfusion.

• In general, young healthy people who are euvolemic can tolerate a hematocrit as low as 20 without serious problems.

Nonpharmacological treatment

For peptic ulcer

• Endoscopic treatment consisting of bipolar cautery, heater probe, laser, and injection (*e.g.*, with epinephrine, saline) have been shown to reduce rebleeding rates, need for surgery, and mortality. The choice of a specific treatment depends on the endoscopist's expertise.

• Repeated endoscopic treatment is usually preferable to surgery, particularly in elderly patients or individuals with other comorbid conditions.

• Surgery: in patients with continued or recurrent bleeding in hospital; if surgery necessary, best done before repeated episodes of hypotension have impaired chances of recovery.

For bleeding varices

• *See* Variceal bleeding.

Endoscopic variceal injection sclerotherapy, using sclerosants such as monoethanolamine, alcohol, sodium tetradecyl sulfate, or sodium morrhuate: has been shown to reduce the incidence of further bleeding and to reduce mortality in patients with recent bleeding from esophageal varices, and it can stop bleeding from varices.

Endoscopic variceal band ligation: less invasive than surgery, has lower rebleeding and complication rates than endoscopic sclerotherapy.

Balloon tamponade: stops bleeding in 85% of patients, but bleeding recurs in 21%–60% and survival not improved; complications include esophageal rupture and aspiration pneumonia, with lethal complications of 10%.

Transjugular intrahepatic portacaval shunt (TIPS): for patients who have recurrent variceal bleeding despite sclerotherapy or ligation therapy.

Surgery: for the few patients who do not respond to endoscopic treatment and TIPS; options include portosystemic shunt, esophageal transection, devascularization, or hepatic transplantation [4].

• Patients with continued bleeding of 6–8 U over 24 hours despite endoscopic attempts at control require an alternative approach (*e.g.*, TIPS).

Complications of treatment

After endoscopy for bleeding peptic ulcer: precipitation of acute bleeding, perforation, infarction of stomach or duodenum (with injection).

After endoscopy for bleeding varices: esophageal ulceration, perforation, septicemia, distant thrombosis, pleural effusion, aspiration.

After surgery: pneumonia, renal or cardiac failure, further bleeding.

Treatment aims

To halt bleeding.

To normalize the patient's volume status and erythrocyte mass.

To prevent further episodes of bleeding.

Prognosis

• 80% of upper gastrointestinal bleeding stops spontaneously.

• For peptic ulcer bleeding, the risk of rebleeding in the hospital is 15%–30%; of these, urgent surgery is required in 15%–20%, and death occurs in 5%–10%.

• The risk of death after admission with first variceal bleeding is 30%.

• 70% of patients with bleeding varices die within 1–4 years.

• Bleeding due to Mallory-Weiss tear, esophagitis, gastritis, and duodenitis has excellent prognosis.

• Most patients with bleeding upper gastrointestinal cancer die within 1 year.

Follow-up and management

• Ulcer patients with major bleeding should have follow-up endoscopy to check healing and eradication of *Helicobacter pylori.*

• Patients with a second major bleed should be considered for surgery.

Key references

1. Consensus Development Panel, National Institutes of Health 1990: Consensus statement on therapeutic endoscopy and bleeding ulcers. *Gastrointest Endosc* 1990, **36**:S62–S63.
2. Cook DJ, *et al.*: Endoscopic therapy for acute nonvariceal upper gastrointestinal hemorrhage: a meta-analysis. *Gastroenterology* 1992, **102**:139–148.
3. Van Dam J, Brugge WR: Endoscopy of the upper gastrointestinal tract. *N Engl J Med* 1999, **341**:1738–1748.
4. Saeed ZA, Woods KL: Gastrointestinal bleeding. *Curr Pract Med* 1998, **1**:785–796.

Urinary incontinence

Diagnosis [1]

Symptoms

• Many affected patients will not spontaneously mention urinary incontinence to their physician; routinely ask all patients >65 years of age (especially women): "Do you have trouble controlling your urine?"

• History should include detailed description of episodes, estimate of voided quantity (often inaccurate or unknown), onset, frequency, fluid intake patterns, change in bowel or sexual function, medications, menopausal status, mental status changes.

• 24-hour voiding record can be very useful in characterizing incontinence; should include time and amount of voids and associated symptoms (urgency, coughing, sense of complete evacuation) and neurologic evalution.

Signs

• Physical examination should include assessment of intravascular fluid status (orthostatic BP), abdominal examination (distended bladder), genital, pelvic, and rectal examinations (cystocele, rectocele) and neurologic evaluation.

Classification

• The relationships of the traditional classification of urge, stress, and overflow incontinence to detrusor and outlet function are shown in the table.

Physiological causes of common types of chronic urinary incontinence

Urge incontinence	Stress incontinence	Overflow incontinence
Usually due to detrusor instability Detrusor hyperreflexia (caused by neurological lesion) Detrusor hyperactivity with impaired bladder contractility (usually in frail, elderly patients)	Urethral hypermobility (most common cause in women) Intrinsic urethral sphincter insufficiency	Due to bladder overdistention Underactive detrusor (often neurologic cause) Bladder outlet or urethral obstruction (more common in men)

Investigations

Postvoid residual (PVR) measurement: indicated in virtually all patients; identifies detrusor underactivity and/or outlet obstruction. Normal PVR is < 50 mL; borderline, 50–200 mL; abnormal >200 mL. PVR can be estimated via ultrasonography if in-and-out catheterization is not feasible.

Urinalysis, serum creatinine, blood urea nitrogen, glucose, calcium.

Other investigations as indicated by initial workup: consider urinary cytology if hematuria and/or irritative voiding symptoms without urinary tract infection (UTI); i.v. pyelogram if hematuria.

Urodynamic examinations usually unnecessary.

Complications

Urinary retention, reflux, renal damage (detrusor underactivity, outlet obstruction), infection.

Social impairment due to limitations in activities.

Differential diagnosis

Transient urinary incontinence (DIAPERS) [1]

Delerium: usually clinically evident.

Infection (if symptomatic): asymptomatic UTI is rarely a cause of incontinence.

Atrophic vaginitis.

Pharmaceutical: sedative/hypnotics, diuretics, anticholinergic agents, alpha-antagonists, alpha-agonists, calcium-channel blockers.

Excessive urine formation: hypercalcemia, hyperglycemia, diabetes insipidus, volume-expanded states (congestive heart failure, lower extremity venous insufficiency).

Restricted mobility: parkinsonism, postcerebrovascular accident (CVA).

Stool impaction.

Etiology

Detrusor overactivity with upper motor neuron (UMN) lesion (*e.g.*, CVA); can be accompanied by external sphincter dyssynergia (simultaneous contraction of external urethral sphincter with detrusor contraction); termed detrusor (external) sphincter dyssynergia (DSD).

Detrusor overactivity without upper motor neuron lesion ("detrusor instability"): causes include physical irritant (*e.g.*, bladder tumor, renal impaction, infection) and detrusor hyperactivity with impaired contractility (DHIC), a common idiopathic condition among the frail elderly characterized by involuntary contractions with high residuals.

Detrusor underactivity: neurological (peripheral neuropathy, sacral irradiation or surgery, spinal cord injury), anticholinergic drugs, B_{12} deficiency.

Outlet overactivity (obstruction): benign prostatic hypertrophy, urethral stricture, DSD (see above), medications (*e.g.*, alpha-agonists).

Outlet underactivity: pelvic relaxation syndrome, medications (*e.g.*, alpha-blockers), postsurgical urethral sphincter insufficiency.

Epidemiology

1%–5% of men, 10%–25% of women age 15–64 years.

• 15%–30% of community-dwelling elders (>60 years of age) have urinary incontinence; two-thirds are women; 25%–30% of those with incontinence have episodes of incontinence at least weekly.

• Conservative estimate of cost of caring for incontinence among community-dwelling adults is $15 billion annually (1990), and among nursing home residents $3.3 billion annually.

Treatment [1]

Diet and lifestyle

Bladder training: conscious delays in voiding; appropriate in detrusor instability (detrusor overactivity without UMN lesion) and stress incontinence.

Habit (timed) or prompted voiding: void on a regular basis, before urge is felt; timing parameters are based on incontinence record; most helpful for cognitively impaired patients with urge incontinence.

• Pelvic muscle ("Kegel") exercises improve stress incontinence among motivated women; they strengthen voluntary periurethral and pelvic muscles, exerting a closing force on the urethra. Exercise performed as 10-second flexion, 10-second relaxation. Target performing exercises 30–80 times a day for at least 6 weeks; can also be used in postsurgical incontinence due to outlet laxity.

Pharmacological treatment

For urge incontinence: anticholinergic medications

Usual dosage Oxybutynin, 2.5–5.0 mg 3–4 times daily. Also has direct smooth muscle relaxant properties.

Probantheline, 7.5–30 mg 3–5 times daily.

Tricyclics should be reserved for carefully evaluated patients.

Contraindications Narrow-angle glaucoma.

Special points Useful for low-PVR detrusor overactivity (urge) incontinence; PVR should be checked after obtaining therapeutic response or maximal tolerated dose, to rule out retention, drowsiness, nausea, tachycardia.

Main drug interactions None.

Main side effects Dry mouth, orthostasis, constipation, urinary retention.

For stress incontinence: phenylpropanolamine

Usual dosage 50 mg twice daily (sustained release form).

Contraindications Use with caution, if at all, in patients with hyperthyroidism, cardiovascular disorders, hypertension, diabetes, glaucoma, or prostatic hypertrophy.

Special points Useful in mild stress incontinence; monitor blood pressure among hypertensive patients; some preparations contain tartrazine (yellow dye no. 5), a potent allergen in some patients.

Main drug interactions Do not use with monoamine oxidase inhibitors; additive effects with other sympathomimetic agents.

Main side effects Usually none or mild at therapeutic doses; can cause nervousness, restlessness, palpitations, elevations in blood pressure.

Conjugated estrogens

Usual dosage 0.3–1.25 mg/day orally or 2 g/day intravaginally.

• Combined therapy with both phenyl propanolamine and estrogen is recommended when therapy with either agent alone is ineffective.

Treatment aims

To minimize or eliminate symptoms.

To maximize social function.

Other treatments

Refer to urologist or gynecologist for further diagnosis and treatment if:

High PVR.

Diagnosis uncertain and *either* no reasonable empiric plan *or* lack of consistent picture from symptoms and signs.

Failure to respond to empiric trial and candidate for further (usually surgical) therapy.

Hematuria without infection.

Other conditions that warrant investigation: suspected new systemic or local neurological condition, prostate nodule, severe symptoms of difficulty emptying bladder (suggests mass lesion), incontinence associated with recurrent UTIs (rule out structural defect), severe and symptomatic pelvic prolapse.

Prognosis

Urge incontinence: 90% of appropriately selected women will show improvement or cure with bladder training; up to 40% of women will be cured, and up to 80% improved, with pharmacological treatment (anticholinergic agents).

Stress incontinence: 15% cured and 60% improved with pelvic muscle or bladder training, 15% cured and up to 60% improved with pharmacological treatment (alpha-agonists), 80% cured with surgery.

Follow-up and management

As appropriate to condition and treatment, routine inquiry regarding recurrence of symptoms is indicated.

Patient support

National Association for Continence
P.O. Box 8310
Spartanburg, SC 29305
(800) BLADDER or www. nafc.org

Key references

1. Urinary Incontinence Guidline Panel. Urinary Incontinence in Adults: Clinical Practice Guideline. AHCPR Pub. No. 92-0038. Rockville, MD: Department of Health and Human Services. March 1996. (800-358-9295 or http://text.nlm.nih.gov/).
2. Winograd CH, Resnick NM: Incontinence. In Scientific American Medicine, vol IX. Edited by Rubenstein E, Federman DD. New York: Scientific American Press; 1991.

Urinary tract infection

Diagnosis

Symptoms and signs

Lower urinary tract infection

Cystitis: dysuria, frequency, and suprapubic tenderness.

Acute prostatitis: dysuria, frequency, fever, perineal pain, obstructive voiding dysfunction, tenderness.

Chronic prostatitis: relapsing infection, voiding dysfunction, abdominal or back pain.

Upper urinary tract infection

Acute pyelonephritis: fever, chills, prostration, back or flank pain and tenderness, dysuria, and frequency.

Renal abscesses: fever and chills, flank pain and tenderness, flank or abdominal mass, dysuria, and frequency.

Symptomatic bacteremia of urinary tract origin: clinical features of bacteremia often overshadow those relating to urinary tract.

Investigations

To establish presence of infection

Urine culture: $>10^2$ colony-forming units (CFU) coliforms/mL or $>10^5$ CFU noncoliforms/mL in symptomatic women, 10^3 CFU bacteria/mL in symptomatic men, $>10^5$ CFU bacteria/mL in asymptomatic patients on two consecutive specimens, $>10^2$ CFU bacteria/mL in catheterized patients, any growth of bacteria from a suprapubic aspirate in symptomatic patients.

Urine microscopy: pyuria (>10 leukocytes/mL unspun urine) supportive evidence of urinary tract infection but not specific; pus cells in "sterile" urine (sterile pyuria) may indicate fastidious organisms or previous antibiotic treatment; microscopic hematuria in 50% of patients.

Dipstick testing of urine: combined leukocyte esterase and nitrite test useful screening procedure, with negative predictive value of 96%–97% at level of 10^5 CFU/mL.

To establish site of infection

- Whether infection is confined to the lower tract or has ascended to the upper tract has important treatment implications; the distinction is usually made clinically.

Radiography

- Radiography is used to identify structural abnormalities of urinary tract, including reflux nephropathy, obstruction, calculi, congenital abnormalities, and, in children, vesicoureteric reflux.
- It is indicated in children and men in first infection and in women with recurrent infections, upper urinary tract infection, unusual infecting organism, fever persisting >48 hours after starting treatment, coexistent hypertension, or persistent microscopic hematuria.

Intravenous urography: investigation of choice in adults (usually delayed until after recovery); ultrasonography may be substituted or added in the case of renal impairment or when renal abscess or pelvic disease is suspected.

^{99m}Tc-DMSA scan and ultrasonography: with either voiding cystourethrography or radionuclide cystography; investigation of choice in children.

Complications

Reflux nephropathy: cortical scarring and clubbing of underlying calyces in infants with bacteriuria associated with vesicoureteric reflux.

Renal damage, perinephric abscess formation, septicemia: due to infection in presence of complicating factors (*e.g.*, obstruction, stones, vesicoureteric reflux).

Differential diagnosis

Urethritis: chlamydia, gonorrhea, herpesvirus.

Vaginitis: bacteria, trichomonas, yeasts.

Perineal lesions: herpesvirus, other sexually transmitted diseases, dermatological conditions, physical or chemical irritants.

Etiology

- The common uropathogens are normal constituents of the colonic flora.
- *Escherichia coli* accounts for 85% of community-acquired urinary tract infection.
- Catheterization, instrumentation, cross infection, and selection of resistant bowel and environmental flora account for the different microbiological spectrum of hospital-acquired urinary tract infection.
- Almost always, infection is due to ascent of microorganisms through the urethra from the colonized perineum.

Epidemiology

- 3.7% of boys and 2% of girls in the first year of life have bacteriuria.
- 4%–7% of pregnant women have bacteriuria, compared with 1%–3% of young, nonpregnant women.
- Urinary tract infection is rare in young men except in practicing homosexuals.
- 10%–20% of elderly people living at home and up to 50% of institutionalized elderly people have bacteriuria.

Complicated or uncomplicated infection

- This distinction is useful for directing treatment.
- The following suggest occult renal involvement in apparent lower urinary tract infection or the presence of complicated urinary tract infection:

Male sex.
History of childhood urinary tract infection.
Symptoms for >7 days at presentation.
Recent antibiotic use.
Pregnancy.
Institutionalization: in elderly patients.
Recent instrumentation.
Indwelling catheter.
Underlying urinary tract abnormality.
Diabetes.
Immunosuppression.
Spinal cord injury.

Treatment

Diet and lifestyle

• A high fluid intake may help to alleviate dysuria during an acute episode; in the long term, it may be useful prophylactically.

• In women, postcoital voiding may be helpful; those using diaphragms and spermicides may benefit from changing to alternative contraceptive methods.

Pharmacological treatment

Indications

For lower urinary tract infections (uncomplicated): 3–5-day courses of trimethoprim, co-trimoxazole, nitrofurantoin, or co-amoxiclav; as effective as 7–14-day course; result in fewer relapses than single-dose treatment.

For lower urinary tract infections (complicated): antibiotic therapy as above continued for 7–14 days; short courses not suitable.

In pregnant women: 7–10-day course of amoxicillin, cephalexin, or nitrofurantoin; early screening and treatment of asymptomatic bacteriuria.

In men with prostatitis: trimethoprim, co-trimoxazole, or a quinolone for 4 weeks (longer for chronic prostatitis); nonbacterial prostatitis may respond to doxycycline or erythromycin.

For upper urinary tract infections (uncomplicated): severity of constitutional upset determines need for hospitalization.

In patients treated at home: oral trimethoprim, co-trimoxazole, co-amoxiclav, or quinolone for 14 days.

In hospitalized patients: initially, i.v. cefuroxime, cefotaxime, ciprofloxacin, co-amoxiclav, or co-trimoxazole; when fever subsides, oral treatment dictated by culture, continued for 14 days; relapses treated for 6 weeks.

For upper urinary tract infection (complicated):

In previously instrumented or catheterized patients: initially i.v. ceftazidime or amoxicillin with ciprofloxacin or gentamicin.

In patients with obstructed, infected upper tract: antibiotic therapy as above, with prompt drainage by percutaneous nephrostomy pending definitive surgery.

In patients with renal abscess: antibiotic therapy as above, with i.v. flucloxacillin, then 4–6-week courses of antibiotics based on cultures; percutaneous drainage usually needed.

Selected regimens

Amoxicillin, 500 mg orally 3 times daily.
Cefotaxime, 1 g i.v. 3 times daily.
Ceftazidime, 1–2 g i.v. twice daily.
Cefuroxime, 750 mg i.v. 3 times daily.
Cephalexin, 500 mg orally 4 times daily.
Ciprofloxacin, 500 mg orally or 200 mg i.v. twice daily.
Co-trimoxazole, 800 mg (sulfamethoxazole) and 160 mg (trimethoprim) orally twice daily.
Flucloxacillin, 500 mg i.v. 4 times daily.
Gentamicin, 80 mg i.v. 3 times daily, follow peak and trough levels.
Nitrofurantoin, 100 mg orally 4 times daily.
Ofloxacin, 200 mg orally twice daily.
Trimethoprim, 200 mg orally twice daily.

Antibiotics: contraindications and side effects

Chronic renal failure: nitrofurantoin ineffective, causes neuropathy; tetracyclines worsen uremia; aminoglycosides can be used but concentrations must be monitored to avoid nephrotoxicity and auditory/vestibular toxicity.

Pregnancy: tetracyclines cause bone or teeth dystrophy; trimethoprim possibly teratogenic; quinolones possibly cause arthropathy; aminoglycosides cause auditory/vestibular toxicity.

Infancy: tetracyclines cause bone or teeth dystrophy; sulfonamides cause hemolysis.

Prophylaxis

• Postcoital or nightly: trimethoprim, 100 mg, nitrofurantoin, 100 mg, or co-trimoxazole, 480 mg, reduces recurrence in women with normal urinary tracts.

• Prophylaxis is also useful after acute pyelonephritis in pregnancy.

Treatment aims

To relieve symptoms.

To prevent increase in prematurity and perinatal mortality.

To prevent and eradicate systemic sepsis.

To prevent progressive renal damage.

Prognosis

• Renal impairment in reflux nephropathy may progress without persisting infection and reflux.

• Adults with uncomplicated infection suffer minimal long-term sequelae if adequately treated.

• Complicated upper tract infections are potentially more damaging and may cause progressive renal scarring.

Follow-up and management

• Follow-up urine cultures are essential in pregnancy, after uncomplicated acute pyelonephritis, and after all complicated urinary tract infections.

• Any predisposing factors should be treated.

• Obstruction must be relieved by surgery or intermittent self-catheterization when indicated; calculi must be removed.

Recurrent infection

Relapse

• Relapse occurs soon after cessation of treatment.

• The same organism is involved.

• Relapse indicates inappropriate drug or duration of treatment, poor compliance, occult renal involvement, or underlying urinary tract abnormality.

Reinfection

• Reinfection occurs >6 weeks after cessation of treatment.

• A different organism is involved.

• Reinfection indicates failure of host defenses.

General references

Childs SJ, Egan RJ: Bacteriuria and urinary infections in the elderly. *Urol Clin North Am* 1996, **23**:43–54.

Funfstuck R, Smith JW, Tschape H, Stein G: Pathogenetic aspects of uncomplicated urinary tract infection: recent advances. *Clin Nephrol* 1997, **47**:13–18.

Rosenfeld DL, *et al.*: Current recommendations for children with urinary tract infections. *Clin Pediatr* 1995, **34**:261–264.

Diagnosis

Symptoms

Itching and swelling of skin.

Painful or burning sensation of the skin: uncommon.

Wheezing, dyspnea, hoarseness, arthralgias, nausea, diarrhea: may accompany severe cases.

Signs

Evanescent, red, elevated papules or plaques: often with blanched centers or annular configurations.

Angioedema of the lips and periorbital regions: not uncommon.

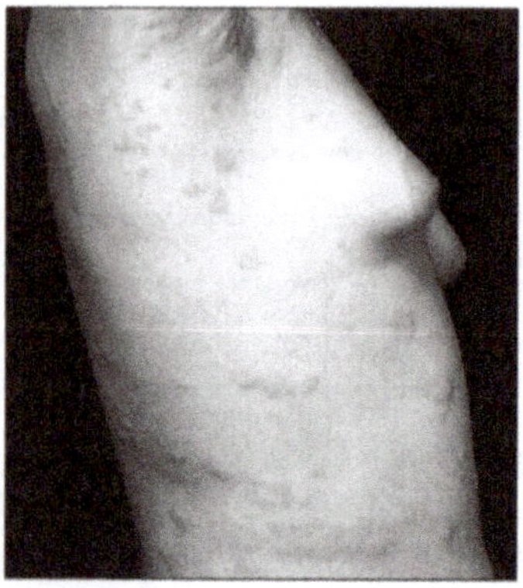

Scattered urticarial wheals on the trunk. (*See* Color Plate.)

Investigations

Acute urticaria (<6 weeks)

• **Standard history and physical examination:** performed with emphasis on recent infections and food and drug ingestion.

Chronic urticaria (>6 weeks)

• **Very challenging;** costly tests are rarely helpful.

• **Thorough history and physical examination:** further laboratory testing should be directed toward any positive findings.

• **Intradermal, radioallergosorbent, or skin patch testing:** of little diagnostic value but may help identify sensitivity to provocative agents in a limited number of cases.

• **Skin biopsy:** may be needed if urticarial vasculitis is suspected.

Complications

Anaphylactic shock: in cases of IgE-mediated acute urticarial reactions.

Sleep disturbances, depression: in chronic urticaria.

Differential diagnosis

Urticarial vasculitis (wheals last >24 hours).

Erythema multiforme.

Erythema chronicum migrans.

Urticarial component of bullous pemphigoid.

Herpes gestationis.

Hereditary angioedema: usually involves only mucous membranes with few urticarial skin lesions; life-threatening laryngeal spasm.

Urticaria pigmentosa.

Etiology

Acute urticaria is often caused by upper respiratory tract infection, drug ingestion, or idiopathic causes.

Chronic urticaria is most often idiopathic.

Many cases of urticaria represent a type I, IgE-mediated hypersensitivity reaction.

There are multiple potential causes:

Drugs: penicillin, NSAIDs, aspirin.

Foods: seafood, strawberries, chocolate, nuts.

Systemic conditions: connective tissue disease, infection (*e.g., Helicobacter pylori*), cancer, serum sickness.

Environmental: heat/cold, exercise, stress, water, pressure, sun exposure, insect bites/stings, contact (e.g., with latex).

Genetic: hereditary angioedema.

Other: autoimmune urticaria (IgG autoantibodies against IgE receptor), autoimmune thyroid disease.

Direct mast cell degranulation may occur: radiocontrast media, opiate analgesics, polymyxin B, curare.

Epidemiology

• Urticaria affects 25% of the population at some point in their lives.

• 25% of those with urticaria develop chronic urticaria.

Treatment

Diet and lifestyle

• Known triggering agents should be identified and avoided.

Patients should avoid aspirin and NSAIDs because these drugs may be exacerbating factors (even if not causative).

Patients with a history of urticaria accompanied by bronchospasm have an increased risk for anaphylactic shock during future episodes and should carry an epinephrine autoinjector (EpiPen) at all times.

Pharmacological treatment

• Antipruritic lotions are often helpful.

• For anaphylactic symptoms (wheezing, dyspnea, chest tightness): epinephrine 1:1000 dilution, 0.5 mL subcutaneously, repeat every 15–20 minutes for 3–4 doses until systemic symptoms resolve. Use with caution in the elderly and patients with coronary artery disease; may cause arrhythmias, hypertension, headache.

H_1 antagonists

Standard dosage — *Nonsedating*: cetirizine, 10 mg once daily to twice daily; loratadine, 10 mg once daily to twice daily; fexofenadine, 60 mg once daily to twice daily.

Sedating: hydroxyzine, 25 mg once daily to four times daily; doxepin, 10–25 mg once daily to three times daily.

Contraindications — The need to drive or operate machinery.

Special points — Nonsedating antihistamines are often used during the daytime in conjunction with sedating antihistamines at bedtime.

Main drug interactions — Alcohol and benzodiazepines may increase sedation.

Main side effects — Sedation, anticholinergic effects (dry mouth, urinary retention).

Systemic corticosteroids

For short-term use, only in severe cases.

Standard doses — Prednisone, 20–30 mg daily for 5 days.

Contraindications — Underlying systemic infection (*e.g.*, tuberculosis); use with caution in patients with a history of diabetes mellitus, hypertension, glaucoma, or peptic ulcer disease.

Main side effects — Unusual with a brief course; increased blood glucose level, hypertension, psychiatric disturbances.

Alternative medicine

Recommended use: relaxation techniques; hypnosis.

Common use: quercetin; vitamin C; vitamin B_{12}.

Caution: none.

Treatment aims

To relieve itching and reduce swelling.

Identify cause to prevent recurrence.

Other treatments

For refractory chronic urticaria:

Histamine-2 antagonists (cimetidine).

Ketotifen fumarate: mast cell stabilizer, not yet available in the United States.

Dapsone.

Colchicine.

Nifedipine.

Stanazolol.

Plasmapheresis.

Prognosis

Excellent for acute urticaria.

• 50% of patients with chronic urticaria are symptom free after 1 year.

• 20% may experience episodes for more than 20 years.

Follow-up and management

Individualized for each patient.

General references

Cooper KD: Urticaria and angioedema: diagnosis and evaluation. *J Am Acad Dermatol* 1991, **25**:166–174.

Friedmann PS: Assessment of urticaria and angio-oedema. *Clin Exp Allergy* 1999, **29(3)**:109–112.

Greaves MW: Chronic urticaria. *N Engl J Med* 1995, **332**:1767–1772.

Greaves MW, Sabroe RA: ABC of allergies. Allergy and the skin. I—Urticaria. *BMJ* 1998, **316**:1147–1150.

Reborah A, Drago F, Parodi A: May *Helicobacter pylori* be important for dermatologists? *Dermatology* 1995, **191**:6–8.

Ring J, Behrendt H: H_1 and H_2 antagonists in allergic and pseudoallergic diseases. *Clin Exp Allergy* 1990, **20**:43–49.

Sabroe RA, Greaves MW: The pathogenesis of chronic idiopathic urticaria. *Arch Dermatol* 1997, **133**:1003–1008.

Variceal bleeding

Diagnosis

Symptoms

Major hematemesis or melena: variceal bleeding is almost always massive; not occult.

Abdominal pain: crampy; cathartic effect of blood.

Confusion: in patients with poorly compensated liver disease.

Loss of consciousness: in acute volume loss, exsanguination.

Signs

Visible blood: from mouth or rectum; almost always present.

Tachycardia: orthostatic changes in blood pressure and pulse.

Skin stigmata of chronic liver disease: palmar erythema, spider angiomata, etc., should raise the suspicion of variceal bleeding in a patient with frank hemorrhage.

Hepatic encephalopathy: aggravated by volume loss, increased protein load to gut bacteria.

Investigations

Complete blood count, prothrombin time, partial thromboplastin time: to help evaluate degree of blood loss and to evaluate clotting measures.

Esophagogastroduodenoscopy: to evaluate varices and gastric mucosa for portal gastropathy.

Doppler ultrasonography: to establish patency of portal vein.

Liver chemistry tests, CT, liver biopsy: to identify cause of underlying liver disease.

Measurement of portal venous, wedged hepatic venous, or intravariceal pressure: Special investigations to evaluate unusual causes of portal hypertension or for use in studies evaluating pharmacological agents; often done when placing a transjugular intrahepatic portosystemic shunt (TIPS) to demonstrate efficacy of shunt.

Complications

Infection: in ~30% of patients during admission.

Renal failure: acute tubular necrosis, hepatorenal syndrome.

Delirium tremens, Wernicke–Korsakoff syndrome: related to alcohol withdrawal.

Ascites: precipitated by fluid overload.

Portal systemic encephalopathy: precipitated by blood in gut and liver hypoxia.

Aspiration pneumonia.

Spontaneous bacterial peritonitis.

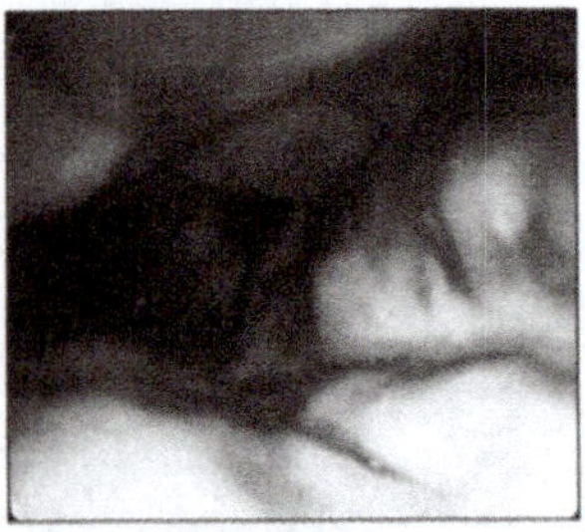

Endoscopic view of the lower esophagus showing nonbleeding esophageal varices.

Differential diagnosis

Peptic ulcer.
Mallory–Weiss tear.
Gastric erosions.
Gastric carcinoma, e.g., NSAID-related.
Portal-hypertensive gastropathy.
Gastric vascular malformations.
Esophagitis, esophageal ulcer.

Etiology

- Precipitants of variceal bleeding include the following:

Infection.
Drugs: e.g., aspirin, NSAIDs.
Development of hepatocellular carcinoma or portal-vein thrombosis in cirrhotic patients.
Heavy alcohol binges in cirrhotic patients.

Epidemiology

- Varices develop in 90% of patients with cirrhosis; the risk of hemorrhage is highest in the first 2 years after identification.
- The risk of bleeding is highest in patients with large esophageal varices (>5 mm diameter), red signs on varices, and poor liver function.

Conditions complicated by variceal bleeding

Precirrhotic severe alcoholic hepatitis/fatty liver.
Cirrhosis.
Schistosomiasis.
Splenic-vein thrombosis: usually causes gastric fundal varices, with no esophageal varices.
Budd–Chiari syndrome.
Congenital hepatic fibrosis.
Idiopathic portal hypertension.
Nodular regenerative hyperplasia of liver.
Partial nodular transformation of liver.

Pugh's modified grading of the severity of liver disease

Points	1	2	3
Encephalopathy	None	Grade 1–2	Grade 3–4
Ascites	Absent	Slight	Moderate
Bilirubin (mg/dL)	<2.0	2.0–3.0	>3.0
Albumin (g/L)	>35	28–35	<28
Prothrombin (secs, prolonged)	1–3	4–10	>10

Pugh's grade A, 5–6; B, 7–9; C, 10–15 points.

Treatment

Diet and lifestyle

- Patients must avoid NSAIDs, such as aspirin.
- Excessive amounts of acetaminophen (e.g, >4 g/day) should be avoided.
- Alcohol should be avoided.
- Patients should have ready access to acute care medical services.

Pharmacological treatment

Emergency drug treatment

- Octreotide is useful when emergency endoscopy is not available or is delayed; octreotide, 25–50 μg/h i.v. for 2–5 days [1].

Vasopressin: not as effective and associated with significant complications, which can be reduced with the concomitant use of nitroglycerin.

Prophylaxis: primary and secondary

- Propranolol reduces the risk of first hemorrhage; the resting pulse rate should be reduced to 60 beats/min or by 25% of the pretreatment rate. Treatment is recommended in cirrhotic patients with large varices and red signs. Beta-blockade also reduces bleeding from portal gastropathy and possibly reduces the risk of recurrent variceal bleeding.
- For prevention of recurrent hemorrhage, endoscopic banding or sclerotherapy should be repeated until varices are obliterated.

Nonpharmacological treatment

Resuscitation

Airway protection to prevent aspiration.

Insertion of large i.v. line (cross-matching of at least 6 units of blood).

Crystalloid and colloid infusion to maintain euvolemia until cross-matched blood is available.

Insertion of central venous line to guide further replacement therapy when systolic blood pressure >100 mm Hg.

Fresh frozen plasma to correct clotting abnormalities.

Platelet transfusion if thrombocytopenia exists.

Emergency treatment

Emergency endoscopy to confirm variceal bleeding.

Local, immediate treatment can be provided, ideally by using endoscopic banding (lower rates of rebleeding and complications), although sclerotherapy may be more readily available. Several studies have now shown that ligation therapy is also useful in patients with large varices but no prior episodes of bleeding.

Balloon tamponade for temporary control of bleeding or bleeding refractory to sclerotherapy, banding; TIPS [1].

Other options

TIPS: if emergency endoscopic treatment fails; also under evaluation for prevention of recurrent hemorrhages, but high rate of shunt occlusion (30% at 1 year) and encephalopathy (10%–20%) [2].

Emergency shunt surgery.

Emergency esophageal transection.

Liver transplantation: can be considered for prevention of recurrent hemorrhage in patients with liver failure.

Treatment aims [3]

- The aims of treatment, in order of importance, are as follows:

To resuscitate the patient.

To control bleeding quickly.

To maintain liver function.

To identify and treat complications.

To prevent rebleeding.

Prognosis

- Esophageal band ligation or sclerotherapy has high success rates, with bleeding controlled in 90% of patients and variceal size reduced after 2–3 sessions.
- 70% of patients rebleed after balloon tamponade, so definitive treatment must be arranged.
- Mortality is 30%–40% with the first variceal bleed, 15%–20% with subsequent bleeds.
- Prognosis depends on the underlying liver function.
- Approximately one-third of deaths in cirrhotic patients are related to bleeding.

Follow-up and management

- Patients should be followed up every 3 months for the first year after the varices have been obliterated by band ligation or sclerotherapy.
- After TIPS placement, Doppler ultrasound should be performed every 6 months to evaluate shunt patency.

Key references

1. Roberts LR, Kamath PS: Pathophysiology and treatment of variceal hemorrhage. *Mayo Clin Proc* 1996, **71**:973–983.
2. Papatheodoridis GV, *et al.*: Transjugular intrahepatic portosystemic shunt compared with endoscopic treatment for prevention of variceal bleedings: a meta-analysis. *Hepatology* 1999, **30**:612–622.
3. Saeed ZA, Woods KL: Gastrointestinal bleeding. *Curr Pract Med* 1998, **1**:785–796.

Diagnosis

Symptoms

Pruritis, pain.

Fever, malaise, arthralgias.

Symptoms of the predisposing disease.

Signs

Painful, palpable purpura: the three "P's."

Crops of violaceous nodules: usually in dependent areas (lower extremities, buttocks, arms).

Lesions: tender; do not blanch; hemorrhagic blisters; black, necrotic, ulcerating in severe disease.

Subcutaneous nodules along arteries: indicating polyarteritis nodosa.

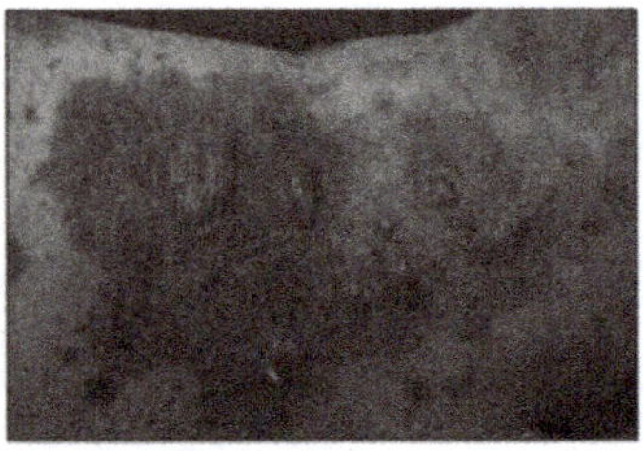

Cutaneous vasculitis on the legs, showing red/purple palpable painful lesions, some of which have overlying hemorrhagic blisters. (*See* Color Plate.)

Investigations

To confirm the diagnosis:

Skin biopsy: may be helpful in identifying infiltrating inflammatory cells, type and size of blood vessels involved, and whether granulomatous changes are present; special stains may identify infectious organisms.

To identify systemic involvement:

Urinalysis, urine microscopy, serum creatinine measurement: to identify renal involvement.

Liver function tests: to identify hepatic involvement.

Other laboratory testing as indicated by thorough history and physical examination.

To identify an underlying cause:

Measurement of rheumatoid factor, antinuclear antibodies, anticardiolipin antibodies: to identify connective tissue disorders.

Blood culture, culture of possible sites of infection: to identify infectious cause.

Cryoglobulin measurement: collected after fasting and taken to laboratory at 37 °C.

Measurement of antineutrophil cytoplasmic antibodies: to identify specific vasculitides.

Complications

Ulceration: particularly on lower limbs.

Secondary infection.

Renal involvement: in 30%–60% of patients.

Joint, gastrointestinal tract, CNS, or lung involvement.

Peripheral neuropathy.

Differential diagnosis

Nonpalpable purpura:

Thrombocytopenic purpura.

Platelet dysfunction.

Corticosteroid treatment.

Disseminated intravascular coagulation.

Skin fragility (age, actinic damage).

Nonaccidental injury in children.

Scurvy.

Kaposi's sarcoma.

Septic emboli.

Etiology

Vasculitis may be of a specific type (Wegener's granulomatosis, polyarteritis nodosa), may be infectious (Rocky Mountain spotted fever, meningococcemia), or may be a nonspecific leukocytoclastic vasculitis.

Leukocytoclastic vasculitis is also known as hypersensitivity vasculitis because, although it may be idiopathic, it often represents a reaction to an underlying stimulus. These include:

Infections: group A streptococcus, hepatitis B, hepatitis C (leading to mixed cryoglobulinemia), leprosy.

Drugs: penicillins, sulfonamides.

Connective tissue disease: rheumatoid arthritis, Sjögren's syndrome, systemic lupus erythematosus.

Malignancy: Hodgkin's lymphoma, leukemia.

Epidemiology

- Vasculitis is a relatively common condition.
- The male:female ratio is equal.
- It can affect people at any age.

Treatment

Diet and lifestyle

- Bed rest during acute episodes.

Pharmacological treatment

- Treatment should center on identification of an underlying cause.
- Drugs that are probable causes of vasculitis should be discontinued.
- Precipitating infections should be treated.

Indomethacin

NSAIDs such as indomethacin may relieve symptoms in acute cutaneous vasculitis.

Standard dosage Indomethacin, 25–50 mg one to three times daily.

Contraindications Active peptic ulcer disease, previous hypersensitivity reaction, renal insufficiency.

Main drug interactions Warfarin may exacerbate active peptic ulcer disease.

Side effects Gastrointestinal.

Dapsone

Dapsone may be used in refractory chronic vasculitis.

Standard dosage Dapsone, 50–200 mg daily.

Contraindications Glucose-6-phosphate dehydrogenase deficiency, severe anemia, poorly compensated congestive heart failure.

Main side effects Gastrointestinal, peripheral motor neuropathy, dose-related hemolysis and methemoglobinemia, idiosyncratic agranulocytosis and hepatotoxicity.

Prednisone

Usage should be limited to patients with severe progressive systemic disease.

Standard dosage Prednisone, 40–60 mg daily initially, then tapered as tolerated.

Contraindications Underlying systemic infection (*e.g.*, tuberculosis); use caution in patients with a history of osteoporosis, diabetes mellitus, hypertension, glaucoma, or peptic ulcer disease.

Main side effects Osteoporosis, increased blood glucose level, hypertension, peptic ulceration, weight gain, psychiatric disturbances.

Treatment aims

To alleviate discomfort.

To minimize cutaneous complications.

To identify and treat any underlying disease.

To detect systemic involvement early.

Other treatments

Antihistamines (symptomatic relief).

Colchicine.

Hydroxychloroquine.

Immunosuppressive agents (azathioprine, methotrexate).

Prognosis

- Individual episodes may clear after 3–6 weeks.
- Relapse and chronic disease are common.
- Patients with infective or drug-induced vasculitis usually recover fully on removal of the cause, although chronic vasculitis or, rarely, fatal systemic necrotizing vasculitis occurs.

Follow-up and management

Dictated by severity and duration of vasculitis, and of any underlying cause.

General references

Berlit P: The spectrum of vasculopathies in the differential diagnosis of vasculitis. *Semin Neurol* 1994, **14**:370–379.

Blanco R, *et al.*: Cutaneous vasculitis in children and adults. Associated diseases and etiologic factors in 303 patients. *Medicine* 1998, **77**:403–418.

Lotti T, *et al.*: Cutaneous small-vessel vasculitis. *J Am Acad Dermatol* 1998, **39** (5 Pt 1):667–687.

Somer T, Finegold SM: Vasculidities associated with infections, immunization, and antimicrobial drugs. *Clin Infect Dis* 1995, **20**:1010–1036.

Watts RA, Scott DG: ABC of rheumatology, rashes, and vasculitis. *BMJ* 1995, **310(6987)**:1128–1132.

Vasculitis, systemic

Diagnosis

Symptoms

• Symptoms depend on the size and site of the vessel involved. The following concentrates particularly on primary systemic vasculitis involving small- and medium-sized arteries.

Malaise, weight loss, fever, diffuse myalgia, arthralgia.
Symptoms of any underlying disease or secondary vasculitis: *e.g.*, rheumatoid arthritis, SLE.
Rash.
Epistaxis, nasal crusting, sinusitis: especially in Wegener's granulomatosis.
Chest pain, hemoptysis, dyspnea, cough, late-onset asthma (normally precedes Churg–Strauss syndrome).
Mouth ulcers, abdominal pain, diarrhea.
Numbness, weakness.

Signs

Pyrexia, lymphadenopathy, muscle wasting, weakness.
Microscopic hematuria or proteinuria, or both.
Skin purpura, ulcer, infarction.
Nasal crusting or collapse, septal perforation: especially in Wegener's granulomatosis.
Crackles, wheeze, cardiomyopathy, pericarditis: especially in Churg–Strauss vasculitis.
Mononeuritis or mononeuritis multiplex, peripheral neuropathy.
Arthritis: usually of large joints.

Investigations

Urinalysis: most urgent investigation because renal involvement influences prognosis.
Plasma urea and creatinine, 24-hour urinary protein and creatinine clearance measurement: to assess renal function.
Complete blood count: shows anemia, leukocytosis (leukocyte count normal or low in vasculitis secondary to rheumatoid arthritis or SLE), eosinophilia (especially in Churg–Strauss vasculitis), thrombocytosis.
ESR, CRP, and liver enzyme (*e.g.*, alkaline phosphatase) measurement: raised values.
Antineutrophil cytoplasmic autoantibody analysis: most useful for diagnosis; diffuse cytoplasmic staining (anti-proteinase III) in 80% of patients with systemic Wegener's granulomatosis, 50% limited Wegener's; perinuclear staining less specific (antimyeloperoxidase) but common in microscopic polyangiitis and idiopathic crescentic glomerulonephritis [1,2].
Other autoantibody tests: antinuclear antibody and rheumatoid factor nonspecific; may reflect underlying disease; C3 and C4 usually increased in primary vasculitis, low or normal in vasculitis associated with SLE and rheumatoid arthritis; high levels of cryoglobulins may indicate need for plasma exchange.
von Willebrand's factor antigen test: measure of vascular damage; also increased in noninflammatory vascular injury (*e.g.*, thrombosis).
Viral studies: for hepatitis B, cytomegalovirus, Epstein–Barr virus.
Chest radiography: shows nodules, fibrosis, infiltrate.
Sinus radiography: shows sinusitis, bone destruction.
Angiography: shows microaneurysms in up to 70% of patients with polyarteritis nodosa; rarely with Wegener's granulomatosis and Churg–Strauss vasculitis.
Two-dimensional echocardiography: to exclude vegetations and atrial myxoma.
Biopsy: of kidney, skin, nose, muscle, sural nerve, rectum, or temporal artery.

Complications

Renal failure: acute, especially if diagnosis or treatment delayed, or chronic (<10% of patients dependent on dialysis).
Gangrene or infarction: can lead to amputation or chronic skin ulcer.
Neuropathy: possibly permanent (*e.g.*, footdrop), although 60% improve on treatment.
Subglottic stenosis: leading to tracheostomy.
Nasal collapse: permanent and may necessitate later plastic surgery.
Severe pulmonary hemorrhage: may cause breathlessness; and unexplained anemia.
Coronary arteritis: may cause myocardial infarction and heart failure.
Hypertension.

Differential diagnosis

Nonspecific systemic illness
Infection: subacute bacterial endocarditis, other chronic and atypical infections.
Connective tissue disease.
Malignancy: especially myeloproliferative, metastatic disease, multiple myeloma.
Sarcoid, HIV, Goodpasture's syndrome.

Vasculopathy and necrotizing granuloma
Lymphomatoid granulomatosis, idiopathic midline granuloma.
Cholesterol atheroembolism.
Cardiac myxoma, antiphospholipid antibody syndrome.

Etiology

• Causes include the following:
Autoimmune: autoantibodies, *e.g.*, antineutrophil cytoplasmic autoantibodies in Wegener's granulomatosis.
Immune complex: particularly secondary vasculitis associated with SLE and rheumatoid arthritis.
Viral infection: *e.g.*, hepatitis B, HIV, cytomegalovirus.
Neoplasms (especially hematological).

Epidemiology

• The annual incidence may be increasing, ~40 per million being affected each year.
• The male:female ratio is 1.5:1.
• The age range is wide, with an increasing incidence with age in women.

Classification

Large-artery
Giant-cell arteritis, Takayasu's arteritis.

Medium-artery
Polyarteritis nodosa, Kawasaki disease.

Medium- or small-artery
Wegener's granulomatosis, Churg–Strauss vasculitis, microscopic polyangiitis.

Small-vessel
Henoch–Schönlein purpura, essential mixed cryoglobulinemia, leukocytoclastic cutaneous vasculitis.

• Secondary vasculitis, *e.g.*, infection, drugs, rheumatoid arthritis, SLE, and Sjögren's syndrome, usually involves either medium or small arteries or pure small vessel.

Treatment

Diet and lifestyle

• Because they are often immunosuppressed, patients should take precautions against possible infections.

Pharmacological treatment [3,4]

Steroids

• Steroids are only used alone in patients with small-vessel or large-artery disease (*see* Classification).

Standard dosage	*Continuous:* prednisolone, 15–60 mg orally depending on severity and type of vasculitis; usually reducing course. *Pulse:* methylprednisolone, 1 g i.v. or 100 mg orally for 3 days; dose and frequency varied according to response.
Contraindications	Infection (*e.g.*, subacute bacterial endocarditis).
Special points	Adrenal suppression may be a problem with long-term treatment.
Main drug interactions	Drugs that induce liver enzymes promote steroid metabolism; prednisolone antagonizes antihypertensive treatment.
Main side effects	Diabetes, hypertension, osteoporosis, mood change, cushingoid appearance.

Immunosuppressants

• Immunosuppressants are indicated for more severe vasculitis, particularly of small or medium artery.

Standard dosage	*Continuous:* cyclophosphamide, 2 mg/kg orally daily. *Pulse:* cyclophosphamide, 15 mg/kg i.v.; alternatively, 5 mg/kg orally daily for 3 days; dose and frequency vary according to response, renal function, and leukocyte count (measured at 7, 10, and 14 days).
Contraindications	Pregnancy (first trimester especially), uncontrolled infection.
Main drug interactions	None.
Main side effects	Bone-marrow suppression, hemorrhagic cystitis (rare with pulse treatment), nausea, alopecia, infertility.

Combination treatment

Pulse i.v. cyclophosphamide, 15 mg/kg, and methylprednisolone, 1 g every 2 weeks for 6 courses (remission induction), then every 3 weeks for 2 pulses, then monthly for 3 pulses (maintenance).

Pulse oral cyclophosphamide, 5 mg/kg daily, and prednisone, 100–200 mg daily for 3 consecutive days; interval between treatments as for pulse i.v. treatment.

Continuous oral cyclophosphamide, 2 mg/kg daily, and prednisone, 40–60 mg daily; prednisolone reduced to 20 mg daily by month 3, to 10 mg daily by month 6.

• Cyclophosphamide should be withdrawn at 9–12 months.

• Longer treatment or change to azathioprine, 2 mg/kg daily, is often needed in patients with Wegener's granulomatosis or rheumatoid vasculitis.

• Methotrexate may be an effective steroid-sparing agent.

Other drugs

Azathioprine: steroid-sparing and immunosuppressive.

Plasmapheresis: for pulmonary hemorrhage and severe renal disease.

Treatment aims

To induce and maintain remission.

To recognize and treat relapses early.

To avoid toxicity and side effects.

Prognosis

• In patients with Wegener's granulomatosis or polyarteritis nodosa, 75% remit and 50% relapse with continuous oral treatment.

• The 2-year survival rate ranges from 10% with no treatment to 80% with cyclophosphamide treatment.

• For patients with small-vessel vasculitis, the prognosis is good.

Follow-up and management

• Long-term follow-up is essential, with regular clinical examination, complete blood count, renal function tests (especially urinalysis), and immunology.

• Daily steroids are more often used for large- and small-vessel vasculitis, with reduction in dose when the patient is in remission, aiming for alternate-day treatment.

• Early recognition of relapse is essential.

Key references

1. Gross WL, Schmitt WH, Caernok E: ANCA associated diseases: a rheumatologist's perspective. *Am J Kidney Dis* 1991, **2**:175–179.
2. Hoffman G: Wegener's granulomatosis: an analysis of 158 patients. *Ann Intern Med* 1992, **116**:488–498.
3. Chakravarty K, Scott DGI: Management of systemic vasculitis. *Rheumatol Rev* 1992, **1**:81–99.
4. Griffith ME, Gaskin G, Pusey CD: Classification, pathogenesis, and treatment of systemic vasculitis. *Ren Fail* 1996, **18**:785–802.

Viral warts

Diagnosis

Symptoms

Most warts are asymptomatic.

Concerns about cosmetic appearance in common or flat warts.

Emotional upset resulting from diagnosis of a sexually transmitted disease in genital warts.

Warts sometimes cause severe pain (especially plantar warts).

Signs

Common wart (verruca vulgaris)

Well-demarcated verrucous papule with "seeds" (*i.e.*, thrombosed capillaries).

Plantar wart (verruca plantaris)

Hyperkeratotic plaque: on the plantar surface of the feet, often painful to pressure.

Flat wart (verruca plana)

1–3-mm flat-topped papules: on face, legs (spread by shaving), or elsewhere.

Genital wart (condyloma acuminatum)

White moist or keratotic papules: occur anywhere on the anogenital skin or mucosa.

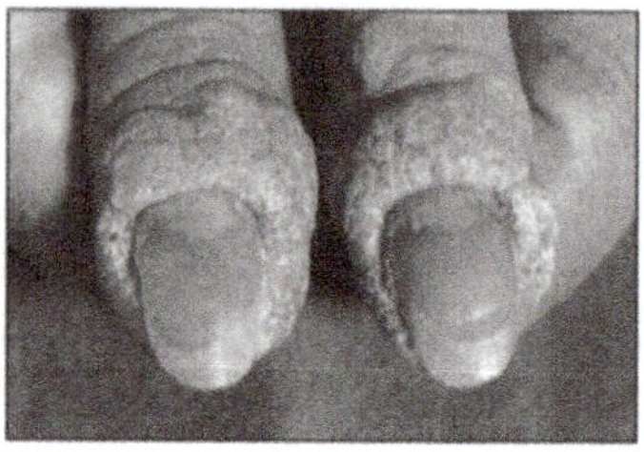

Periungual viral warts. (See Color Plate.)

Investigations

- A viral wart is a clinical diagnosis.

Rapid plasma reagin test: to rule out secondary syphilis if condyloma latum is considered.

Biopsy: in select cases to rule out verrucous carcinoma.

Colposcopy: indicated in female patients with condyloma and an abnormal Papanicolauo smear or an obvious cervical lesion.

Proctoscopy and cytoscopy.

Screening for chlamydia, gonorrhea, HIV: patients with genital warts are at risk for other sexually transmitted diseases.

Virus typing: to identify human papillomavirus types with an increased incidence of malignancy and facilitate aggressive treatment. Not yet available for widespread use.

Complications

- Extensive involvement in immunosuppressed patients.

Oncogenic potential: squamous cell carcinoma of cervix or glans penis secondary to human papillomavirus subtypes 16, 18, 31, 33, and 35.

Urogenital dysplasia and carcinoma: associated with anogenital and laryngeal warts and cervical condylomata.

Obstruction of urethral meatus: by urethral condyloma, making treatment extremely difficult.

Laryngeal condyloma: can develop in children born to mothers with condyloma acuminatum, causing respiratory difficulty in the infant; laryngeal condyloma can also occur in surgeons after treating condyloma with carbon dioxide laser.

Differential diagnosis

Corn/callus

Stucco keratosis (form of seborrheic keratosis resembling verruca planae).

Condyloma latum.

Arsenical keratosis.

Molluscum contagiosum.

Acrochordon (skin tag).

Epidermodysplasia verruciformis.

Etiology

Cause

Human papillomavirus infections; sensitive DNA hybridization techniques have identified more than 60 types of viral DNA.

Spread

- Spread of viral warts is by contact (*i.e.*, skin to skin in verruca vulgaris; sexual contact with condyloma acuminatum; maternal genital tract for neonates).

Epidemiology

- Anogenital warts occur most often in young sexually active patients.
- Common warts occur most often in children and young adults.

Treatment

Diet and lifestyle

Condyloma acuminatum

- Close prenatal care and counseling is recommended for pregnant women.
- Education and the importance of examination and treatment of sexual partners should be emphasized.
- Condoms should be used.

Pharmacological treatment

- Treatment should be individualized, as treatment is difficult and no one method can be used in all patients with equal success.

For cutaneous warts

Standard dosage Salicylic acid as ointments, plasters, gels (concentration from 10%–50%) applied nightly for 3–4 months.
Tretinoin solution applied daily to flat warts.

Contraindications Local hypersensitivity.

Special points The main objective is to cause inflammation but not infection or scarring.

Main drug interactions None.

Main side effects Skin irritation and pain.

For anogenital warts

Standard dosage Podofilox: 0.5% gel, applied twice daily on 3 consecutive days per week for 4 weeks.

Podophyllin: 25% solution, applied biweekly only in a physician's office.

Imiquimod: 5% cream, applied three times per week.

Contraindications Widespread areas of involvement due to possible systemic absorption.

Special points Treatment is individualized with respect to severity of disease.

Main side effects Local irritation, burning, ulceration, pain, and blistering.

Second-line treatment

Liquid nitrogen: either applied or sprayed onto the wart in order to cause a blister; repeated at 2–4-week intervals.

Electrodesiccation and curettage: often results in scarring.

CO_2 laser: may result in scarring.

Pulsed dye laser.

Cantharidin: a blistering agent that is painless to apply and is indicated for children who cannot tolerate cryotherapy; applied only in a physician's office and to limited areas of the body.

Intralesional bleomycin: for refractory warts; leads to hemorrhagic blisters.

Intralesional or systemic interferon-alpha therapy: for refractory anogenital warts; side effects include fever, chills, myalgia, headache, and leukopenia.

- Cimetidine therapy at a dose of 30–40 mg/kg/day is a useful adjuvant therapy for multiple viral warts in children. The mechanism of action is unknown but appears to up-regulate the immune system against the wart virus. Therapy should be continued for 3 months.

Alternative medicine

Recommended use: None.

Common use: ceder (*Thuja occidentalis*); dandelion latex (*Taraxacum officinale*); hypnotherapy; lemon; multiple folk remedies.

Caution: folk remedies may include caustic substances, such as bleach or drain cleaners.

Treatment aims

To clear clinical disease without causing scarring.

Other treatments

Hypnosis, particularly in children.

Contact sensitization.

Prognosis

No treatment definitively eradicates the virus; warts may recur after successful treatment.

Follow-up and management

- Routine cervical cytology in women with anogenital warts is warranted because of the oncogenic potential (colposcopy if indicated).

General references

Benton EC: Therapy of cutaneous warts. *Clin Dermatol* 1997, **15**:449–455.

Drake LA, *et al.*: Guidelines for care of warts: human papillomavirus. Committee on Guidelines of Care. *J Am Acad Dermatol* 1995, **32**:98–103.

Edwards L, *et al.*: Self administered topical 5% imiquimod cream for external anogenital warts. *Arch Dermatol* 1998, **134**:25–30.

Ewin DM: Hypnotherapy for warts (verruca vulgaris): 41 consecutive cases with 33 cures. *Am J Clin Hypn* 1992, **35**:1–10.

Reichman RC, *et al.*: Treatment of condyloma acuminatum with three different interferon-alpha preparations administered parenterally: a double-blind placebo-controlled trial. *J Infect Dis* 1990, **162**:1270.

Rogers CJ, *et al.*: Cimetidine therapy for recalcitrant warts in adults: is it any better than placebo? *J Am Acad Dermatol* 1999, **41**:123–127.

Tyring S, *et al.*: Safety and efficacy of 0.5% podofilox gel in the treatment of anogenital warts. *Arch Dermatol* 1998, **134**:33–38.

Waldenström's macroglobulinemia

Diagnosis

Symptoms

Fatigue, weakness, weight loss: in >80% of patients.

Bleeding tendency: in 60%.

Sensorimotor peripheral neuropathy: in 15%.

Headache, dizziness, vertigo, confusion, stroke, drowsiness, breathlessness, dependent edema: features of hyperviscosity syndrome in 20%.

Epistaxis, gastrointestinal hemorrhage, dependent purpura.

Signs

Lymphadenopathy: in 40%.

Splenomegaly: in 30%.

Hepatomegaly: in 30%.

Peripheral neuropathy: in 15%.

Ataxia; nystagmus; hemiplegia; dementia; coma; signs of congestive cardiac failure; dependent purpura; hemorrhage; dilated, tortuous retinal veins with "sausage-like" segmentation; retinal hemorrhage; papilledema: signs of hyperviscosity syndrome.

Investigations [1]

Complete blood count: shows normocytic, normochromic anemia in 80% of patients; rouleaux, sometimes spuriously raised mean cell volume, neutropenia, thrombocytopenia; lymphocytes may be increased but seldom $>5 \times 10^9$/L.

Cell marker analysis: surface immunoglobulin of single light chain class (κ or λ); $CD19^+$, $CD20^+$, $CD37^+$, $CD38^+$, $CD5^-$, $CD10^-$.

Bone-marrow aspiration: increase in small lymphocytes and plasmacytoid lymphocytes, sometimes in plasma cells.

Serum electrophoresis: monoclonal spike in β- or γ-globulins; identifiable as IgM by immunoelectrophoresis; serum IgG and IgA often reduced.

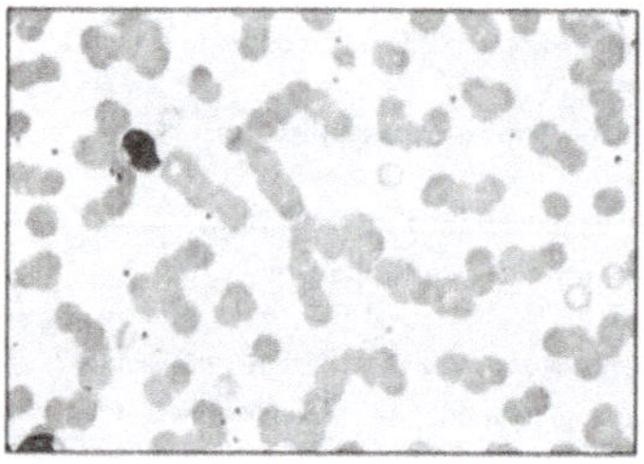

Rouleaux on Romanowsky-stained blood film. (*See* Color Plate.)

Plasma viscosity measurement: raised; hyperviscosity syndrome only if relative serum viscosity >4 times water, and patient is symptomatic.

Cryoglobulin analysis: proteins that precipitate at 4°C found in 15% of patients.

Cold agglutinin analysis: erythrocyte autoantibodies (anti-I or anti-i) agglutinate erythrocytes in the cold; idiopathic acquired variety monoclonal IgM.

• Clotting studies may indicate a pseudo-von Willebrand's state with prolonged activated partial thromboplastin time, bleeding time, and abnormal platelet function.

Complications

Amyloid: in <10%.

IgM monoclonal protein autoantibody activity: occasionally.

Peripheral neuropathy, cold agglutination syndrome, acquired hemophilia: due, respectively, to antimyelin, antierythrocyte, and anti-factor VIII antibodies.

Differential diagnosis

Diseases associated with IgM monoclonal proteins:

Essential (benign) monoclonal macroglobulinemia (27%).

Cold agglutinin syndrome (3%).

Chronic lymphocytic leukemia (10%).

Other B-cell lymphomas (30%).

IgM myeloma (3%).

Extramedullary plasmacytoma (2%).

Waldenström's macroglobulinemia (25%).

Etiology

• Presumably, a mutation event occurs in a susceptible clone.

• Proliferation of antibody-producing cells in response to antigenic stimulation may become autonomous when a mutation leads to a lack of control of the cell cycle.

Epidemiology

• Waldenström's macroglobulinemia is predominantly a disease of the elderly, the median age at presentation being 65 years.

• The annual incidence is 1 in 200 000.

• It occurs more often in men than women.

• Familial incidence is slightly increased.

Bleeding abnormalities

• The IgM paraprotein interferes with the formation of the platelet plug.

• Platelet adhesiveness is reduced, as is the release of platelet factor 3.

• The paraprotein also interferes with the coagulation cascade and may be an antibody against factor VIII.

• Some paraproteins bind to fibrin and inhibit fibrin monomer aggregation, resulting in a bulky gelatinous clot with impaired clot retraction.

• Factor X deficiencies may be seen in patients who develop amyloidosis.

Treatment

Diet and lifestyle

• The patient should be encouraged to live as normal a life as possible.

Pharmacological treatment

• Chlorambucil, given under specialist supervision, is the mainstay of treatment, but only ~50% of patients respond.

• Other alkylating agents give similar responses and probably could be used interchangeably.

• Recent reports have suggested that fludarabine and 2-chlorodeoxyadenasine [2,3] are useful drugs. Reports indicate that α-interferon may be of value [2].

Standard dosage	Chlorambucil orally daily for 2 weeks every 4 weeks.
Contraindications	No absolute contraindications.
Special points	Full blood count essential because chlorambucil may cause bone-marrow suppression.
Main drug interactions	No major interactions known.
Main side effects	Bone-marrow suppression, nausea and vomiting, diarrhea, oral ulcers, hypersensitivity rashes, occasionally myelodysplasia, acute leukemia.

Treatment aims

To relieve symptoms.

To prolong life.

Other treatments

• Plasma exchange should be instituted urgently for hyperviscosity syndrome; one plasma volume exchanged at regular intervals until relative viscosity <4 times that of water.

• Maintenance plasmapheresis alone may be sufficient to control the disease; viscosity need not be restored to normal.

Prognosis

• The disease is not curable.

• Median survival is 4 years in patients who respond to treatment, 2 years in non-responders; the peripheral neuropathy is frequently unresponsive.

Follow-up and management

• Patients should be followed up at regular intervals.

• Full blood count and IgM concentrations should be monitored.

• Plasma viscosity indicates whether plasmapheresis is indicated.

• No large controlled trials are available to guide the physician. By analogy with other low-grade lymphomas, it is reasonable to withhold treatment in asymptomatic patients.

Key references

1. Pangalis GA, Angelopoulou MK, Vassilakopoulos TP, *et al.*: B-chronic lymphocytic leukemia, small lymphocytic lymphoma, and lymphoplasmacytic lymphoma, including Waldenström's macroglobulinemia: a clinical, morphologic, and biologic spectrum of similar disorders. *Semin Hematol* 1999, **36**:104–114.
2. Dimopoulos MA, O'Brien S, Kantarjian HM, *et al.*: Fludarabine therapy in Waldenström's macroglobulinemia. *Am J Med* 1993, **95**:49–52.
3. Dimopoulos MA, Kantarjian HM, Estey E, *et al.*: Treatment of Waldenström macroglobulinemia with 2-chloro-deoxyadenosine. *Ann Intern Med* 1993, **118**:195–198.

Wolff–Parkinson–White syndrome

Diagnosis

Definition

• Myocardial activation from atrial to ventricular myocardium occurs over an accessory connection (accessory to the normal His-Purkinje system).

• If conduction occurs in sinus rhythm, pre-excitation is apparent on the ECG; the combination of short PR interval and a delta wave is the electrocardiographic signature of this condition.

• The substrate for atrioventricular re-entry tachycardia is present; conduction in tachycardia from ventricle to atrium over the accessory connection is orthodromic (90%) or from atrium to ventricle is antidromic.

Symptoms

Palpitation: most common symptom; caused by re-entry tachycardia (sudden onset and termination; regular, rapid—often >200 beats/min); may also be caused by paroxysmal atrial fibrillation (in ~5% of patients).
Chest pain: during tachycardia; pain or discomfort similar to angina; rarely indicates coronary artery disease.
Impaired consciousness: dizziness or faintness common; syncope less frequent (5%) and usually follows vasodilatation occurring as a secondary response to tachycardia.
Polyuria: accompanying sustained episodes of tachycardia.

Sudden death: although unusual, may be the first clinical manifestation of this syndrome.

Signs

• In sinus rhythm, no clinical signs indicate the presence of the condition. During tachycardia, clinical signs associated with the impaired circulation and abnormal cardiac action may be found, including: rapid pulse, hypotension, alteration in the venous form.

Investigations

Pre-excitation ECG: the QRS configuration (*i.e.*, pre-excitation) is generated by fusion of ventricular activation from the normal His-Purkinje system and accessory atrioventricular connection—the myocardium activated through the accessory pathway gives rise to the delta wave (slurred initial QRS); precise delta wave pattern depends on the location of accessory connection on atrioventricular ring. Pre-excitation changes depend on the balance of activation between the normal and accessory pathways (both influenced by autonomic tone). The short PR interval results from myocardial activation through the accessory connection, which lacks decremental conduction properties

ECG during tachycardia: in 90% narrow complex tachycardia; no delta wave because during orthodromic tachycardia the ventricles are depolarized over the normal atrioventricular conduction system. Broad QRS complex tachycardia in antidromic conduction or rate-related bundle branch block (aberrancy).

Ambulatory monitoring: paroxysms of tachycardia may be seen on 24- or 48-hour monitoring; usually too infrequent for capture of tachycardia to be probable; self-activated recording devices (cardiac memo/wrist recorder) with transtelephonic transmission to a recording center may be useful.

Electrophysiologic study: the most reliable method of determining the refractory period of the accessory pathway and the number of pathways present. Such a study is recommended as part of the routine evaluation of all *symptomatic* patients, *even in the absence of documented tachycardia.* The anterograde effective refractory period of the accessory pathway is probably the most important factor in determining the risk of ventricular fibrillation during atrial fibrillation. A value below 250 msec has been used to segregate patients who are at particular risk.

Complications

Atrial fibrillation and atrial flutter: are particularly hazardous and result in ventricular rates that approach or exceed 300 beats/min and ventricular fibrillation can occur under such circumstances; it may be a particular risk in patients with multiple accessory pathways. In atrial fibrillation ECG is irregularly irregular; variable QRS configuration.

Sudden death: rare

Differential diagnosis

Atrioventricular nodal re-entry tachycardia: tachycardia due to dual atrioventricular node physiology allowing re-entry within the atrioventricular node; other types of supraventricular tachycardia (*e.g.*, atrial flutter, atrial fibrillation, ectopic atrial tachycardia, Mahaim re-entry).

Ventricular tachycardia: broad QRS complexes (due to antidromic tachycardia or aberrant conduction) may be misdiagnosed as tachycardia arising from a ventricular focus.

Etiology

• Wolff–Parkinson–White syndrome is not inherited. However, when associated with hypertrophic cardiomyopathy, it maps to a locus on chromosome 7q3.

• Accessory connections appear microscopically to be normal myocardial muscle bundles bridging atrial and ventricular myocardium; they may have subepicardial or subendocardial locations; they are multiple in ~10% of patients with the condition.

• Ebstein's anomaly is associated with their presence, and multiple pathways are more common in these patients.

Epidemiology

• Early studies have suggested that ECG evidence of pre-excitation can be found in 0.3% of the population; probably only a few of such patients are symptomatic, but the evidence is conflicting.

• Depending on the nature of the population studies, documentation of tachycardia has varied from 5% to 90% of patients.

Treatment

Diet and lifestyle

• In patients with frequent symptoms, lifestyle is restricted by the occurrence of palpitations (often apparently related to stress or exertion) or by the side effects of drug treatment.

Pharmacological treatment

• Drugs are now considered second-line treatment.

• Asymptomatic patients need no drug treatment unless their occupation demands removal of all risk of tachycardia (*e.g.*, airline pilots, certain military, police, and fire-brigade personnel).

• Symptomatic patients who need treatment but who do not wish to have radiofrequency catheter ablation can be given antiarrhythmic drugs; these exert their effect by altering atrioventricular nodal conduction, accessory connection conduction, or both, so that re-entry tachycardia will less probably be sustained.

• Drugs that slow atrioventricular nodal conduction but enhance accessory pathway conduction (*e.g.*, digoxin, calcium channel blockers, adenosine) should not be used in isolation.

• Antiarrhythmic drugs often have unacceptable side effects, and some have been shown to have dangerous proarrhythmic effects.

• Drugs must be taken continuously, and not on an ad-hoc basis, to give optimal control of symptoms; even then, abolition of symptoms is rare.

• Atrial fibrillation in these patients is best treated with intravenous procainamide, which slows the ventricular rate by blocking conduction over the accessory pathways. Electrical cardioversion may also be used when necessary.

• The choice of maintenance therapy should be made only after electrophysiologic study to assess the anterograde refractory period of the accessory pathway(s) and the risk of hazardous rates during atrial fibrillation.

• Class I antiarrhythmic agents that lengthen the refractory period of the accessory pathway and reduce ventricular rates during atrial fibrillation are agents of choice for maintenance therapy. Flecainide, propafenone (in those with no associated heart disease), quinidine, procainamide, and disopyramide can be used.

Nonpharmacological treatment

Catheter ablation

• Catheter ablation is technically demanding but is associated with very low mortality and morbidity rates in skilled hands.

• Apposition of an ablation electrode to the endocardial location nearest the accessory connection results in cessation of accessory connection conduction on delivery of radiofrequency energy through the electrode.

• This is a low-voltage, high-frequency energy source, which results in heating of the electrode tip, in turn producing a small endocardial lesion (5–7 mm) that extends into the myocardium.

• Primary success is >90%.

Successful ablation results in the disappearance of the delta wave and further episodes of tachycardia.

• In approximately 10% of patients, accessory conduction will return within 2 months after apparently successful ablation, requiring a second procedure.

• Radiofrequency catheter ablation is the treatment of choice because it is curative; other energy sources are available but are associated with various disadvantages.

• Complete atrioventricular block requiring a permanent pacemaker may occur in 0.3% of patients, all of whom have septal accessory pathways.

Surgery

• Although curative, surgical division of accessory connections needs major cardiac surgery and so is associated with higher morbidity and mortality rates than catheter ablation.

• It should be reserved for patients in whom catheter ablation has failed repeatedly.

Treatment aims

To abolish accessory connection conduction and therefore risk of tachycardia and palpitation.

To remove risk of sudden cardiac death.

To assess risk in asymptomatic patients.

Prognosis

• The prognosis is probably that of the normal population after successful catheter ablation.

• Lesions induced by radiofrequency catheter ablation have not been associated with impairment of ventricular function or arrhythmogenic complications except in infant hearts, when lesions may grow with heart size.

• Untreated asymptomatic Wolff–Parkinson–White syndrome carries a good prognosis; the risk of sudden death in asymptomatic patients is probably very small.

Follow-up and management

• Recurrence of pre-excitation may occur early after a primarily successful catheter ablation (within 6 weeks) in as many as 10% of patients; occasionally, recurrence is not accompanied by symptom recurrence because of modification of the connection conduction properties.

• Late recurrence after successful catheter ablation (>3 months) is rare; patients usually experience short-lived episodes of palpitation or rhythm irregularity for some months after successful ablations, which may relate to a learning effect through which individuals have become sensitized to any short-lived change in heart rhythm (*e.g.*, ectopic activity) because before treatment, these heralded onset of tachycardia; these symptoms resolve with time and reassurance.

• After surgical treatment, standard follow-up is needed.

• Follow-up of patients treated by antiarrhythmic drugs is determined by their symptoms and drug side effects.

General reference

Ganz LI, Friedman PL: Supraventricular tachycardia. *N Engl J Med* 1995, **332**:162.

Appendix A: Health screening

Basis of recommendations

Beginning in the 1970s, three groups, the US Preventive Services Task Force (USPSTF) [1], the American College of Physicians (ACP) [2], and the Canadian Task Force on the Periodic Health Exam [CTF] [3], produced disease screening and prevention recommendations for a wide spectrum of diseases based on explicit criteria that measure and report the strength of scientific evidence to support each recommendation. Practitioners should monitor the recommendations of these evidence-based groups in determining optimal disease screening and prevention practices for their patients.

Searchable full-text versions of many clinical guidelines for health screening are available through the National Guidelines Clearinghouse (www.guideline.gov).

Recommended practices for asymptomatic, low-risk adults

The table summarizes the recommendations for disease screening and prevention developed at The University of Michigan's health maintenance organization (M-CARE) in 1998, based primarily on the recommendations of the CTF, USPSTF, and ACP.

Breast cancer

USPSTF: screening for breast cancer every 1–2 years (mammography ± clinical breast examination [CBE]) for women aged 50–69 years. Recommendations for or against routine mammography or CBE in women aged 40-49 years cannot be made based on current evidence.

ACP: mammography yearly for women aged 50-74 years.

CTF: annual CBE and mammography for women aged 50–69 years only.

Other: American Cancer Society, American College of Radiology, American Medical Association, and American College of Obstetrics and Gynecology recommend screening with annual CBE and biannual mammography beginning at age 40 years, and annual CBE and mammography beginning at age 50 years.

Hyperlipidemia

USPSTF: total cholesterol levels (nonfasting) should be measured in men aged 35–65 years and women aged 45–65 years.

ACP: total cholesterol levels (nonfasting) should be considered in men aged 35–65 years and women aged 45–65 years with fewer than two additional risk factors and without a strong family history of coronary artery disease [4].

CTF: total cholesterol measurement should be considered in men aged 30–59 years.

Other: National Cholesterol Education Program (NCEP) [5] advocates screening all adults for hyperlipidemia.

Cervical cancer

USPSTF: Papanicolaou (Pap) smears at least every 3 years beginning with onset of sexual activity; discontinue testing after age 65 years in women who have had regular previous screenings in which the smears have been consistently normal.

ACP: Pap smears every 3 years for women aged 20–65 years and every 2 years for women at high risk; screening is recommended for women aged 66–75 years every 3 years if they have not been screened from age 56–66 years.

CTF: annual Pap smears beginning at age 18 years or the onset of sexual activity. After two normal smears, screen every 3 years to age 69 years.

Colorectal cancer

USPSTF: annual fecal occult blood testing (FOBT) or sigmoidoscopy (interval unspecified), or both, for all persons aged 50 years and older.

ACP: screening options for patients aged 50–70 years include flexible sigmoidoscopy, colonoscopy, or air-contrast barium enema, repeated at 10-year intervals; FOBT is recommended for patients who decline these screening tests.

CTF: there is insufficient evidence to support screening of asymptomatic individuals over age 40 years.

Other: The Agency for Health Care Policy and Research, in conjunction with several specialty societies, released a consensus statement in 1997 that included colonoscopy every 10 years (among other alternatives endorsed by other groups) as a recommended screening method [6].

Prostate cancer

USPSTF: routine screening for prostate cancer not recommended.

ACP: individualized screening based on patient and physician preferences.

CTF: the routine use of prostate-specific antigen (PSA) is not recommended. Qualified support for digital rectal examination (DRE) in men aged 50–70 years.

Key references

1. U.S. Preventive Services Task Force: Guide to Clinical Preventive Services, edn 2. Baltimore: Williams & Wilkins; 1996.
2. Sox HC: Preventive health services in adults. *N Engl J Med* 1994, **330**:1589-1595.
3. Canadian Task Force on the Periodic Health Examination: Canadian Guide to Clinical Preventive Health Care. Ottawa: Canada Communication Group; 1994.
4. Guidelines for using serum cholesterol, high-density lipoprotein cholesterol, and triglyceride levels as screening tests for preventing coronary heart disease in adults. *Ann Intern Med* 1996, **124**:515-517.
5. Summary of the second report of the National Cholesterol Education Program (NCEP) Expert Panel on Detection, Evaluation, and Treatment of High Blood Cholesterol in Adults (Adult Treatment Panel II). *JAMA* 1993, **269**:3015-3023.
6. Winawer SJ, Fletcher RH, Miller L, et al.: Colorectal cancer screening: clinical guidelines and rationale. *Gastroenterology* 1997, **112**:594-642.

M-CARE Preventive Care Guidelines, 1998 (minimum levels of preventive care for asymptomatic, low-risk adults)

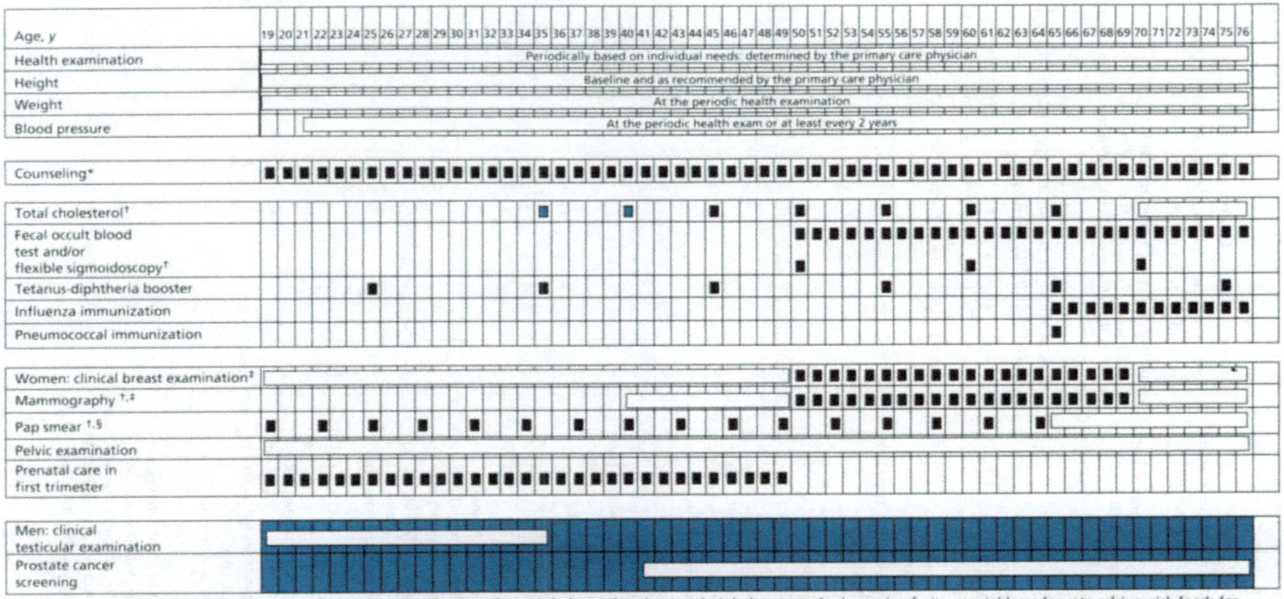

* Counseling topics include tobacco cessation, alcohol/drug use, diet (limit fat and cholesterol; maintain caloric balance; emphasize grains, fruits, vegetables; adequate calcium-rich foods for women; recommend breast-feeding, if appropriate), regular physical activity, injury prevention (lap/shoulder belts, appropriate helmet use, smoke detector use, safe storage/removal of firearms, violence prevention, poison control, fall prevention), sexual behavior (sexually transmitted disease prevention, unintended pregnancy), dental health, multivitamin with folic acid for women of childbearing age, hormone prophylaxis in peri- and postmenopausal women, and skin cancer counseling if family history of skin cancer and fair skin, eyes, or hair.

† More frequently and/or at an earlier age, based on risk factors.

‡ Screen every 1 to 2 years with mammography alone or with mammography and clinical breast examination.

§ Regular screening may be discontinued after age 65 years in women who have had regular screenings that have been consistently normal.

Green boxes indicate men only; white boxes indicate as recommended by the primary care physician.

M-CARE— University of Michigan's health maintenance organization.

Appendix B: Total parenteral & enteral nutrition

Indications for nutritional support

Malnourished patients unable to maintain adequate oral intake of nutrients (*e.g.*, surgical patients with prolonged ileus, medical patients with pancreatitis, or patients with severe diabetic gastroparesis).

Well-nourished patients who will be NPO for >10–14 days.

Patients who are not able to maintain adequate oral intake when full nutrition is required (*e.g.*, burn patients, trauma patients, Crohn's disease patients.)

Patients with portasystemic encephalopathy recceiving nutritional therapy, such as providing branched-chain amino acids (BCAAs).

Nutritional requirements

Fluid

• ~35 mL/kg/day or 1 mL/kcal is required for patients without excess fluid loss; additional fluid is needed to replace losses from nasogastric suction, diarrhea, third-spaced fluid, and burns.

Caloric requirements

Maintenance requirements: 25 kcal/kg/day.

• Patients generally require 100%–120% of basal energy expenditure (kcal/day) as prescribed by Harris-Benedict formula.

Trauma, febrile, pancreatitis: 30 kcal/kg/day.

Minor burns, sepsis: 35 kcal/kg/day; major burns: 40 kcal/kg/day.

Carbohydrate

• Glucose (8%–25% solution) is the main source of calories in parenteral formulas. Although glucose can provide all nonprotein calories, this requires large fluid volumes for delivery, resulting in edema, fluid overload, hyperglycemia, and fatty liver.

Protein

• A positive nitrogen balance is maintained by adequate protein intake (amino acid infusion) and sufficient nonprotein calories to prevent protein breakdown (gluconeogenesis). The recommended dietary protein intake is 0.8 g/kg/day but can be increased to 1.5 g/kg/day in stressed patients (*e.g.*, burn, trauma, postoperative patients).

Fat

• Lipids are emulsions of soybean or safflower oil and contain linoleic acid, an essential fatty acid. In standard formulas, lipids provide ~30% of nonprotein calories. Patients with respiratory failure can be given a higher percentage of lipid calories to decrease CO_2 production. Excessive use of lipids can result in hyperlipidemia and increased risk of infection via impairment of neutrophilic function.

Electrolytes

• Electrolyte replacement should be closely monitored, particularly in patients with renal disease, cirrhosis with ascites, congestive heart failure, diarrheal states, nasogastric suction, and third spacing of fluids. Potassium and phosphorus requirements may be high in malnourished patients beginning total parenteral nutrition (TPN).

Minerals and vitamins

• Commercial multivitamin products (*e.g.*, MVI-12), which typically do not include vitamin K, are required. Trace elements (*e.g.*, zinc, copper, and selenium) should also be added for patients who require prolonged nutritional support. Iron cannot be given with lipids and may need to be given separately. Patients with diarrhea may need extra zinc replacement.

Assessment of nutritional status

• Often the clinician's overall assessment of the patient's nutritional status is most accurate.

• Helpful indicators of poor nutrition include the following:

Ideal body weight 15% below ideal.

Signs of muscle wasting, decreased hand grip strength.

Serum albumin <3.0 g/dL.

Anthropomorphic measurements:
Triceps skin fold: female <15 mm; male <11.4 mm.
Midarm muscle circumference: female <25.8 mm; male <26.4 mm.

Calculation of basal energy expenditure (BEE): Harris-Benedict formula

Male: BEE (kcal) = 66.5 + 13.7 × weight (kg) + 5 × height (cm) − 6.8 × age (years)

Female: BEE (kcal) = 65.5 + 9.6 × weight (kg) + 1.7 × height (cm) − 4.7 × age (years)

Central TPN

• Patients needing complete nutrition parenterally require central TPN. To provide total calories intravenously requires a large osmotic load that must be given through a large central vein, where the mixture is quickly diluted. Solutions with up to 25% glucose can be used. In peripheral veins, osmolality must be kept <900 mOsmL with glucose concentration <10% to prevent unacceptable phlebitis.

Standard TPN solution/24 hours

Volume: 2600 mL.

Total calories: 2000.

Calorie to nitrogen ratio: 131:1.

Macronutrients

Glucose (15% solution): 350 g (60% of total calories).

Amino acids: 80 g (16% of total calories).

Lipid emulsion (20%): 240 mL (24% of total calories).

Electrolytes

Sodium: 120 mEq.

Potassium: 80 mEq.

Chloride: 140 mEq.

Acetate: 20 mEq.

Phosphorus: 30 mmol.

Calcium gluconate: 9.2 mEq (2 g).

Magnesium sulfate: 16.8 mEq (2 g).

Vitamins

MVI-12: daily.

Vitamin K: 5 mg/week (do not use in patients requiring anticoagulation with warfarin).

Peripheral parenteral nutrition (PPN)

• Patients who require additional calories to supplement oral intake or patients who are not malnourished and require short-term nutritional support may use PPN. Roughly 1000 kcal/day can be delivered via PPN. Isotonic fat emulsions have greatly increased the amount of calories that can be delivered peripherally, but exclusive reliance on these products would result in hyperlipidemia.

Laboratory monitoring

• Before starting parenteral nutrition, a complete blood count, electrolytes, blood urea nitrogen, creatinine, albumin, total protein, liver chemistries, triglycerides, weight, and 24-hour urine for urea and creatinine should be obtained. After initiation of parenteral nutrition, electrolytes/creatinine/blood urea nitrogen and weight should be obtained daily to detect significant electrolyte shifts for the first 2 weeks. Glucose should be monitored closely, including every-6-hour bedside monitoring until the serum glucose is <200 g/dL. Liver function tests, triglycerides, and renal function should be followed weekly. Stable patients receiving long-term parenteral nutrition are followed at less frequent intervals.

Complications

Electrolyte abnormalities.
Hyperglycemia.
Hypoglycemia.
Elevated transaminases.
Fatty liver.
Hyperlipidemia.
Fluid overload.
Hyperosmotic coma.
Gallstones.
Cholecystitis.
Sepsis.
Pneumothorax.
Air embolus.
Broken catheter embolus.
Catheter/venous thrombosis.
Mineral deficiences.

Enteral nutrition

• If the patient's gastrointestinal tract is functional, this is the preferred method of nutritional support. Supplements include standard formulas with complex carbohydrates, intact protein, and fat such as vegetable oil. Some are modified- to high-calorie (2 kcal/mL), high-fiber, high-protein, low-protein, or volume-restricted formulations. Elemental dietary supplements are expensive preparations designed for patients with impaired digestion, short gut syndrome, or as a possible therapeutic modality in Crohn's disease.

Oral supplementation

• If patients are able to eat without aspiration but are not taking an adequate amount of food, liquid supplements such as Ensure (1 kcal/mL) can raise caloric intake enough to maintain weight.

Nasogastric tube

• Nasogastric bolus tube feeding can be used in patients with normal gastric emptying. Patients should be placed in the upright position during administration and over the subsequent hour. Complications include aspiration, gastric ulcers, perforation, bleeding, and gastroesophageal reflux.

Small-bore nasoduodenal tube

• Small-bore nasoduodenal tubes are moderately well tolerated and can be used for long-term feeding. A pump is required to deliver a continuous infusion because the small bowel cannot tolerate bolus feeding. Complications include tube occlusion, accidental removal, difficulty replacing the tube, diarrhea, aspiration.

Percutaneous gastric tube

• Percutaneous gastric tubes have the advantage of using a large-bore tube that is not easily clogged and cannot be pulled out accidentally during sleep. Patients should have a normally functioning stomach. Care should be taken in patients with a history of aspiration pneumonia and significant gastroesophageal reflux. Complications include gastric ulcers, gastric bleeding, gastric outlet obstruction, wound infection, necrotizing fasciitis, and rapid closure of the fistula if the tube falls out.

Surgical jejunostomy tube

• In patients who have a nonfunctioning stomach, recurrent aspiration pneumonia, recent gastric surgery, or duodenal and gastric outlet obstruction, a surgical jejunostomy-tube may be necessary. A pump and continuous infusion is required. Complications include diarrhea, wound infection, small bowel obstruction, and jejunal ulcers.

General references

Alpers DH, Stenson WF, Bier D: *Manual of Nutrition Therapeutics*. edn 3. Boston: Little, Brown; 1995.

Souba WW, Nutritional support. *N Engl J Med* 1997, **336**:41–48.

Stenson WF, Eisenberg P: Parenteral and enteral nutrition. In *Textbook of Internal Medicine*, edn 3. Philadelphia: Lippincott-Raven; 1997.

Appendix C: Viral hepatitis, immunization

Indications for immunization

Hepatitis A virus (HAV)

• HAV vaccine is recommended for travelers to endemic areas and should replace the use of immunoglobulin for foreign travelers. It is recommended for adults and children living in communities with high rates of HAV infection or periodic outbreaks of HAV infection, staff and clients of group homes for disabled persons, daycare centers, homosexual men, and illicit i.v. drug users.

Serum immunoglobulin: for postexposure prophylaxis (*e.g.*, outbreaks in daycare centers or household contacts), the vaccine does not offer acceptable protection and immune globulin should be given. For short trips to endemic regions, immunoglobulin alone is still an acceptable alternative (vaccine is preferred), and for those who must depart on short notice, a combination of immunoglobulin and vaccine can be given.

• Patients who are already serum IgM HAV antibody-positive (indicating acute HAV infection) or serum IgG HAV antibody-positive (indicating past exposure to HAV) will not benefit from vaccination or serum immunoglobulin.

Hepatitis B virus (HBV)

• HBV vaccine is recommended for all children as part of childhood immunization series and previously unvaccinated adolescents. It is recommended for household contacts of HBV carriers, infants born to HBsAg-positive mothers, health care workers, homosexual men, illicit i.v. drug users, people living or traveling in endemic areas; and people requiring postexposure prophylaxis.

• Patients who are serum HBsAg positive are chronic carriers (or acutely infected) and will not benefit from vaccination. Patients who are HBsAb positive have either been exposed to HBV in the past or have been vaccinated previously. In either instance vaccination is not needed.

Hepatitis C virus (HCV)

• No vaccine is available. Serum immunoglobulin is not recommended for postexposure prophylaxsis.

Hepatitis D virus (HDV)

• Because HDV infection requires previous or simultaneous infection with HBV, vaccination against HBV effectively prevents infection with HDV.

Investigations

• Preimmunization testing to determine if recipient has already been exposed to HAV or HBV is not routinely recommended. Patients who are already HBsAg positive or HBsAb positive do not need to be vaccinated. Postimmunization testing is not recommended but may be indicated in patients who are immunocompromised, those suspected of having a poor response to immunization, or in those considered to be at high risk for exposure (*e.g.*, a surgeon or phlebotomist).

Complications of immunization

Soreness, erythema at the sight of the injection: common.

Fever: rare.

Anaphylactic reactions, Guillain-Barré syndrome: rare.

Immunization dosage and schedule

HAV

Standard dosage

Adults: 1440 ELISA U/1 mL (Havrix) or 50 U/0.5 mL given at 0 and 6–12 months.

Children (2–18 years): 720 ELISA U/0.5 mL or 25 U/0.5 mL (Vaqta) given at 0 and 6–12 months.

Newborns: neither vaccine is approved for children <2 years of age.

Serum immunoglobulin: 0.02 mL/kg i.m. for postexposure prophylaxis or foreign travel lasting <3 months; for longer trips 0.06 mL/kg provides protection for up to 6 months.

HBV

Standard dosage

Adults: one 1-mL dose given at 0, 1–2, and 4–6 months for a total of three doses.

Children: one dose given at 0, 1–2, and 4–6 months for a total of three doses

Newborns: one dose given at 0–2, 1–4, and 6–18 months for a total of three doses.

For newborns of HBsAg-positive mothers: within 12 hours of birth give HBIG along with first dose of vaccine given at a separate site.

Postexposure prophylaxis

For needle-stick injuries from a patient who is HBsAg positive, if the injured person has not been vaccinated previously, give hepatitis B immunoglobulin and first dose of vaccine at a separate site, then complete vaccine schedule. If the injured person has been vaccinated consider checking HBsAb level and give vaccine booster if undetectable.

Immunocompromised patients

One dose given at 0, 1, and 6 months.

Causes of pharmacological treatment failure

Gluteal injections associated with decreased response to HBV vaccination; immunocompromised patients such as renal transplant patients and AIDS patients; HBV mutants.

General references

Health Information for International Travel 1999–2000. U. S. Department of Health and Human Services, Edited by Koplan JP, *et al.*, Atlanta: Centers for Disease Control and Prevention: 1999:93–102.

Lemon SM, Thomas DL: Vaccines to prevent viral hepatitis. *N Engl J Med* 1997, **336**:196–204.

Color plates

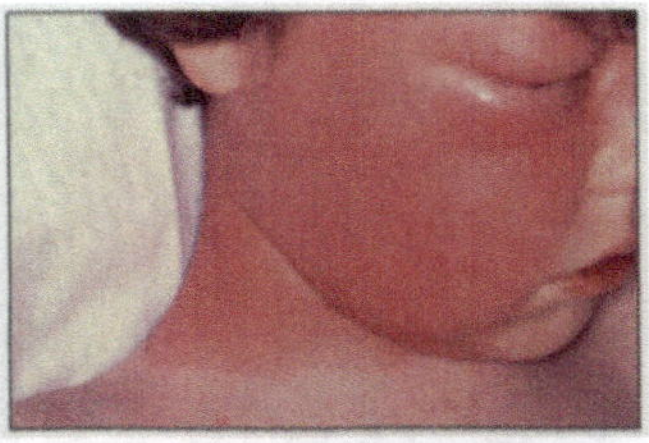

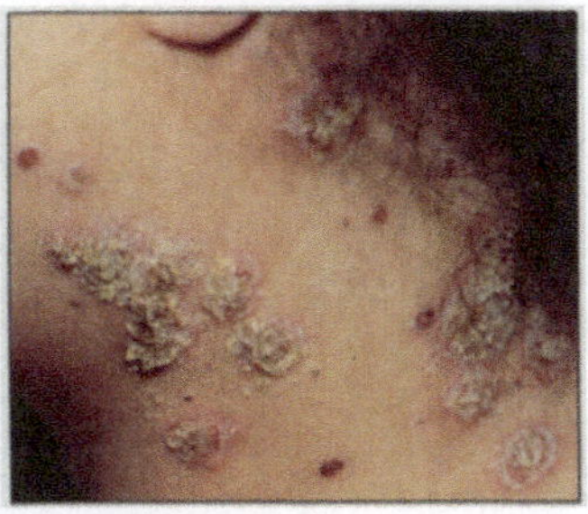

Skin infections, page 404.

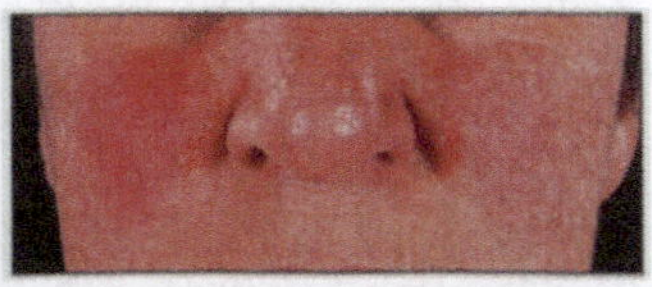

Systemic lupus erythematosus, page 424.

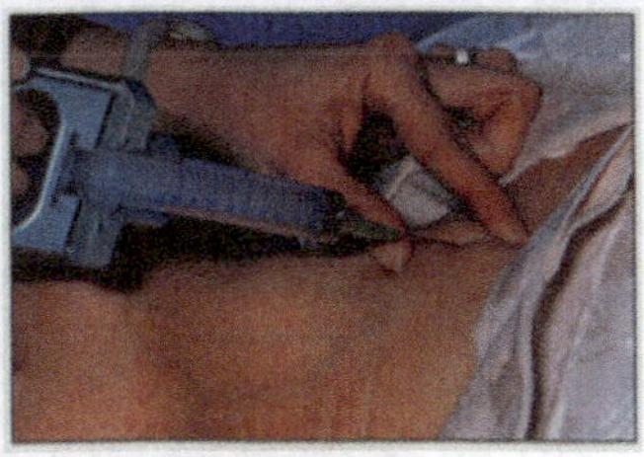

Thyroid carcinoma, page 434.

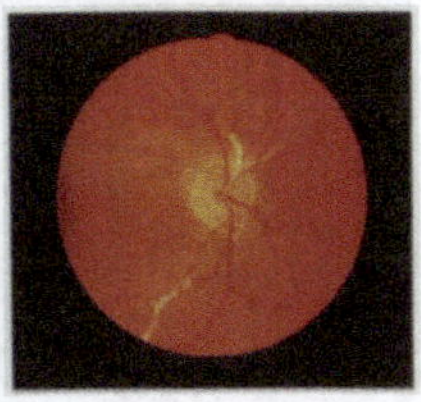

Transient ischemic attacks, page 444.

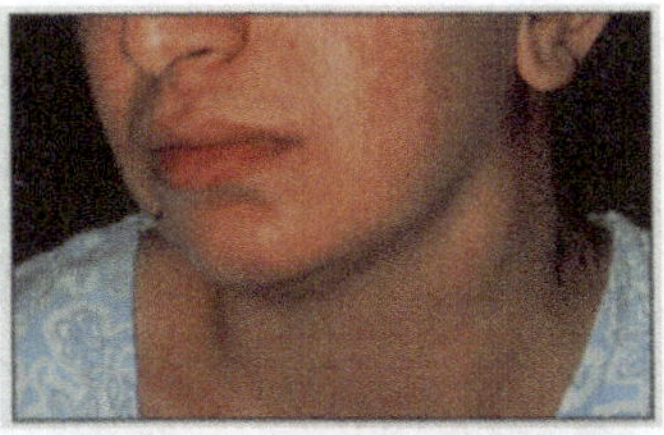

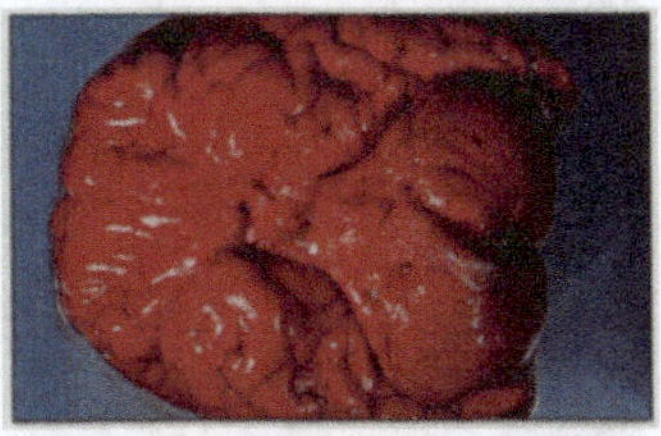

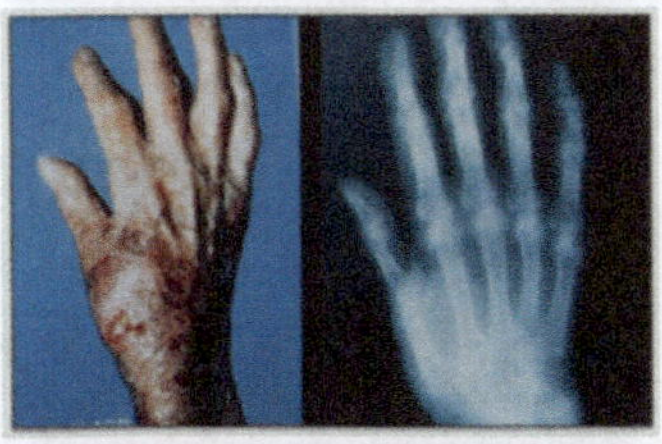

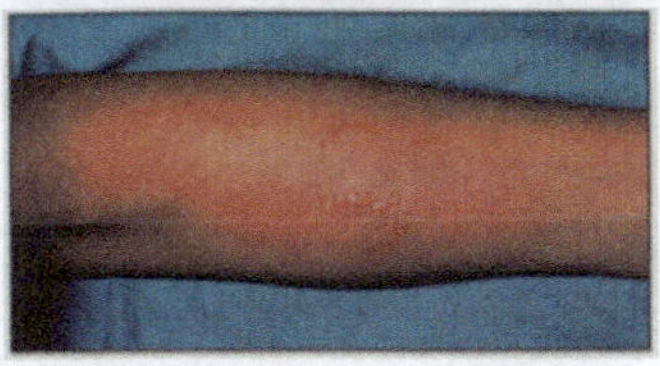

Tuberculosis, extrapulmonary; page 448.

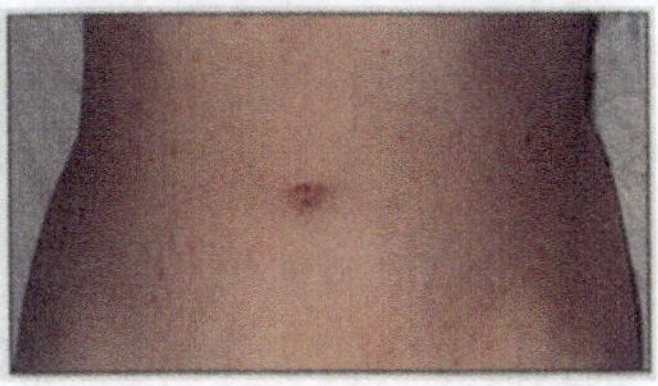

Typhoid and paratyphoid fevers, page 452.

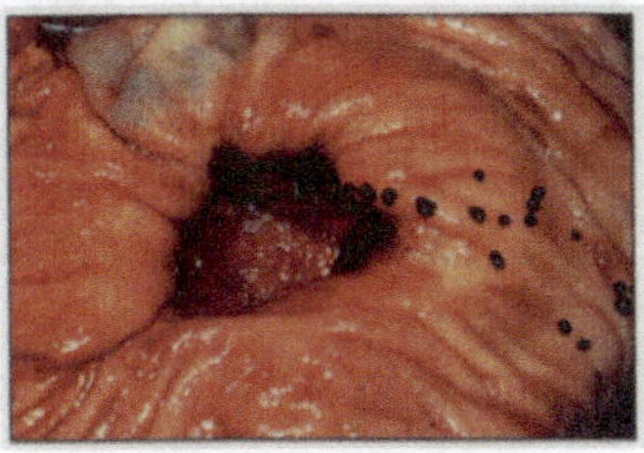

Upper gastrointestinal tract bleeding, page 456.

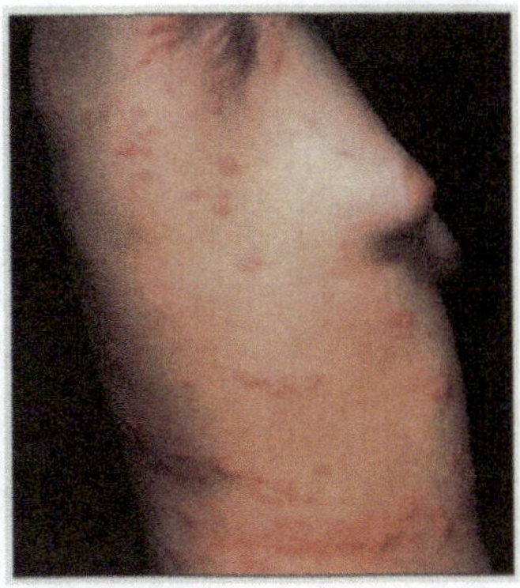

Urticaria, page 462.

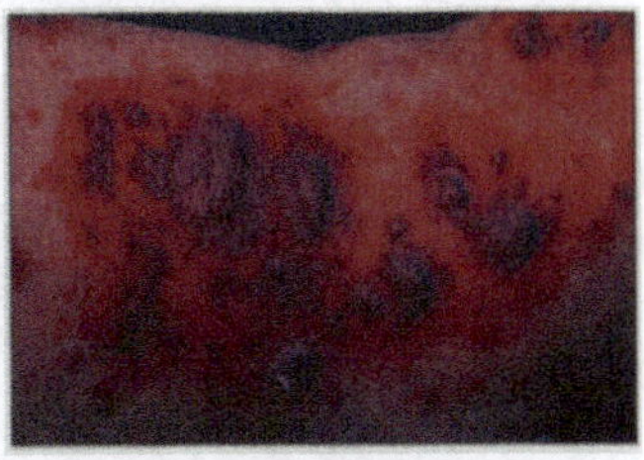

Vasculitis, skin manifestations; page 466.

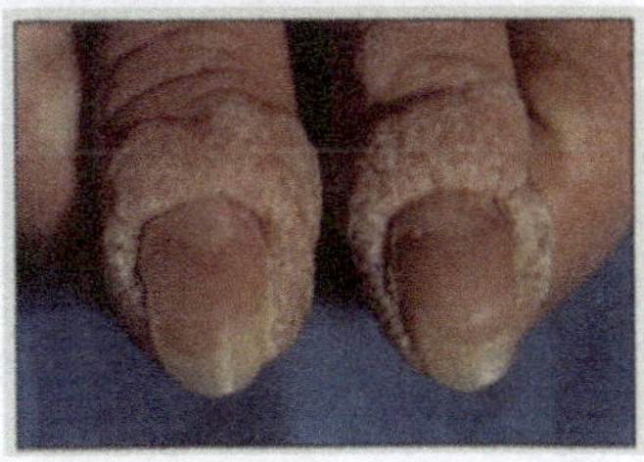

Viral warts, page 470.

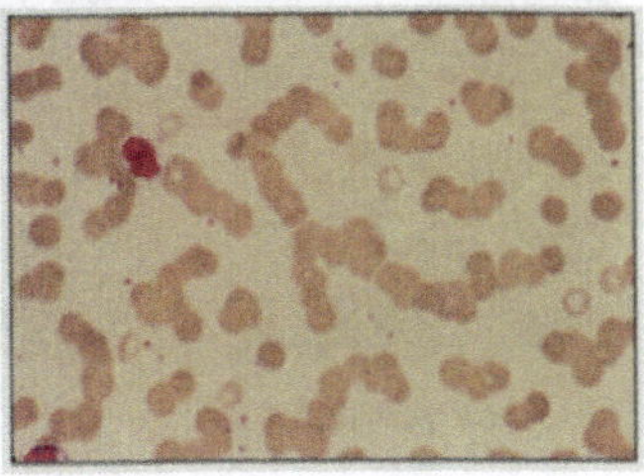

Waldenström's macroglobulinemia, page 472.

Color plates

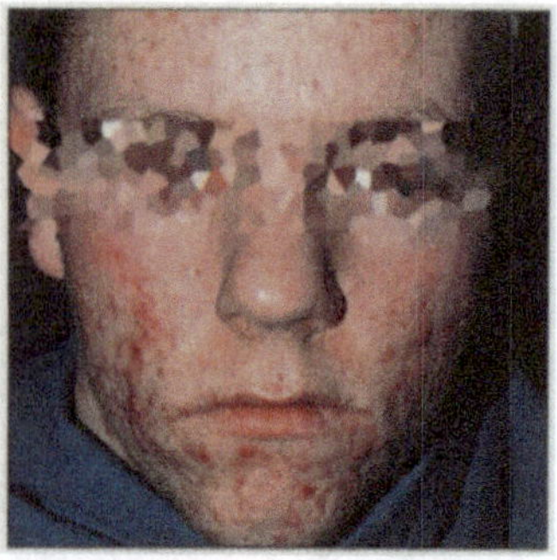

Acne, page 6.

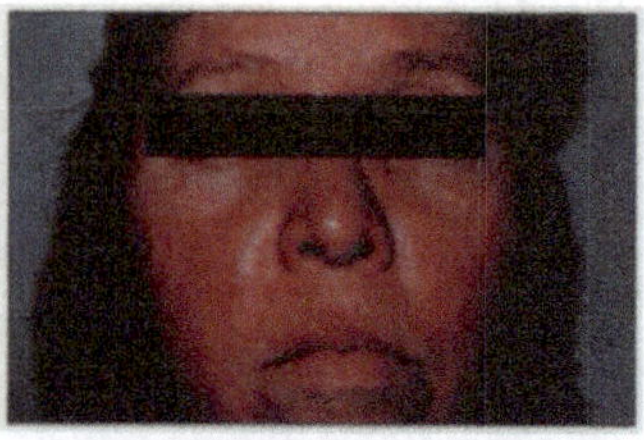

Acne rosacea, page 8.

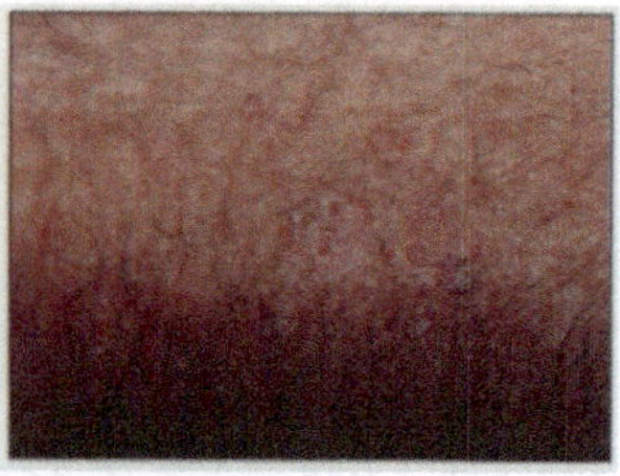

Actinic keratoses, page 10.

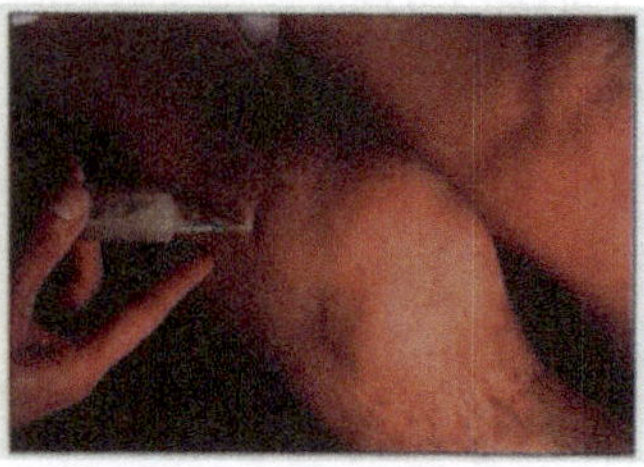

Acute crystal synovitis, page 12.

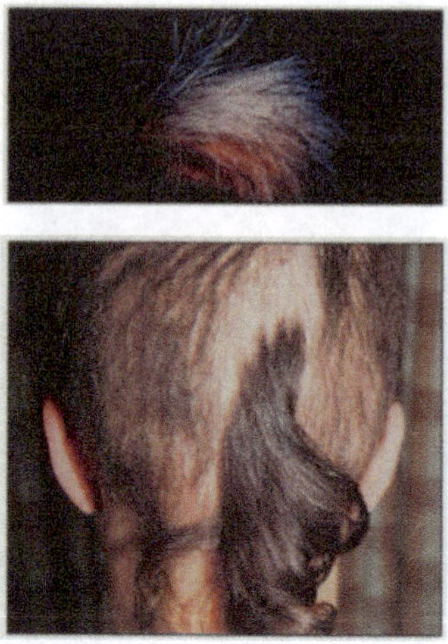

Alopecia, page 26.

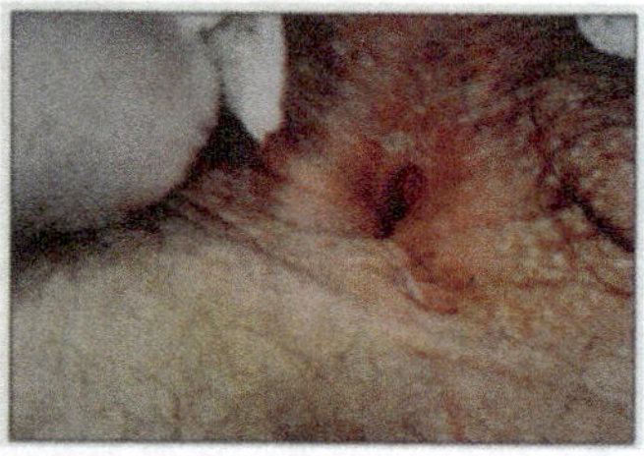

Anal fissure, page 28.

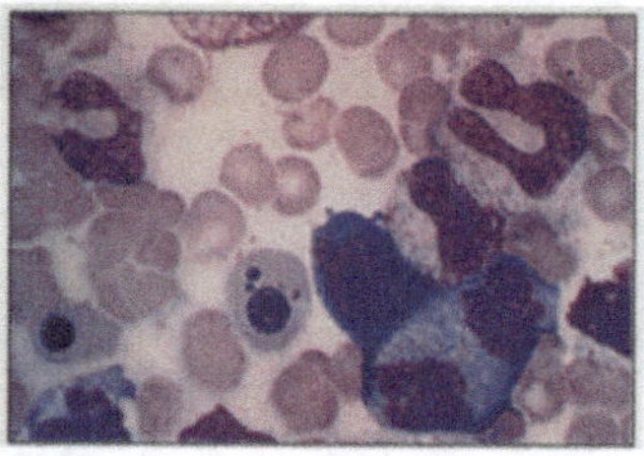

Anemia, megaloblastic; page 32.

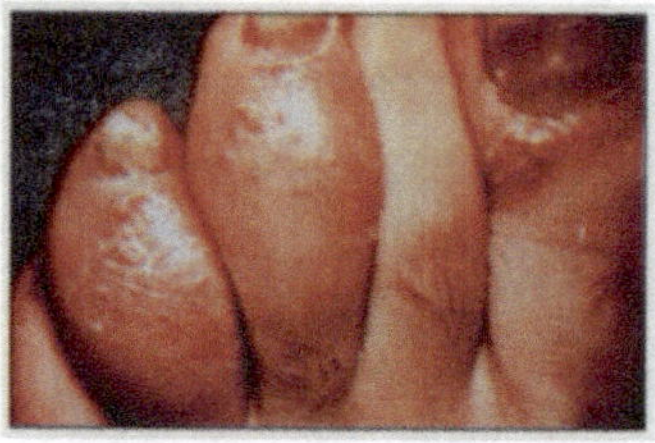

Arthritis, psoriatic; page 52.

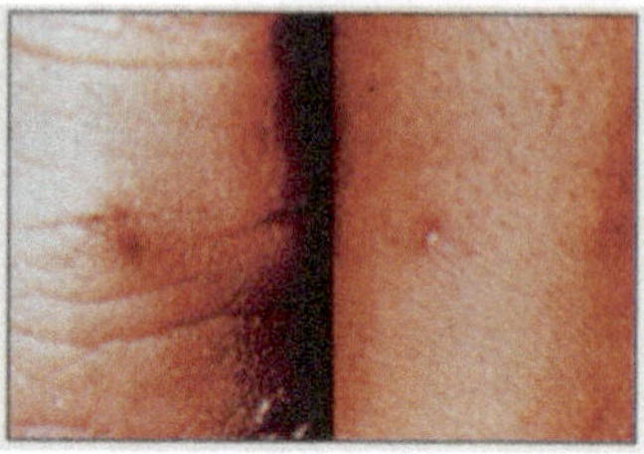

Arthritis, septic; page 56.

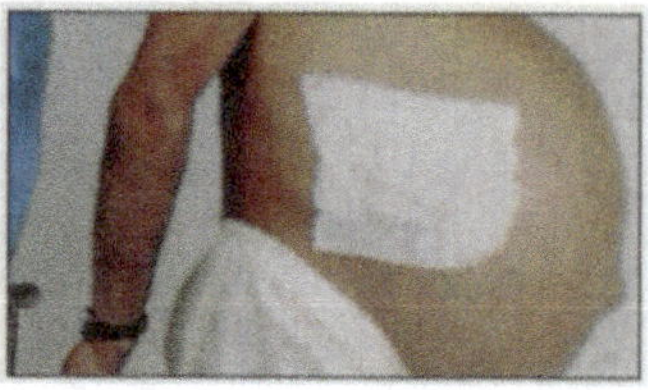

Ascites, page 58.

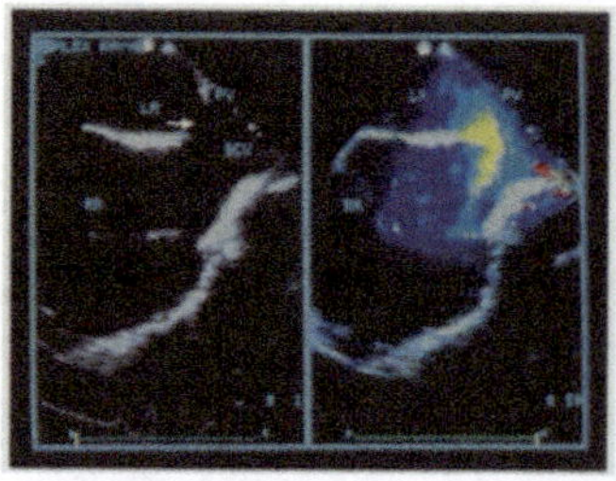

Atrial septal defect, page 66.

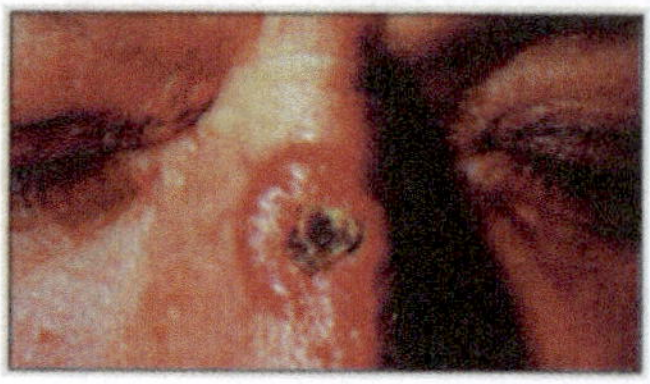

Basal cell carcinoma, page 70.

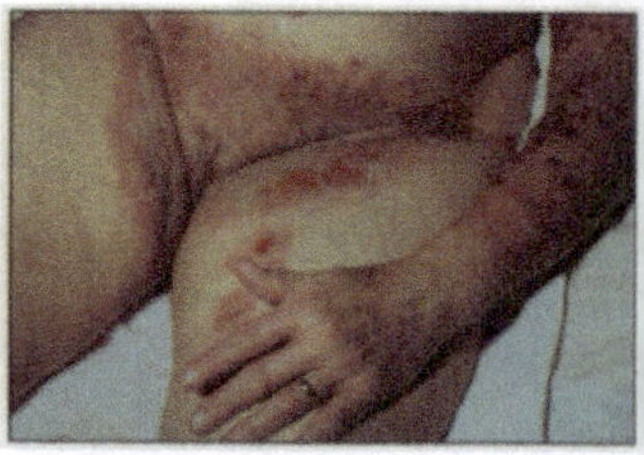

Bullous disorders, page 78.

Color plates

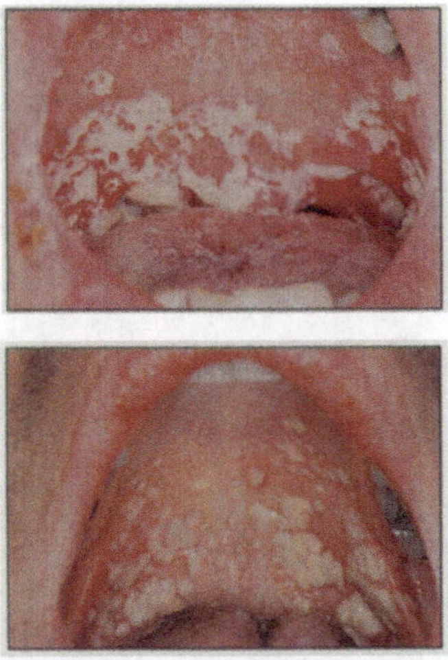

Candidiasis, buccal and esophageal in AIDS; page 80.

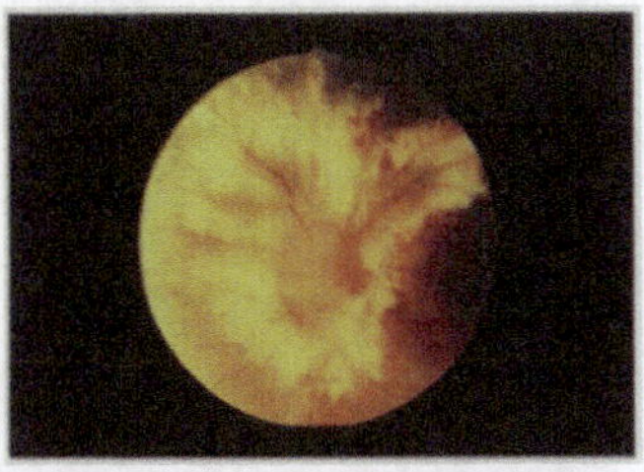

Cytomegalovirus infection in AIDS, page 114.

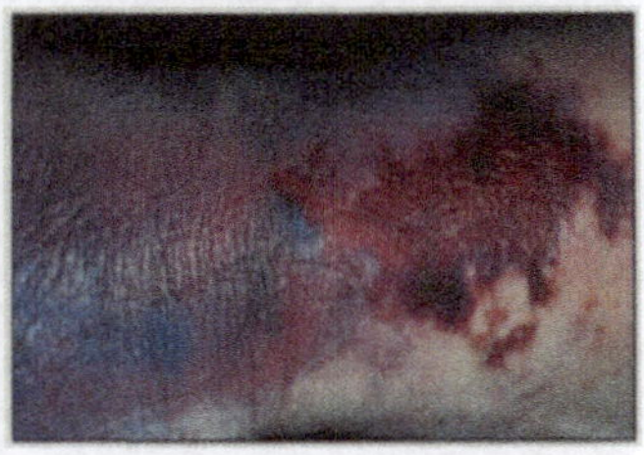

Disseminated intravascular coagulation, page 136.

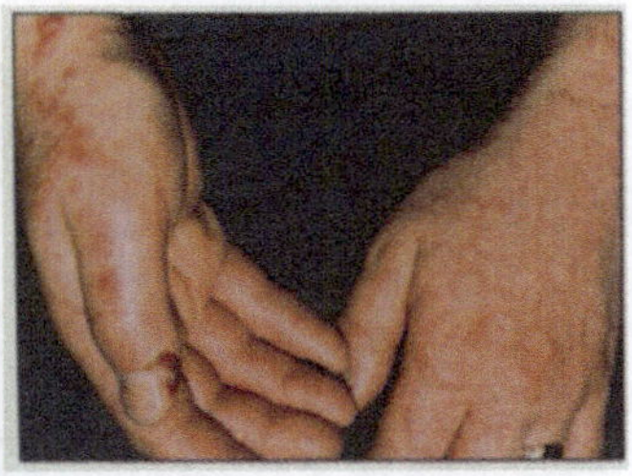

Erythema multiforme and Stevens–Johnson syndrome, page 156.

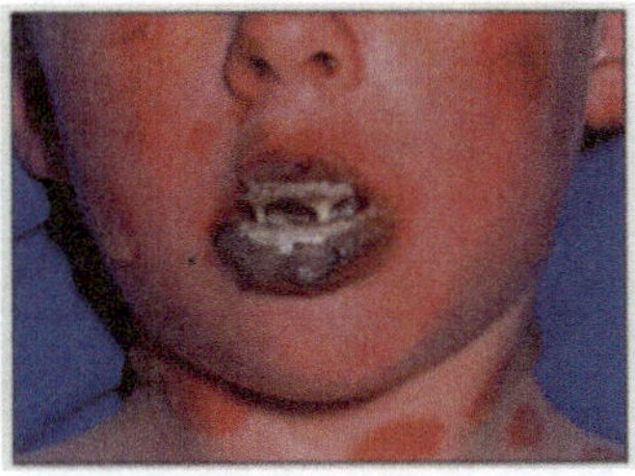

Erythema multiforme and Stevens–Johnson syndrome, page 156.

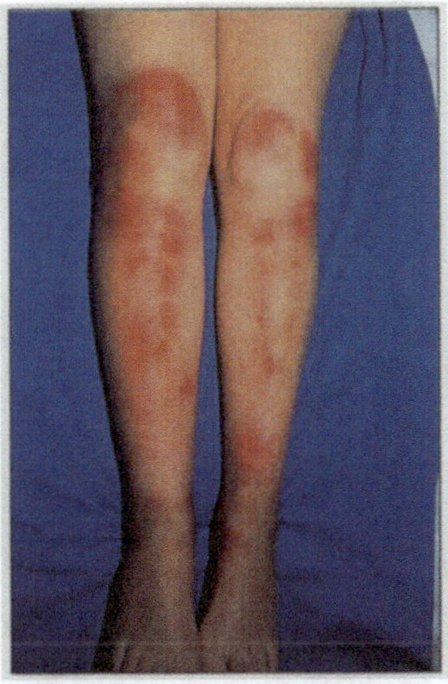

Erythema nodosum, page 158.

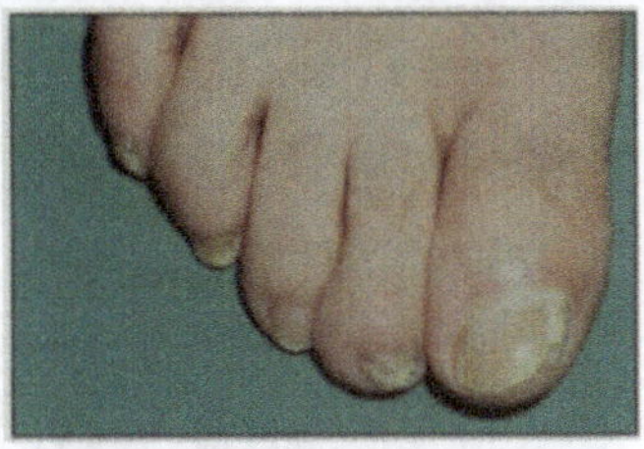

Fungal nail infection, page 168.

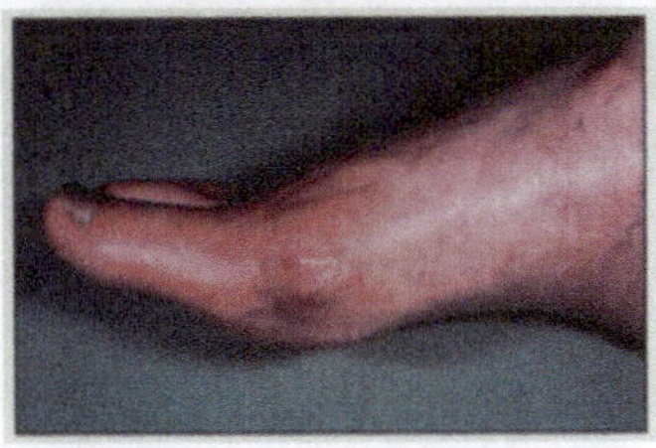

Gout, page 178.

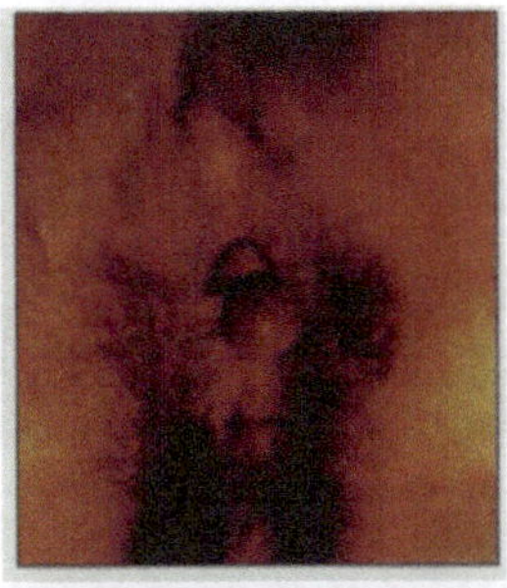

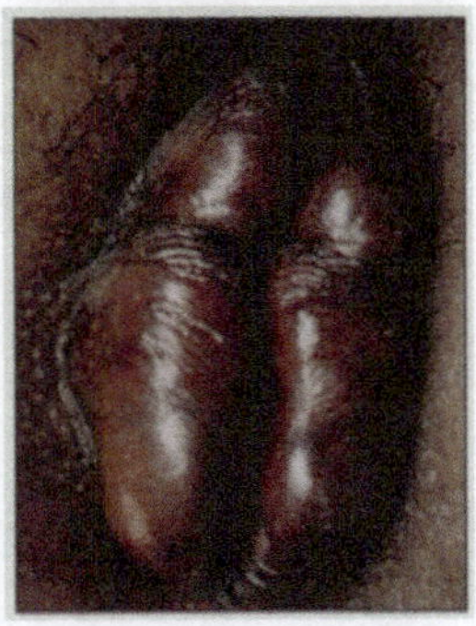

Hemorrhoidal disease, page 194.

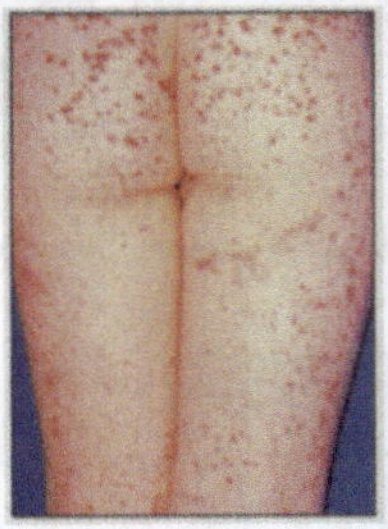

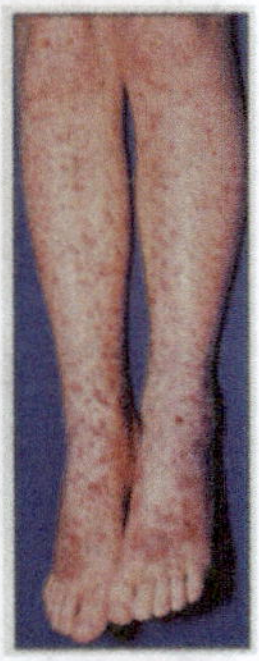

Henoch-Schönlein purpura, page 196.

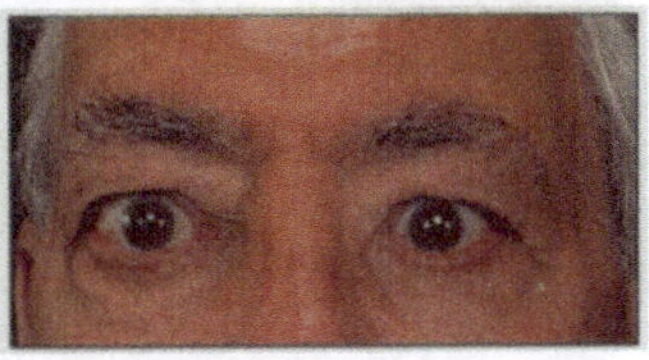

Hyperthyroidism, page 226.

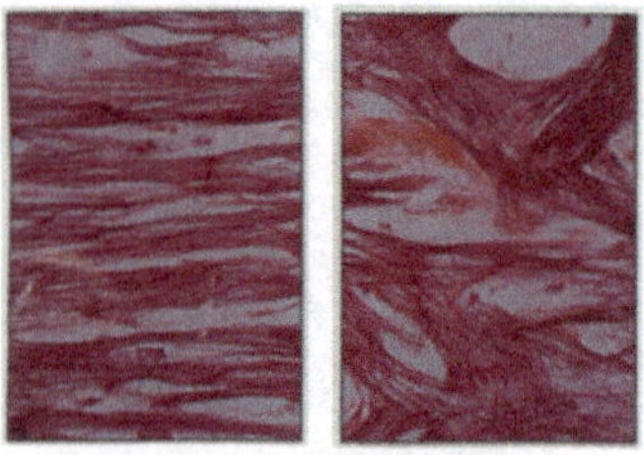

Hypertrophic cardiomyopathy, page 228.

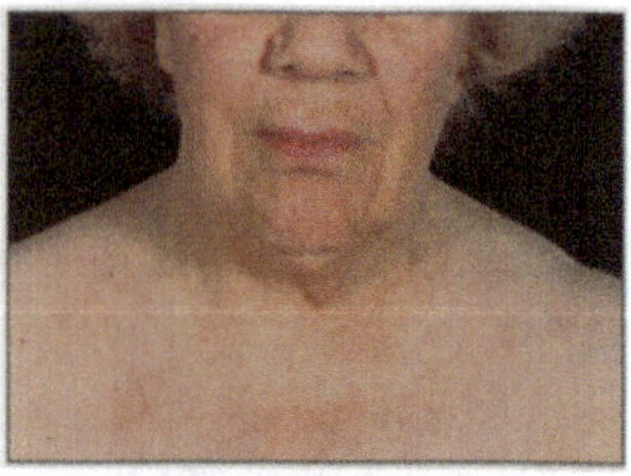

Hypothyroidism, page 236.

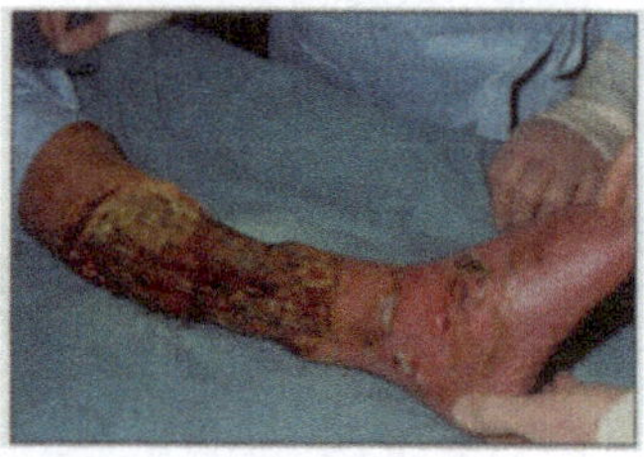

Infections in hematological malignancy, page 238.

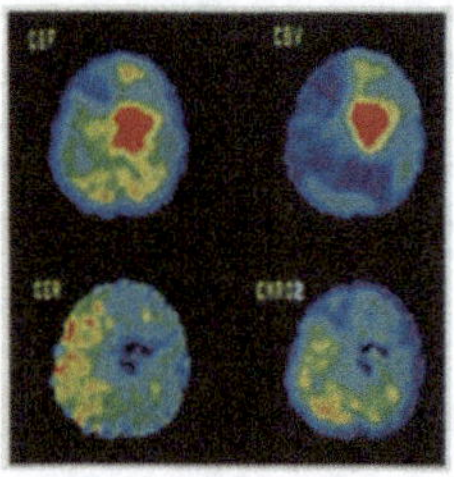

Intracerebral hemorrhage, page 242.

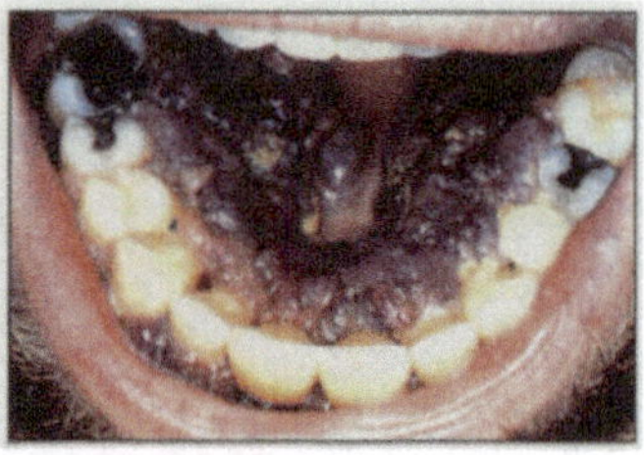

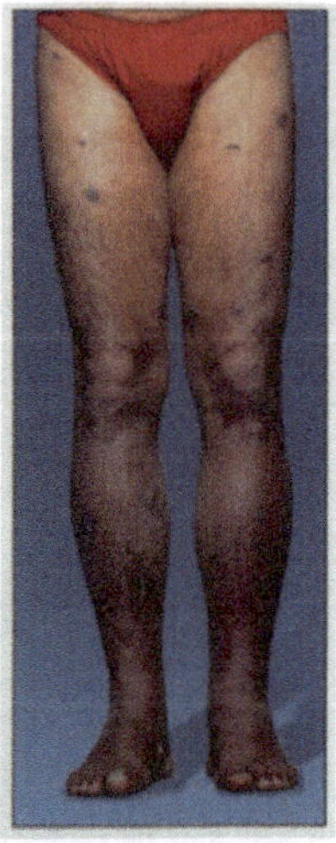

Kaposi's sarcoma in AIDS, page 246.

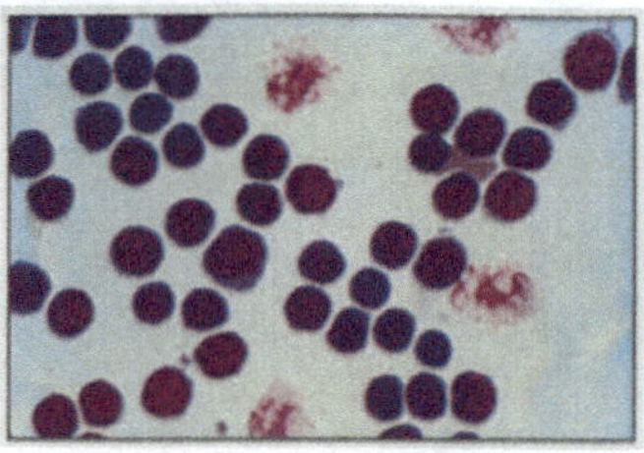

Leukemia, chronic lymphocytic; page 258.

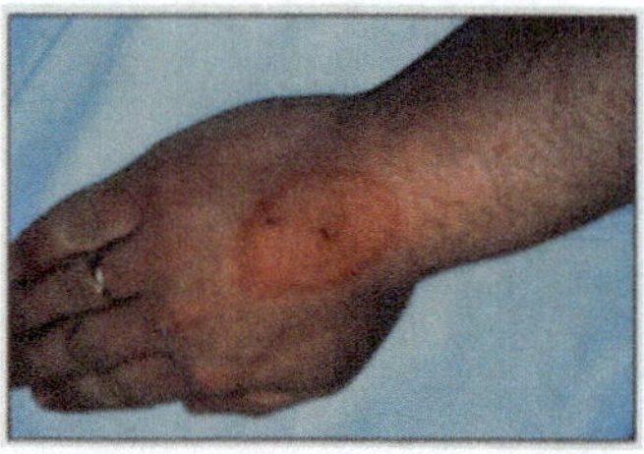

Lyme disease, page 270.

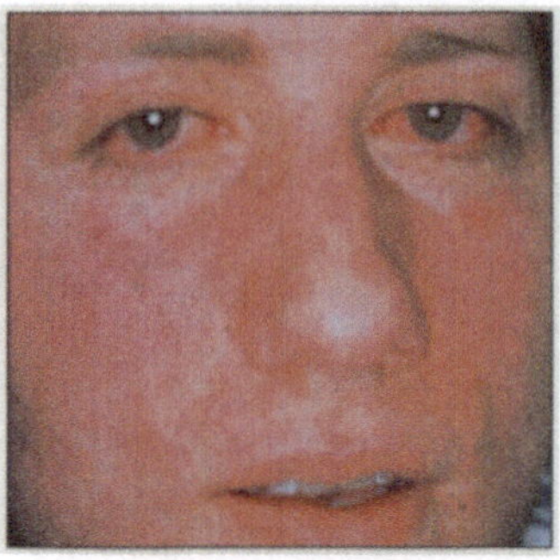

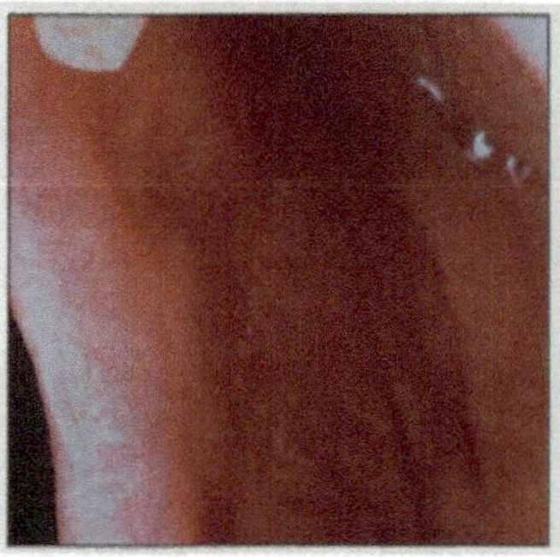

Measles, page 272.

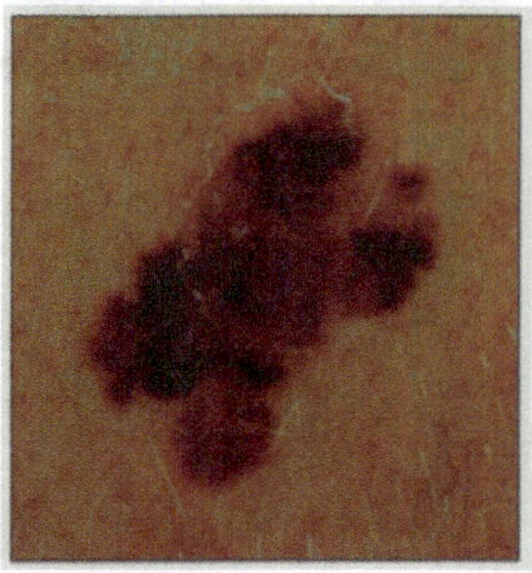

Melanoma, page 274.

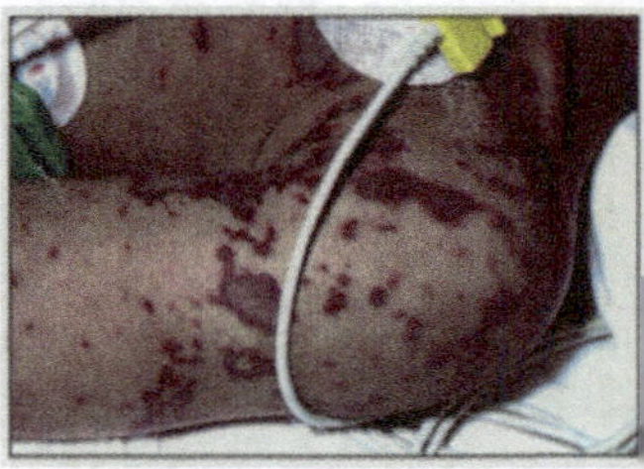

Meningitis, bacterial; page 276.

Color plates

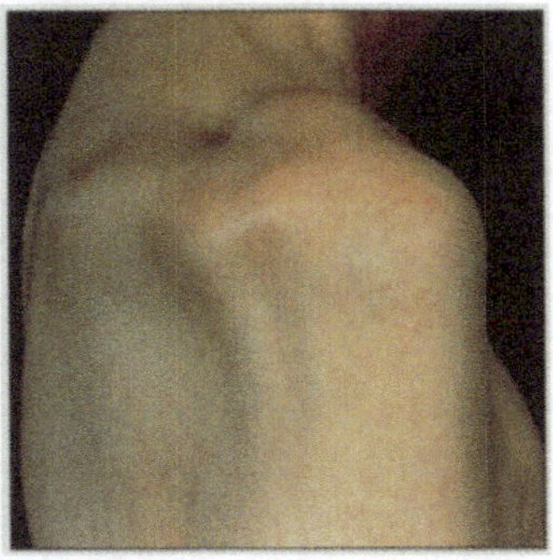

Motor neuron disease, page 288.

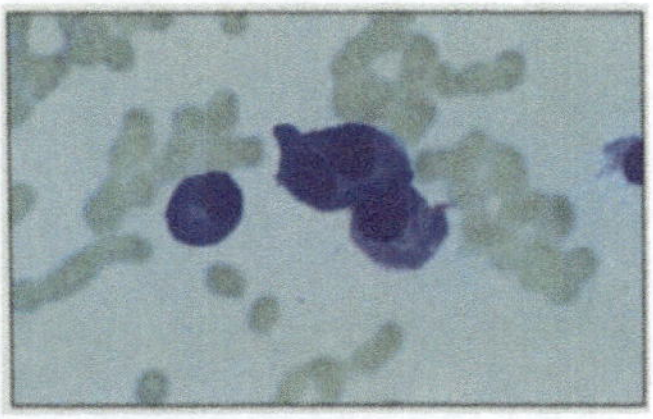

Multiple myeloma, page 290.

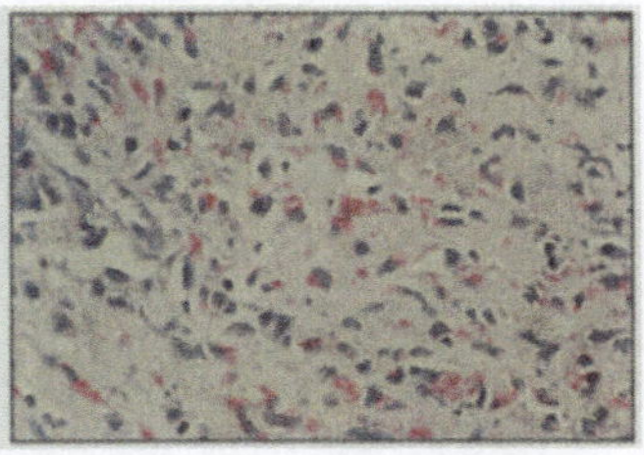

Mycobacterium avium complex infection in AIDS, page 296.

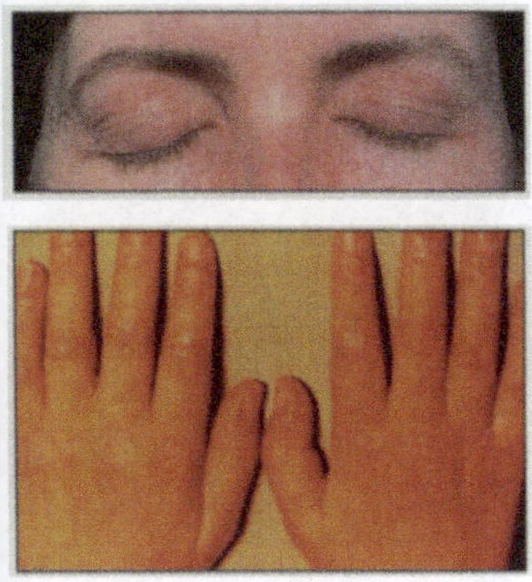

Myositis, inflammatory; page 302.

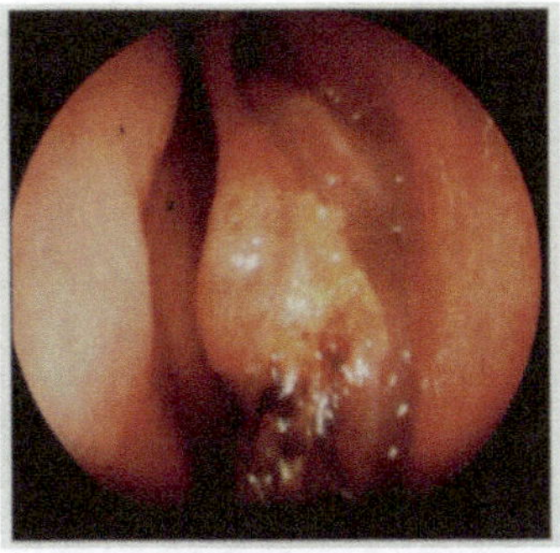

Nasal polyposis, page 304.

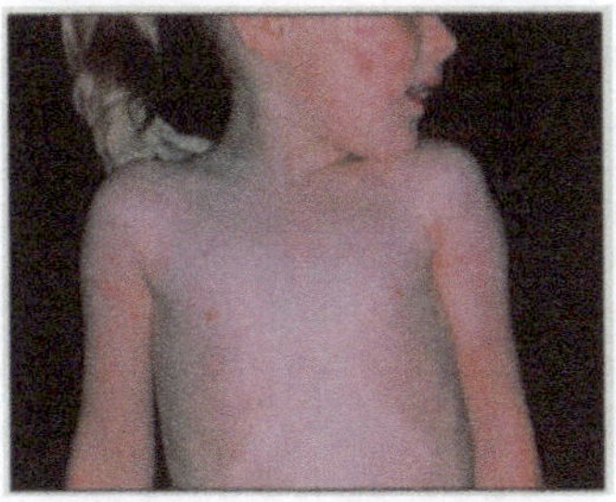

Parvovirus B19 infection, page 334.

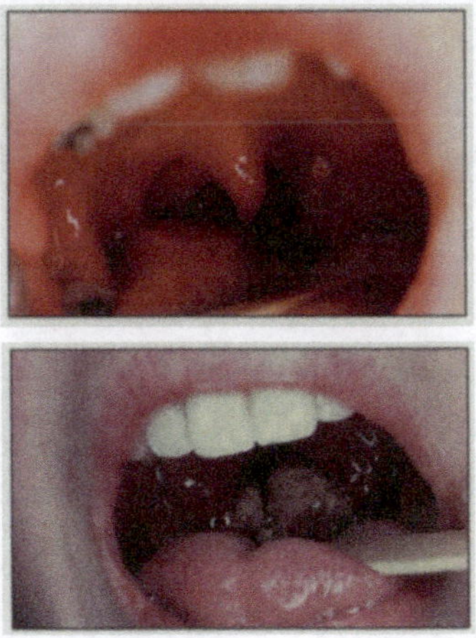

Pharyngitis, page 340.

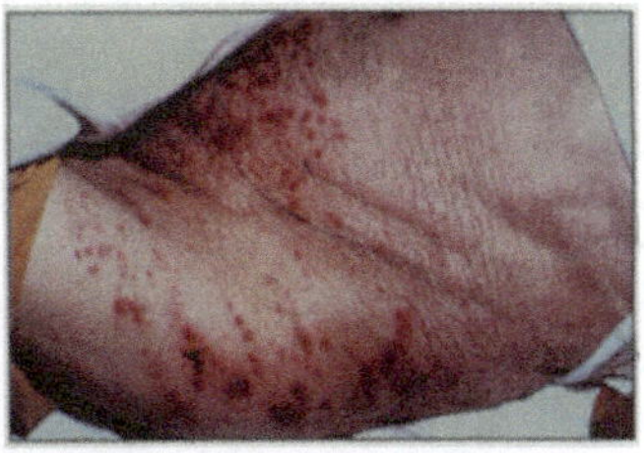

Platelet disorders, page 344.

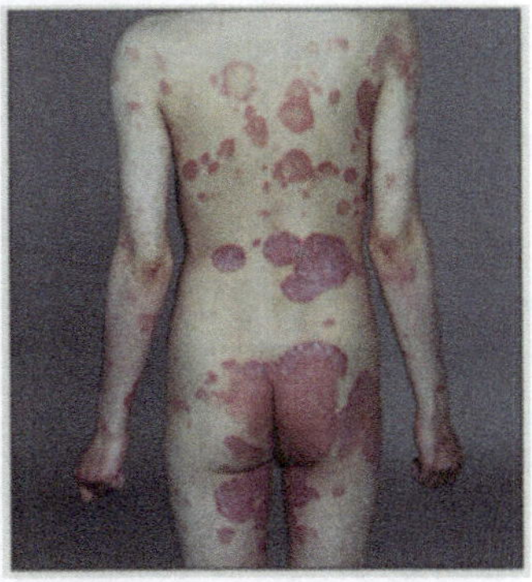

Psoriasis, page 368.

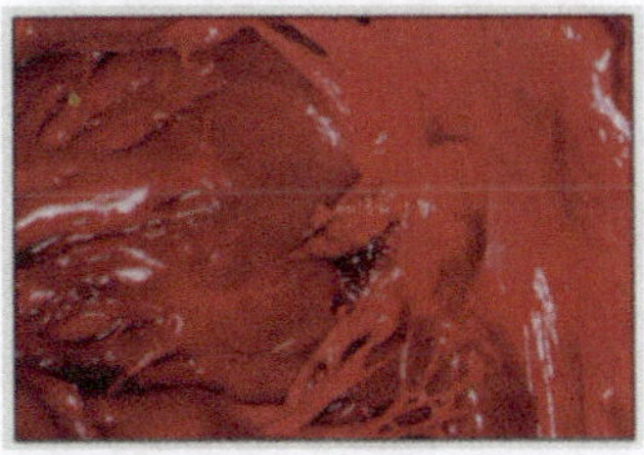

Rheumatic fever, acute; page 390.

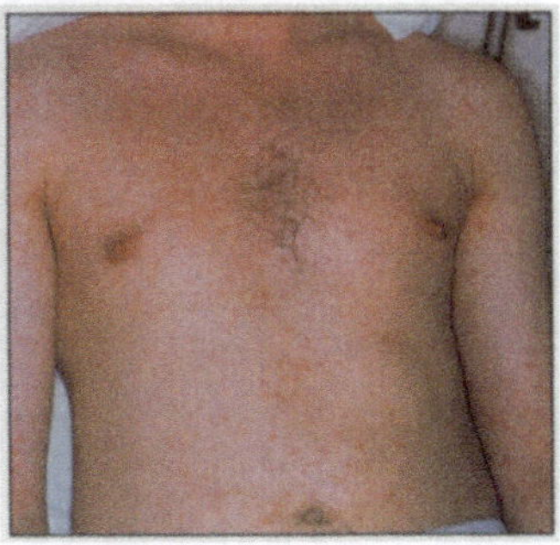

Rubella (German measles), page 394.

GPSR Compliance

The European Union's (EU) General Product Safety Regulation (GPSR) is a set of rules that requires consumer products to be safe and our obligations to ensure this.

If you have any concerns about our products, you can contact us on ProductSafety@springernature.com

In case Publisher is established outside the EU, the EU authorized representative is:

Springer Nature Customer Service Center GmbH
Europaplatz 3
69115 Heidelberg, Germany

Batch number: 10712230

Printed by Printforce, the Netherlands